THE
NETTER COLLECTION
OF MEDICAL ILLUSTRATIONS

3rd Edition

Endocrine System

A compilation of paintings prepared by **FRANK H. NETTER, MD**

VOLUME 2

Edited by

William F. Young, Jr, MD, MSc
Tyson Family Endocrinology Clinical Professor
Professor of Medicine, Mayo Clinic College of Medicine and Science
Division of Endocrinology, Diabetes, Metabolism, and Nutrition
Mayo Clinic
Rochester, Minnesota

Additional Illustrations by
Carlos A.G. Machado, MD

CONTRIBUTING ILLUSTRATORS
John A. Craig, MD
Tiffany S. DaVanzo, MA, CMI
DragonFly Media
Paul Kim, MS
Kristen W. Marzejon, CMI
James A. Perkins, MS, MFA

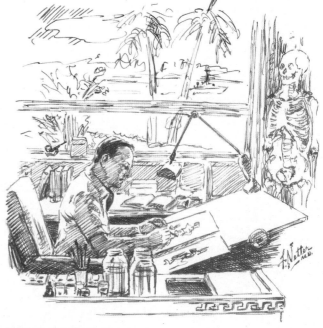

Self portrait by Dr. Netter

ELSEVIER

Elsevier
1600 John F. Kennedy Blvd.
Suite 1600
Philadelphia, Pennsylvania

THE NETTER COLLECTION OF MEDICAL ILLUSTRATIONS:
ENDOCRINE SYSTEM, VOLUME 2, THIRD EDITION   ISBN: 978-0-323-88126-5

Publisher: Elyse O'Grady
Senior Content Strategist: Marybeth Thiel
Publishing Services Manager: Catherine Jackson
Project Manager: Rosanne Toroian
Book Design: Patrick Ferguson

Printed in India

Last digit is the print number: 9 8 7 6 5 4 3 2

Working together
to grow libraries in
developing countries

www.elsevier.com • www.bookaid.org

"Clarification is the goal. No matter how beautifully it is painted, a medical illustration has little value if it does not make clear a medical point."

Frank H. Netter, MD

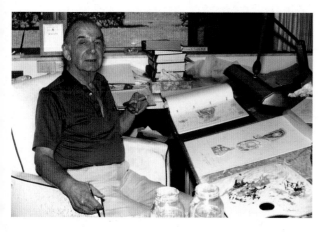

Dr. Frank Netter at work.

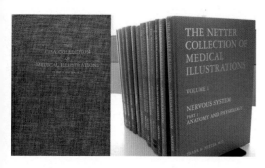

The single-volume "Blue Book" that preceded the multivolume Netter Collection of Medical Illustrations series, affectionately known as the "Green Books."

The Netter Collection
OF MEDICAL ILLUSTRATIONS
3rd Edition

Dr. Frank Netter created an illustrated legacy unifying his perspectives as physician, artist, and teacher. Both his greatest challenge and greatest success was charting a middle course between artistic clarity and instructional complexity. That success is captured in *The Netter Collection,* beginning in 1948 when the first comprehensive book of Netter's work was published by CIBA Pharmaceuticals. It met with such success that over the following 40 years the collection was expanded into an 8-volume series—with each title devoted to a single body system. Between 2011 and 2016, these books were updated and rereleased. Now, after another decade of innovation in medical imaging, renewed focus on patient-centered care, conscious efforts to improve inequities in healthcare and medical education, and a growing understanding of many clinical conditions, including multisystem effects of COVID-19, we are happy to make available a third edition of Netter's timeless work enhanced and informed by modern medical knowledge and context.

Inside the classic green covers, students and practitioners will find hundreds of original works of art. This is a collection of the human body in pictures—Dr. Netter called them *pictures,* never paintings. The latest expert medical knowledge is anchored by the sublime style of Frank Netter that has guided physicians' hands and nurtured their imaginations for more than half a century.

Noted artist-physician Carlos Machado, MD, the primary successor responsible for continuing the Netter tradition, has particular appreciation for the Green Book series. "*The Reproductive System* is of special significance for those who, like me, deeply admire Dr. Netter's work. In this volume, he masters the representation of textures of different surfaces, which I like to call 'the rhythm of the brush,' since it is the dimension, the direction of the strokes, and the interval separating them that create the illusion of given textures: organs have their external surfaces, the surfaces of their cavities, and texture of their parenchymas realistically represented. It set the style for the subsequent volumes of *The Netter Collection*—each an amazing combination of painting masterpieces and precise scientific information."

This third edition could not exist without the dedication of all those who edited, authored, or in other ways contributed to the second edition or the original books, nor, of course, without the excellence of Dr. Netter. For this third edition, we also owe our gratitude to the authors, editors, and artists whose relentless efforts were instrumental in adapting these classic works into reliable references for today's clinicians in training and in practice. From all of us with the Netter Publishing Team at Elsevier, thank you.

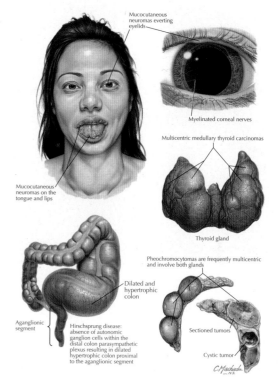

An illustrated plate painted by Carlos Machado, MD.

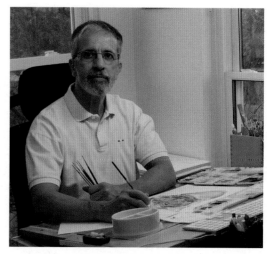

Dr. Carlos Machado at work.

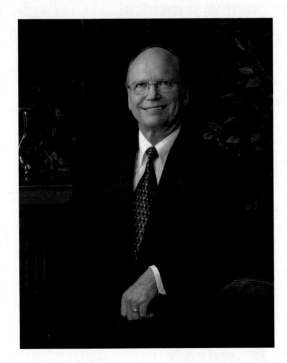

William F. Young, Jr, MD, MSc, is Professor of Medicine at Mayo Clinic College of Medicine and Science, Rochester, Minnesota. He holds the Tyson Family Endocrinology Clinical Professorship in Honor of Vahab Fatourechi, MD. He received his bachelor degree and his medical degree from Michigan State University and his master of science degree from the University of Minnesota. Dr. Young trained in internal medicine at William Beaumont Hospital in Royal Oak, Michigan, and completed a fellowship in endocrinology and metabolism at Mayo Clinic in Rochester, Minnesota. He has been a member of the staff at Mayo Clinic since 1984. Dr. Young is the recipient of multiple education awards, including the Mayo Fellows Association Teacher of the Year Award in Internal Medicine, the Mayo Clinic Endocrinology Teacher of the Year Award, the Mayo School of Continuing Medical Education Outstanding Faculty Member Award, the Delbert A. Fisher Research Scholar Award/Clark T. Sawin Memorial History of Endocrinology Lecturer from the Endocrine Society, and the H. Jack Baskin, MD, Endocrine Teaching Award from the American Association of Clinical Endocrinologists in recognition of his profound impact in teaching fellows in training. He is a past president of the Endocrine Society and past chair of the Division of Endocrinology at Mayo Clinic.

Professional honors include being a recipient of the Distinguished Mayo Clinician Award, the Distinction in Clinical Endocrinology Award from the American College of Endocrinology, the Distinguished Physician Laureate Award from the Endocrine Society, and the Outstanding Leadership in Endocrinology Laureate Award from the Endocrine Society. Dr. Young's clinical research focuses on primary aldosteronism and pheochromocytoma. He has published more than 300 articles on endocrine hypertension and adrenal and pituitary disorders. Dr. Young has delivered more than 800 presentations at national and international meetings and has been an invited visiting professor at more than 160 medical institutions.

The third edition of the *Endocrine System* volume of the *Netter Collection of Medical Illustrations* is designed to provide physicians at all stages of training and practice with a visual guide to the anatomy, physiology, and pathophysiology of the endocrine glands. The first edition was published in 1965 and the second edition in 2011. In 2011 the text was entirely rewritten, but most of the anatomic and clinical artwork of Frank H. Netter, MD, stood the test of time. Because new endocrine disorders and treatment approaches had been recognized, new artwork was added in every section. The accompanying text serves to illuminate and expand on the concepts demonstrated in the images.

The book is organized in eight sections, which correspond to the glands and components of the endocrine system: pituitary and hypothalamus, thyroid, adrenal, reproduction, pancreas, bone and calcium, lipids and nutrition, and genetics and endocrine neoplasia. In some cases, the Netter drawings are supplemented with modern diagnostic images (e.g., computed tomography and magnetic resonance imaging). The original Netter edition and the new illustrations focus on embryology, gross anatomy, histology, physiology, pathology, clinical manifestations of disease, diagnostic modalities, and surgical and therapeutic techniques. The third edition is a complete update of each section, reflecting the latest advances in endocrinology. New artwork and topics include pituitary stalk lesions, empty sella, thyroid biopsy, metastatic pheochromocytoma and paraganglioma, adrenocortical carcinoma, diabetes-related dermatologic manifestations, McCune-Albright syndrome, and the Carney triad. This work is not a complete textbook of endocrinology, but rather it is a visual tour of the highlights of this medical discipline. I hope readers find the artwork and accompanying text useful guides as they navigate the world of endocrinology.

I gratefully acknowledge my colleagues and patients at Mayo Clinic who have provided me with the clinical experience, perspective, and insights to address the broad field of endocrinology. The editorial and production staffs at Elsevier have been very supportive at every step from initial general concepts to final publication. I am indebted to the incredible second generation of Netter artists.

William F. Young, Jr, MD, MSc
January 2023

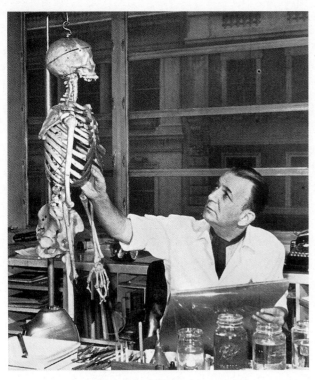

Many readers of the CIBA COLLECTION have expressed a desire to know more about Dr. Netter. In response to these requests this summary of Dr. Netter's career has been prepared.

Frank Henry Netter, born in 1906 in Brooklyn, New York, received his M.D. degree from New York University in 1931. To help pay his way through medical school and internship at Bellevue, he worked as a commercial artist and as an illustrator of medical books and articles for his professors and other physicians, perfecting his natural talent by studying at the National Academy of Design and attending courses at the Art Students' League.

In 1933 Dr. Netter entered the private practice of surgery in New York City. But it was the depth of the Depression, and the recently married physician continued to accept art assignments to supplement his income. Soon he was spending more and more time at the drawing board and finally, realizing that his career lay in medical illustration, he decided to give up practicing and become a full-time artist.

Soon, Dr. Netter was receiving requests to develop many unusual projects. One of the most arduous of these was building the "transparent woman" for the San Francisco Golden Gate Exposition. This 7-foot-high transparent figure depicted the menstrual process, the development and birth of a baby, and the physical and sexual development of a woman, while a synchronized voice told the story of the female endocrine system. Dr. Netter labored on this project night and day for 7 months. Another interesting assignment involved a series of paintings of incidents in the life of a physician. Among others, the pictures showed a medical student sitting up the night before the osteology examination, studying away to the point of exhaustion; an emergency ward; an ambulance call; a class reunion; and a night call made by a country doctor.

During World War II, Dr. Netter was an officer in the Army, stationed first at the Army Institute of Pathology, later at the Surgeon General's Office, in charge of graphic training aids for the Medical Department. Numerous manuals were produced under his direction, among them first aid for combat troops, roentgenology for technicians, sanitation in the field, and survival in the tropics.

After the war, Dr. Netter began work on several major projects for CIBA Pharmaceutical Company, culminating in THE CIBA COLLECTION OF MEDICAL ILLUSTRATIONS. To date, five volumes have been published and work is in progress on the sixth, dealing with the urinary tract.

Dr. Netter goes about planning and executing his illustrations in a very exacting way. First comes the study, unquestionably the most important and most difficult part of the entire undertaking. No drawing is ever started until Dr. Netter has acquired a complete understanding of the subject matter, either through reading or by consultation with leading authorities in the field. Often he visits hospitals to observe clinical cases, pathologic or surgical specimens, or operative procedures. Sometimes an original dissection is necessary.

When all his questions have been answered and the problem is thoroughly understood, Dr. Netter makes a pencil sketch on a tissue or tracing pad. Always, the subject must be visualized from the standpoint of the physician; is it to be viewed from above or below, from the side, the rear, or the front? What area is to be covered, the entire body or just certain segments? What plane provides the clearest understanding? In some pictures two, three, or four planes of dissection may be necessary.

When the sketch is at last satisfactory, Dr. Netter transfers it to a piece of illustration board for the finished drawing. This is done by blocking the back of the picture with a soft pencil, taping the tissue down on the board with Scotch tape, then going over the lines with a hard pencil. Over the years, our physician-artist has used many media to finish his illustrations, but now he works almost exclusively in transparent water colors mixed with white paint.

In spite of the tremendously productive life Dr. Netter has led, he has been able to enjoy his family, first in a handsome country home in East Norwich, Long Island, and, after the five children had grown up, in a penthouse overlooking the East River in Manhattan.

Alfred W. Custer

In the early days the endocrine glands were looked upon as an isolated group of structures, secreting substances which, in some strange way, influenced the human organism. The thyroid gland was known to be an organ of considerable significance. The clinical syndromes of hyper- and hypothyroidism and the therapeutic effects of thyroid administration and thyroidectomy were recognized. Insulin had become available, and its use in controlling diabetes was being explored. It was known generally that the pituitary gland exerted some influence over the growth and sex life of mankind. Nonetheless, the endocrine glands were still considered as a system apart, secreting mysterious and potent substances. In the light of modern knowledge, however, this is not an isolated system at all but, rather, an essential and controlling mechanism of all the other systems; indeed, together with the nervous system, the integrator of biochemistry and physiology in the living organism.

Thus although this volume was originally planned as an atlas on the endocrine glands, it was impossible to execute it intelligently without becoming involved in such basic and related subjects as carbohydrate, protein, and fat metabolism; the major vitamins; enzyme chemistry; genetics; and inborn metabolic errors. As a matter of fact, as I now survey the entire subject, it seems to me that the growth of our understanding of the function of the endocrine glands has come about as much or more from the study of the basic physiology of the glandular secretions as from study of the morphologic effects of the endocrine system itself. I have also been tremendously impressed and awed by the painstaking, patient, and unrelenting work of the men and women who have, bit by bit, unraveled and correlated the mysteries of these various fields. It has been my great pleasure, in creating this volume, to have worked with some of these pioneers or with their disciples. No words of appreciation for the help and encouragement I received from all my collaborators can completely convey the satisfaction I obtained from getting to know each of them and becoming their friend.

In finding my way through the uncharted space of the endocrine universe, I sorely needed a guide—one who could plot a course among the biochemical constellations, yet at all times would know his way back to earthly clinical considerations. Such a one I found in Dr. Peter H. Forsham, who took over the editorship of this volume upon the death of Dr. Ernst Oppenheimer, about whom I have written in the preceding pages. I shall always cherish the stimulating hours Dr. Forsham and I spent together in work and, occasionally, in play.

A creative effort such as that which this volume has demanded absorbs a great deal of one's time, effort, and dreams. In short, it tends to detach the artist from his surroundings and personal relationships and to make him difficult to live with! For these reasons I must express special appreciation to my wife, Vera, for patiently bearing with me through these tribulations. She always managed to return me to reality when I became too detached, bring a smile to my face when I was distressed, and help me in so many other ways during this challenging but rather awesome assignment.

Frank H. Netter, MD

CONTENTS

PITUITARY AND HYPOTHALAMUS

Plate 1.1   Endocrine System: VOLUME 2

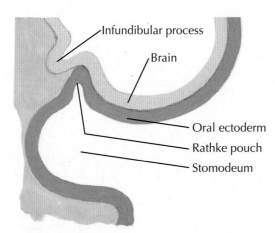

1. Beginning formation of Rathke pouch and infundibular process

- Infundibular process
- Brain
- Oral ectoderm
- Rathke pouch
- Stomodeum

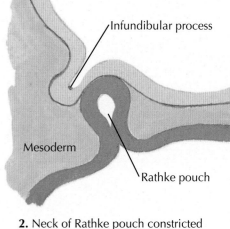

2. Neck of Rathke pouch constricted by growth of mesoderm

- Infundibular process
- Mesoderm
- Rathke pouch

DEVELOPMENT OF THE PITUITARY GLAND

The pituitary gland, also termed the *hypophysis,* consists of two major components, the adenohypophysis and the neurohypophysis. The adenohypophysis (anterior lobe) is derived from the oral ectoderm, and the neurohypophysis (posterior lobe) is derived from the neural ectoderm of the floor of the forebrain.

A pouchlike recess—Rathke pouch—in the ectodermal lining of the roof of the stomodeum is formed by the fourth to fifth week of gestation and gives rise to the anterior pituitary gland. Rathke pouch extends upward to contact the undersurface of the forebrain and is then constricted by the surrounding mesoderm to form a closed cavity. The original connection between Rathke pouch and the stomodeum—known as the *craniopharyngeal canal*—runs from the anterior part of the pituitary fossa to the undersurface of the skull. Although it is usually obliterated, a remnant may persist in adult life as a "pharyngeal pituitary" embedded in the mucosa on the dorsal wall of the pharynx. The pharyngeal pituitary may give rise to ectopic hormone-secreting pituitary adenomas later in life.

Behind Rathke pouch, a hollow neural outgrowth extends toward the mouth from the floor of the third ventricle. This neural process forms a funnel-shaped sac—the infundibular process—that becomes a solid structure, except at the upper end where the cavity persists as the infundibular recess of the third ventricle. As Rathke pouch extends toward the third ventricle, it fuses on each side of the infundibular process and subsequently obliterates its lumen, which sometimes persists as Rathke cleft. The anterior lobe of the pituitary is formed from Rathke pouch, and the infundibular process gives rise to the adjacent posterior lobe (neurohypophysis). The neurohypophysis consists of the axons and nerve endings of neurons whose cell bodies reside in the supraoptic and paraventricular nuclei of the hypothalamus, forming a hypothalamic-neurohypophysial nerve tract that contains approximately 100,000 nerve fibers. Remnants of Rathke pouch may persist at the boundary of the neurohypophysis, resulting in small colloid cysts.

The anterior lobe also gives off two processes from its ventral wall that extend along the infundibulum as the pars tuberalis, which fuses to surround the upper end of the pituitary stalk. The cleft is the remains of the original cavity of the stomodeal diverticulum. The dorsal (posterior) wall of the cleft remains thin and fuses with the adjoining posterior lobe to form the pars intermedia. The pars intermedia remains intact in some species, but in humans, its cells become interspersed

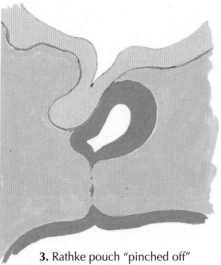

3. Rathke pouch "pinched off"

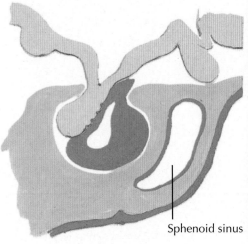

Sphenoid sinus

4. "Pinched off" segment conforms to neural process, forming pars distalis, pars intermedia, and pars tuberalis.

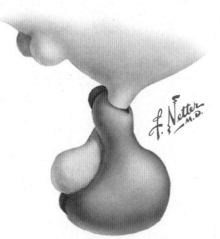

5. Pars tuberalis encircles infundibular stalk (lateral surface view).

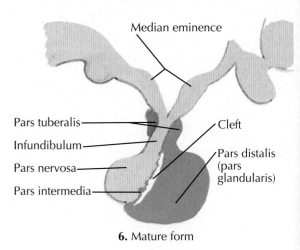

Median eminence

- Pars tuberalis
- Infundibulum
- Pars nervosa
- Pars intermedia
- Cleft
- Pars distalis (pars glandularis)

6. Mature form

with those of the anterior lobe, and it develops the capacity to synthesize and secrete proopiomelanocortin (POMC) and adrenocorticotropic hormone (ACTH; corticotropin). The part of the tuber cinereum that lies immediately above the pars tuberalis is termed the *median eminence.*

Both the adenohypophysis and the neurohypophysis are subdivided into three parts. The adenohypophysis consists of the pars tuberalis, a thin strip of tissue that surrounds the median eminence and the upper part of the neural stalk; the pars intermedia, the portion posterior to the cleft and in contact with the neurohypophysis; and the pars distalis (pars glandularis), the major secretory part of the gland. The neurohypophysis is composed of an expanded distal portion termed the *infundibular process;* the infundibular stem (neural stalk); and the expanded upper end of the stalk, the median eminence of the tuber cinereum.

Plate 1.2

Pituitary and Hypothalamus

DIVISIONS OF THE PITUITARY GLAND AND RELATIONSHIP TO THE HYPOTHALAMUS

The pituitary gland (hypophysis) is composed of the neurohypophysis (posterior pituitary lobe) and adenohypophysis (anterior pituitary lobe). The neurohypophysis consists of three parts: the median eminence of the tuber cinereum, infundibular stem, and infundibular process (neural lobe). The adenohypophysis is likewise divided into three parts: the pars tuberalis, pars intermedia, and pars distalis (glandularis). The infundibular stem, together with portions of the adenohypophysis that form a sheath around it, is designated as the hypophysial (pituitary) stalk. The extension of neurohypophysial tissue up the stalk and into the median eminence of the tuber cinereum constitutes approximately 15% of the neurohypophysis. A low stalk section may leave enough of the gland still in contact with its higher connections in the paraventricular and supraoptic nuclei to prevent the onset of diabetes insipidus (DI). Atrophy and disappearance of cell bodies in the supraoptic and paraventricular nuclei follow damage to their axons in the supraopticohypophysial tract. If the tract is cut at the level of the diaphragma sellae, only 70% of these cells are affected; if the tract is severed above the median eminence, about 85% of the cells will atrophy. Thus approximately 15% of the axons terminate between these levels.

The main nerve supply, both functionally and anatomically, of the neurohypophysis is the hypothalamohypophysial tract in the pituitary stalk. It consists of two main parts: the supraopticohypophysial tract, running in the anterior or ventral wall of the stalk, and the tuberohypophysial tract in the posterior, or dorsal, wall of the stalk. The tuberohypophysial tract originates in the central and posterior parts of the hypothalamus from the paraventricular nucleus (PVN) and from scattered cells and nuclei in the tuberal region and mamillary bodies. The supraopticohypophysial tract arises from the supraoptic and paraventricular nuclei. On entering the median eminence, it occupies a very superficial position, where it is liable to be affected by basal infections of the brain and granulomatous inflammatory processes. The tuberohypophysial tract in the dorsal region of the median eminence is smaller and consists of finer fibers. In the neural stalk, all the fibers congregate into a dense bundle lying in a central position, leaving a peripheral zone in contact with the pars tuberalis, which is relatively free of nerve elements. The hypothalamohypophysial tract terminates mainly in the neurohypophysis.

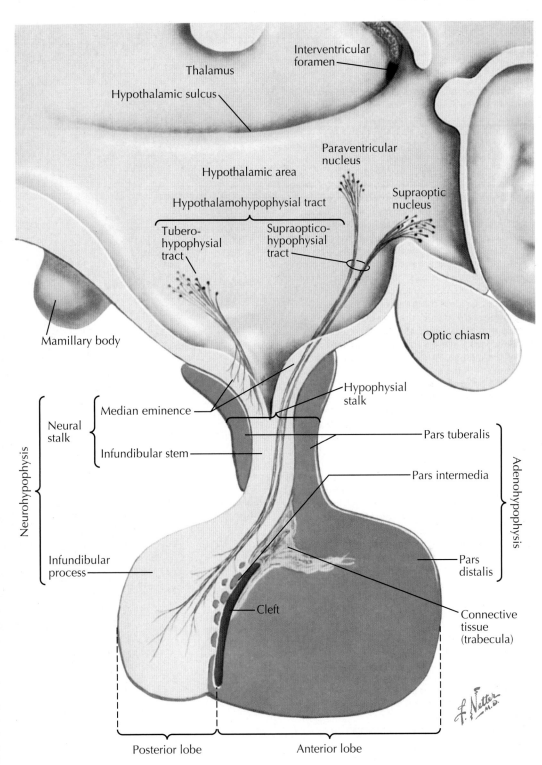

The hypothalamus has ill-defined boundaries. Anteroinferiorly, it is limited by the optic chiasm and optic tracts; passing posteriorly, it is bounded by the posterior perforated substance and the cerebral peduncles. On sagittal section, it can be seen to be separated from the thalamus by the hypothalamic sulcus on the wall of the third ventricle. Anteriorly, it merges with the preoptic septal region, and posteriorly, it merges with the tegmental area of the midbrain. Its lateral relations are the subthalamus and the internal capsule.

A connective tissue trabecula separates the posterior and anterior lobes of the pituitary; it also extends out into the anterior pituitary lobe for a variable distance as a vascular bed for the large-lumened artery of the trabecula. The embryonic cleft, which marks the site of the Rathke pouch within the gland, may be contained, in part, in this trabecula. It is easier to see in newborns and tends to disappear in later life. Colloid-filled follicles in the adult gland mark the site of the pars intermedia at the junction between the pars distalis and the neurohypophysis. This boundary may be quite irregular because fingerlike projections of adenohypophysial tissue are frequently found in the substance of the neurohypophysis.

Plate 1.3

Endocrine System: VOLUME 2

BLOOD SUPPLY OF THE PITUITARY GLAND

The pituitary gland receives its arterial blood supply from two paired systems of vessels: from above come the right and left superior hypophysial arteries, and from below arise the right and left inferior hypophysial arteries. Each superior hypophysial artery divides into two main branches—the anterior and posterior hypophysial arteries passing to the hypophysial stalk. Communicating branches between these anterior and posterior superior hypophysial arteries run on the lateral aspects of the hypophysial stalk; numerous branches arise from this arterial circle. Some pass upward to supply the optic chiasm and the hypothalamus. Other branches, called *infundibular arteries,* pass either superiorly to penetrate the stalk in its upper part or inferiorly to enter the stalk at a lower level. Another important branch of the anterior superior hypophysial artery on each side is the artery of the trabecula, which passes downward to enter the pars distalis. The trabecula is a prominent, compact band of connective tissue and blood vessels lying within the pars distalis on either side of the midline. At its central end the trabecula is contiguous with the mass of connective tissue, which is interposed between the pars distalis and the lower infundibular stem. Peripherally, the components of the trabecula spread out to form a fibrovascular tuft. On approaching the lower infundibular stem, the artery of the trabecula gives off numerous straight parallel vessels to the superior portion of this area and thus constitutes the "superior artery of the lower infundibular stem." The "inferior artery of the lower infundibular stem" is derived from the inferior hypophysial arterial system. The artery of the trabecula is of large caliber throughout its course; it gives off no branches to the epithelial tissue through which it passes. It is markedly tortuous and is always surrounded by connective tissue.

The inferior hypophysial arteries arise as a single branch from each internal carotid artery in its intracavernous segment. Near the junction of the anterior and posterior lobes of the pituitary, the artery gives off one or more tortuous vessels to the dural covering of the pars distalis and finally divides into two main branches—a medial and a lateral inferior hypophysial artery. The infundibular process is surrounded by an arterial ring formed by the medial and lateral branches of the paired inferior hypophysial arteries. From this arterial ring, branches are given off to the posterior lobe and to the lower infundibular stem. Components of the superior and inferior hypophysial arterial systems anastomose freely.

The epithelial tissue of the pars distalis receives no direct arterial blood. The sinusoids of the anterior lobe receive their blood supply from the hypophysial portal vessels, which arise from the capillary beds within the median eminence and the upper and lower portions of the infundibular stem. Blood is conveyed from this primary capillary network through hypophysial portal veins to the epithelial tissue of the anterior lobe. Here, a secondary plexus of the pituitary portal system is formed, leading to the venous dural sinuses, which surround the pituitary, and to the general circulation. Some of the long hypophysial portal veins run along the surface of the stalk, chiefly on its anterior and lateral aspects. Most of the long hypophysial portal vessels leave the neural tissue to run down within the pars tuberalis, but a few remain deep within the stalk until they reach the pars distalis. The short hypophysial portal veins are embedded in the tissue surrounding the lower infundibular stem. They supply the sinusoidal

Superior hypophysial artery

Hypothalamic vessels

Artery of trabecula

Efferent hypophysial vein to cavernous sinus

Trabecula (fibrous tissue)

Adenohypophysis (anterior lobe of pituitary gland)

Secondary plexus of hypophysial portal system

Efferent hypophysial veins to cavernous sinus

Primary plexus of hypophysial portal system

Long hypophysial portal veins

Short hypophysial portal veins

Efferent hypophysial vein to cavernous sinus

Neurohypophysis (posterior lobe of pituitary gland)

Efferent hypophysial vein to cavernous sinus

Capillary plexus of infundibular process

Inferior hypophysial artery

bed of the posterior part of the pars distalis, and the long portal veins supply its anterior and lateral regions.

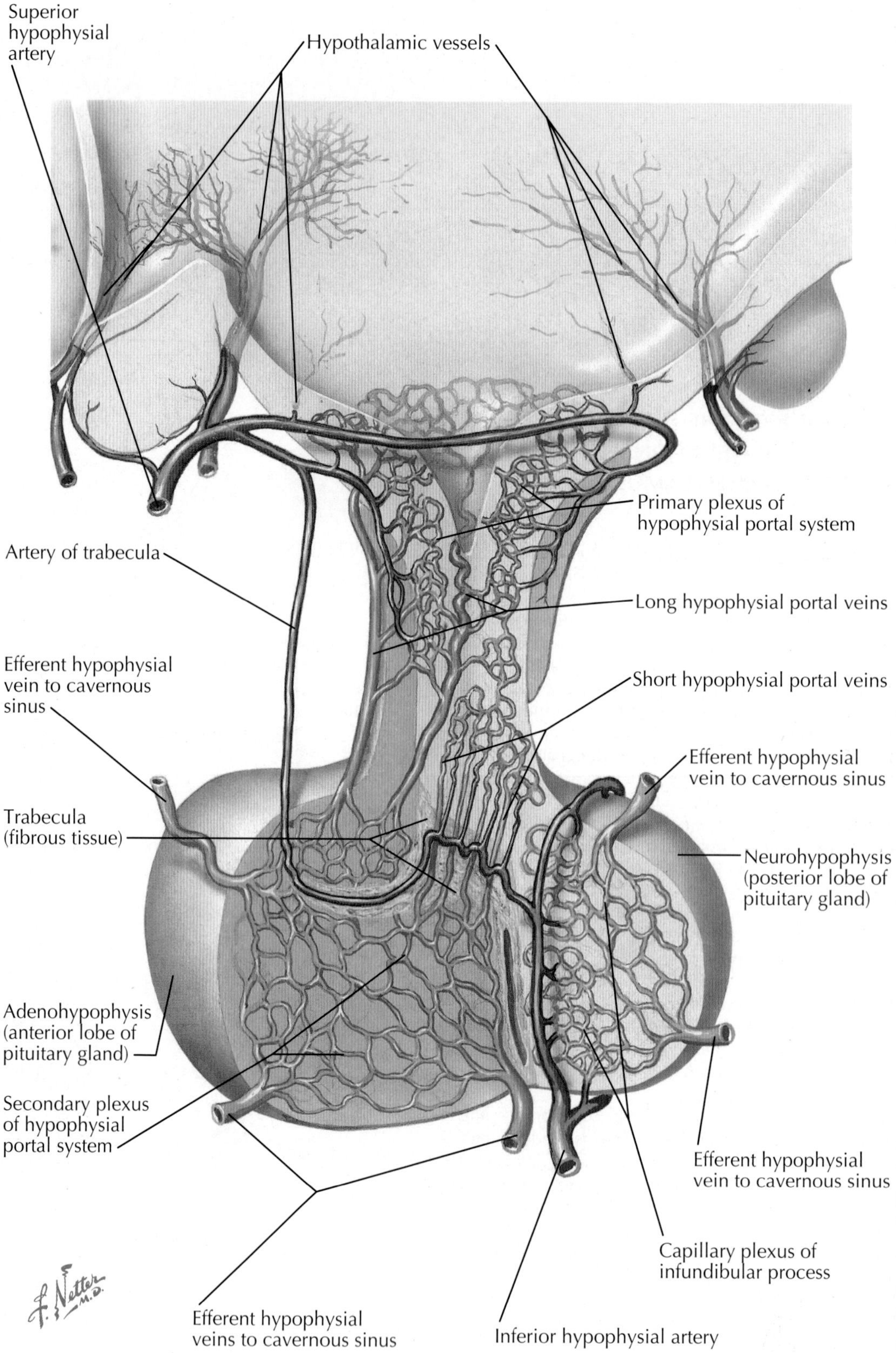

Vascular tufts, comprising the primary capillary network in the median eminence and infundibular stem, are intimately related to the great mass of nerve fibers of the hypothalamohypophysial tract running in this region. On excitation, these nerve fibers liberate into the portal vessels, releasing hormones (e.g., growth hormone-releasing hormone [GHRH], corticotropin-releasing hormone [CRH], gonadotropin-releasing hormone [GnRH], thyrotropin-releasing hormone [TRH]) and inhibitory factors (e.g., somatostatin, prolactin-inhibitory factor [dopamine]), which are conveyed to the sinusoids of the pars distalis. Extensive occlusion of the hypophysial portal vessels or of the capillary beds of the hypophysial stalk may lead to ischemic necrosis of the anterior pituitary because these hypophysial portal vessels are the only afferent channels to the sinusoids of the pars distalis.

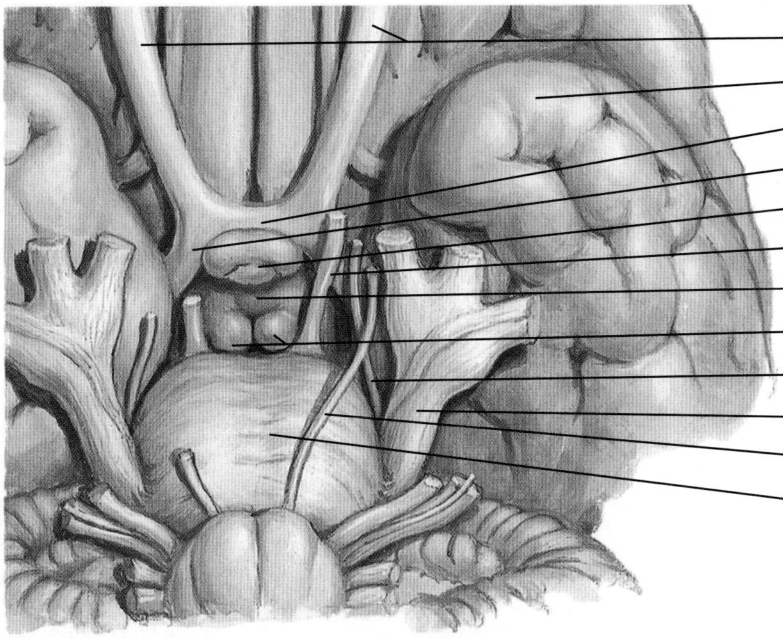

Plate 1.4   Pituitary and Hypothalamus

Optic nerves
Temporal pole of brain
Optic chiasm
Right optic tract
Pituitary gland
Oculomotor nerve (III)
Tuber cinereum
Mamillary bodies
Trochlear nerve (IV)
Trigeminal nerve (V)
Abducens nerve (VI)
Pons

ANATOMY AND RELATIONSHIPS OF THE PITUITARY GLAND

The pituitary gland is reddish-gray and ovoid, measuring about 12 mm transversely, 8 mm in its anterior-posterior diameter, and 6 mm in its vertical dimension. It weighs approximately 500 mg in males and 600 mg in females. It is contiguous with the end of the infundibulum and is situated in the hypophysial fossa of the sphenoid bone. A circular fold of dura mater, the diaphragma sellae, forms the roof of this fossa. In turn, the floor of the hypophysial fossa forms part of the roof of the sphenoid sinus. The diaphragma sellae is pierced by a small central aperture through which the pituitary stalk passes, and it separates the anterior part of the upper surface of the gland from the optic chiasm. The hypophysis is bound on each side by the cavernous sinuses and the structures that they contain. Inferiorly, it is separated from the floor of the fossa by a large, partially vacuolated venous sinus, which communicates freely with the circular sinus. The meninges blend with the capsule of the gland and cannot be identified as separate layers of the fossa. However, the subarachnoid space often extends a variable distance into the sella, particularly anteriorly, and may be referred to as a *partially empty sella* when seen on magnetic resonance imaging (MRI) (see Plate 1.12). In some cases of subarachnoid hemorrhage, the dorsal third of the gland may be covered with blood that has extended down into this space.

The hypothalamus is an important relation of the pituitary gland, both anatomically and functionally. This designation refers to the structures contained in the anterior part of the floor of the third ventricle and to those constituting the lateral wall of the third ventricle below and in front of the hypothalamic sulcus. The mamillary bodies are two round, white, pea-sized masses located side by side below the gray matter of the floor of the third ventricle in front of the posterior perforated substance. They form the posterior limits of the hypothalamus. At certain sites at the base of the brain, the arachnoid is separated from the pia mater by wide intervals that communicate freely with one another; these are called *subarachnoid cisterns*. As the arachnoid extends across between the two temporal lobes, it is separated from the cerebral peduncles by the interpeduncular cistern. Anteriorly, this space is continued in front of the optic chiasm as the chiasmatic cistern. Space-occupying lesions distort these cisterns.

The optic chiasm is an extremely important superior relation of the pituitary gland. It is a flat, somewhat quadrilateral bundle of optic nerve fibers situated at the junction of the anterior wall of the third ventricle with its floor. Its anterolateral angles are contiguous with the optic nerves, and its posterolateral angles are

Fornix
Choroid plexus of 3rd ventricle
Thalamus
Pineal gland
Interventricular foramen
Corpus callosum
Hypothalamic sulcus
Anterior commissure
Lamina terminalis
Tuber cinereum
Mamillary body
Chiasmatic cistern
Optic chiasm
Diaphragma sellae
Interpeduncular cistern
Pituitary gland
Sphenoidal sinus
Nasal septum
Nasopharynx
Pontine cistern

contiguous with the optic tracts. The lamina terminalis, which represents the cephalic end of the primitive neural tube, forms a thin layer of gray matter stretching from the upper surface of the chiasm to the rostrum of the corpus callosum. Inferiorly, the chiasm rests on the diaphragma sellae just behind the optic groove of the sphenoid bone. A small recess of the third ventricle, called the *optic recess,* passes downward and forward over its upper surface as far as the lamina

terminalis. A more distant relationship is the pineal gland, which is a small, conical, reddish-gray body lying below the splenium of the corpus callosum. Rarely, ectopic pineal tissue occurs in the floor of the third ventricle and gives rise to tumors of that region. Compression of neighboring cranial nerves, other than the optic nerves, may occur if there is extensive cavernous sinus extension from a pituitary neoplasm (see Plate 1.24).

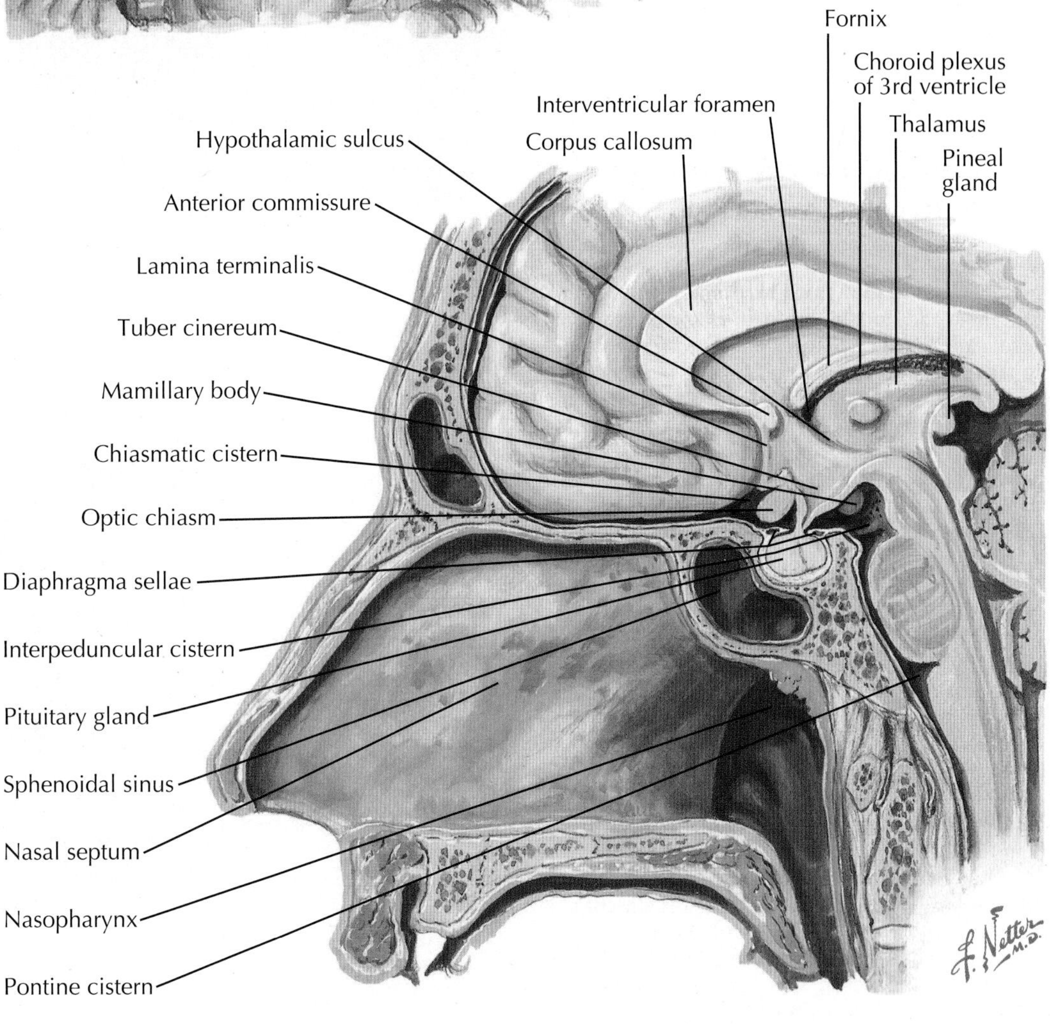

Plate 1.5

Endocrine System: VOLUME 2

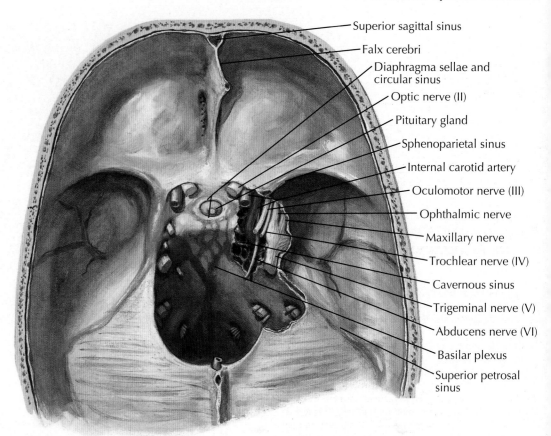

- Superior sagittal sinus
- Falx cerebri
- Diaphragma sellae and circular sinus
- Optic nerve (II)
- Pituitary gland
- Sphenoparietal sinus
- Internal carotid artery
- Oculomotor nerve (III)
- Ophthalmic nerve
- Maxillary nerve
- Trochlear nerve (IV)
- Cavernous sinus
- Trigeminal nerve (V)
- Abducens nerve (VI)
- Basilar plexus
- Superior petrosal sinus

RELATIONSHIP OF THE PITUITARY GLAND TO THE CAVERNOUS SINUS

The sinuses of the dura mater are venous channels that drain the blood from the brain. The cavernous sinuses are so named because of their reticulated structure, being traversed by numerous interlacing filaments that radiate out from the internal carotid artery extending anteroposteriorly in the center of the sinuses. They are located astride and on either side of the body of the sphenoid bone and adjacent to the pituitary gland. Each opens behind into the superior and inferior petrosal sinuses (see Plate 3.10). On the medial wall of each cavernous sinus, the internal carotid artery is in close contact with the abducens nerve (VI). On the lateral wall are the oculomotor (III) and trochlear (IV) nerves and the ophthalmic and maxillary divisions of the trigeminal nerve (V). These structures are separated from the blood flowing along the sinus by the endothelial lining membrane. The two cavernous sinuses communicate with each other by means of two intercavernous sinuses. The anterior sinus passes in front of the pituitary gland and the posterior behind it. Together they form a circular sinus around the hypophysis. These channels are found between the two layers of dura mater that make up the diaphragma sellae and are responsible for copious bleeding when this structure is incised when a transcranial surgical approach to the pituitary gland is used. Sometimes profuse bleeding from an inferior circular sinus is encountered in the transsphenoidal approach to the pituitary gland (see Plate 1.33).

The superior petrosal sinus is a small, narrow channel that connects the cavernous sinus with the transverse sinus. It runs backward and laterally from the posterior end of the cavernous sinus over the trigeminal nerve (V) and lies in the attached margin of the tentorium cerebelli and in the superior petrosal sulcus of the temporal bone. The cavernous sinus also receives the small sphenoparietal sinus, which runs anteriorly along the undersurface of the lesser wing of the sphenoid.

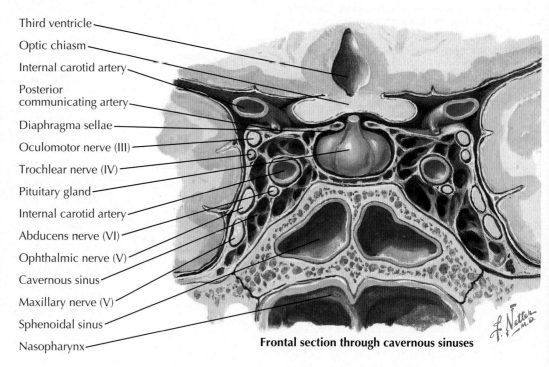

- Third ventricle
- Optic chiasm
- Internal carotid artery
- Posterior communicating artery
- Diaphragma sellae
- Oculomotor nerve (III)
- Trochlear nerve (IV)
- Pituitary gland
- Internal carotid artery
- Abducens nerve (VI)
- Ophthalmic nerve (V)
- Cavernous sinus
- Maxillary nerve (V)
- Sphenoidal sinus
- Nasopharynx

Frontal section through cavernous sinuses

The intercavernous portion of the internal carotid artery runs a complicated course. At first, it ascends toward the posterior clinoid process; then it passes forward alongside the body of the sphenoid bone and again curves upward on the medial side of the anterior clinoid process. It perforates the dura mater that forms the roof of the sinus. This portion of the artery is surrounded by filaments of sympathetic nerves as it passes between the optic and oculomotor nerves. The hypophysial arteries are branches of the intercavernous segment of the internal carotid artery. The inferior branch supplies the posterior lobe of the pituitary gland, and the superior branch leads into the median eminence to start the hypophysial portal system to the anterior lobe.

The surgical approaches to the pituitary gland are designed to circumvent the major vascular channels and to avoid injury to the optic nerves and to the optic chiasm (see Plate 1.33).

Plate 1.6

Pituitary and Hypothalamus

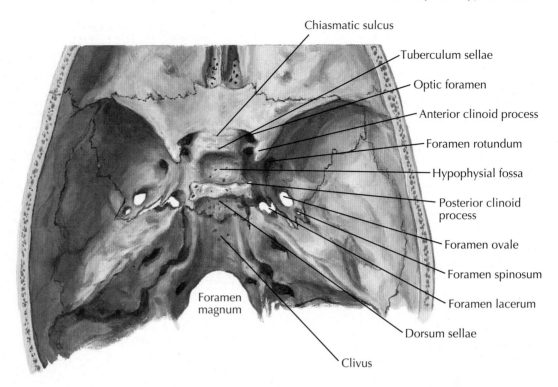

Chiasmatic sulcus
Tuberculum sellae
Optic foramen
Anterior clinoid process
Foramen rotundum
Hypophysial fossa
Posterior clinoid process
Foramen ovale
Foramen spinosum
Foramen lacerum
Dorsum sellae
Foramen magnum
Clivus

RELATIONSHIPS OF THE SELLA TURCICA

The sella turcica—where the pituitary gland is located—is the deep depression in the body of the sphenoid bone. In adults, the normal mean anterior-posterior length is less than 14 mm, and the height from the floor to a line between the tuberculum sellae and the tip of the posterior clinoid is less than 12 mm.

To understand its relations, a more general description of the sphenoid bone is needed. Situated at the base of the skull in front of the temporal bones and the basilar part of the occipital bone, the sphenoid bone somewhat resembles a bat with its wings extended. It is divided into a median portion, or body, two great and two small wings extending outward from the sides of the body, and two pterygoid processes projecting below. The cubical body is hollowed out to form two large cavities, the sphenoidal air sinuses, which are separated from each other by a septum that is often oblique. The superior surface of the body articulates anteriorly with the cribriform plate of the ethmoid and laterally with the frontal bones. Most of the frontal articulation is with the small wing of the sphenoid bone. Behind the ethmoidal articulation is a smooth surface, slightly raised in the midline and grooved on either side, for the olfactory lobes of the brain. This surface is bound behind by a ridge, which forms the anterior border of a narrow transverse groove, the chiasmatic sulcus, above and behind which lies the optic chiasm. The groove ends on either side in the optic foramen, through which the optic nerve and ophthalmic artery enter into the orbital cavity.

Behind the chiasmatic sulcus is an elevation, the tuberculum sellae. Immediately posterior there is a deep depression, the sella turcica, the deepest part of which is called the *hypophysial fossa*. The anterior boundary of the sella turcica is completed by two small prominences, one on each side, called the *middle clinoid processes*. The posterior boundary of the sella is formed by an elongated plate of bone, the dorsum sellae, which ends at its superior angles as two tubercles, the posterior clinoid processes.

Behind the dorsum sellae is a shallow depression, the clivus, which slopes obliquely backward to continue as a groove on the basilar portion of the occipital bone. The lateral surfaces of the sphenoid body are united with the great wings and the medial pterygoid plates. Above the attachment of each great wing is a broad

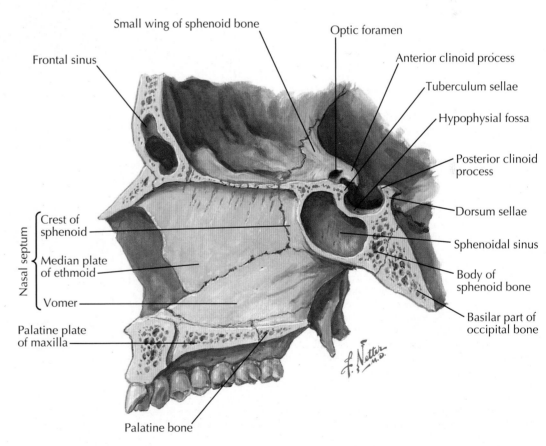

Small wing of sphenoid bone
Optic foramen
Frontal sinus
Anterior clinoid process
Tuberculum sellae
Hypophysial fossa
Posterior clinoid process
Dorsum sellae
Sphenoidal sinus
Body of sphenoid bone
Basilar part of occipital bone
Nasal septum
Crest of sphenoid
Median plate of ethmoid
Vomer
Palatine plate of maxilla
Palatine bone

groove that contains the internal carotid artery and the cavernous sinus. The superior surface of each great wing forms part of the middle fossa of the skull. The internal carotid artery passes through the foramen lacerum, a large, somewhat triangular aperture bound in the front by the great wing of the sphenoid, behind by the apex of the petrous portion of the temporal bone, and medially by the body of the sphenoid and the basilar portion of the occipital bone. The nasal relations of the pituitary fossa are the crest of the sphenoid bone and the median, or perpendicular, plate of the ethmoid.

Since the introduction of the operating microscope in 1969 by Jules Hardy, the sublabial transseptal transsphenoidal approach to the pituitary has been the standard in the treatment of pituitary adenomas. However, improved endoscopes have led to development of endoscopic transnasal applications in many pituitary surgical centers (see Plate 1.33).

Plate 1.7

Endocrine System: VOLUME 2

ANTERIOR PITUITARY HORMONES AND FEEDBACK CONTROL

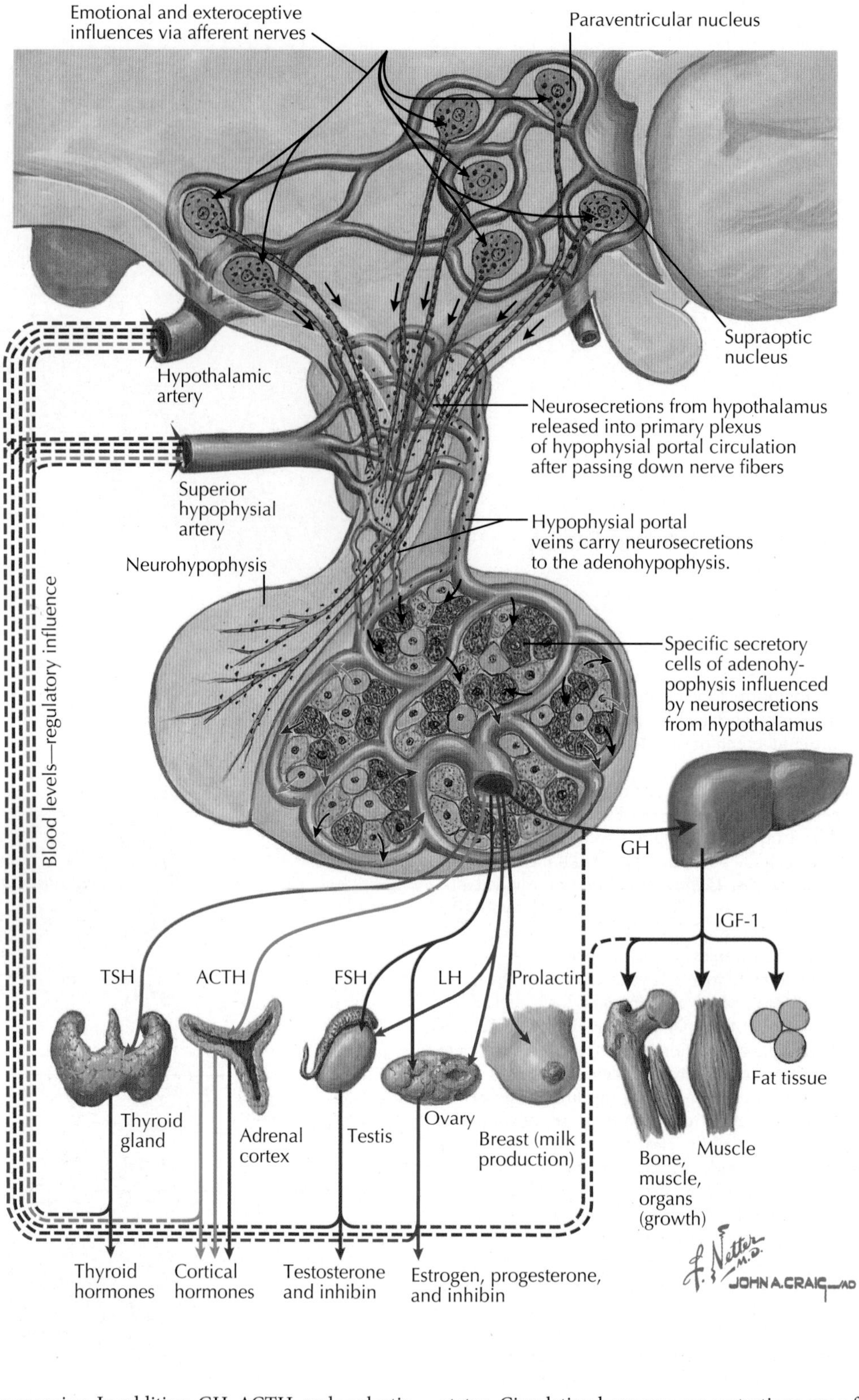

The quantitative and temporal secretion of the pituitary trophic hormones is tightly regulated and controlled at three levels. (1) Adenohypophysiotropic hormones from the hypothalamus are secreted into the portal system and act on pituitary G-protein-linked cell surface membrane binding sites, resulting in either positive or negative signals mediating pituitary hormone gene transcription and secretion. (2) Circulating hormones from the target glands provide negative feedback regulation of their trophic hormones. (3) Intrapituitary autocrine and paracrine cytokines and growth factors act locally to regulate cell development and function. The hypothalamic-releasing hormones include GHRH, CRH, TRH, and GnRH. The two hypothalamic inhibitory regulatory factors are somatostatin and dopamine, which suppress the secretion of growth hormone (GH) and prolactin, respectively. The six anterior pituitary trophic hormones—ACTH, GH, thyroid-stimulating hormone (TSH; thyrotropin), follicle-stimulating hormone (FSH), luteinizing hormone (LH), and prolactin—are secreted in a pulsatile fashion into the cavernous sinuses and circulate systemically.

Hypothalamic-pituitary-target gland hormonal systems function in a feedback loop, where the target gland blood hormone concentration—or a biochemical surrogate—determines the rate of secretion of the hypothalamic factor and pituitary trophic hormone. The feedback system may be "negative," in which the target gland hormone inhibits the hypothalamic-pituitary unit, or "positive," in which the target gland hormone or surrogate increases the hypothalamic-pituitary unit secretion. These two feedback control systems may be closed loop (regulation is restricted to the interacting trophic and target gland hormones) or open loop (the nervous system or other factors influence the feedback loop). All hypothalamic-pituitary-target gland feedback loops are in part open loop—they have some degree of nervous system (emotional and exteroceptive influences) inputs that either alter the setpoint of the feedback control system or can override the closed-loop controls. Feedback inhibition to the hypothalamus and pituitary is also provided by other target gland factors. For example, inhibin, a heterodimeric glycoprotein product of the Sertoli cell of the testes and the ovarian granulosa cell, provides negative feedback on the secretion of FSH from the pituitary. Synthesis and secretion of gonadal inhibin is induced by FSH.

Blood levels of trophic and target gland hormones are also affected by endogenous secretory rhythms. Most hormonal axes have an endogenous secretory rhythm of 24 hours—termed *circadian* or *diurnal rhythms*—and are regulated by retinal inputs and hypothalamic nuclei. The retinohypothalamic tract affects the circadian pulse generators in the hypothalamic suprachiasmatic nuclei. Rhythms that occur more frequently than once a day are termed *ultradian rhythms*, and those that have a period longer than a day are termed *infradian rhythms* (e.g., menstrual cycle). Examples of circadian rhythms of pituitary and target gland hormones include the following: GH and prolactin secretion is highest shortly after the onset of sleep; cortisol secretion is lowest at 11 pm and highest between 2 and 6 AM; and testosterone secretion is highest

in the morning. In addition, GH, ACTH, and prolactin are also secreted in brief regular pulses, reflecting the pulsatile release of their respective hypothalamic releasing factors.

The circadian and pulsatile secretion of pituitary and target gland hormones must be considered when assessing endocrine function. For example, because of pulsatile secretion, a single blood GH measurement is not a good assessment of either hyperfunction or hypofunction of pituitary somatotropes; the serum concentration of the GH-dependent peptide insulin-like growth factor 1 (IGF-1)—because of its much longer serum half-life—provides a better assessment of GH secretory

status. Circulating hormone concentrations are a function of circadian rhythms and hormone clearance rates; laboratories standardize the reference ranges for hormones based on the time of day. For example, the reference range for cortisol changes depending on whether it is measured in the morning or afternoon. Normal serum testosterone concentrations are standardized based on samples obtained from morning venipuncture. Disrupted circadian rhythms should clue the clinician to possible endocrine dysfunction—thus, the loss of circadian ACTH secretion with high midnight concentrations of cortisol in the blood and saliva is consistent with ACTH-dependent Cushing syndrome.

Plate 1.8

Pituitary and Hypothalamus

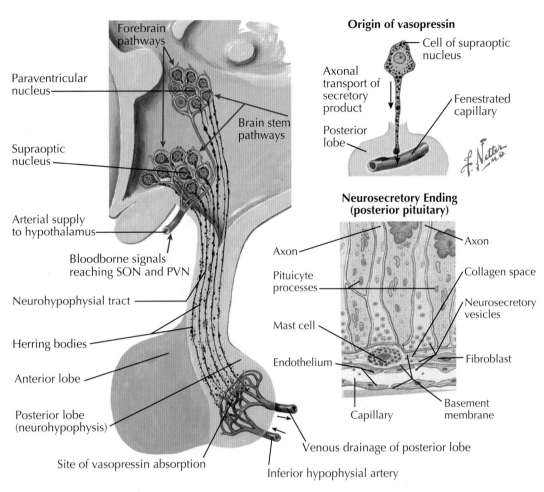

Origin of vasopressin

Cell of supraoptic nucleus

Axonal transport of secretory product

Posterior lobe

Fenestrated capillary

Forebrain pathways

Paraventricular nucleus

Supraoptic nucleus

Brain stem pathways

Arterial supply to hypothalamus

Bloodborne signals reaching SON and PVN

Neurohypophysial tract

Herring bodies

Anterior lobe

Posterior lobe (neurohypophysis)

Site of vasopressin absorption

Inferior hypophysial artery

Venous drainage of posterior lobe

Neurosecretory Ending (posterior pituitary)

Axon

Pituicyte processes

Mast cell

Endothelium

Axon

Collagen space

Neurosecretory vesicles

Fibroblast

Basement membrane

Capillary

POSTERIOR PITUITARY GLAND

The posterior pituitary is neural tissue and is formed by the distal axons of the supraoptic nucleus (SON) and the PVN of the hypothalamus. The axon terminals store neurosecretory granules that contain antidiuretic hormone (ADH; vasopressin) and oxytocin—both are nonapeptides consisting of a six-amino acid ring with a cysteine-to-cysteine bridge and a three-amino acid tail. In embryogenesis, neuroepithelial cells of the lining of the third ventricle migrate laterally to and above the optic chiasm to form the SON and to the walls of the third ventricle to form the PVN. The blood supply for the posterior pituitary is from the inferior hypophysial arteries, and the venous drainage is into the cavernous sinus and internal jugular vein.

The posterior pituitary serves to store and release vasopressin and oxytocin. The posterior pituitary stores enough vasopressin to sustain basal release for approximately 30 days and to sustain maximum release for approximately 5 days. Whereas approximately 90% of the SON neurons produce vasopressin, and all its axons end in the posterior pituitary, the PVN has five subnuclei that synthesize other peptides in addition to vasopressin (e.g., somatostatin, CRH, TRH, and opioids). The neurons of the PVN subnuclei project to the median eminence, brainstem, and spinal cord. The major stimulatory input for vasopressin and oxytocin secretion is glutamate, and the major inhibitory input is γ-aminobutyric acid. When a stimulus for secretion of vasopressin or oxytocin acts on the SON or PVN, an action potential is generated that propagates down the long axon to the posterior pituitary. The action potential triggers an influx of calcium that causes the

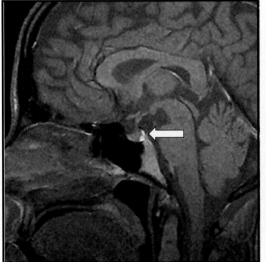

Posterior pituitary bright spot. Sagittal T1-weighted MRI image showing hyperintensity (*arrow*) in the posterior aspect of the sella turcica.

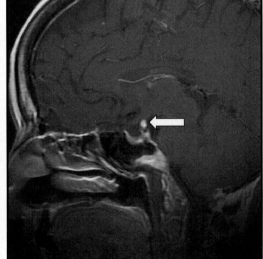

Ectopic posterior pituitary. Sagittal T1-weighted MRI image showing hyperintensity (*arrow*) along the posterior aspect of the pituitary infundibulum.

neurosecretory granules to fuse with the cell membrane and release the contents of the neurosecretory granule into the perivascular space and subsequently into the fenestrated capillary system of the posterior pituitary.

The stored vasopressin in neurosecretory granules in the posterior pituitary produces a bright signal on T1-weighted MRI—the "posterior pituitary bright spot." The posterior pituitary bright spot is present in most healthy individuals and is absent in individuals with

central DI. In addition, this bright spot may be located elsewhere in individuals with congenital abnormalities such that the posterior pituitary is undescended—it may appear at the base of the hypothalamus or along the pituitary stalk. Although posterior pituitary function is usually intact, this "ectopic posterior pituitary" may be associated with a hypoplastic anterior pituitary gland and with varying degrees of anterior pituitary dysfunction.

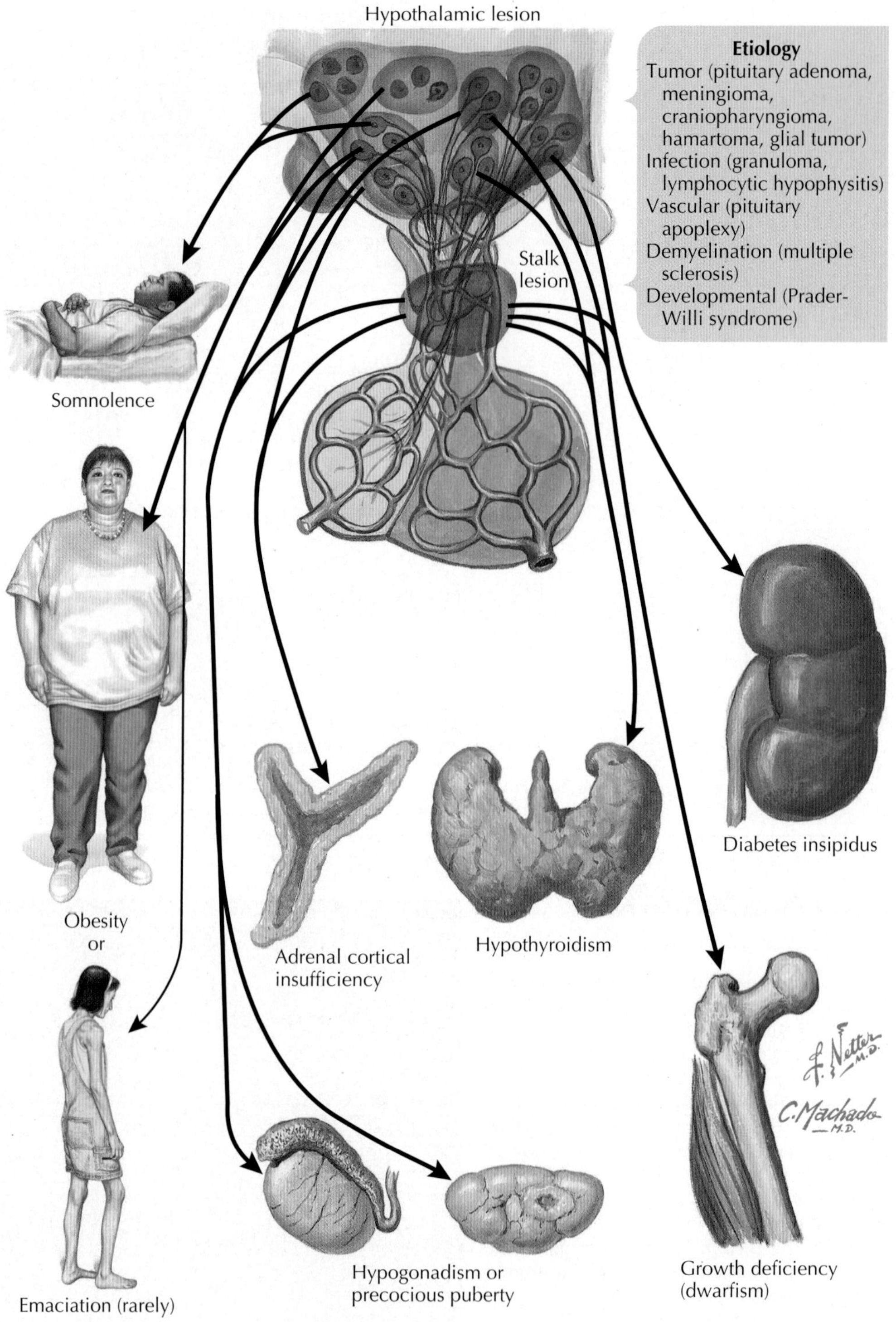

Plate 1.9

Endocrine System: VOLUME 2

Hypothalamic lesion

Stalk lesion

Etiology
Tumor (pituitary adenoma, meningioma, craniopharyngioma, hamartoma, glial tumor)
Infection (granuloma, lymphocytic hypophysitis)
Vascular (pituitary apoplexy)
Demyelination (multiple sclerosis)
Developmental (Prader-Willi syndrome)

Somnolence

Obesity or

Emaciation (rarely)

Adrenal cortical insufficiency

Hypothyroidism

Hypogonadism or precocious puberty

Diabetes insipidus

Growth deficiency (dwarfism)

MANIFESTATIONS OF SUPRASELLAR DISEASE

Suprasellar lesions that may lead to hypothalamic dysfunction include craniopharyngioma, dysgerminoma, granulomatous diseases (e.g., sarcoidosis, tuberculosis, Langerhans cell histiocytosis [LCH]), lymphocytic hypophysitis, metastatic neoplasm, suprasellar extension of a pituitary tumor, glioma (e.g., hypothalamic, third ventricle, optic nerve), sellar chordoma, meningioma, hamartoma, gangliocytoma, suprasellar arachnoid cyst, and ependymoma.

Endocrine and nonendocrine sequelae are related to hypothalamic mass lesions. Because of the proximity to the optic chiasm, hypothalamic lesions are frequently associated with vision loss. An enlarging hypothalamic mass may also cause headaches and recurrent emesis. The hypothalamus is responsible for many homeostatic functions such as appetite control, the sleep-wake cycle, water metabolism, temperature regulation, anterior pituitary function, circadian rhythms, and inputs to the parasympathetic and sympathetic nervous systems. The clinical presentation is more dependent on the location within the hypothalamus than on the pathologic process. Mass lesions may affect only one or all of the four regions of the hypothalamus (from anterior to posterior: preoptic, supraoptic, tuberal, and mammary regions) or one or all of the three zones (from midline to lateral: periventricular, medial, and lateral zones). For example, hypersomnolence is a symptom associated with damage to the posterior hypothalamus (mammary region) where the rostral portion of the ascending reticular activating system is located. Patients with lesions in the anterior (preoptic) hypothalamus may present with hyperactivity and insomnia, alterations in the sleep-wake cycle (e.g., nighttime hyperactivity and daytime sleepiness), or dysthermia (acute hyperthermia or chronic hypothermia).

The appetite center is located in the ventromedial hypothalamus, and the satiety center is localized to the medial hypothalamus. Destructive lesions involving the more centrally located satiety center lead to hyperphagia and obesity, a relatively common presentation for patients with a hypothalamic mass. Destructive lesions of both of the more laterally located feeding centers may lead to hypophagia, weight loss, and cachexia.

Destruction of the vasopressin-producing magnocellular neurons in the supraoptic and paraventricular nuclei in the tuberal region of the hypothalamus results in central DI (see Plate 1.27). In addition, DI may be caused by lesions (e.g., high pituitary stalk lesions) that interrupt the transport of vasopressin through the magnocellular axons that terminate in the pituitary stalk and posterior pituitary. Polydipsia and hypodipsia

are associated with damage to central osmoreceptors located in anterior medial and anterior lateral preoptic regions. The impaired thirst mechanism results in dehydration and hypernatremia.

Anterior pituitary function control emanates primarily from the arcuate nucleus in the tuberal region of the hypothalamus. Thus lesions that involve the floor of the third ventricle and median eminence frequently result in varying degrees of anterior pituitary dysfunction (e.g., secondary hypothyroidism, secondary adrenal insufficiency, secondary hypogonadism, and GH deficiency).

Hypothalamic hamartomas, gangliocytomas, and germ cell tumors may produce peptides normally

secreted by the hypothalamus. Thus patients may present with endocrine hyperfunction syndromes such as precocious puberty with GnRH expression by hamartomas; acromegaly or Cushing syndrome with GHRH expression or CRH expression, respectively, by hypothalamic gangliocytomas; and precocious puberty with β-human chorionic gonadotropin (β-hCG) expression by suprasellar germ cell tumors.

Because of the close microanatomic continuity of the hypothalamic regions and zones, patients with suprasellar disease typically present with not one but many of the dysfunction syndromes discussed.

Plate 1.10

Pituitary and Hypothalamus

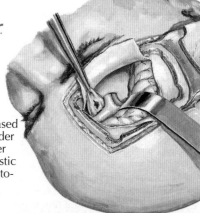

Large cystic suprasellar craniopharyngioma compressing optic chiasm and hypothalamus, filling third ventricle up to interventricular foramen (of Monro), thus causing visual impairment, diabetes insipidus, and hydrocephalus

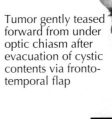

Tumor gently teased forward from under optic chiasm after evacuation of cystic contents via fronto-temporal flap

Intrasellar cystic craniopharyngioma compressing pituitary gland to cause hypopituitarism

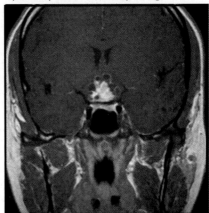

MRI (sagittal view) showing cystic suprasellar craniopharngioma

CRANIOPHARYNGIOMA

Craniopharyngioma is the most common tumor found in the region of the pituitary gland in children and adolescents and constitutes about 3% of all intracranial tumors and up to 10% of all childhood brain tumors. Craniopharyngiomas—histologically benign epithelioid tumors arising from embryonic squamous remnants of Rathke pouch—may be large (e.g., >6 cm in diameter) and invade the third ventricle and associated brain structures. This tumorous process is usually located above the sella turcica, depressing the optic chiasm and extending up into the third ventricle. Less frequently, craniopharyngiomas are located within the sella, causing compression of the pituitary gland and frequently eroding the bony confines of the sella turcica. Signs and symptoms—primarily caused by mass effect—typically occur in the adolescent years and rarely after age 40 years. The mass effect symptoms include vision loss by compression of the optic chiasm; DI by invasion or disruption of the hypothalamus or pituitary stalk; hypothalamic dysfunction (e.g., obesity with hyperphagia, hypersomnolence, disturbance in temperature regulation); various degrees of anterior pituitary insufficiency (e.g., GH deficiency with short stature in childhood, hypogonadism, adrenal insufficiency, hypothyroidism); hyperprolactinemia caused by compression of the pituitary stalk or damage to the dopaminergic neurons in the hypothalamus; signs and symptoms of increased intracranial pressure (e.g., headache, projectile emesis, papilledema, optic atrophy); symptoms of hydrocephalus (e.g., mental dullness and confusion) when large tumors obstruct the flow of cerebrospinal fluid (CSF); and cranial nerve palsies caused by cavernous sinus invasion.

The findings on radiologic imaging are quite characteristic. Plain skull radiographs and computed tomography (CT) show irregular calcification in

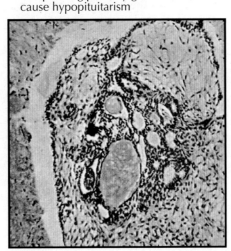

Histologic section: craniopharyngioma (H&E stain, ×125)

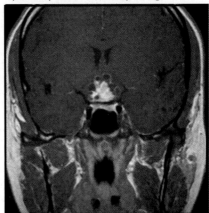

MRI (coronal view) showing suprasellar craniopharngioma

the suprasellar region. MRI typically shows a multilobulated cystic structure that is usually suprasellar in location, but it may also appear to arise from the sella. The cystic regions are usually filled with a turbid, cholesterol-rich, viscous fluid. The walls of the cystic and solid components are composed of whorls and cords of epithelial cells separated by a loose network of stellate cells. If there are intercellular epithelial bridges and keratohyalin, the tumor is classified as an adamantinoma.

Treatment options for patients with craniopharyngiomas include observation, endonasal transsphenoidal surgery for smaller intrasellar tumors, craniotomy for larger suprasellar tumors, stereotactic radiotherapy, or a combination of these modalities. Most of these treatment approaches result in varying degrees of anterior or posterior pituitary hormone deficits (or both). In addition, recurrent disease after treatment is common (~40%) because of tumor adherence to surrounding structures, and long-term follow-up is indicated.

Plate 1.11

Endocrine System: VOLUME 2

EFFECTS OF PITUITARY TUMORS ON THE VISUAL APPARATUS

The optic chiasm lies above the diaphragma sellae. The most common sign that a pituitary tumor has extended beyond the confines of the sella turcica is a visual defect caused by the growth pressing on the optic chiasm. The most frequent disturbance is a bitemporal hemianopsia, which is produced by the tumor pressing on the crossing central fibers of the chiasm and sparing the uncrossed lateral fibers. The earliest changes are usually enlargement of the blind spot; loss of color vision, especially for red; and a wedge-shaped area of defective vision in the upper-temporal quadrants, which gradually enlarges to occupy the whole quadrant and subsequently extends to include the lower temporal quadrant as well.

The type of visual defect produced depends on the position of the chiasm in relation to the pituitary gland and the direction of tumor growth. In about 10% of the cases, the chiasm may be found almost entirely anterior or posterior to the diaphragma sellae instead of in its usual position, which is directly above the diaphragma. There are also lateral displacements of the chiasm, which may cause either its right or its left branch to lie above the diaphragma. If the chiasm is abnormally fixed, the adenoma may grow upward for a long time before it seriously disturbs vision. Bilateral central scotomas are caused by damage to the posterior part of the chiasm, and their occurrence suggests that the chiasm is prefixed and that the tumor is large. In other cases of prefixed chiasm, the tumor may extend in such a direction as to compress the optic tract rather than the chiasm, thus producing a homonymous hemianopsia. However, homonymous defects do not always indicate a prefixed chiasm; they may also be produced by lateral extension into the temporal lobe below a normally placed chiasm. Other visual defects that may occur include unilateral central scotoma; dimness of vision (amblyopia) in one eye caused by compression of one optic nerve; and an inferior quadrantal hemianopsia, presumably resulting from a large tumor causing the anterior cerebral arteries to cut into the dorsal surface of a normally placed chiasm.

Primary optic atrophy is present in most cases, but it may be absent when the lesion is behind the chiasm. Although papilledema is rare, it may occur with large tumors that cause increased intracranial pressure. If pressure on the visual pathway is relieved (e.g., with surgery or pharmacotherapy), the visual fields may return to normal. However, vision recovery is caused partly by the degree and duration of the optic tract deformation. Field defects can be detected on gross examination by observing the angle at which an object, such as the examiner's finger, becomes visible when the patient looks straight ahead. Quantitative perimetry is necessary for exact plotting of the size and shape of the field defect.

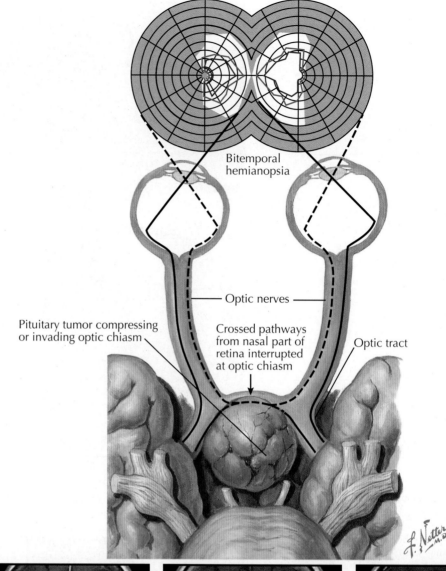

Bitemporal hemianopsia

Pituitary tumor compressing or invading optic chiasm

Optic nerves

Crossed pathways from nasal part of retina interrupted at optic chiasm

Optic tract

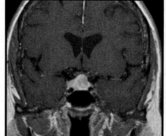

MRI showing pituitary macroadenoma with suprasellar and right cavernous sinus extension. Optic chiasm is raised slightly, but visual fields are normal.

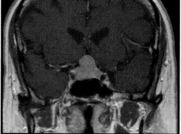

MRI showing pituitary macroadenoma with suprasellar and bilateral cavernous sinus extension. The optic chiasm is compressed, causing bitemporal superior quadrant vision loss.

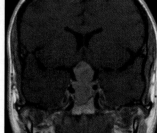

MRI showing pituitary macroadenoma with suprasellar, bilateral cavernous, and sphenoid extensions. The optic chiasm is markedly compressed, causing complete bitemporal hemianopsia.

In some cases of pituitary tumor showing expansive growth sufficient to enlarge the sella, the visual pathway escapes damage because the sellar diaphragm is tough and prevents expansion toward the chiasm. In these cases, the pituitary tumor may extend laterally into the cavernous sinus or inferiorly into the sphenoid sinus. This structure shows considerable variation, from a dense, closely knit membrane to a small rim with a wide infundibular opening. In most cases, the diaphragm does yield to pressure from below. Usually, the chiasm lies directly on the diaphragm and is separated from it by only a potential cleft. Frequently, particularly where there is a well-developed chiasmatic cistern, the optic chiasm may be as high as 1 cm above the diaphragm, which allows an invading tumor considerable room for expansion before it presses on the visual pathway.

Plate 1.12   Pituitary and Hypothalamus

NONTUMOROUS LESIONS OF THE PITUITARY GLAND

The nontumorous lesions of the pituitary gland that can affect function include lymphocytic hypophysitis, granulomatous disorders (e.g., sarcoidosis, tuberculosis, LCH, Wegener granulomatosis), immune checkpoint inhibitor-induced hypophysitis, xanthomatous hypophysitis, hemorrhage (see Plate 1.18), infarction (see Plate 1.17), head trauma with skull base fracture, iron overload states (e.g., hemochromatosis, hemosiderosis), intrasellar carotid artery aneurysm, primary empty sella (see Plate 1.31), infection (e.g., encephalitis, pituitary abscess), mutations in genes encoding pituitary transcription factors, and developmental midline anomalies.

Lymphocytic hypophysitis is an autoimmune disorder characterized by lymphocytic infiltration and enlargement of the pituitary gland followed by selective destruction of pituitary cells. The most common clinical setting is in late pregnancy or in the postpartum period. Patients typically present with headaches and signs and symptoms of deficiency of one or more pituitary hormones. Frequently, there is a curious preferential destruction of corticotrophs. However, these patients may have panhypopituitarism (including DI). MRI usually shows a homogeneous, contrast-enhancing sellar mass with pituitary stalk involvement. The pituitary hormone deficits are usually permanent, but recovery of both anterior and posterior pituitary function may occur.

Granulomatous hypophysitis can be caused by sarcoidosis, tuberculosis, LCH, or Wegener granulomatosis. The granulomatous inflammation may involve the hypothalamus, pituitary stalk, and pituitary gland and cause hypopituitarism, including DI.

Immune checkpoint inhibitor-induced hypophysitis is caused by drugs that enhance the immune system. Checkpoint inhibition is associated with a unique spectrum of side effects termed immune-related adverse events. Ipilimumab is a T-lymphocyte antigen 4 antibody and frequently used to treat metastatic melanoma. Hypophysitis occurs in approximately 8% of patients at a median time of 4 months after ipilimumab initiation. Pituitary deficits are limited to the anterior pituitary gland and most commonly secondary adrenal insufficiency. Hypophysitis is less common in those treated with antiprogrammed cell death 1 (PD-1) antibodies (e.g., nivolumab) and antiprogrammed cell death 1 ligand (PD-L1) antibodies (e.g., atezolizumab).

Head trauma that results in a skull base fracture may cause hypothalamic hormone deficiencies, resulting in deficient secretion of anterior and posterior pituitary hormones. Head trauma may lead to direct pituitary damage by a sella turcica fracture, pituitary stalk section, trauma-induced vasospasm, or ischemic infarction after blunt trauma.

Iron overload states of hemochromatosis and hemosiderosis of thalassemia may involve the pituitary, resulting in iron deposition (siderosis) in pituitary cells. Iron overload most commonly results in selective gonadotropin deficiency.

Hypopituitarism is also associated with mutations in genes that encode the transcription factors whose expression is necessary for the differentiation of anterior pituitary cells (e.g., *HESX1, LHX3, LHX4, PROP1, POU1F1* [formerly *PIT1*], *TBX19* [also known as *TPIT*]). Mutations in *PROP1* are the most common cause of familial and sporadic congenital hypopituitarism. *PROP1* is necessary for the differentiation of a cell

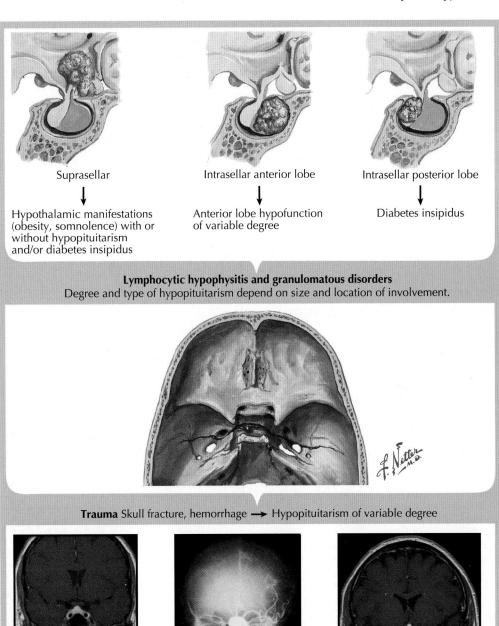

Suprasellar → Hypothalamic manifestations (obesity, somnolence) with or without hypopituitarism and/or diabetes insipidus

Intrasellar anterior lobe → Anterior lobe hypofunction of variable degree

Intrasellar posterior lobe → Diabetes insipidus

Lymphocytic hypophysitis and granulomatous disorders
Degree and type of hypopituitarism depend on size and location of involvement.

Trauma Skull fracture, hemorrhage → Hypopituitarism of variable degree

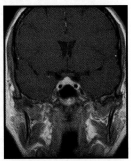
MRI showing diffusely enhancing lymphocytic hypophysitis filling the sella and extending toward the optic chiasm

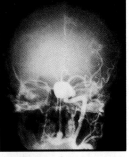
Angiogram showing intrasellar carotid artery aneurysm

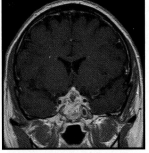
Pituitary abscess due to nocardia farcinica

Imaging is key in the diagnosis of and in determining the type of nontumorous sellar process.

type that is a precursor of somatotroph, lactotroph, thyrotroph, and gonadotroph cells. The protein encoded by *POU1F1*, which acts temporally just after the protein encoded by *PROP1*, is necessary for the differentiation of a cell type that is a precursor of somatotroph, lactotroph, and to a lesser degree, thyrotroph cells. *TBX19* is required for specific differentiation of the corticotroph cells. Because the proteins encoded by *HEXS1, LHX3*, and *LHX4* act early in pituicyte differentiation, mutations in these genes cause combined pituitary hormone

deficiency, which refers to deficiencies of GH, prolactin, TSH, LH, and FSH (see Plate 1.13).

Developmental midline anomalies may lead to structural pituitary anomalies (e.g., pituitary aplasia or hypoplasia). Craniofacial developmental anomalies may result in cleft lip and palate, basal encephalocele, hypertelorism, and optic nerve hypoplasia, with varying degrees of pituitary dysplasia and aplasia. Congenital basal encephalocele may cause the pituitary to herniate through the sphenoid sinus roof, resulting in pituitary failure and DI.

Plate 1.13

Endocrine System: VOLUME 2

Growth hormone absent

Pituitary, anterior lobe

Growth hormone

Pituitary gonadotropins (FSH and LH) absent

No androgen

No androgen

Panhypopituitarism
(pituitary dwarf)

Selective pituitary gonadotropic deficiency
(pituitary eunuchoid)

Unstimulated; therefore, infantile testes

Pituitary Anterior Lobe Deficiency in Childhood and Adolescence in Boys

The most common deficient hormones in children and adolescents with anterior pituitary failure are the gonadotropins, LH, and FSH. Gonadotropin deficiency may occur in isolation or in concert with other anterior pituitary hormone deficiencies. In the absence of gonadotropins in boys, puberty is delayed, and secondary sex characteristics do not develop (see Plate 4.7). The penis and prostate gland remain small, and the scrotum fails to develop rugae; the larynx fails to enlarge, and the voice maintains the high pitch of childhood. Some pubic hair appears, but it is usually sparse and fine. Axillary hair either does not appear or is sparse. Beard growth is absent.

Lack of androgens leads to prolonged persistence of open epiphysial plates and—in the presence of intact GH and IGF-1—linear growth continues for longer than normal. The linear growth is particularly prominent in the extremities, and the arms and legs become disproportionately long. Eunuchoid proportions develop; lower body length (from the soles of the feet to the pubis) exceeds upper body length (from the pubis to the top of the cranium). In addition, the arm span exceeds the standing height (normally, these dimensions should be equal). Eventually, the epiphyses close in the third decade of life, even in untreated eunuchoid males. Administration of testosterone leads to prompt epiphysial closure. Excessive linear growth is not seen in adults with anterior pituitary deficiency after epiphysial closure.

The presentation of secondary hypogonadism in adolescence may be affected by the presence or absence of other anterior pituitary hormone deficiencies. If GH is also deficient in childhood, short stature is evident. Short stature occurs when a child is two standard deviations or more below the mean height for children of that gender and chronologic age—typically below the 3rd percentile for height. The three phases of growth are infantile, childhood, and pubertal. Infantile growth is a rapid but decelerating growth pattern during the first 2 years of life with an average growth of 30 cm. A statistically significant and positive correlation exists between the height at age 2 years and final adult height. The childhood growth phase progresses at a relatively constant velocity of 5 to 7 cm per year. The pubertal growth phase refers to the growth spurt of 8 to 14 cm per year that occurs during puberty. The most common

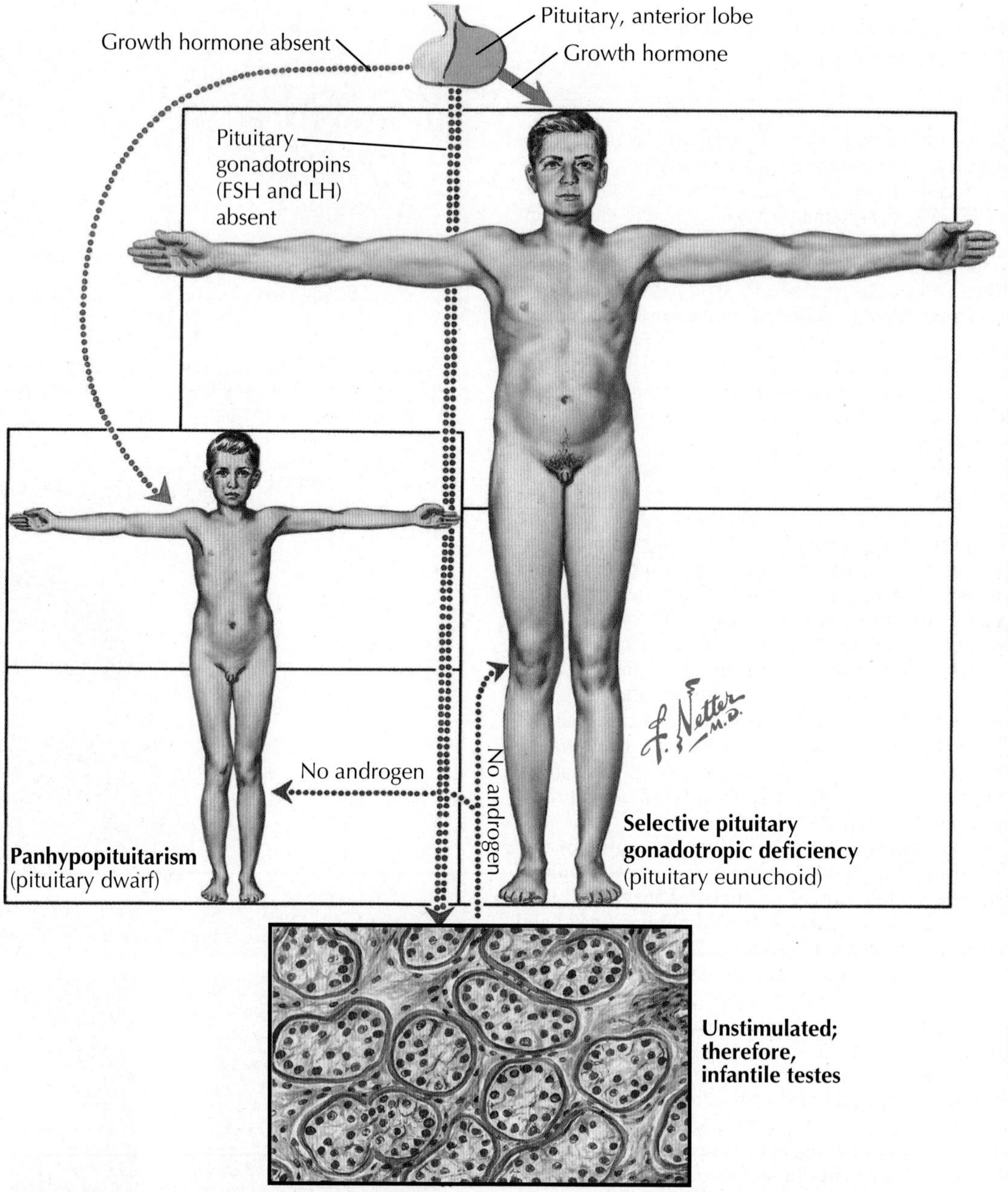

Pituitary causes:
▶ Pituitary adenoma
▶ Pituitary cyst
▶ Pituitary surgery
▶ Infiltrative lesion
    (e.g., lymphocytic hypophysitis)
▶ Infarction (e.g., Sheehan syndrome)
▶ Apoplexy
▶ Genetic disorder (e.g., *POU1F1* mutation)
▶ Primary empty sella syndrome
▶ Metastatic disease to the sella

Hypothalamic causes:
▶ Mass lesion (e.g., craniopharyngioma)
▶ Radiation (e.g., for brain malignancy)
▶ Infiltrative lesion (e.g., sarcoidosis)
▶ Trauma with skull base fracture
▶ Infection (e.g., viral encephalitis)

causes of short stature are genetic short stature and delayed growth. In addition to GH deficiency, the disorders that are most often associated with short stature are renal disease, cancer (and its treatment), glucocorticoid therapy, pulmonary diseases (e.g., cystic fibrosis), cardiac disorders (e.g., congenital heart disease), gastrointestinal disorders (e.g., celiac disease, inflammatory bowel disease), poorly controlled diabetes mellitus, vitamin D deficiency, hypothyroidism, and Cushing syndrome.

Additional anterior pituitary hormone deficiencies may contribute to the clinical presentation. For example, corticotropin deficiency may cause signs and symptoms of postural hypotension, tachycardia, fatigue, anorexia, weight loss, hyponatremia, and hypoglycemia. Thyrotropin deficiency may contribute signs and symptoms of fatigue, cold intolerance, constipation, facial puffiness with periorbital edema, dry skin, bradycardia, and delayed relaxation phase of the deep tendon reflexes.

Plate 1.14

Pituitary and Hypothalamus

PITUITARY ANTERIOR LOBE DEFICIENCY IN ADULTS

Anterior pituitary deficiency is decreased secretion of pituitary hormones caused by a disorder of the pituitary or hypothalamus. Compression of a normal pituitary gland by a pituitary adenoma is the most common cause. Other causes of anterior pituitary failure include pituitary cyst, pituitary surgery, pituitary radiation, infiltrative lesion (e.g., lymphocytic hypophysitis, hemochromatosis), infarction (e.g., Sheehan syndrome), apoplexy, genetic disorder (e.g., pit-1 mutation, *POU1F1* mutation), primary empty sella syndrome, and metastatic disease to the sella. Hypothalamic diseases that may cause varying degrees of hypopituitarism include mass lesions (e.g., craniopharyngioma, germinoma, metastatic disease), radiation (e.g., for brain or nasopharyngeal malignancies), infiltrative lesions (e.g., sarcoidosis, LCH), trauma with skull base fracture, and infection (e.g., viral encephalitis, tuberculous meningitis).

The signs and symptoms related to anterior pituitary insufficiency may occur slowly or suddenly; may be mild or severe; and may affect the secretion of a single, several, or all pituitary hormones. Whereas pituitary apoplexy (see Plate 1.18) is an example of a sudden onset presentation dominated by abrupt loss of corticotropin secretion, the effects of slow-growing nonfunctioning pituitary adenomas or radiation therapy on pituitary function develop over years. *Panhypopituitarism* is the term used to describe deficiency of all pituitary hormones. Partial hypopituitarism is more common. In general, the secretion of GH and gonadotropins is more likely to be affected than corticotropin and thyrotropin.

The clinical picture may be dominated by secondary hypogonadism from gonadotropin deficiency. With long-standing gonadal steroid deficiency, individuals develop fine facial wrinkles around the eyes, mouth, and cheeks. Pallor, out of proportion to the moderate anemia usually present, is observed. There is loss of axillary and pubic hair. In females, amenorrhea, infertility, vaginal dryness and atrophy, hot flashes, breast atrophy, osteoporosis, and loss of libido occur. In males, secondary gonadal failure may cause infertility, decreased libido, decreased vitality, decreased testicular size, erectile dysfunction, and osteoporosis.

GH deficiency in adults may be associated with decreased sense of well-being, increased fat mass, decreased muscle mass, increased risk of cardiovascular disease, and decreased bone mineral density.

Prolactin deficiency may result in the inability to lactate postpartum.

Thyroid deficiency produces a subnormal temperature, cold intolerance, a low metabolic rate, fatigue, dry skin, periorbital puffiness (myxedema facies), bradycardia,

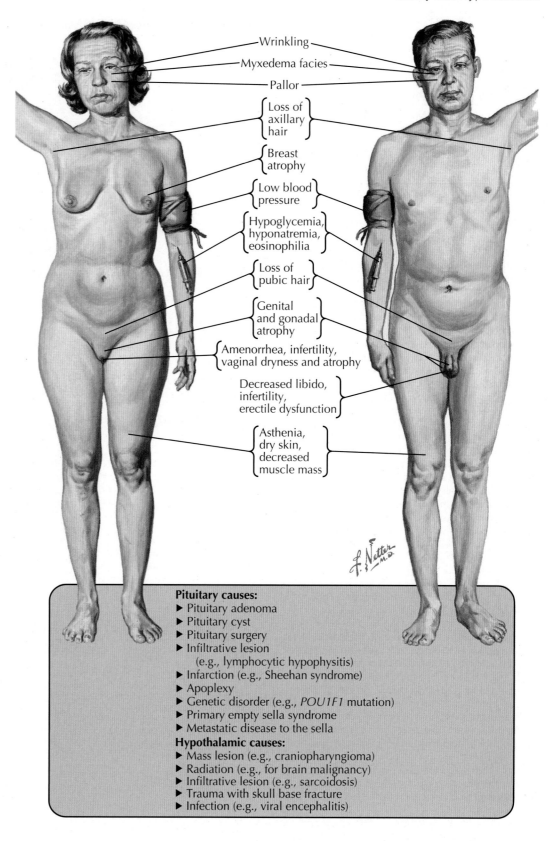

Pituitary causes:
▶ Pituitary adenoma
▶ Pituitary cyst
▶ Pituitary surgery
▶ Infiltrative lesion
   (e.g., lymphocytic hypophysitis)
▶ Infarction (e.g., Sheehan syndrome)
▶ Apoplexy
▶ Genetic disorder (e.g., *POU1F1* mutation)
▶ Primary empty sella syndrome
▶ Metastatic disease to the sella
Hypothalamic causes:
▶ Mass lesion (e.g., craniopharyngioma)
▶ Radiation (e.g., for brain malignancy)
▶ Infiltrative lesion (e.g., sarcoidosis)
▶ Trauma with skull base fracture
▶ Infection (e.g., viral encephalitis)

anemia, delayed relaxation phase of the deep tendon reflexes, and constipation (see Plates 2.14 and 2.15). Also, the combined decrease of thyroid hormone and testosterone may result in loss of the lateral third of the eyebrows.

Adrenal insufficiency is responsible for low blood pressure, asthenia, weight loss, eosinophilia, and crises of nausea and vomiting, which may be associated with spontaneous hypoglycemia. Because the adrenal secretion of aldosterone is preserved, secondary adrenal failure does not cause salt wasting or hyperkalemia (see Plate 3.24). Also, the hyperpigmentation characteristic of primary adrenal failure (see Plate 3.22) is absent. However, both primary and secondary adrenal failure may cause hyponatremia, a result of inappropriate secretion of vasopressin and a lack of permissive effect of cortisol for the kidneys to excrete free water.

Plate 1.15

Endocrine System: VOLUME 2

SELECTIVE AND PARTIAL HYPOPITUITARISM

Selective and partial hypopituitarism refers to the loss of at least one but not all pituitary hormones. The term *panhypopituitarism* is reserved for the syndrome resulting from the loss of all the hormonal functions of the pituitary, including those of the neurohypophysis (see Plates 1.16 and 1.27). The clinical presentation depends on the rapidity of hormone loss (e.g., sudden with pituitary apoplexy [see Plate 1.18] vs. slow with a slowly growing pituitary tumor) and the number of pituitary hormones affected.

The gonadotropic function of the pituitary is usually the first to fail, probably because the gonadotrophs are more sensitive to adverse conditions than are the other anterior pituitary cell types. In children with mild pituitary destruction, puberty is delayed or does not occur. If GH is present in normal quantities and the other functions of the pituitary are not impaired, then overgrowth of the long bones will occur, and a eunuchoid body habitus will develop (see Plate 1.13). Adults with acquired secondary hypogonadism typically present with slowly progressive symptoms (see Plate 1.14). Blood concentrations of testosterone in males and estradiol in females are below the reference ranges, and concentrations of the gonadotropins LH and FSH are inappropriately normal or low.

GH deficiency also tends to occur early in patients with hypopituitarism, and the potential symptoms in adults (e.g., decreased sense of well being, increased fat mass, decreased muscle mass) may be attributed to other causes, but with GH deficiency in childhood, a slowing of linear growth is typically evident. GH deficiency is evaluated by blood measurement of IGF-1 and GH response to provocation (e.g., insulin-induced hypoglycemia, arginine infusion, glucagon, GH secretagogues [such as macimorelin], or GHRH administration).

With more severe insults to the pituitary gland, thyrotroph function and subsequently corticotroph function may be affected. Blood concentrations of thyroxine (total and free) are below the reference range, and thyrotropin is inappropriately normal or low. The symptoms of primary hypothyroidism (see Plates 2.14–2.16) are indistinguishable from those of secondary hypothyroidism. In some instances, hypothyroidism-related symptoms may dominate the clinical picture, and treatment with levothyroxine in patients with concurrent secondary adrenal insufficiency may increase the clearance of the limited cortisol being produced, create an additional metabolic strain on the patient, and precipitate an adrenal crisis.

Secondary adrenal insufficiency differs from primary adrenal insufficiency in two important ways: (1) because of the loss of corticotropin and melanocyte-stimulating hormone (MSH), pallor may be present that is not proportional to the moderate anemia sometimes seen, and (2) adrenal aldosterone secretion remains intact because the main regulators (angiotensin II and blood potassium) are not dependent on normal pituitary function. The blood concentrations of cortisol and dehydroepiandrosterone-sulfate measured at 8 AM are below the reference ranges, and corticotropin is typically undetectable (see Plate 3.24).

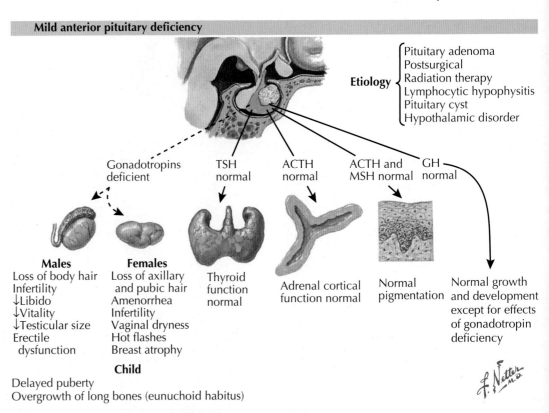

Mild anterior pituitary deficiency

Etiology
- Pituitary adenoma
- Postsurgical
- Radiation therapy
- Lymphocytic hypophysitis
- Pituitary cyst
- Hypothalamic disorder

Gonadotropins deficient — TSH normal — ACTH normal — ACTH and MSH normal — GH normal

Males
Loss of body hair
Infertility
↓Libido
↓Vitality
↓Testicular size
Erectile dysfunction

Females
Loss of axillary and pubic hair
Amenorrhea
Infertility
Vaginal dryness
Hot flashes
Breast atrophy

Thyroid function normal

Adrenal cortical function normal

Normal pigmentation

Normal growth and development except for effects of gonadotropin deficiency

Child
Delayed puberty
Overgrowth of long bones (eunuchoid habitus)

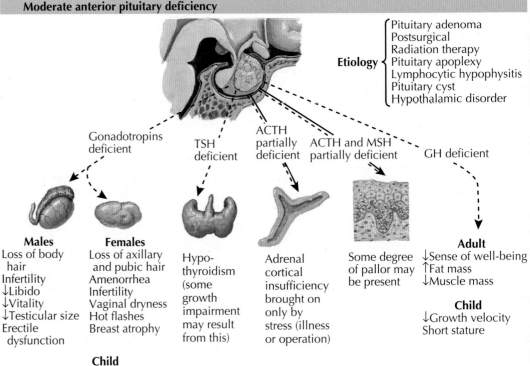

Moderate anterior pituitary deficiency

Etiology
- Pituitary adenoma
- Postsurgical
- Radiation therapy
- Pituitary apoplexy
- Lymphocytic hypophysitis
- Pituitary cyst
- Hypothalamic disorder

Gonadotropins deficient — TSH deficient — ACTH partially deficient — ACTH and MSH partially deficient — GH deficient

Males
Loss of body hair
Infertility
↓Libido
↓Vitality
↓Testicular size
Erectile dysfunction

Females
Loss of axillary and pubic hair
Amenorrhea
Infertility
Vaginal dryness
Hot flashes
Breast atrophy

Hypothyroidism (some growth impairment may result from this)

Adrenal cortical insufficiency brought on only by stress (illness or operation)

Some degree of pallor may be present

Adult
↓Sense of well-being
↑Fat mass
↓Muscle mass

Child
↓Growth velocity
Short stature

Child
Delayed puberty
Overgrowth of long bones (eunuchoid habitus)

Prolactin is frequently the most preserved pituitary hormone in patients with progressive hypopituitarism, and its absence may only be evident by the inability to lactate after delivery.

Selective loss of one pituitary hormone may also occur with lymphocytic hypophysitis—for example, these patients may present with selective corticotropin deficiency. If the partial hypopituitarism is attributable to a pituitary or sellar mass, patients may also have symptoms related to tumor-specific pituitary hormone hypersecretion (e.g., acromegaly, hyperprolactinemia, or Cushing syndrome) or related to mass effect (e.g., vision loss, diplopia, or headache).

Typically, patients with single or multiple pituitary hormone deficiencies respond well to target hormone replacement therapy. If the causative lesion is not progressive, the prognosis for a long and active life is excellent.

Plate 1.16

Pituitary and Hypothalamus

SEVERE ANTERIOR PITUITARY DEFICIENCY OR PANHYPOPITUITARISM

Severe symptoms of anterior pituitary insufficiency appear only when destruction of the adenohypophysis is nearly complete. With progressive destruction (>75%), mild hypogonadism becomes more severe, and general symptoms attributable to thyroid and adrenal cortical hypofunction, such as asthenia, fatigue, loss of appetite, and cold intolerance, appear and progress. Complete anterior pituitary failure may occur after surgery for a pituitary macroadenoma.

Atrophy of the gonads is a constant finding in this disease. A regression of secondary sexual characteristics also occurs. In females, the ovaries become small and fibrous, and the uterus regresses to infantile proportions with an extremely thin layer of endometrium. The external genitalia shrink, as does the vagina, which develops a smooth, atrophic epithelium. The breasts regress, and the areolae lose pigmentation. In males, the penis is small, the testes are shrunken and devoid of rugae, and the prostate is markedly atrophied. In both sexes, the thyroid gland is small, with follicles lined with low cuboidal epithelium. Shrinkage of the adrenal cortex is most obvious in the zona fasciculata and zona reticularis. The zona glomerulosa, which is the site of aldosterone production, does not depend on ACTH secretion, in contrast to the other two layers. The general architectural pattern of the adrenal cortex is maintained, but the cells are poor in lipid content.

Pallor that is not proportional to the moderate anemia is typically present and is probably attributable to a deficiency of ACTH and MSH. There is a loss of muscle mass—although multifactorial, the lack of GH is a main contributor. Children have a tendency to have hypoglycemia, which is associated with deficiency of adrenal glucocorticoids as well as lack of GH together with poor food intake.

The term *panhypopituitarism* should be reserved for cases in which all the functions of the adenohypophysis and neurohypophysis are affected. Patients with slowly progressive destructive lesions of this region may first manifest DI, which disappears when involvement of the adenohypophysis becomes extreme enough to cause secondary adrenal cortical insufficiency. This antagonism between vasopressin and glucocorticoids is further demonstrated by the reappearance of DI when these patients are treated with replacement doses of cortisol.

The treatments for ACTH, TSH, LH, and FSH deficiencies are the same as the treatments for primary deficiencies of the respective target glands. For example, for ACTH deficiency, hydrocortisone (or other glucocorticoid) is administered to mimic the normal pattern of cortisol secretion with regard to timing and amount, and the patient is instructed on the need for higher doses in times of illness and other stresses. The goal of therapy is resolution of signs and symptoms of adrenal insufficiency and avoidance of excess glucocorticoid effect (e.g., Cushing syndrome).

Patients with TSH deficiency are treated with levothyroxine. The goal of therapy is a midnormal serum free thyroxine concentration. In patients with panhypopituitarism, levothyroxine should not be administered until glucocorticoid replacement has been initiated.

Treatment of patients with LH and FSH deficiency depends on whether fertility is desired. In males, transdermal testosterone replacement is the treatment of choice for those not interested in fertility. The dosage of testosterone is adjusted for midnormal blood total and bioavailable testosterone concentrations. If fertility is desired, males are treated with gonadotropins. Females can be treated with estrogen-progestin replacement therapy. Females who wish to become fertile can undergo ovulation induction.

Although the role for GH replacement in children with hypopituitarism is clear, GH replacement in adults is optional. Adults with GH deficiency can be treated with GH to optimize body fat, muscle mass, bone mineral density, and a sense of well-being. The dosage of GH is titrated to reach a midnormal IGF-1 concentration.

The only symptom related to prolactin deficiency is the inability to breastfeed. Recombinant human prolactin for the treatment of lactation insufficiency is in development.

Patients with DI can be treated with desmopressin—a two-amino acid modification of vasopressin that has potent antidiuretic but no vasopressor activity. The goals of therapy are to reduce nocturia to provide adequate sleep and to control excess urination during the day. Desmopressin can be administered as a nose spray or an oral tablet.

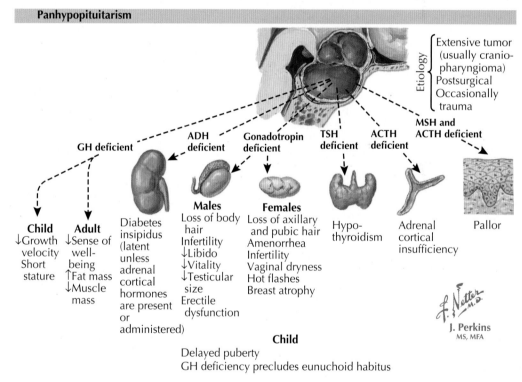

Severe anterior pituitary deficiency

Etiology: Extensive destructive macroadenoma or craniopharyngioma / Postpartum necrosis / Occasionally trauma / Postsurgical

GH deficient
- **Child** ↓Growth velocity, Short stature
- **Adult** ↓Sense of well-being, ↑Fat mass, ↓Muscle mass

Gonadotropins deficient
- **Males** Loss of body hair, Infertility, ↓Libido, ↓Vitality, ↓Testicular size, Erectile dysfunction
- **Females** Loss of axillary and pubic hair, Amenorrhea, Infertility, Vaginal dryness, Hot flashes, Breast atrophy
- **Child** Delayed puberty. GH deficiency precludes eunuchoid habitus

TSH deficient Hypothyroidism

ACTH deficient Adrenal cortical insufficiency

MSH deficient Pallor

Panhypopituitarism

Etiology: Extensive tumor (usually craniopharyngioma) / Postsurgical / Occasionally trauma

GH deficient
- **Child** ↓Growth velocity, Short stature
- **Adult** ↓Sense of well-being, ↑Fat mass, ↓Muscle mass

ADH deficient Diabetes insipidus (latent unless adrenal cortical hormones are present or administered)

Gonadotropin deficient
- **Males** Loss of body hair, Infertility, ↓Libido, ↓Vitality, ↓Testicular size, Erectile dysfunction
- **Females** Loss of axillary and pubic hair, Amenorrhea, Infertility, Vaginal dryness, Hot flashes, Breast atrophy
- **Child** Delayed puberty. GH deficiency precludes eunuchoid habitus

TSH deficient Hypothyroidism

ACTH deficient Adrenal cortical insufficiency

MSH and ACTH deficient Pallor

J. Netter M.D.

J. Perkins MS, MFA

Plate 1.17

Endocrine System: VOLUME 2

POSTPARTUM PITUITARY INFARCTION (SHEEHAN SYNDROME)

The pituitary gland enlarges during pregnancy (primarily because of lactotroph hyperplasia), and because of its portal venous blood supply, it is uniquely vulnerable to changes in arterial blood pressure. In 1937 Sheehan suggested that in the setting of severe postpartum uterine hemorrhage, spasm of the infundibular arteries, which are drained by the hypophysial portal vessels, could result in pituitary infarction. If the lack of blood flow continued for several hours, most of the tissues of the anterior pituitary gland infarcted; when blood finally started to flow, stasis and thrombosis occurred in the stalk and the adenohypophysis. The necrotic areas of the adenohypophysis underwent organization and formed a fibrous scar. Sheehan speculated that variations in the extent and duration of the spasm account for variations in the extent of the necrosis. Today it is recognized that the basic mechanism is infarction secondary to a lack of blood flow to the adenohypophysis. However, it is actually not clear if the infarction is a result of vasospasm, thrombosis, or vascular compression.

In about half of postpartum pituitary infarction cases, the process involves approximately 97% of the anterior lobe, but the pars tuberalis and a small portion of the superior surface of the adenohypophysis are preserved. This remnant retains its structural connections with the hypothalamus and receives portal blood supply from the neural portion of the stalk. Another type of anterior lobe remnant that is sometimes found in these cases is a small area of parenchyma at the lateral pole of the gland without vascular or neural connections with the stalk and hypothalamus. In other instances, a thin layer of parenchyma remains up against the wall of the sella under the capsule. Presumably, these peripheral remnants are nourished by a small capsular blood supply. Normal pituitary function can be maintained by approximately 50% of the gland, but partial and complete anterior pituitary failure results in losses of 75% and 90%, respectively, of the adenohypophysis cells. If more than 30% of the gland is preserved, there is usually sufficient function to forestall the development of acute pituitary failure.

The clinical presentation may range from hypovolemic shock (associated with both the uterine hemorrhage and glucocorticoid deficiency) to gradual onset of partial to complete anterior pituitary insufficiency, only recognized when the patient is unable to breastfeed and has postpartum amenorrhea. These patients may have all of the signs and symptoms of partial or complete hypopituitarism (see Plates 1.15 and 1.16). The acute loss of glucocorticoids can be fatal if not recognized. These patients require lifelong pituitary target gland replacement therapy. DI in this setting is rare.

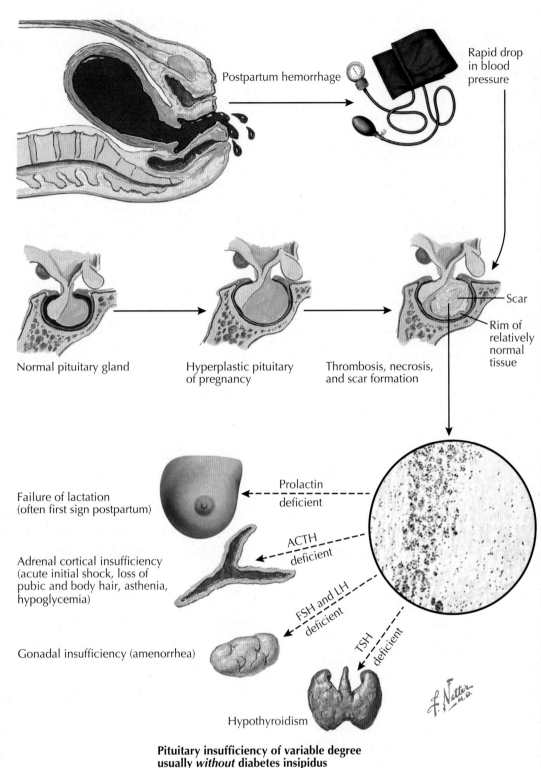

Postpartum hemorrhage

Rapid drop in blood pressure

Normal pituitary gland

Hyperplastic pituitary of pregnancy

Thrombosis, necrosis, and scar formation

Scar

Rim of relatively normal tissue

Failure of lactation (often first sign postpartum) — Prolactin deficient

Adrenal cortical insufficiency (acute initial shock, loss of pubic and body hair, asthenia, hypoglycemia) — ACTH deficient

Gonadal insufficiency (amenorrhea) — FSH and LH deficient

TSH deficient

Hypothyroidism

Pituitary insufficiency of variable degree usually *without* diabetes insipidus

Sheehan syndrome should be suspected in females who have a history of postpartum hemorrhage—severe enough to require blood transfusion—and who develop postpartum lethargy, anorexia, weight loss, inability to lactate, amenorrhea, or loss of axillary and pubic hair. The evaluation involves measuring blood concentrations of the pituitary-dependent target hormones— 8 AM cortisol, free thyroxine, prolactin, estradiol, and IGF-1. Sheehan syndrome is one of the few conditions in which hypoprolactinemia may be found. MRI shows evidence of ischemic infarct in the pituitary gland with enlargement followed by gradual shrinkage over several months and eventual pituitary atrophy and the appearance of an empty sella.

Because of the improvements in obstetric care, Sheehan syndrome is no longer the most common cause of postpartum hypopituitarism. Lymphocytic hypophysitis is the most common cause of postpartum pituitary dysfunction (see Plate 1.12).

Very rarely, a normal nonparturient pituitary may become infarcted in association with hemorrhagic shock.

Plate 1.18   Pituitary and Hypothalamus

PITUITARY APOPLEXY

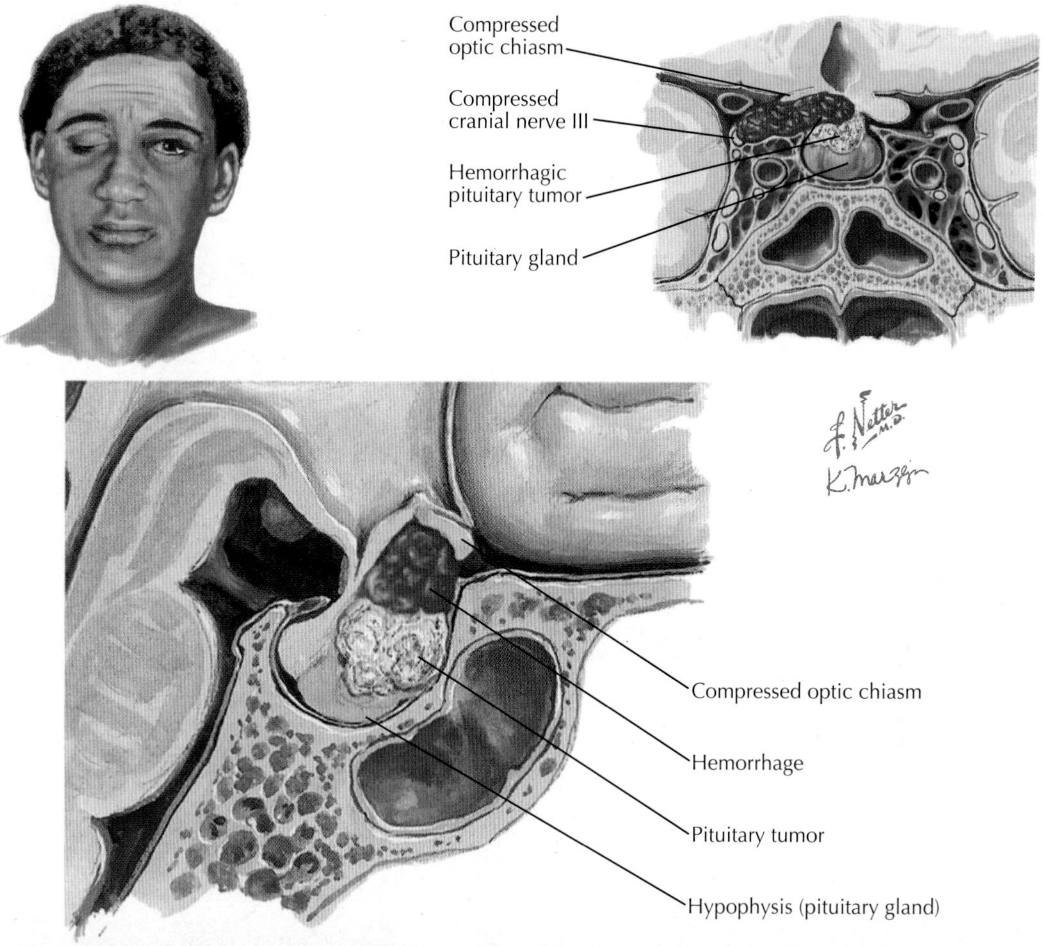

Although pituitary apoplexy, acute hemorrhage of the pituitary gland, is an uncommon event, it is an endocrine emergency, and prompt diagnosis and treatment are critical. The typical presentation is acute onset of severe headache (frequently described as "the worst headache of my life"), vision loss (the hemorrhagic expansion takes the path of least resistance and extends superiorly and compresses the optic chiasm), facial pain, nausea and vomiting, or ocular nerve palsies (e.g., ptosis, diplopia) caused by impingement of the third, fourth, and sixth cranial nerves in the cavernous sinuses. In addition, patients may have signs of meningeal irritation and an altered level of consciousness. Increased intracranial pressure may result in increasing drowsiness and stupor and may mandate surgical intervention and decompression. Hypothalamic involvement may lead to disorders of sympathetic autoregulation, resulting in dysrhythmia and disordered breathing. Erythrocytes and an increased protein concentration are found in the CSF of many patients with pituitary apoplexy. This may be a potential source of confusion in differentiating pituitary apoplexy from meningitis or subarachnoid hemorrhage.

The most immediate hormonal deficiency is secondary adrenal insufficiency, which may lead to hypotension and adrenal crisis. Pituitary apoplexy occurs most often in the setting of a preexisting pituitary macroadenoma or cyst, and the hemorrhage may be spontaneous or triggered by head trauma, coagulation disorders (e.g., idiopathic thrombocytopenic purpura), or anticoagulant (e.g., heparin, warfarin, factor Xa inhibitors) administration. Rarely, the pituitary tumor apoplexy may be induced by the administration of a hypothalamic-releasing hormone (e.g., GnRH agonist in a patient with a gonadotropin-secreting adenoma) or by the administration of an agent used to treat the pituitary tumor (e.g., bromocriptine for a prolactin-secreting pituitary tumor). The rapid expansion of the sellar contents results in the immediate mass-effect symptoms. In more than 50% of cases of pituitary apoplexy, the apoplectic event is the initial clinical presentation of a pituitary tumor. The risk of pituitary apoplexy is not related to age or gender.

Pituitary imaging with MRI is diagnostic and typically shows signs of intrapituitary or intraadenoma hemorrhage, fluid-fluid level, and compression of normal pituitary tissue. Hormonal evaluation typically shows complete anterior pituitary failure (including prolactin). Because of the anatomy of the pituitary circulation and the sparing of the infundibular circulation (inferior hypophysial arteries), the posterior pituitary is infrequently affected by pituitary apoplexy. Thus DI is rare in patients with pituitary apoplexy.

The clinical course of pituitary apoplexy varies widely in duration and severity. Thus the appropriate intervention may be difficult to determine. Treatment is aimed at alleviating or relieving local compression that compromises adjacent structures such as the visual individualized pathways.

In addition to anatomic considerations, the endocrine status of the patient must be considered and treated accordingly. The timing of therapy must be individualized on the basis of the symptoms and the severity of the apoplectic event. Neurosurgical intervention is often the most rapid and effective method of decompressing the sella turcica and the surrounding structures and is indicated in the event of mental status changes and other symptoms attributable to increased intracranial pressure. Surgical decompression is also indicated in the absence of these symptoms when the visual pathways are

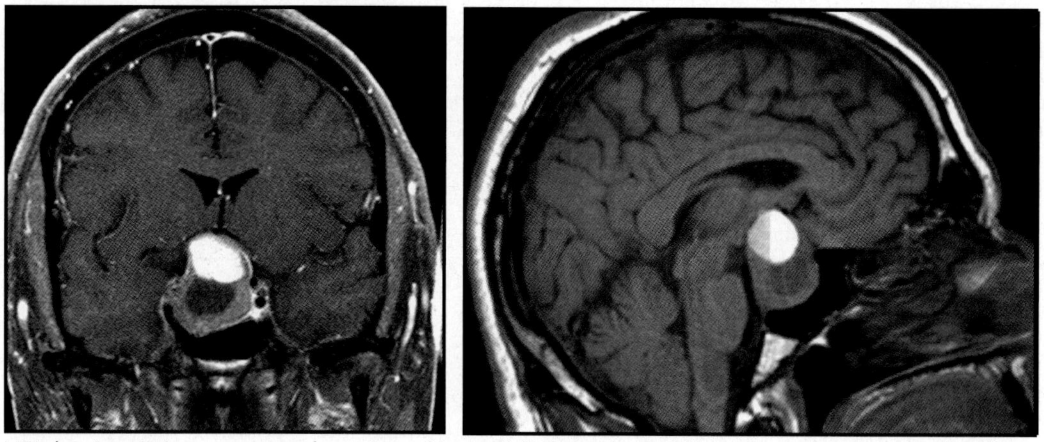

MRI showing pituitary tumor apoplexy. Coronal image (*left*) shows the partially cystic pituitary tumor in the sella with the hemorrhagic component extending above the sella. Sagittal image (*right*) shows fluid-fluid level within the area of recent hemorrhage.

compromised to prevent prolonged ischemia leading to irreversible nerve dysfunction. Although the timing of the surgical intervention does not seem to affect the recovery of ocular palsies, an operation within 1 week after apoplexy in a conscious patient whose condition is stable improves recovery of visual acuity more than an operation performed with a delay of more than 1 week after the event. Although hemorrhagic areas of the pituitary are absorbed over time, reabsorption alone may not occur fast enough for recovery of visual acuity. Therefore waiting for spontaneous resolution of a visual field defect in a patient whose condition is otherwise stable may not be optimal management. In patients with normal visual

fields who lack cranial nerve palsies, observation is a reasonable treatment approach. Stress dosages of glucocorticoids should be initiated in all patients with pituitary apoplexy. Pituitary function may not recover, and long-term pituitary target gland hormone replacement therapy may be needed.

It should be noted that necrosis and hemorrhage within a pituitary tumor occur much more frequently than the clinical syndrome of pituitary apoplexy, especially in silent corticotroph adenomas, in which hemorrhage occurs in more than 50% of the tumors. Overall, hemorrhage occurs in 10% to 15% of pituitary adenomas, and it is usually clinically silent.

Plate 1.19

Endocrine System: VOLUME 2

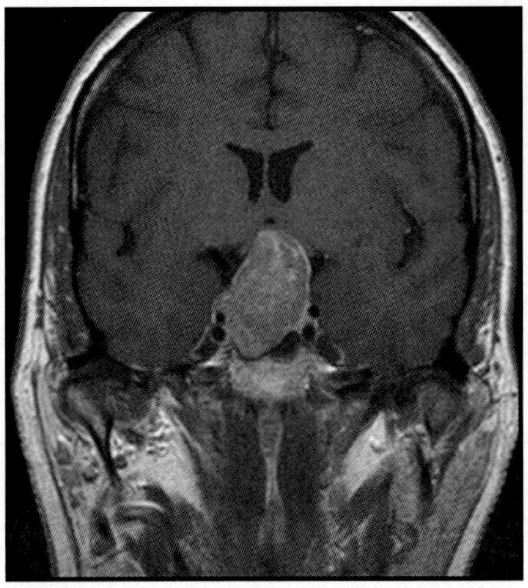

MRI (coronal view) shows a large GH-secreting pituitary tumor in a 16-year-old adolescent boy with gigantism.

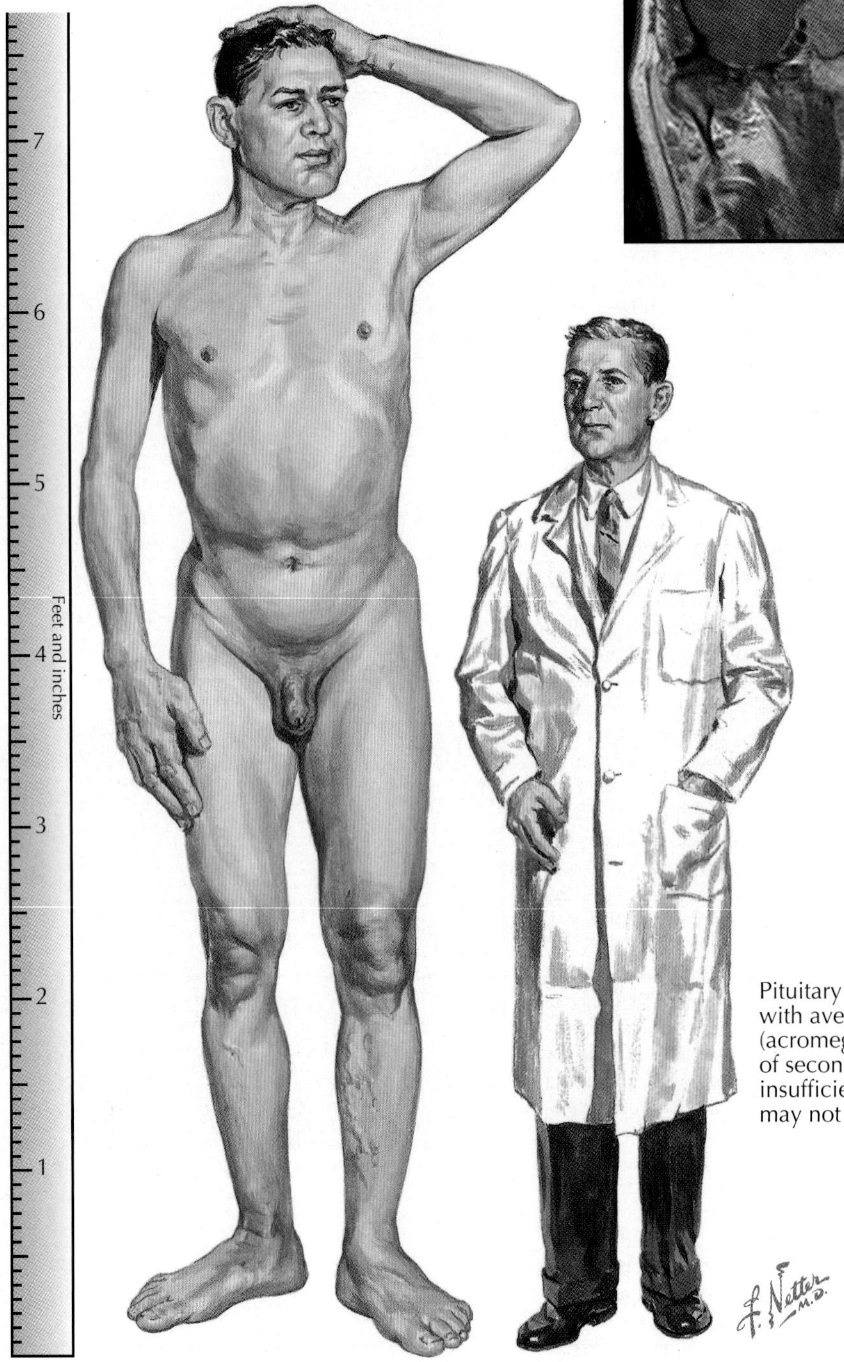

Pituitary Gigantism

Pituitary gigantism occurs when a GH-secreting pituitary tumor develops before fusion of the epiphyseal growth plates in a child or adolescent. In contrast, when GH-secreting pituitary tumors develop in an adult (after complete epiphyseal fusion), there is no linear growth, but there are acral changes, and the condition is termed *acromegaly* (see Plate 1.20).

Pituitary gigantism is rare. When it starts in infancy, it may lead to exceptional height. The tallest well-documented person with pituitary gigantism measured 8 ft, 11 in (272 cm). When untreated, pituitary giants are typically taller than 7 ft (213 cm). The GH-secreting pituitary tumors in individuals with pituitary gigantism are usually sporadic, but they may arise as part of a syndrome such as multiple endocrine neoplasia type 1 (see Plate 8.1), McCune-Albright syndrome (see Plates 4.11 and 8.8), and the Carney complex (see Plate 3.12). In addition, pathogenic variants in aryl hydrocarbon receptor interacting protein (*AIP*) gene and chromosome Xq26.3 microduplications in the *GPR101* gene (referred to as *X-linked acro-gigantism* [*X-LAG*]) have been documented in patients with gigantism. Male predominance is seen among *AIP*-mutated gigantism, whereas X-LAG has a strong female predilection.

Although usually caused by a pituitary GH-secreting adenoma, pituitary gigantism may also be caused by an ectopic tumor secreting GHRH or by hypothalamic dysfunction with hypersecretion of GHRH.

In addition to the accelerated linear growth, patients with pituitary gigantism may slowly develop many of those features seen in adults with acromegaly—for example, soft tissue overgrowth, progressive dental malocclusion (underbite), a low-pitched voice, headaches, malodorous hyperhidrosis, oily skin, proximal muscle weakness, diabetes mellitus, hypertension, obstructive sleep apnea, and cardiac dysfunction. The mass effects of GH-producing pituitary macroadenomas (>10 mm) are similar to those of other pituitary macroadenomas—they include visual field defects, oculomotor pareses, headaches, and pituitary insufficiency.

It is important to note that most children with accelerated linear growth do not have pituitary gigantism. More common causes of tall stature include precocious puberty, genetic tall stature, and hyperthyroidism.

High plasma GH levels are not diagnostic of pituitary gigantism. The diagnosis of pituitary gigantism should be considered in patients after other causes of accelerated linear growth have been excluded. The biochemical diagnosis is based on two criteria: a GH level that is not suppressed to less than 0.4 ng/mL after an oral glucose load (75–100 g) and an increased serum concentration (based on normal range adjusted for age and gender) of IGF-1. Serum prolactin concentrations should also be measured because the pituitary neoplasm in children frequently arises from the mammosomatotroph, so co-hypersecretion of prolactin may occur. The laboratory assessment of pituitary gigantism is supplemented with MRI of the pituitary and visual field examination by quantitative perimetry. If imaging of the pituitary fails to detect an adenoma, then plasma GHRH concentration and CT of the chest and abdomen are indicated in search of an ectopic GHRH-producing tumor (e.g., pancreatic or small cell lung neoplasm).

Treatment is indicated for all patients with confirmed pituitary gigantism. The goals of treatment are to prevent the long-term consequences of GH excess, remove the sellar mass, and preserve normal pituitary tissue and function. Treatment options include surgery, targeted irradiation, and medical therapy. Surgery—transsphenoidal adenectomy by an experienced neurosurgeon—is the treatment of choice and should be supplemented, if necessary, with Gamma Knife radiotherapy, pharmacotherapy, or both.

Pituitary giant contrasted with average-size man (acromegaly and signs of secondary pituitary insufficiency may or may not be present)

Plate 1.20

Pituitary and Hypothalamus

ACROMEGALY

Chronic GH excess from a GH-producing pituitary tumor results in the clinical syndrome of acromegaly. Acromegaly was the first pituitary syndrome to be recognized, described by Pierre Marie in 1886. If untreated, this syndrome is associated with increased morbidity and mortality. Although the annual incidence is estimated to be only 3 per 1 million persons in the general population, a GH-secreting pituitary adenoma is the second most common hormone-secreting pituitary tumor. The effects of the chronic GH excess include acral and soft tissue overgrowth, progressive dental malocclusion (underbite), degenerative arthritis related to chondral and synovial tissue overgrowth within joints, a low-pitched sonorous voice, headaches, malodorous hyperhidrosis, oily skin, perineural hypertrophy leading to nerve entrapment (e.g., carpal tunnel syndrome), proximal muscle weakness, carbohydrate intolerance (the initial presentation may be diabetes mellitus), hypertension, colonic neoplasia, obstructive sleep apnea, and cardiac dysfunction. The mass effects of GH-producing pituitary macroadenomas (>10 mm) are similar to those of other pituitary macroadenomas and include visual field defects, oculomotor pareses, headaches, and pituitary insufficiency.

Patients with acromegaly have a characteristic appearance with coarsening of the facial features, prognathism, frontal bossing, spadelike hands, and wide feet. Often there is a history of progressive increase in shoe, glove, ring, or hat size. These changes may occur slowly and may go unrecognized by the patient, family, and physician. The average delay in diagnosis from the onset of the first symptoms to the eventual diagnosis is 8.5 years. Comparison with earlier photographs of the patient is helpful in confirming the clinical suspicion of acromegaly.

High plasma GH levels are not diagnostic of acromegaly. Basal plasma GH levels are increased in patients with poorly controlled diabetes mellitus, chronic hepatic or renal failure, or conditions characterized by protein-calorie malnutrition such as anorexia nervosa. The diagnosis of acromegaly depends on two criteria: a GH level that is not suppressed to less than 0.4 ng/mL after an oral glucose load (75–100 g) and an increased serum concentration (based on normal range adjusted for age and gender) of IGF-1 (a GH-dependent growth factor responsible for many of the effects of GH and previously known as *somatomedin C*). Serum IGF-1 levels are rarely falsely elevated. IGF-1 levels do rise in pregnancy two- to threefold above the upper limit of gender- and age-adjusted normal values. The laboratory assessment of acromegaly is supplemented with MRI of the pituitary and with visual field examination by quantitative perimetry. If imaging of the pituitary fails to detect an adenoma, then plasma GHRH concentration and CT of the chest and abdomen are indicated in search of an ectopic GHRH-producing tumor (e.g., pancreatic or small cell lung neoplasm). Gallium-68 (^{68}Ga) 1,4,7,10-tetraazacyclododecane-1,4,7,10-tetraacetic acid (DOTA)-octreotate (DOTATATE) positron emission tomography (PET) CT scan may be needed in selected cases to confirm the neuroendocrine nature of the suspected GHRH-producing neoplasm found on cross-sectional imaging.

Treatment is indicated for all patients with acromegaly. The goals of treatment are to prevent the long-term consequences of GH excess, remove the sellar mass, and preserve normal pituitary tissue and function. Treatment options include surgery, targeted irradiation, and medical therapy. Surgery—transsphenoidal adenectomy by an experienced neurosurgeon—is the treatment of choice and should be supplemented, if necessary, with Gamma Knife radiotherapy, pharmacotherapy, or both.

After successful surgical treatment, there is a marked regression of the soft tissue excess, but the bone changes are permanent. After the soft tissue changes have stabilized, combined oral and plastic surgery may be indicated (e.g., mandibular osteotomies, recession of the supraorbital ridges, rhinoplasties, and reduction of tongue size). Disabling hypertrophic osteoarthropathy of the hip or other large joints may require joint replacement. Because of the increased risk of colorectal adenomas and cancer, patients with acromegaly should be offered regular colonoscopic screening.

The effects of the chronic GH excess include acral and soft tissue overgrowth, coarsening of facial features, prognathism, frontal bossing, and progressive dental malocclusion (underbite).

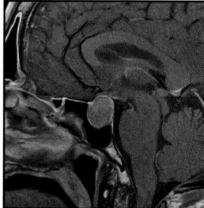

MRI (coronal view) shows a 2.1-cm pituitary macroadenoma eroding the sellar floor on the right, extending into the right cavernous sinus, and extending to the optic chiasm above the sella turcica.

MRI (midline sagittal view) shows pituitary macroadenoma extending into the sphenoid sinus and suprasellar region.

Plate 1.21

Endocrine System: VOLUME 2

PROLACTIN-SECRETING PITUITARY TUMOR

Prolactin-secreting pituitary tumors (prolactinomas) are the most common hormone-secreting pituitary tumor. They are monoclonal lactotroph cell adenomas that appear to result from sporadic mutations. Although most prolactinomas are sporadic, they are the most frequent pituitary tumor in persons with multiple endocrine neoplasia type 1 (see Plate 8.1). In addition, more than 99% of prolactinomas are benign. Approximately 10% of prolactin-secreting pituitary tumors cosecrete GH because of a somatotroph or mammosomatotroph component.

In females, the typical clinical presentation of a prolactin-secreting microadenoma (≤10 mm in largest diameter) is secondary amenorrhea with or without galactorrhea. But in males, because of the lack of symptoms related to small prolactinomas, a prolactinoma is not usually diagnosed until the tumor has enlarged enough to cause mass-effect symptoms. This late diagnosis is also the typical clinical scenario in postmenopausal females. Mass-effect symptoms of prolactin-secreting macroadenomas include visual field defects with suprasellar extension, cranial nerve palsies with lateral (cavernous sinus) extension (e.g., diplopia, ptosis), headaches, and varying degrees of hypopituitarism with compression of the normal pituitary tissue.

Hyperprolactinemia results in decreased gonadotropin secretion. In males, hypogonadotropic hypogonadism causes testicular atrophy, low serum testosterone concentrations, decreased libido, sexual dysfunction, decreased facial hair growth, and decreased muscle mass. Because males lack the estrogen needed to prepare breast glandular tissues, they rarely present with galactorrhea. In premenopausal females, however, hyperprolactinemia may cause bilateral spontaneous or expressible galactorrhea (see Plate 4.26). In addition, prolactin-dependent hypogonadotropic hypogonadism in females results in secondary amenorrhea and estrogen deficiency symptoms. Long-standing hypogonadism in both males and females may lead to osteopenia and osteoporosis.

In general, the blood concentration of prolactin is proportionate to the size of the prolactinoma. For example, a 5-mm prolactinoma is associated with serum prolactin concentrations of 50 to 250 ng/mL (reference ranges, 4.0–15.2 ng/mL in males and 8–23.3 ng/mL in females), but prolactinomas larger than 2 cm in diameter are associated with serum prolactin concentrations greater than 1000 ng/mL. However, there are exceptional cases of small prolactinomas that have extremely efficient prolactin secretory capacity (e.g., serum prolactin concentration > 1000 ng/mL) and cases of the converse—very inefficient prolactin-secreting macroadenomas (e.g., serum prolactin concentrations < 200 ng/mL).

Treatment decisions in patients with prolactin-secreting pituitary tumors are guided by the signs and symptoms related to hyperprolactinemia and mass-effect symptoms related to the sellar mass. For example, a 4-mm prolactin-secreting microadenoma detected incidentally in an asymptomatic postmenopausal woman may be observed without treatment. However, because prolactin-secreting pituitary macroadenomas grow over time, treatment is almost always indicated for macroprolactinomas even if the patient lacks tumor-related symptomatology. When treatment is indicated (e.g., if secondary hypogonadism is present in males or in premenopausal females or if a macroadenoma is present), an orally administered dopamine agonist (e.g., cabergoline or

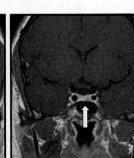
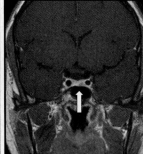

In premenopausal females, hyperprolactinemia causes bilateral spontaneous galactorrhea.

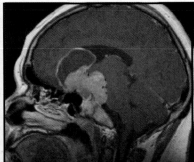

Mass-effect symptoms of prolactin-secreting macroadenomas include visual field defects with suprasellar extension, cranial nerve palsies with lateral (cavernous sinus) extension (e.g., diplopia, ptosis), headaches, and varying degrees of hypopituitarism.

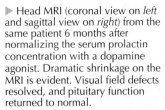

Serial head MRI scans (coronal views) from a patient with a 9-mm prolactin-secreting pituitary micro-adenoma (arrows). At the time of diagnosis (image on left), the serum prolactin concentration was 280 ng/mL. The image on the right was obtained 6 months after normalizing the serum prolactin concentration with a dopamine agonist. The size of the prolactinoma decreased more than 50% (image on right).

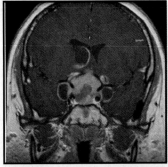

Head MRI (coronal view on left and sagittal view on right) from a patient with a 6.5-cm prolactin-secreting pituitary macroadenoma. There are scattered cystlike areas within the mass; the largest in the right inferior frontal region deforms the frontal horn, resulting in mild midline shift to the left. The mass wraps around the superior and lateral margins of the cavernous sinuses. The patient presented with visual field defects and secondary hypogonadism. Baseline serum prolactin concentration was 6100 ng/mL.

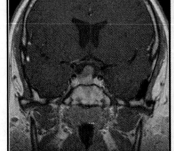
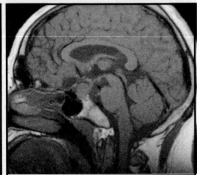

Head MRI (coronal view on left and sagittal view on right) from the same patient 6 months after normalizing the serum prolactin concentration with a dopamine agonist. Dramatic shrinkage on the MRI is evident. Visual field defects resolved, and pituitary function returned to normal.

bromocriptine) is the treatment of choice. Dopamine agonists are very effective in promptly normalizing the serum prolactin concentration and reducing the size of the lactotroph adenoma. After initiating a dopamine agonist, the serum prolactin concentration should be monitored every 2 weeks, and the dosage of bromocriptine or cabergoline should be increased until the prolactin levels decrease into the reference range. Approximately 3 to 6 months after achieving a normal serum prolactin concentration, pituitary-directed MRI should be performed to document tumor shrinkage. The minimal dosage of the dopamine agonist that results in normoprolactinemia should be continued indefinitely. In a small percentage of patients, prolactin-secreting adenomas may be cured

with long-term dopamine agonist therapy. Thus a periodic (e.g., every 2 years) 2-month holiday off the dopamine agonist is indicated to determine whether hyperprolactinemia recurs. Patients with macroprolactinomas that have sphenoid sinus extension should be cautioned about the potential for CSF rhinorrhea that may occur as the tumor shrinks. CSF rhinorrhea requires an urgent neurosurgical procedure to prevent the development of pneumocephalus and bacterial meningitis. When patients are intolerant of the dopamine agonist (e.g., nausea, lightheadedness, mental fogginess, or vivid dreams) or if the tumor is resistant to this form of therapy, transsphenoidal surgery or Gamma Knife radiation therapy may be considered.

Plate 1.22

Pituitary and Hypothalamus

CORTICOTROPIN-SECRETING PITUITARY TUMOR

Corticotropin-secreting pituitary adenomas stimulate excess adrenal secretion of cortisol, resulting in the signs and symptoms characteristic of Cushing syndrome (see Plate 3.9). Corticotropin-secreting pituitary tumors are typically benign microadenomas (≤10 mm in largest diameter); occasionally they are macroadenomas, and very rarely they are carcinomas. Treatment of choice for a corticotropin-secreting pituitary adenoma is transsphenoidal selective adenectomy. Surgical success is defined as cure of Cushing syndrome and intact anterior and posterior pituitary function.

The most common operative approach is an endonasal approach (with use of an endoscope), traversing the sphenoid sinus (transsphenoidal) and through the floor of the sella (see Plate 1.31). Corticotroph adenomas are basophilic and stain positively for corticotropin on immunohistochemistry. Tissue adjacent to the adenoma usually shows Crooke hyaline change, a result of atrophy of normal corticotrophs. Cure rates are 80% to 90% when a microadenoma can be localized preoperatively with either MRI or inferior petrosal sinus sampling (see Plate 3.10). A lack of cure in patients with microadenomas is attributable to either their small size, so they cannot be seen at surgery, or to an inaccessible location (e.g., cavernous sinus). MRI should be performed with a gadolinium enhanced dynamic imaging protocol and a high-strength magnet (e.g., ≥3 tesla). Only about half of corticotropin-secreting pituitary tumors are large enough to be detected by MRI. In addition, approximately 10% of healthy individuals have an apparent microadenoma on MRI; thus in a patient with Cushing syndrome, an apparent small sellar adenoma on MRI is not specific for a corticotroph adenoma. The lower cure rate (~60%) for macroadenomas is usually because of cavernous sinus involvement that prevents complete resection.

On the day of surgery, these patients should receive an intravenous dose of glucocorticoid (e.g., hydrocortisone, 100 mg). The serum cortisol concentration should be measured the morning after surgery (before additional exogenous glucocorticoid administration) to document a short-term cure, defined as a low serum cortisol concentration (e.g., <1.8 μg/dL). If the patient develops symptoms of acute glucocorticoid withdrawal before the serum cortisol laboratory result is available, stress dosages of glucocorticoids should be administered (e.g., hydrocortisone, 100 mg intravenously twice daily). The glucocorticoid dosage is then decreased daily, and patients are typically discharged from the hospital on dosages of exogenous orally administered glucocorticoids twofold above the standard replacement therapy dosage (e.g., prednisone, 10 mg in the morning and 5 mg at 4 PM daily). However, this dosage should be adjusted according to the severity of hypercortisolism preoperatively to prevent severe steroid withdrawal symptoms. Then the dosage of exogenous glucocorticoid is slowly tapered to a standard replacement dosage over 4 to 6 weeks after operation. The hypothalamic CRH neurons and the atrophic anterior pituitary corticotrophs take months to recover from chronic suppression. Most patients tolerate a single dose of a short-acting glucocorticoid (e.g., 15–20 mg of hydrocortisone every morning) starting 8 to 12 weeks after surgical cure. The 8 AM serum cortisol concentration should be measured every 6 weeks; venipuncture should be performed before taking a morning dose of hydrocortisone. The serum cortisol concentration will

slowly increase from undetectable levels to a concentration higher than 10 μg/dL; when this occurs, the hydrocortisone dosage can be tapered and discontinued over 2 weeks. With this postoperative management protocol, the patient with typical pituitary-dependent Cushing syndrome requires exogenous administration of glucocorticoids for approximately 12 months after curative pituitary surgery. The signs and symptoms related to Cushing syndrome resolve very slowly over the first 6 months after surgery.

However, even when the postoperative serum cortisol concentration is low, a risk for recurrent disease remains—if a small number of viable adenomatous corticotroph cells are not resected at surgery, they multiply over time and eventually have the corticotropin secretory mass to cause recurrent Cushing

syndrome. The average time to clinically evident recurrence is 3 to 4 years. Thus all patients should be followed up annually and assessed for recurrent disease.

Patients with Cushing syndrome are at increased thromboembolic risk perioperatively, and prophylactic measures to prevent deep venous thrombosis (including starting ambulation the day after surgery) are encouraged.

When transsphenoidal surgery fails to cure a patient with pituitary-dependent Cushing syndrome, the two main treatment options are to perform another transsphenoidal surgery or to perform bilateral laparoscopic adrenalectomy. Less frequently used options are radiation therapy to the sella or pharmacotherapy to decrease adrenal cortisol production.

Corticotroph adenoma

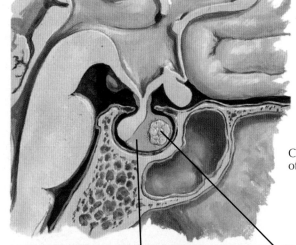

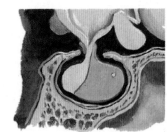

Minute adenoma

Corticotroph adenoma of moderate size

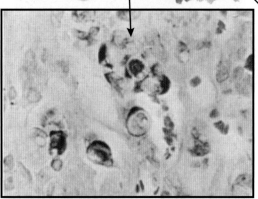

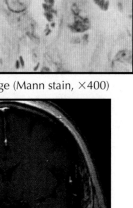

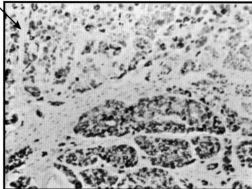

Crooke hyaline change (Mann stain, ×400)

Basophil adenoma (Mann stain, ×125)

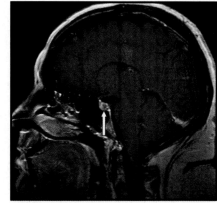

Head MRI (coronal view) with a 4-mm corticotroph adenoma (*arrow*) seen as a rounded, hypodense nodule on left side of the sella

Head MRI (sagittal view) with a 4-mm corticotroph adenoma (*arrow*) located between the anterior and posterior lobes of the pituitary gland

Plate 1.23

Endocrine System: VOLUME 2

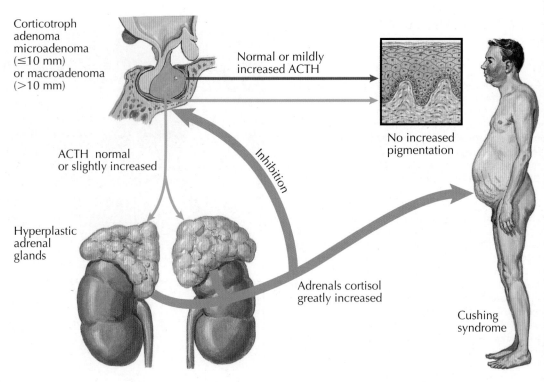

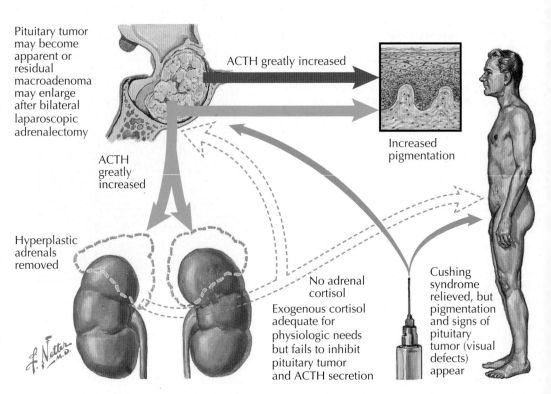

NELSON SYNDROME

Nelson syndrome is progressive pituitary corticotroph tumor enlargement after bilateral adrenalectomy is performed for the treatment of pituitary-dependent Cushing syndrome. Although the treatment of choice for a corticotroph adenoma is selective adenectomy at the time of transsphenoidal surgery (see Plate 1.22), bilateral laparoscopic adrenalectomy is indicated when pituitary surgery is not successful. When bilateral adrenalectomy cures hypercortisolism, there is less negative feedback on the corticotroph tumor cells with physiologic glucocorticoid replacement, and the adenoma may grow. Nelson syndrome occurs in a minority of patients who follow the treatment sequence of failed transsphenoidal surgery and bilateral adrenalectomy. Most corticotroph microadenomas do not enlarge over time in this setting. However, when pituitary-dependent Cushing syndrome is caused by a corticotroph macroadenoma (>10 mm in largest diameter), the risk of tumor enlargement after bilateral adrenalectomy is high.

The clinical features of Nelson syndrome are skin hyperpigmentation related to the markedly increased blood levels of POMC and corticotropin and symptoms related to mass effects of an enlarging pituitary tumor (e.g., visual field defects, oculomotor nerve palsies, hypopituitarism, and headaches). As in Addison disease (see Plate 3.22), generalized hyperpigmentation is caused by corticotropin-driven increased melanin production in the epidermal melanocytes. The extensor surfaces (e.g., knees, knuckles, elbows) and other friction areas (e.g., belt line, bra straps) tend to be even more hyperpigmented. Other sites of prominent hyperpigmentation include the inner surface of the lips, buccal mucosa, gums, hard palate, recent surgical scars, areolae, freckles, and palmar creases (the latter may be a normal finding in individuals with darker skin). The fingernails may show linear bands of darkening arising from the nail beds. Suspected Nelson syndrome can be confirmed by MRI of the sella that demonstrates an enlarging sellar mass. In addition, blood corticotropin concentrations are markedly increased in this setting (e.g., >1000 pg/mL; reference range, 10–60 pg/mL).

Patients with pituitary-dependent Cushing syndrome who are treated with bilateral adrenalectomy should be monitored annually with pituitary MRI for approximately 10 years. Tumor-directed radiation therapy should be considered if tumor growth is documented on serial MRI. If feasible, Gamma Knife radiosurgery is the treatment of choice for Nelson corticotroph tumors. However, unlike most pituitary adenomas, these neoplasms may demonstrate aggressive growth despite radiotherapy. Extensive cavernous sinus involvement may result in multiple cranial nerve palsies. Temozolomide is an effective treatment option for aggressive pituitary tumors or carcinoma. Immune checkpoint inhibitors are being investigated as additional treatment options.

Despite the concern about potential development of Nelson syndrome, clinicians should never hesitate to cure Cushing syndrome with bilateral laparoscopic adrenalectomy when transsphenoidal surgery has not been curative. Untreated Cushing syndrome can be fatal, but Nelson syndrome is usually manageable.

Plate 1.24

Pituitary and Hypothalamus

CLINICALLY NONFUNCTIONING PITUITARY TUMOR

Clinically nonfunctioning pituitary tumors are identified either incidentally (e.g., on head MRI to evaluate unrelated symptoms) or because of sellar mass-related symptoms (e.g., visual field defect). On the basis of autopsy studies, pituitary microadenomas (≤10 mm in largest dimension) are relatively common, present in approximately 11% of all pituitary glands examined. However, pituitary macroadenomas (>10 mm in largest dimension) are uncommon. Immunohistochemical studies on resected pituitary adenomas can determine the adenohypophyseal cell of origin. The most frequent type of pituitary macroadenoma is the gonadotroph cell adenoma; most do not hypersecrete gonadotropins; thus patients who are affected do not present with a hormone excess syndrome. The second most common clinically nonfunctioning pituitary macroadenoma is the null cell adenoma that is not basophilic or acidophilic (chromophobe adenoma); this is a benign neoplasm of adenohypophyseal cells that stains negatively for any anterior pituitary hormone on immunohistochemistry. Rarely, lactotroph, somatotroph, and corticotroph pituitary adenomas may be clinically silent.

The mass-effect symptoms in patients with clinically nonfunctioning pituitary macroadenomas usually prompt evaluation with head MRI. Suprasellar extension of the pituitary adenoma causes compression of the optic chiasm, resulting in the gradual onset of superior bitemporal quadrantopia that may progress to complete bitemporal hemianopsia (see Plate 1.11). Because the onset is gradual, patients may not recognize vision loss until it becomes marked. Additional mass-effect symptoms from an enlarging sellar mass include diplopia (with cavernous sinus extension and oculomotor nerve compression), varying degrees of pituitary insufficiency (related to compression of the normal pituitary gland by the macroadenoma), and headaches.

MRI is the imaging of choice to evaluate the sella and surrounding structures. MRI clearly shows the degree of suprasellar and parasellar extension of pituitary macroadenomas. All patients with pituitary macroadenomas should be assessed for tumoral hyperfunction, compression-related hypopituitarism, and visual field defects. Nonfunctioning pituitary macroadenomas are often associated with mild hyperprolactinemia (e.g., serum prolactin concentration between 30 and 200 ng/mL) because of pituitary stalk compression and prevention of hypothalamic dopamine (prolactin inhibitory factor) from reaching all of the anterior pituitary lactotrophs. Pituitary lactotrophs are the only anterior pituitary cells that are under continuous inhibitory control from the hypothalamus. Additional pituitary-related hormones that should be measured in all patients with pituitary macroadenomas include LH, FSH, α-subunit of glycoprotein hormones, target gonadal hormone (estrogen in females and testosterone in males), IGF-1, corticotropin, cortisol, thyrotropin, and free thyroxine. DI is rare in patients with benign tumors of the adenohypophysis.

The goals of treatment are to correct mass-effect symptoms (e.g., vision loss) and to preserve pituitary

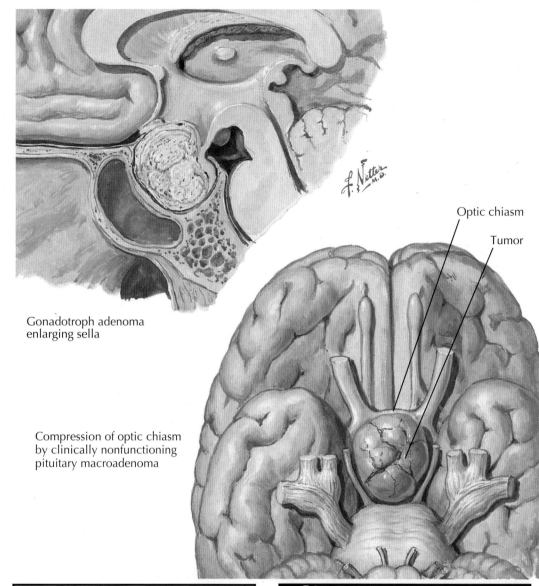

Gonadotroph adenoma enlarging sella

Optic chiasm

Tumor

Compression of optic chiasm by clinically nonfunctioning pituitary macroadenoma

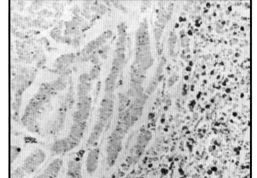

Null cell adenoma (Mann stain, ×100)

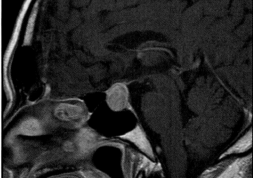

MRI (sagittal view) showing suprasellar extension of a clinically nonfunctioning pituitary macro-adenoma

function. Currently, no effective pharmacologic options are available to treat patients with clinically nonfunctioning pituitary tumors. Observation is a reasonable management approach in elderly patients who have normal visual fields. However, intervention should be considered in all patients with vision loss. Transsphenoidal surgery (see Plate 1.33) can provide prompt resolution of visual field defects and a permanent cure. If present preoperatively, pituitary insufficiency may

recover in some patients after operation. Effectiveness of transsphenoidal surgery is assessed by the findings on postoperative MRI (typically performed 3 months after surgery) and by blood levels of adenoma secretory products that may have been increased before surgery (e.g., α-subunit of glycoprotein hormones). Recurrence of the pituitary adenoma after transsphenoidal surgery can be treated with stereotactic Gamma Knife radiotherapy.

Plate 1.25

Endocrine System: VOLUME 2

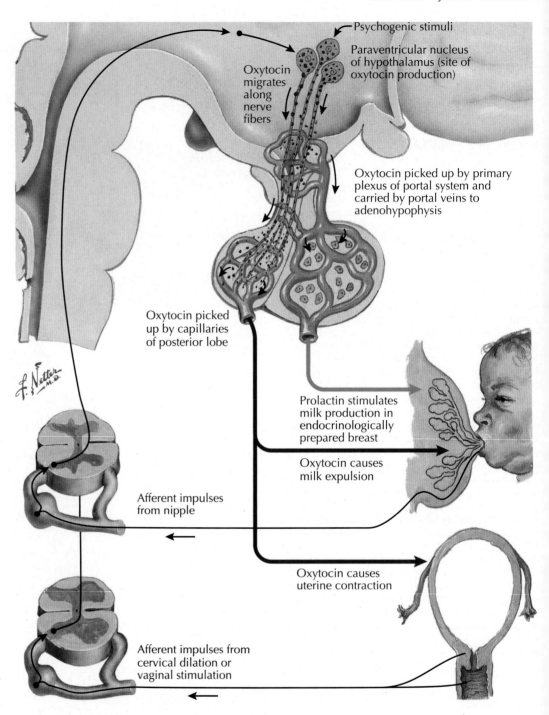

Psychogenic stimuli

Paraventricular nucleus of hypothalamus (site of oxytocin production)

Oxytocin migrates along nerve fibers

Oxytocin picked up by primary plexus of portal system and carried by portal veins to adenohypophysis

Oxytocin picked up by capillaries of posterior lobe

Prolactin stimulates milk production in endocrinologically prepared breast

Oxytocin causes milk expulsion

Afferent impulses from nipple

Oxytocin causes uterine contraction

Afferent impulses from cervical dilation or vaginal stimulation

SECRETION AND ACTION OF OXYTOCIN

The physiologic roles of oxytocin are smooth muscle activation promoting milk letdown with breastfeeding and uterine myometrial contraction at parturition. The milk-producing compartments of the breast are composed of multiple alveolar clusters of milk-producing (glandular) cells surrounded by specialized myoepithelial cells. Prolactin stimulates milk production in endocrinologically prepared breasts. The alveoli are connected to ductules that lead to large ducts and on to the nipple. The glandular cells have receptors for oxytocin and cause myoepithelial contraction when activated. In addition, oxytocin acts on ductal myoepithelial cells to enhance milk flow to the nipple. Activation of nipple tactile and mechanoreceptors by suckling sends an afferent signal to the spinal cord and from the spinal cord to the oxytocinergic neurons in the supraoptic and paraventricular nuclei. Oxytocin is then released from the posterior pituitary in a pulsatile fashion that effects a pumping action on the alveoli, promoting emptying of milk from the alveoli. In the

absence of oxytocin, only approximately 30% of stored milk is released during nursing. There is a latent period of approximately 30 seconds between the onset of suckling and commencement of milk flow. Psychogenic stimuli can also trigger milk letdown in lactating mothers. Changes in estrogen and progesterone at the time of parturition help modulate the lactation response both by affecting oxytocin synthesis and secretion and by affecting oxytocin receptors.

Oxytocin is a powerful uterotonic stimulant for contractions, and oxytocin secretion increases with the expulsive phase of parturition. During pregnancy, the uterus is maintained in a quiet state by the actions of progesterone and relaxin. The initiation of labor is accomplished by a relative increase in estrogen activation and a decrease in progesterone activation. There is

a 200-fold increase in the responsiveness of the uterus to oxytocin as parturition approaches.

Synthetic oxytocin administration is a clinically proven method of labor induction. Oxytocin is administered intravenously at an escalating dose until there is normal progression of labor, strong contractions occurring at 2- to 3-minute intervals, or uterine activity reaching 150 to 350 Montevideo units (the peak strength of contractions in mm Hg measured by an internal monitor multiplied by their frequency over 10 minutes). When uterotonic drugs are administered, continuous monitoring of fetal heart rate and uterine activity helps prevent induction of excessive or inadequate uterine activity. Other methods used to induce labor include "membrane stripping," amniotomy, intravaginal administration of prostaglandins E_2 or E_1, and breast stimulation.

Plate 1.26

Pituitary and Hypothalamus

SECRETION AND ACTION OF VASOPRESSIN

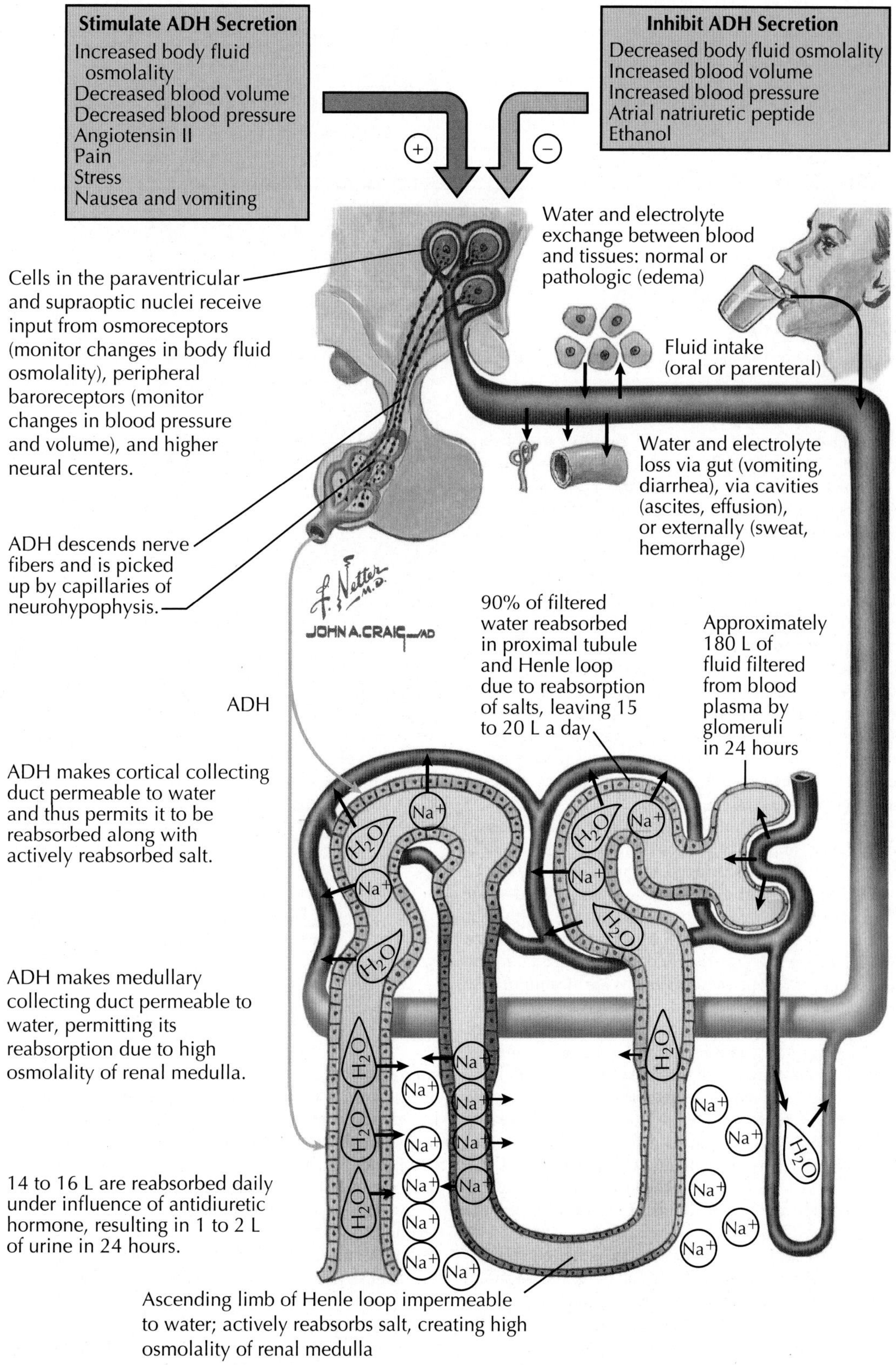

Vasopressin is the key hormone involved in the regulation of water homeostasis and osmolality of body fluids. The secretion and action of vasopressin are regulated by osmotic and pressure/volume factors. Osmoreceptors continuously monitor plasma osmolality. The osmoreceptors are outside the blood-brain barrier, are located in the organum vasculosum of the lamina terminalis (adjacent to the anterior hypothalamus near the anterior wall of the third ventricle), and are perfused by fenestrated capillaries. The normal extracellular fluid osmolality—determined to a major degree by serum sodium concentration—varies from 282 to 287 mOsm/kg in healthy individuals. The keys to maintaining this narrow normal range are (1) the very sensitive osmoreceptor-regulated response of vasopressin secretion to changes in plasma osmolality, (2) the prompt response of urine osmolality to changes in plasma vasopressin, and (3) the short plasma half-life of vasopressin (~15 minutes). Thus small increases in plasma osmolality result in a prompt increase in urine concentration, and small decreases in osmolality result in prompt water diuresis.

Over 24 hours, glomerular filtration presents 180 L of isoosmotic fluid to the proximal convoluted renal tubules. Ninety percent of the filtered water is reabsorbed in the proximal tubule without the help of vasopressin. This passive transfer of water is determined by the active reabsorption of solutes (e.g., sodium and chloride) taking along water by osmotic forces. Thus proximal tubular urine remains isoosmotic with plasma. Distal collecting duct reabsorption of water is controlled by vasopressin. The loop of Henle and the collecting duct in the kidney are critical to water conservation. The countercurrent multiplier system in the loop of Henle generates a high osmolality in the renal medulla. The ascending, or distal, limb of Henle loop actively transports sodium without water from the tubular urine to the interstitial fluid of the renal medulla, making it very hypertonic. The water impermeability of this limb of Henle loop renders the urine entering the distal tubule hypotonic with respect to plasma. In the absence of vasopressin, the distal tubule and collecting ducts remain largely impermeable to water, and very dilute urine leaves the kidney. With maximum vasopressin secretion, urine osmolality plateaus at approximately 1000 to 1200 mOsm/kg, limited by the maximal osmolality of the inner renal medulla. When vasopressin is absent, 14 to 16 L of urine is excreted per day.

The site of action of vasopressin is the V2 receptor on the epithelial principal cells of the collecting ducts. Activation of the collecting duct V2 receptor increases water permeability to allow for osmotic equilibration between the urine and the hypertonic medullary interstitium. Thus water is extracted from the urine into the medullary interstitial blood vessels, causing an increased urine concentration and decreased urine volume. Aquaporins are intracellular organelles, or water channels, that mediate rapid water transport across collecting duct cell membranes. V2-receptor activation by vasopressin increases intracellular cyclic adenosine monophosphate (cAMP) levels by activating adenylate cyclase. cAMP activates protein kinase A, which phosphorylates aquaporin-2 and induces a fusion of aquaporin-2-containing intracytoplasmic vesicles with the apical plasma membranes of the principal cells, thus

Stimulate ADH Secretion
Increased body fluid osmolality
Decreased blood volume
Decreased blood pressure
Angiotensin II
Pain
Stress
Nausea and vomiting

Inhibit ADH Secretion
Decreased body fluid osmolality
Increased blood volume
Increased blood pressure
Atrial natriuretic peptide
Ethanol

Cells in the paraventricular and supraoptic nuclei receive input from osmoreceptors (monitor changes in body fluid osmolality), peripheral baroreceptors (monitor changes in blood pressure and volume), and higher neural centers.

ADH descends nerve fibers and is picked up by capillaries of neurohypophysis.

Water and electrolyte exchange between blood and tissues: normal or pathologic (edema)

Fluid intake (oral or parenteral)

Water and electrolyte loss via gut (vomiting, diarrhea), via cavities (ascites, effusion), or externally (sweat, hemorrhage)

ADH

90% of filtered water reabsorbed in proximal tubule and Henle loop due to reabsorption of salts, leaving 15 to 20 L a day.

Approximately 180 L of fluid filtered from blood plasma by glomeruli in 24 hours

ADH makes cortical collecting duct permeable to water and thus permits it to be reabsorbed along with actively reabsorbed salt.

ADH makes medullary collecting duct permeable to water, permitting its reabsorption due to high osmolality of renal medulla.

14 to 16 L are reabsorbed daily under influence of antidiuretic hormone, resulting in 1 to 2 L of urine in 24 hours.

Ascending limb of Henle loop impermeable to water; actively reabsorbs salt, creating high osmolality of renal medulla

increasing apical water permeability by markedly increasing the number of water-conducting pores in the apical plasma membrane. The aquaporin-containing vesicles are shuttled into and out of the membrane in response to changes in intracellular cAMP levels, resulting in a minute-to-minute regulation of renal water excretion in response to changes in circulating vasopressin.

Water intake is also a key factor in maintaining water homeostasis. Increases in plasma osmolality of the extracellular fluid or decreases in intravascular volume stimulate thirst. Thirst is regulated by osmoreceptors in the anterior hypothalamus and baroreceptors in the chest. The sensation of thirst is typically triggered by a 2% increase in plasma osmolality. Because of unregulated fluid ingestion (e.g., coffee, tea, soft drinks, and water from metabolized food), thirst does not represent a major regulatory mechanism and, in a typical healthy person, excess water is excreted daily by the osmoregulated secretion of vasopressin.

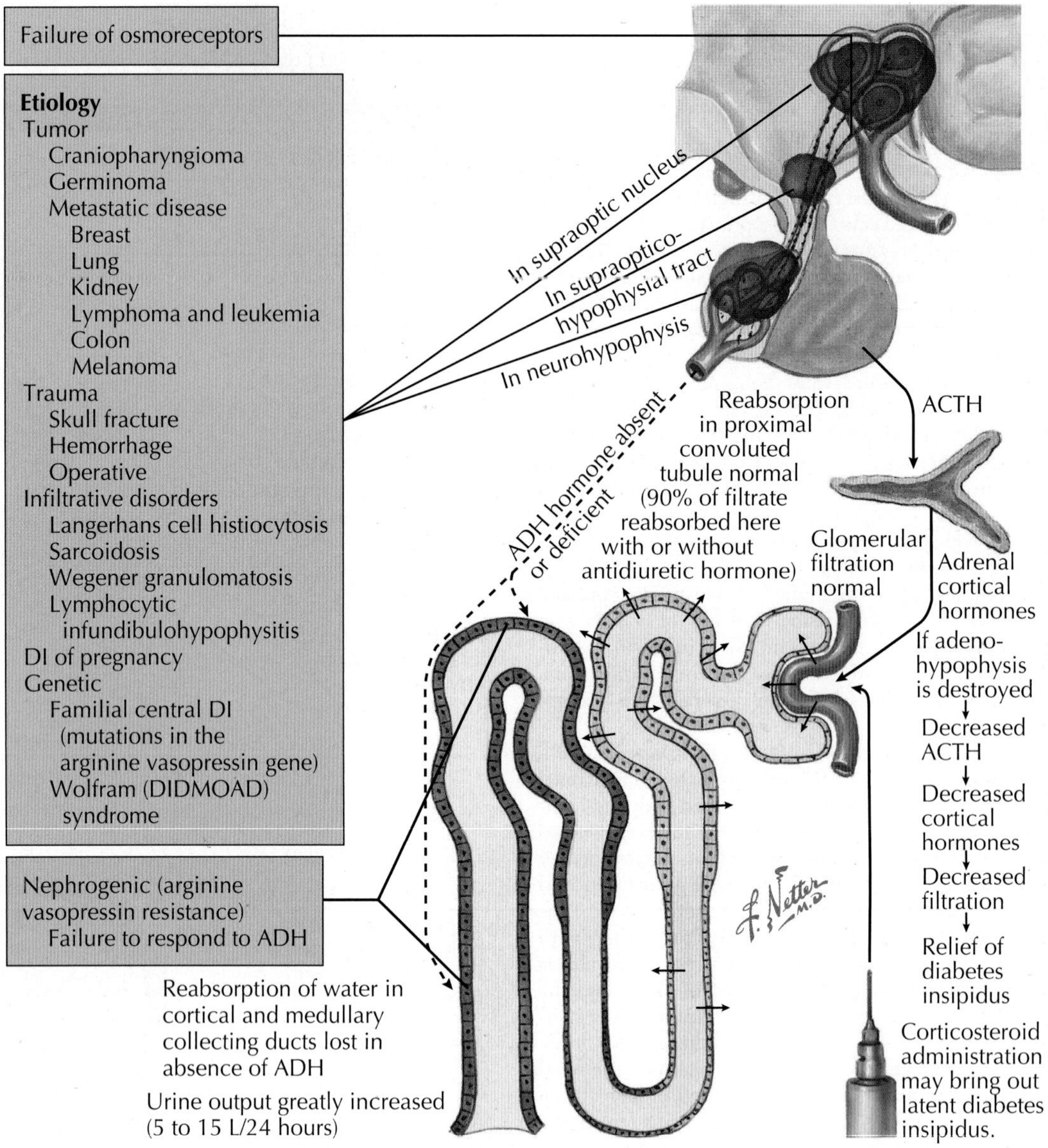

Plate 1.27

Endocrine System: VOLUME 2

CENTRAL DIABETES INSIPIDUS (ARGININE VASOPRESSIN DEFICIENCY)

DI literally means a large volume of urine (diabetes) that is tasteless (insipid). Central DI is characterized by a decreased release of vasopressin, resulting in polydipsia and polyuria. Vasopressin deficiency may be a result of disorders or masses that affect the hypothalamic osmoreceptors, the supraoptic or paraventricular nuclei, or the superior portion of the supraopticohypophyseal tract. Approximately 90% of the vasopressinergic neurons must be destroyed to cause symptomatic DI. Because the posterior pituitary gland stores but does not produce vasopressin, damage by intrasellar pituitary tumors usually does not cause DI. The most common causes of central DI are trauma (e.g., neurosurgery, closed-head trauma), primary or metastatic tumors, and infiltrative disorders. Central DI can be exacerbated by or first become apparent during pregnancy, during which vasopressin catabolism is increased by placental hyperproduction of the enzyme cysteine aminopeptidase (vasopressinase).

Persons with central DI typically have a sudden onset of polyuria and thirst for cold liquids. They usually wake multiple times through the night because of the need to urinate and drink fluids—often ice-cold water from the refrigerator. When seen in the outpatient clinic, these patients usually have a large thermos of ice water by their side. The degree of polyuria is dictated by the degree of vasopressin deficiency—urine output may range from 3 L/day in mild partial DI to more than 10 to 15 L/day in severe DI. In patients with concurrent anterior pituitary failure, secondary adrenal insufficiency is associated with decreased glomerular filtration (associated with decreased blood pressure, cardiac output, and renal blood flow), leading to decreased urine output. Glucocorticoid deficiency also increases vasopressin release in patients with partial DI. These effects are reversed when glucocorticoid replacement is administered and DI is "unmasked," resulting in the rapid onset of polyuria.

Neurosurgery in the sellar region (either by craniotomy or transsphenoidal routes) or blunt head trauma that affects the hypothalamus and posterior pituitary may result in DI. As many as 50% of patients experience transient central DI within 24 hours of pituitary surgery; it resolves over several days. With the minimally invasive endoscopic transnasal transsphenoidal approach to pituitary surgery, the rate of postoperative permanent DI is less than 5%; however, with transcranial operations and with larger tumors that have hypothalamic involvement (e.g., craniopharyngioma), up to 30% of patients develop permanent DI. Damage to the hypothalamus by neurosurgery or trauma often results in a triphasic response: (1) an initial polyuric phase—related to decreased vasopressin release because of axon shock and lack of action potential propagation—beginning within 24 hours of surgery and lasting

Etiology
Tumor
   Craniopharyngioma
   Germinoma
   Metastatic disease
      Breast
      Lung
      Kidney
      Lymphoma and leukemia
      Colon
      Melanoma
Trauma
   Skull fracture
   Hemorrhage
   Operative
Infiltrative disorders
   Langerhans cell histiocytosis
   Sarcoidosis
   Wegener granulomatosis
   Lymphocytic
      infundibulohypophysitis
DI of pregnancy
Genetic
   Familial central DI
   (mutations in the
      arginine vasopressin gene)
   Wolfram (DIDMOAD)
      syndrome

Failure of osmoreceptors

In supraoptic nucleus
In supraoptico-hypophysial tract
In neurohypophysis

ADH hormone absent or deficient

Reabsorption in proximal convoluted tubule normal (90% of filtrate reabsorbed here with or without antidiuretic hormone)

Glomerular filtration normal

ACTH

Adrenal cortical hormones
If adenohypophysis is destroyed
↓
Decreased ACTH
↓
Decreased cortical hormones
↓
Decreased filtration
↓
Relief of diabetes insipidus

Corticosteroid administration may bring out latent diabetes insipidus.

Nephrogenic (arginine vasopressin resistance)
   Failure to respond to ADH

Reabsorption of water in cortical and medullary collecting ducts lost in absence of ADH

Urine output greatly increased (5 to 15 L/24 hours)

approximately 5 days; (2) an antidiuretic phase (days 6–12), during which stored vasopressin is slowly released from the degenerating posterior pituitary, and hyponatremia may develop if excess fluids are administered; and (3) a permanent DI after the posterior pituitary vasopressin stores are depleted. In 10% to 25% of all patients who undergo pituitary surgery, only the second of these three phases is seen, and DI never develops because surgical trauma only damages some of the axons; this results in inappropriate vasopressin release, but the intact axons continue to function and prevent the onset of DI. However, this transient, inappropriate release of vasopressin can have serious consequences, with marked hyponatremia that peaks approximately 7 days after surgery and that may be associated with headaches, nausea, emesis, and seizures. This sequence of events can be avoided by advising the patient to "drink for thirst only for the first 2 weeks" after a pituitary operation.

Primary (e.g., craniopharyngioma, germinoma) or metastatic (e.g., breast, lung, kidney, lymphoma, leukemia, colon, or melanoma) disease in the brain can involve the hypothalamic-pituitary region and lead to central DI. Polyuria and polydipsia may be the presenting symptoms of metastatic disease.

Patients with LCH are at high risk of developing central DI because of hypothalamic-pituitary infiltration. Additional infiltrative disorders that may cause central DI include sarcoidosis, Wegener granulomatosis, and autoimmune lymphocytic infundibulohypophysitis.

Familial central DI is an autosomal dominant disorder caused by mutations in the arginine vasopressin gene, AVP. The incorrectly folded and mutant AVP prohormone accumulates in the endoplasmic reticulum of the supraoptic and paraventricular nuclei and results in cell death. Thus children with autosomal dominant disease progressively develop AVP deficiency, and symptoms usually do not appear until several months or years after birth. Indeed, the posterior pituitary bright spot on MRI (see Plate 1.8) is present early and then slowly disappears with age and advancing damage to the vasopressinergic neurons.

Wolfram syndrome (also known as DIDMOAD) is characterized by central DI, diabetes mellitus, optic atrophy, and deafness. Diabetes mellitus typically occurs before central DI. This syndrome is inherited in an autosomal recessive manner with incomplete penetrance and is caused by pathogenic variants in the gene WFS1, coding for the protein wolframin.

Plate 1.28

Pituitary and Hypothalamus

Langerhans Cell Histiocytosis in Children

LCH is a disorder of the Langerhans cell, a bone marrow-derived dendritic cell that has a key role in antigen processing. Normal Langerhans cells—located in the epidermis, lymph nodes, thymic epithelium, and bronchial mucosa—process antigens and then migrate to lymphoid tissues, where they function as effector cells stimulating T-cell responses. Although the cause of the defect in LCH is unknown, it is a result of immunologic dysfunction. In LCH, the Langerhans cell loses its ability to present antigens.

LCH in children is rare, affecting 3 to 5 children per million each year. LCH may present as a localized or diffuse disorder. When localized, the presenting findings may include bone, skin, or lymph node involvement. In infants, brown-purplish papules may be evident, which are usually associated with a benign and self-healing course in the first year of life. However, multisystem disease may become evident later in childhood. When skin-limited LCH is suspected, it should be confirmed with CT imaging of the chest and abdomen and bone marrow biopsy to verify that there are no other abnormalities. Later in infancy, skin-limited LCH presents as a red papular rash variably involving the neck, axilla, abdomen, back, groin, and scalp.

The most common site of involvement in childhood LCH is bone, typically presenting as a lytic skull lesion identified in the evaluation of localized pain and erythema. Other bones that may be involved include ribs, cervical vertebral bodies, humerus, and femur. LCH lesions can extend from the bone and cause mass-effect presentations. For example, skull base, maxillofacial bone, and sellar involvement may lead to hearing loss, exophthalmos, cranial nerve palsies, and DI. On skull radiographs, extensive involvement of the skull may be observed with irregularly shaped, lucent lesions—"geographic skull." DI is the most common endocrine manifestation of LCH, and it may be the initial presenting symptom complex (see Plate 1.27). These patients also have varying degrees of anterior pituitary insufficiency. In patients with pituitary dysfunction, thickening of the pituitary stalk is usually evident.

LCH may present as isolated lymphadenopathy, usually of the cervical or mediastinal lymph nodes.

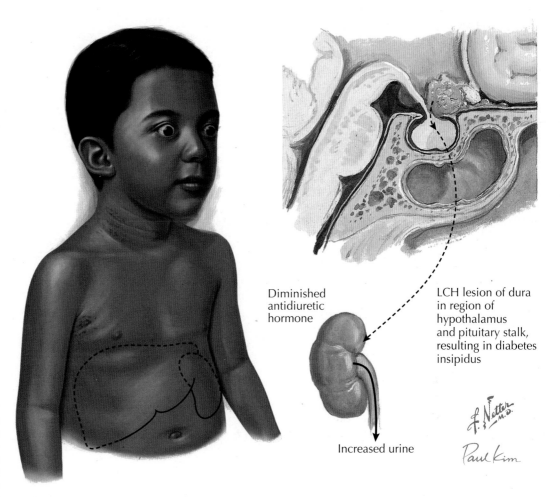

Diminished antidiuretic hormone

LCH lesion of dura in region of hypothalamus and pituitary stalk, resulting in diabetes insipidus

Increased urine

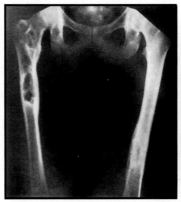
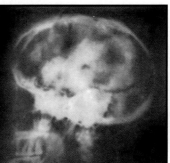
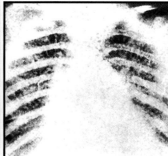

Osteolytic lesions of bones

Osteolytic LCH lesions of skull (geographic skull)

Lung involvement

Diffuse multisystem disease often involves the liver and spleen. Patients with hepatic involvement may present with signs and symptoms related to clotting factor deficiencies, increased bilirubin, and low serum albumin. Cytopenias may result from the splenomegaly. When the lungs are involved, LCH appears in a cystic and nodular pattern; the first sign of pulmonary involvement may be pneumothorax (see Plate 1.29). LCH in the lung can cause diffuse fibrosis with symptoms of dyspnea. Bone marrow involvement is common in patients with diffuse disease. Ataxia and

cognitive dysfunction sometimes result from LCH lesions involving the cerebellum or basal ganglia.

In the past, LCH was referred to as histiocytosis X, or *Hand-Schüller-Christian disease* if the triad of skull defects, DI, and exophthalmos was prominent. *Letterer-Siwe disease* was the term used to describe the presentation of LCH with extensive multiorgan involvement (e.g., skin, lungs, liver, spleen, lymph nodes, bone marrow, lymph nodes). *Eosinophilic granuloma* was the term used to describe localized lesion(s) confined to bone.

Plate 1.29

Endocrine System: VOLUME 2

LANGERHANS CELL HISTIOCYTOSIS IN ADULTS

LCH—previously known as *histiocytosis-X, eosinophilic granuloma, Hand-Schüller-Christian disease,* or *Letterer-Siwe disease*—is a disorder of the Langerhans cell, a bone marrow-derived dendritic cell that has a key role in antigen processing. Normal Langerhans cells—located in the epidermis, lymph nodes, thymic epithelium, and bronchial mucosa—process antigens and then migrate to lymphoid tissues, where they function as effector cells stimulating T-cell responses. LCH is caused by myeloid dendritic cells with activation of the MAP2 kinase pathway. Sixty-five percent of patients with LCH have a *BRAF V600E* mutation in the pathologic dendritic cells.

LCH in adults is rare, affecting 1 to 2 persons per million each year. The mean age at the time of diagnosis is 32 years. The most common presentation is dermatologic symptomatology (rash) followed by pulmonary symptoms (e.g., cough, dyspnea, tachypnea), pain (e.g., bone pain), DI, systemic symptoms (e.g., fever, weight loss), lymphadenopathy, ataxia, and gingival hypertrophy. Because of the diverse presentation and the rarity of this disorder, LCH may not be accurately diagnosed for many years. In some cases, apparent isolated DI is diagnosed in childhood, and the other sites of involvement and associated symptoms do not develop until later in life. DI, caused by Langerhans cell infiltration of the hypothalamus and pituitary stalk, occurs in approximately 25% of patients with LCH and is irreversible.

The skin rash of LCH is papular and pigmented (red, brown). Papule size ranges from 1 mm to 1 cm. Some of the skin lesions may become ulcerated, especially in intertriginous areas.

The most common sites of bone involvement in LCH are the mandible, skull, long bones, pelvic bones, scapula, vertebral bodies, and ribs. Thus the initial presenting symptoms in a patient with LCH may be jaw pain and loose teeth. Dental radiographs may show erosion of the lamina dura and the appearance of "floating teeth." Solitary or polyostotic eosinophilic granuloma, representing 75% of all cases of LCH, typically occur in children or young adults. These lesions present as areas of tenderness and swelling. Radiographs show round lesions with a beveled edge.

Isolated pulmonary involvement may present with pneumothorax. Pulmonary LCH is exacerbated by cigarette smoking. Chest radiographs show a diffuse infiltrate with a "honeycomb lung" appearance. CT shows typical nodules and cysts of LCH.

The diagnosis of LCH should be confirmed with a biopsy of a lesion. Pathologic examination shows a mixed cellular infiltrate with proliferation of immature clonal Langerhans cells. Other inflammatory cells (e.g., eosinophils, macrophages, granulocytes, and lymphocytes) are frequently seen in the specimen. Multinucleated giant cells may be present. The macrophages and multinucleated giant cells are phagocytic and can accumulate cholesterol and have the appearance of "foam cells." Immunohistochemical studies are confirmatory with positive staining for S100 protein, vimentin, CD1a, CD163, and antilangerin (anti-CD207). Quantitative polymerase chain reaction *BRAF V600E* testing on tissue biopsy and circulating cells is also supportive of the diagnosis.

A full laboratory and imaging evaluation is indicated to determine the extent of disease in newly diagnosed patients. Typical laboratory tests include a complete blood cell count, liver function tests, coagulation studies, and simultaneous fasting urine and serum osmolalities. Imaging should include a skeletal survey, skull radiography, and chest radiography. Signs and symptoms should guide whether additional tests are needed (e.g., dental radiographs, head MRI, chest CT, pulmonary function tests, bone marrow biopsy).

The prognosis for patients with LCH can be predicted in part by the age of onset, number of organs involved, and degree of organ dysfunction (e.g., hyperbilirubinemia). For example, whereas an adult with a solitary bone lesion (eosinophilic granuloma) has an excellent prognosis, an infant with marked multiorgan involvement has a worse prognosis. Thus, in general, a better prognosis is associated with an age of onset older than 2 years and involvement of fewer than four organ systems.

Treatment based on prognosis stratification may include cladribine (2-chlorodeoxyadenosine) or a combination of chemotherapeutic agents (e.g., vinblastine, etoposide, methotrexate, and 6-mercaptopurine), corticosteroids (topical or systemic), BRAF inhibitors, and radiotherapy. Solitary bone lesions may be treated with surgical curettage, localized radiation therapy, or both. Bone marrow transplantation may be considered for patients whose disease does not respond to standard therapies.

Disseminated LCH lesions in axilla and on neck and trunk

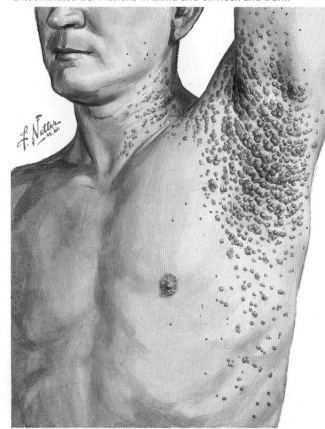

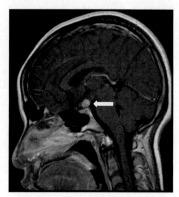

Sagittal head MRI showing a 1-cm enhancing suprasellar lesion (*arrow*) of LCH. Also note the lack of the posterior pituitary bright spot in this patient with diabetes insipidus.

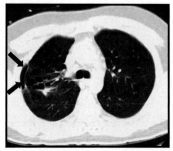

Chest CT showing multiple pulmonary cysts typical of pulmonary LCH. Also note the small pneumothorax on the right lateral chest (*arrows*).

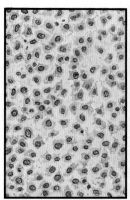

Sheets of Langerhans cell histiocytes with abundant pink cytoplasm and folded nuclei with prominent nuclear grooves

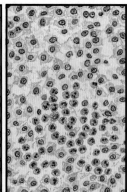

Nests of eosinophils among Langerhans cell

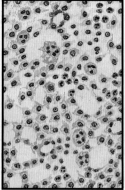

Multinucleated giant cells in granulation tissue

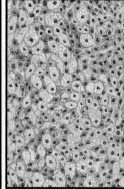

Lipid accumulation within macrophages and giant cells

Plate 1.30

Pituitary and Hypothalamus

Congenital (10%)	Inflammatory (30%)	Neoplastic (60%)
Ectopic neurohypophysis Pituitary cyst Rathke cleft cyst Septo-optic dysplasia	Erdheim Chester disease Immune checkpoint inhibitor induced hypophysitis Langerhans cell histiocytosis Lupus cerebritis Lymphocytic hypophysitis Neurosarcoidosis Granulomatous hypophysitis Xanthoma disseminatum	Astrocytoma Craniopharyngioma Ganglioglioma Germinoma Granular cell tumor Metastasis Neuronal neoplasms Pituicytoma Pituitary adenoma

Imaging configurations of pituitary stalk abnormalities on MRI

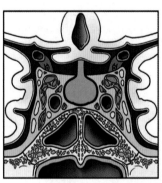
Normal

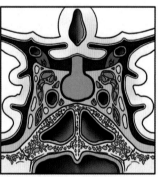
Uniform thickening

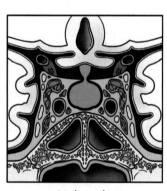
V-shaped

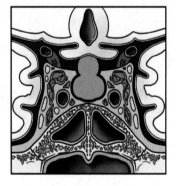
Round/Diamond

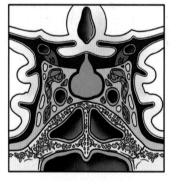
Pyramid

From Turcu AF, Erickson BJ, Lin E, Guadalix S, Schwartz K, Scheithauer BW, Atkinson JL, Young WF Jr. Pituitary stalk lesions: the Mayo Clinic experience. J Clin Endocrinol Metab. 2013 May;98(5):1812-8.

PITUITARY STALK LESIONS

Lesions of the pituitary stalk provide the clinician with a challenging diagnostic conundrum. Due to advances in MRI technology, pituitary stalk lesions may be identified either incidentally or during evaluation for symptoms related to hypothalamic-pituitary dysfunction. Pathologic processes that involve the hypophyseal stalk may extend from the hypothalamus and/or the pituitary gland, or may be limited to the stalk itself. The etiologic spectrum of these lesions is broad and can be divided in three categories: neoplastic, inflammatory, and congenital. Because of the critical location and role of the pituitary stalk, mass lesions in this area are not often biopsied, and the diagnosis may be based on clinical evaluation and imaging clues.

Most congenital pituitary stalk lesions appear round on MRI. The most frequently encountered diagnosis in this category is ectopic neurohypophysis (see Plate 1.8). The characteristic bright signal of the neurohypophysis on MRI in these cases is typically detected in the floor of the third ventricle or along the infundibulum. The sella turcica and anterior pituitary may be small, and the infundibular stalk is absent or hypoplastic.

Most cases of neurosarcoidosis have a uniformly thickened pituitary stalk on MRI. Contrast-enhanced MRI is the preferred imaging test in central nervous system sarcoidosis because other clues leading to this diagnosis are usually evident (e.g., meningeal enhancement, multiple white-matter lesions, hypothalamic infiltration).

Xanthoma disseminatum involving the hypophyseal stalk frequently has a pyramidal pattern of enhancement on MRI.

Lymphomatous involvement of the pituitary stalk most frequently enhances in a V-shaped pattern on MRI. The majority of the metastatic solid cancers are either V-shaped or round on contrast-enhanced MRI.

All patients with pituitary stalk lesions should be evaluated for pituitary deficiencies. Frequently the clinical setting will guide the diagnosis and management. For example, patients presenting with DI and a thickened pituitary stalk in the immediate postpartum period will most likely have lymphocytic hypophysitis (see Plate 1.12). In addition, the MRI imaging phenotype can help guide the evaluation as to the etiology of the stalk lesion. For example, if the MRI findings are suggestive of a congenital lesion, a follow-up MRI in 3 to 6 months to confirm stability would be reasonable approach. If the MRI findings are nonspecific, then screening tests should be completed for inflammatory disorders (e.g., chest CT, bone scan, serum angiotensin converting enzyme level, respiratory and renal evaluations) and neoplastic disorders (e.g., serum and CSF α-fetoprotein and β-hCG). On the other hand, if other similar intracranial lesions are found on MRI, then search for a primary malignancy would be indicated (e.g., 18F-fluorodeoxyglucose PET, biopsy).

Plate 1.31

Endocrine System: VOLUME 2

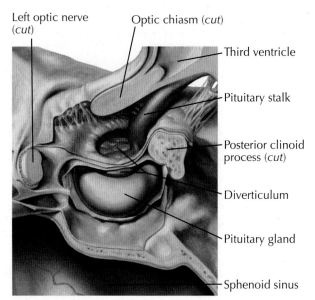

Left optic nerve (*cut*)
Optic chiasm (*cut*)
Third ventricle
Pituitary stalk
Posterior clinoid process (*cut*)
Diverticulum
Pituitary gland
Sphenoid sinus

1. Herniation of arachnoid basal membrane (in red), floor of the chiasmatic cistern, forming a diverticulum into the sella turcica through the diaphragma sellae.

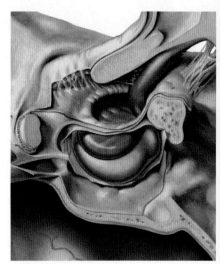

2. Partially empty sella.

Empty Sella

Empty sella is a radiologic finding on MRI or CT and is caused by the herniation of an arachnoid diverticulum into the sella turcica. With expansion of the arachnoid diverticulum, the pituitary gland is flattened on the sellar floor and the infundibulum is elongated. This finding is termed *complete empty sella* when more than 50% of the sellar space is filled with CSF and the pituitary gland is less than 2 mm thick; the term *partial empty sella* is used when less than 50% of sellar space is filled with CSF. The empty sella is termed *primary* if no pathologic process in the sellar region preceded the diagnosis or *secondary* if it is consequent to a pathologic process (e.g., after resection of a pituitary macroadenoma). Primary empty sella is usually discovered incidentally on MRI or CT performed for other reasons and may be the result of increased intracranial pressure and a congenitally incompetent diaphragma sellae. Rarely, there can be bony erosion of the sellar floor and CSF rhinorrhea may occur. Increased intracranial pressure is associated with obesity, obstructive sleep apnea, arterial hypertension, pregnancy, labor, and primary intracranial hypertension.

In autopsy studies, empty sella has been found in 5.5% to 12% of cases—a prevalence replicated on MRI studies. The differential diagnosis includes pituitary cysts and congenital pituitary abnormalities. In primary empty sella, the pituitary stalk is usually thinned and located in the midline. With both primary and secondary empty sella, the optic chiasm may herniate into the sella resulting in visual field loss, and a chiasmal transsphenoidal elevation surgical procedure may be needed. Mild hyperprolactinemia (e.g., <50 ng/mL) is present in approximately 10% of patients with primary empty sella, likely due to compression of the pituitary stalk and decreased dopamine transmission to the normal pituitary lactotrophs.

Although varying degrees of hypopituitarism are common in patients with secondary empty sella, rarely primary empty sella may be associated with pituitary hypofunction. GH deficiency and secondary hypogonadism are most common deficits detected in patients with primary empty sella. Thus hormonal assessment is indicated in all patients with either secondary or primary empty sella.

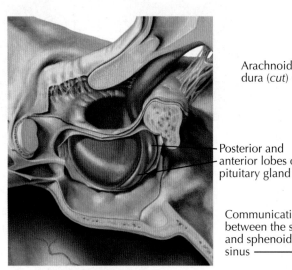

Posterior and anterior lobes of pituitary gland

3. Complete empty sella.

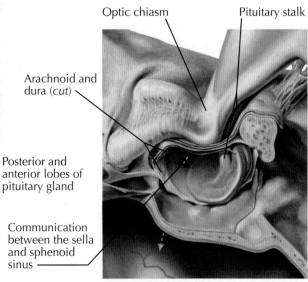

Optic chiasm
Pituitary stalk
Arachnoid and dura (*cut*)
Communication between the sella and sphenoid sinus

4. Herniation of optic chiasm into the sella and erosion of the sellar floor resulting in CSF rhinorrhea are two rare but possible finds.

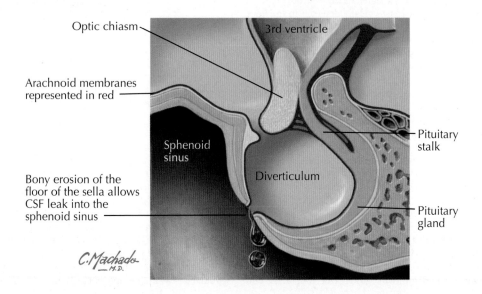

Optic chiasm
3rd ventricle
Arachnoid membranes represented in red
Pituitary stalk
Sphenoid sinus
Diverticulum
Bony erosion of the floor of the sella allows CSF leak into the sphenoid sinus
Pituitary gland

C. Machado M.D.

Plate 1.32   Pituitary and Hypothalamus

Tumors Metastatic to the Pituitary

Metastasis to the pituitary gland is a rare cause of an intrasellar mass discovered during life. When the pituitary gland of patients with cancer is examined at autopsy, pituitary metastases are found in about 3.5% of patients. Most metastases to the pituitary are clinically silent and may be too small to be detected on computed imaging. When detected during life, the most common clinical presentations are DI, visual impairment (e.g., bitemporal hemianopsia), headaches, cranial nerve deficits (e.g., palsies of cranial nerves III or IV), and varying degrees of hypopituitarism. Mild hyperprolactinemia (i.e., serum prolactin concentrations are usually <200 ng/mL) may be present and associated with an interruption of the pituitary stalk delivery of dopamine to suppress normal lactotroph production of prolactin. The most common locations for the primary malignancy (in order of frequency) are the breast, lung, kidney, colon, skin (melanoma), prostate, thyroid, stomach, pancreas, nasopharynx, lymph nodes, uterus, and liver. Breast and lung cancer account for most metastases to the pituitary. In approximately 80% of cases, the pituitary metastasis is discovered after or concurrent with the primary malignancy—the average interval is 3 years. The longest interval between the diagnosis of primary cancer and the discovery of the pituitary metastasis is found in patients with breast cancer, and the shortest interval is found in those with lung cancer. Most of these patients have metastatic disease to five or more sites in addition to the sellar region. The most common sites of extrapituitary metastases are the lymph nodes, lung, and bone.

The routes by which metastases reach the pituitary include hematogenous spread, spread from a hypothalamohypophyseal metastasis though the portal vessels, direct extension from parasellar sites or skull base, or meningeal spread from the suprasellar cistern. Most metastases involve the posterior lobe, presumably because of its direct arterial blood supply from the hypophyseal arteries. Because the anterior lobe does not have a direct arterial supply (see Plate 1.3), metastases that involve the anterior lobe are usually attributable to direct extension from the posterior lobe nidus.

A pituitary metastasis may closely mimic pituitary adenoma. Indeed, the clinical presentation and the neuroimaging and endocrinologic data usually suggest a nonfunctioning pituitary adenoma. Thus metastatic

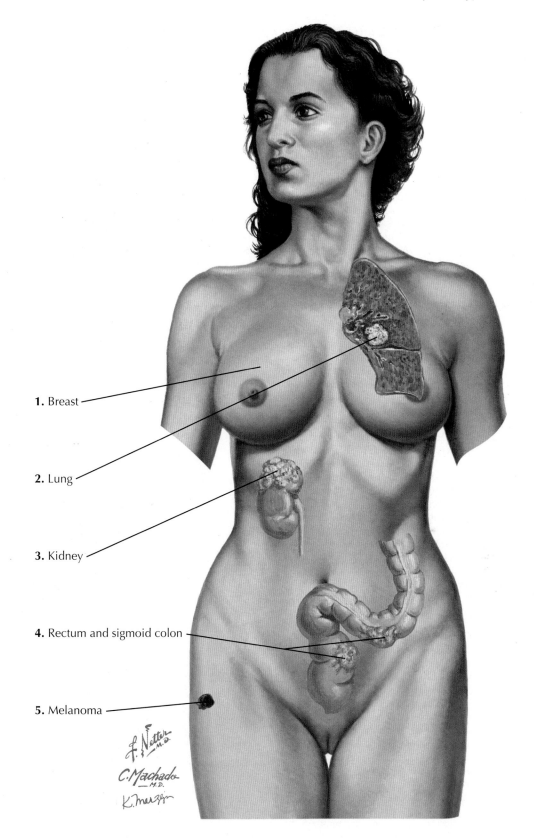

1. Breast

2. Lung

3. Kidney

4. Rectum and sigmoid colon

5. Melanoma

disease should always be considered in the differential diagnosis of a pituitary mass. Because DI is a very unusual (<1%) component of the presentation of benign pituitary adenomas, sellar metastasis should be highly suspected when patients present with DI and a rapidly growing pituitary mass. Tissue diagnosis is required to confirm metastatic disease.

Metastatic disease to the pituitary is a poor prognostic sign; the 1-year mortality rate is 70%. Because of the poor prognosis associated with sellar metastases, the most reasonable therapeutic approaches are palliative radiotherapy, pituitary target hormone replacement therapy when indicated, and primary tumor-directed chemotherapy. Total resection is usually not possible because metastases are usually diffuse, invasive, vascular, and hemorrhagic. Surgical debulking of the sellar metastasis may be beneficial in patients with visual field defects caused by compression of the optic chiasm.

Plate 1.33

Endocrine System: VOLUME 2

SURGICAL APPROACHES TO THE PITUITARY

The three primary goals of pituitary surgery are to (1) completely resect the pituitary adenoma so that visual field defects are corrected and the hormone excess syndrome (e.g., acromegaly, Cushing disease) is cured, (2) avoid complications (e.g., CSF rhinorrhea, neurologic damage), and (3) preserve viable pituitary tissue and avoid hypopituitarism. The ability to meet these three objectives depends on the expertise of the pituitary surgeon and on the size, location, and consistency of the pituitary tumor. For example, whereas the cure rate for pituitary microadenomas (≤10 mm in diameter) is 80% to 90%, the cure rate for pituitary macroadenomas (>10 mm in diameter) is 50% to 60%. When pituitary tumors are larger than 20 mm in diameter, the surgical cure rate decreases to 20%. In addition, the location of the pituitary tumor is an important determinant of the cure rate; invasion of the cavernous sinuses usually prevents complete removal. Some tumors with marked suprasellar extension may adhere to the optic chiasm, the hypothalamus, or both, and attempting complete removal risks vision loss or hypothalamic damage. Most pituitary adenomas are soft in consistency and can be easily curetted. However, when very fibrous, complete resection is difficult.

The sublabial transseptal transsphenoidal surgical approach to the pituitary was developed in the early 1900s but was abandoned because of the high mortality rate related to infection. Up until 1969, the most common surgical approach to the sella was transfrontal craniotomy, an approach associated with clinically significant morbidity and mortality. With the development of the operative microscope and the availability of antibiotics, the sublabial transseptal transsphenoidal surgical approach to the pituitary was reintroduced in the 1970s. This approach to the sphenoid sinus involved making a sublabial incision for access to the nasal cavity and then removing the nasal septum. The sphenoid sinus was entered, allowing access to the sella turcica. After resection of the tumor, the nasal septum was replaced, requiring nasal packing postoperatively. Complications included nasal septal perforation and permanent numbness of the front teeth and upper lip. The sublabial transseptal transsphenoidal surgical approach to the sella has been replaced by the direct transnasal approaches.

The direct transnasal transsphenoidal approach, introduced in the 1990s, requires no external incision. This surgical approach can be completed with an operating microscope or with an endoscope. With the microscope-based procedure, a long, narrow speculum is placed directly into the nostril and extended to the sphenoid ostia. The mucosal incision is made at the posterior aspect of the nasal airway passage, and there is no disruption of the nasal septum. On entering the sphenoid sinus, the anterior wall of the sella is seen and opened under microscopic vision. The tumor is removed under direct microscopic view. The transnasal technique may also be completed with an endoscope. The nasal endoscope is advanced through a nostril to the anterior wall of the sphenoid sinus. The sphenoid ostium is enlarged, and the posterior portion of the vomer is removed, allowing access to the sphenoid sinus. After placement of a self-retaining nasal speculum, the sella turcica is entered, and the neurosurgical portion of the procedure is undertaken as with the sublabial transseptal approach. After resection of the tumor, the nasal speculum is withdrawn, the nasal

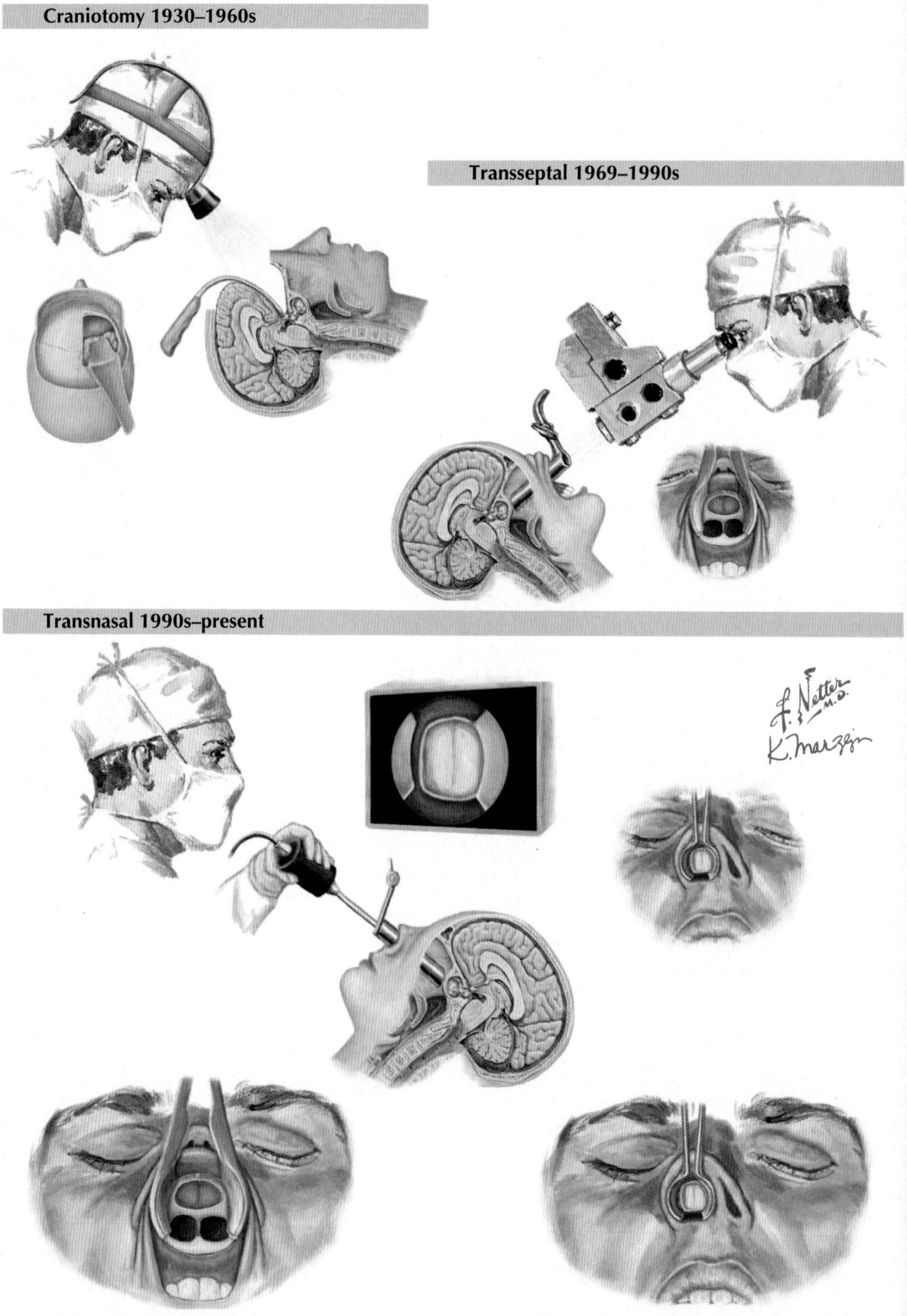

Craniotomy 1930–1960s

Transseptal 1969–1990s

Transnasal 1990s–present

Sublabial transseptal transsphenoidal surgical approach

Endoscopic transnasal transsphenoidal surgical approach

septum is adjusted to midline if necessary, and a mustache nasal dressing is applied. The operative time, anesthesia time, and hospital length of stay are shorter in patients who undergo the endoscopic transnasal approach to pituitary surgery than in those who undergo the sublabial transseptal procedure. Most patients are in the hospital for 1 night.

Although intraoperative complications are rare, they can be serious, and they include injury to the cavernous

carotid artery; injury to the optic pathways; injury to cranial nerves III, IV, V, and VI; and CSF leakage. Postoperatively, the potential complications include sellar hematoma, CSF rhinorrhea, meningitis, pneumocranium, and hypopituitarism.

More than 90% of sellar and parasellar tumors can be removed with the transnasal approach. The transcranial approach is reserved for lesions that extend into the middle fossa or have a large, complex suprasellar component.

THYROID

Plate 2.1

Endocrine System: VOLUME 2

ANATOMY OF THE THYROID AND PARATHYROID GLANDS

Located between the larynx and the trachea medially and the carotid sheath and the sternomastoid muscles laterally, the thyroid gland weighs 15 to 25 g. The lateral thyroid lobes are 3 to 4 cm long and 1.5 to 2 cm wide; the isthmus is 1.2 to 2 cm long and 2 cm wide and crosses the trachea between the I and II rings. In Plate 2.1 (upper image), the skin, subcutaneous fat, and platysma muscle have been excised, exposing, on the right half of the neck, the anterior or first cervical fascia. This fascia envelops the external and anterior jugular veins and the transverse cervical nerves. The subcutaneous fat and platysma muscle contain a rich blood supply, so that wide surgical exposures may be obtained, without sacrificing skin, by raising flaps of skin, subcutaneous fat, and platysma. The veins and nerves thus exposed are left initially in situ to be moved later with the muscles beneath.

On the left side of the neck (Plate 2.1, upper image), the first cervical fascia, the external jugular vein, the transverse nerves, and the sternocleidomastoid muscle have been excised. This excision shows the positions of the omohyoid muscle, the ansa hypoglossal nerve, the important limiting insertion of the shorter inner pretracheal muscle, the sternothyroid muscle, and the entire course of the longer thyrohyoid muscle. The same fascial layer has been incised down the midline, exposing the medial borders of the sternohyoid muscle. These muscles, normally meeting together in the midline, have been partially retracted to expose the thyroid and cricoid cartilages, the isthmus of the thyroid, and the upper trachea lying beneath.

The anterior jugular veins supplement the external jugular vein in returning the blood from the pharynx and upper neck. They also receive tributaries throughout their length: first, from the platysma superficial to them; second, from the pretracheal muscles (sternohyoid, sternothyroid, and omohyoid) deep to them; and third, at the level of the larynx, particularly at the notch, from several fine tributaries from the upper larynx near the midline. In exposing the thyroid and parathyroid glands and the trachea, it is important to save as many of these vessels as possible by retracting them, rather than dividing them, to avoid unnecessary edema of the upper neck and larynx. These anterior veins may be greatly dilated when tumors of the thyroid or other organs deep in the neck have pressed on either internal jugular vein.

The sensory transverse cervical nerves may be severed because they will regenerate. However, this is not true for the two lower branches of the facial nerve—transection of the marginal mandibular branch is followed by drooping of the lower lip on the paralyzed side. The ansa hypoglossal nerve, lying along the anterior medial aspect of the carotid sheath, should be preserved. In exposing the nerve, it is helpful to remember that a small branch of the superior thyroid artery comes down just in front of the nerve, delivering branches to the posterior edge of the muscle as well as supplying the nerve. Division of this nerve renders swallowing more difficult after operation.

The lymphatic vessels in the superficial fascia, anterior to the prethyroid muscles, are not prominent. Lymph nodes are rare; the first one consistently encountered lies immediately in front of the thyroid isthmus in the midline between the pretracheal muscles, deep to the anterior fasciae and superficial to the second or middle cervical fasciae, the false capsule of

the thyroid. This node drains the pharynx or larynx but not the thyroid gland or deeper tissues beneath. It is thus enlarged in patients with acute pharyngitis and laryngitis but not in those with thyroiditis or tracheitis.

Exposure of the thyroid, parathyroid, and thymus glands is achieved by retracting the pretracheal or prethyroid muscles. The widest exposure is obtained if the muscles are cut transversely and the ends retracted up and down. A good view of the upper thyroid pole often requires transection of the inner muscle.

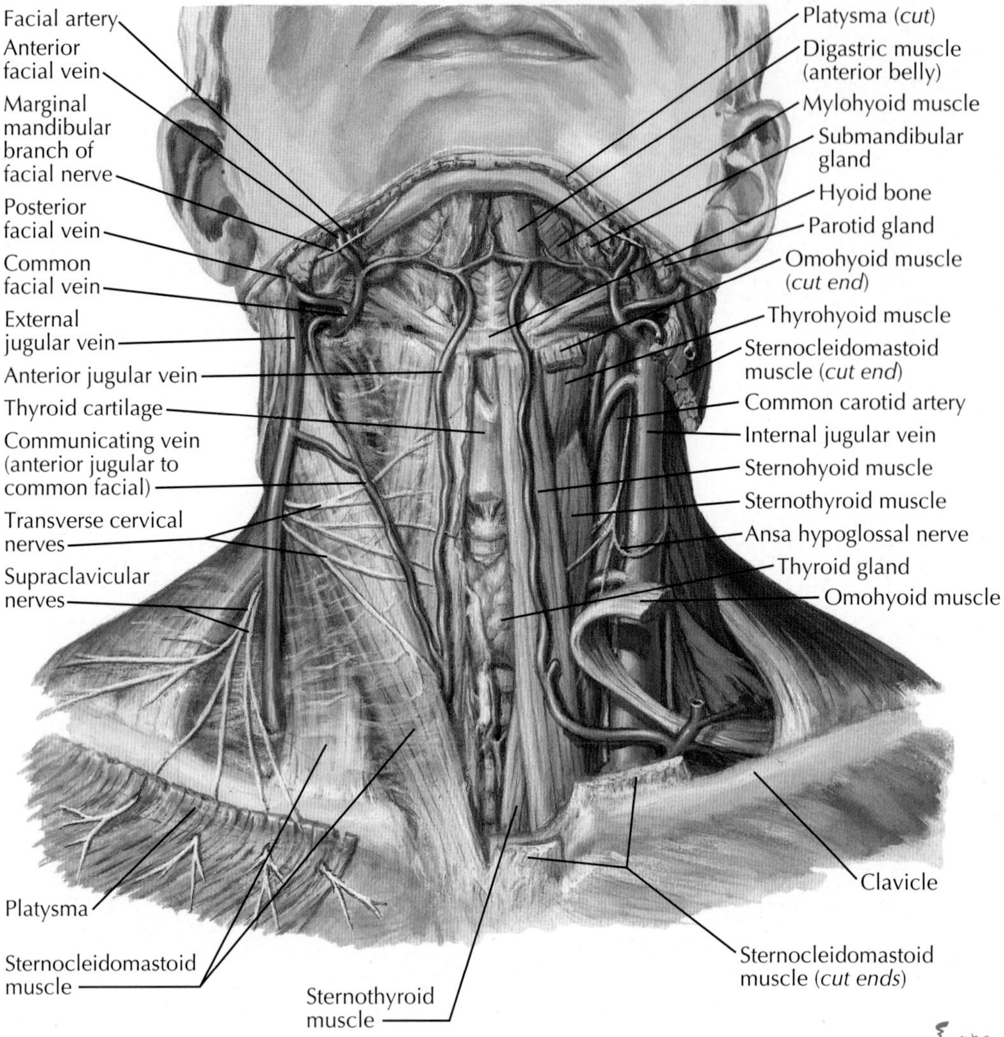

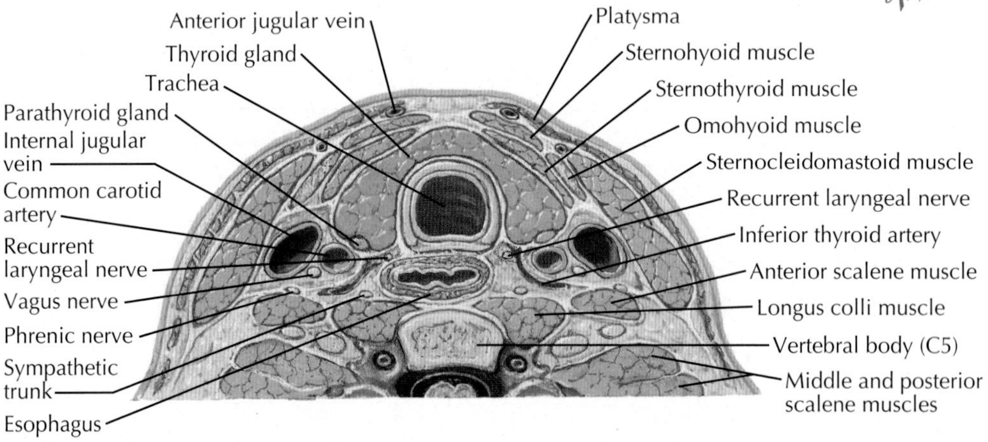

The position of the esophagus, shown slightly to the right of midline (Plate 2.1, lower image), is adjacent to the usually larger right lobe of the thyroid.

Plate 2.2 (upper image) depicts the organs of the neck and anterior superior mediastinum with the anterior neck muscles and the bones of the upper thorax removed. When the thyroid, parathyroid, and thymus glands are first exposed, they lie enveloped on their anterior, lateral, and posterior surfaces by an ill-defined loose areolar fascia (also called the false capsule of the thyroid), which permits the glands, larynx, and trachea to rise and fall with swallowing. Indeed, nearly the

Plate 2.2

Thyroid

ANATOMY OF THE THYROID AND PARATHYROID GLANDS (Continued)

entire anterior surface of both thyroid lobes can be palpated when the patient is instructed to swallow.

The normal thyroid gland is nearly always asymmetric. The right lobe may be even twice as large as the left lobe. The right upper pole extends higher up in the neck, and the lower pole extends lower. In a patient with dextrocardia, the lobe size is reversed.

Four developmental anomalies are to be noted. A pyramidal lobe persists in at least 15% of the population, becoming enlarged if the thyroid is enlarged by a diffuse process. It is occasionally the site or origin of thyroid neoplasia. The second anomaly is the failure of thyroid tissue to be contained within the main thyroid mass posteriorly, which occurs in at least 5% of people. The noncontiguous nature may be palpable on physical examination, giving rise to suspicion of a tumor. The third and fourth anomalies are the failure of the isthmus to fuse in the midline and the absence of a substantial part of the lateral lobe, notably the lower half of the left lobe. These anomalies are rare, occurring in less than 1% of the population. When the isthmus fails to fuse, the medial aspects of the lateral lobes may feel like tumors, but palpating the tracheal rings where the isthmus should be will give the clue. Similarly, absence of the lower half of a lateral lobe may lead to the mistaken impression that the upper half is a thyroid nodule.

The lower image on Plate 2.2 is a lateral view of the organs of the right side of the neck, with the neck muscles, right clavicle, and sternum removed. The position and size of the normal parathyroids are variable. Usually, there are four glands, two upper and two lower. Rarely, there is a fifth, which the surgeon may need to find if it is adenomatous and the source of parathyroid hormone hypersecretion or if it is involved in hyperplasia (e.g., in multiple endocrine neoplasia type 1). The upper glands are more constant and circumscribed in position than the lower glands, often significantly larger, and therefore easier to find. They lie in the plane behind the thyroid, from the upper thyroid pole to the lower branches of the inferior thyroid artery. When enlarged by disease, they may be displaced downward into the posterior mediastinum. The lower glands, arising from a branchial cleft higher than the upper glands and associated, in their embryologic descent, with the thymus, are found over a much wider extent—above or behind the thyroid and down into the anterior mediastinum as far as thymic tissue is found.

The lymphatic vessels and nodes, in the *upper image* on Plate 2.2, follow a consistent pattern. The most readily felt and the first encountered are those in the midline in front. The uppermost, just above the thyroid isthmus, in front of the cricoid cartilage, and medial to a pyramidal lobe, if present, is a constant node group of one to five nodes, which has been termed the *Delphian node*. If involved in thyroid cancer or Hashimoto thyroiditis, it may be felt preoperatively. The pretracheal nodes below the thyroid isthmus are harder to identify because they are embedded in fat and not so constant in position as the Delphian. The other node groups, in order of operative importance, are those on the lateral thyroid surface along the lateral thyroid vein, the nodes along the upper stretch of the recurrent laryngeal nerve behind the thyroid lobe, those at the angle of the jaw, those along the carotid sheath (jugular chain), and the

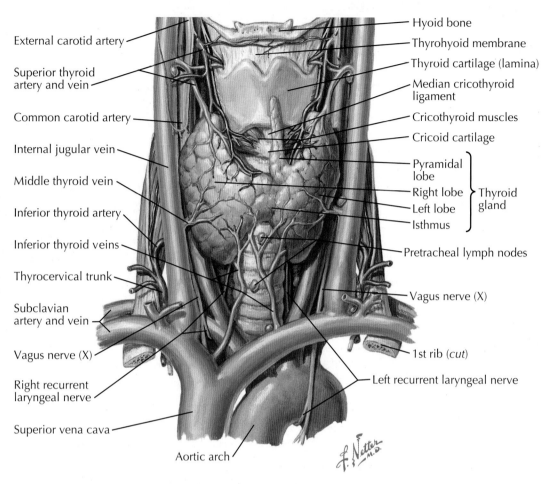

Anterior view

External carotid artery
Superior thyroid artery and vein
Common carotid artery
Internal jugular vein
Middle thyroid vein
Inferior thyroid artery
Inferior thyroid veins
Thyrocervical trunk
Subclavian artery and vein
Vagus nerve (X)
Right recurrent laryngeal nerve
Superior vena cava
Aortic arch

Hyoid bone
Thyrohyoid membrane
Thyroid cartilage (lamina)
Median cricothyroid ligament
Cricothyroid muscles
Cricoid cartilage
Pyramidal lobe
Right lobe
Left lobe } Thyroid gland
Isthmus
Pretracheal lymph nodes
Vagus nerve (X)
1st rib (*cut*)
Left recurrent laryngeal nerve

f. Netter M.D.

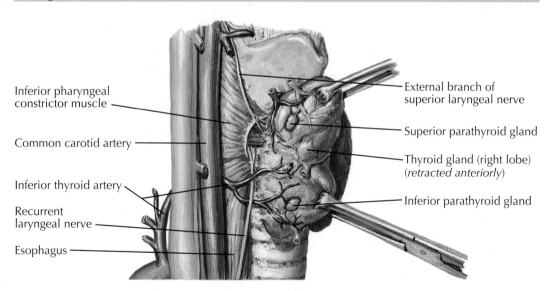

Right lateral view

Inferior pharyngeal constrictor muscle
Common carotid artery
Inferior thyroid artery
Recurrent laryngeal nerve
Esophagus

External branch of superior laryngeal nerve
Superior parathyroid gland
Thyroid gland (right lobe) (*retracted anteriorly*)
Inferior parathyroid gland

more lateral nodes in the supraclavicular fossa. The sentinel nodes of Virchow are the lowermost of the jugular chain at the upper end of the thoracic duct. These nodes may be involved with thyroid and parathyroid carcinoma, as well as with metastases from carcinomas localized outside of the neck.

The laryngeal motor nerves are well depicted in both images on Plate 2.2. The superior nerve carries the motor branch to the cricothyroid muscle. This muscle tenses the vocal cord by drawing the front of the thyroid cartilage

down on the cricoid. Fuzziness of the voice follows section of the nerve, particularly if the injury is bilateral.

The different sites of origin of the two inferior or recurrent laryngeal nerves induce a different course for the nerve on either side. The right nerve passes diagonally from lateral to medial on its upward course, but the left is thrown by the aortic arch, at its inception, against the trachea and esophagus and comes straight up in the tracheoesophageal groove. This constant course makes it the easier of the two to find.

Plate 2.3

Endocrine System: VOLUME 2

DEVELOPMENT OF THE THYROID AND PARATHYROID GLANDS

PHARYNX

By the beginning of the second month of embryonic development, the portion of the originally tubular entodermal foregut caudal to the buccopharyngeal (oral) membrane has differentiated into the pharynx. At this time, the pharynx is relatively wide; compressed dorsoventrally; and has on each side a series of four lateral outpocketings, the pharyngeal pouches (see A and B at right). Each pouch is in close relationship to an aortic arch and is situated opposite a branchial cleft (gill furrow) (see A).

In certain aquatic species, the tissue in the depths of the branchial clefts and at the extremities of the pharyngeal pouches disintegrates to produce communications (the gill slits) between the pharyngeal cavity and the surface of the body. Persistent gill slits can occur in humans; the anomaly may be a slender, epithelially lined tract (branchial or cervical fistula) that extends from the pharyngeal cavity to an opening near the auricle (first pouch) or onto the neck (second and third pouches) (see Plate 2.4). When the anomaly is less extensive, it is either a cervical diverticulum or an epithelially lined cervical cyst. A blind diverticulum may extend either outward from the pharynx, for a variable distance, or inward from the neck. A cyst may be located at one site or another in the depths of the neck, causing no trouble unless it becomes infected or filled with fluid in postnatal life.

The central lumen of the embryonic pharynx gives rise to the adult pharynx (see Plate 2.4). The first, or most cephalic, pair of pharyngeal pouches gives rise to the auditory (eustachian) tubes, to the tympanic (middle ear) cavities, and to the mucous membrane lining the inner surface of each tympanum. The first branchial clefts, located opposite the first pouches, give rise to the external acoustic (auditory) meatuses and to the outer epithelial lining of each eardrum. The second pouches give rise to the epithelium lining the palatine tonsils. The latter pouches are, for the most part, absorbed into the pharyngeal wall, persisting only as pharyngeal outpocketings by contributing to the formation of the supratonsillar fossae (see Plate 2.4).

THYROID GLAND

At a level between the first and second pharyngeal pouches, a saclike entodermal diverticulum (the thyroid sac) appears in the midline of the ventral surface of the pharynx. This sac, destined to give rise to the parenchyma of the thyroid gland (see A), is the first glandular derivative of the pharynx. When it appears, near the end of the fourth gestational week, it almost immediately becomes bilobated, and a narrow, hollow neck connects the two lobes. This neck is known as the *thyroglossal duct* because its pharyngeal attachment is located where the ventral floor of the pharynx contributes to the formation of the tongue. The duct becomes a solid stalk and begins to atrophy by the sixth gestational week; however, its pharyngeal connection results in a permanent pit, the foramen cecum, at the apex of the V-shaped sulcus terminalis on the dorsum of the tongue (see C at right and Plate 2.4).

The thyroid sac is converted into a solid mass of cells by the time the thyroglossal stalk disappears. By the end of the seventh week, the developing thyroid becomes crescentic in shape and is relocated to a position at the level of the developing trachea (see C). This relocation occurs because the thyroid is left behind as the pharynx grows forward. At this time, the thyroid's two (lateral) lobes, one on each side of the trachea, are connected in the midline by a very narrow isthmus of developing thyroid tissue (see C).

The formation of thyroid follicles begins during the eighth week of development. They acquire colloid by the third month. By the end of the fourth month, new follicles arise only by the budding and subdivision of those already present. The mesenchyma, surrounding the thyroid primordium, differentiates into the stroma of the gland and its thin proper fiber-elastic capsule.

The thyroglossal duct may persist either as an epithelial tract, which is open from the foramen cecum of the tongue to the level of the larynx, or as a series of blind pockets (thyroglossal duct cysts) (see Plates 2.4 and 2.5).

A. Pharynx and related structures: 4th week

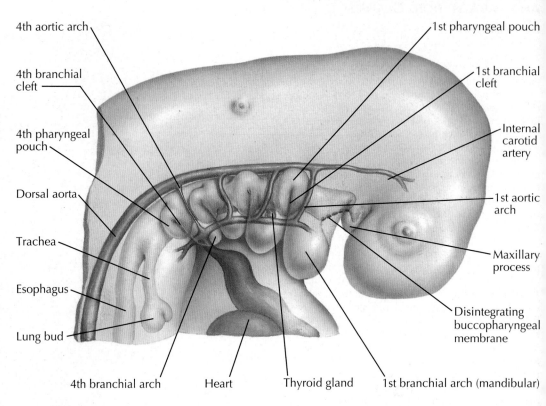

4th aortic arch
4th branchial cleft
4th pharyngeal pouch
Dorsal aorta
Trachea
Esophagus
Lung bud
4th branchial arch
Heart
Thyroid gland
1st branchial arch (mandibular)
1st pharyngeal pouch
1st branchial cleft
Internal carotid artery
1st aortic arch
Maxillary process
Disintegrating buccopharyngeal membrane

B. Pharynx (ventral view) 4th week

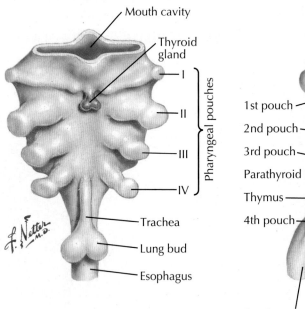

Mouth cavity
Thyroid gland
I
II
III
IV
Pharyngeal pouches
Trachea
Lung bud
Esophagus

C. Pharynx and derivatives (between 6th and 7th weeks)

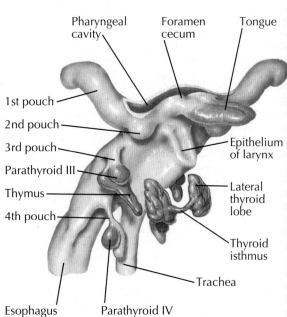

Pharyngeal cavity
Foramen cecum
Tongue
1st pouch
2nd pouch
3rd pouch
Parathyroid III
Thymus
4th pouch
Esophagus
Parathyroid IV
Epithelium of larynx
Lateral thyroid lobe
Thyroid isthmus
Trachea

Plate 2.4

Thyroid

DEVELOPMENT OF THE THYROID AND PARATHYROID GLANDS (Continued)

Persistent portions of the duct or stalk may give rise to accessory thyroids or to a median fistula that opens onto the neck. When a portion of thyroglossal duct persists at the level of the hyoid bone, it passes through the body of the bone.

The variably occurring "pyramidal lobe of the thyroid" results from the retention and growth of the lower end of the stalk. A ligament or a band of muscle, usually located to the left of the midline, may connect the pyramidal lobe either to the thyroid cartilage or to the hyoid bone. The pyramidal lobe undergoes gradual atrophy; therefore it is found more often in children than in adults.

Other variations of the thyroid gland are found. For example, the isthmus may be voluminous, rudimentary, or absent. The lateral lobes may be of different sizes, or both may be absent, with only the isthmic portion present. The shape of the gland may be more like that of an "H" than that of a "horseshoe." Rarely, the gland may be located at the base of the tongue (lingual thyroid) or deep to the sternum. Complete absence of the gland or failure of the gland to function is seldom noticed until a few weeks after birth because fetuses are supplied, through the placenta, with sufficient maternal thyroid hormone to permit normal development. If proper hormonal treatment is not instituted after birth, the result is congenital hypothyroidism.

PARATHYROID AND THYMUS GLANDS

During the fifth and sixth weeks of development, the entodermal epithelium of the dorsal portions of the distal ends of the third and fourth pharyngeal pouches differentiates into the primordia of the parathyroid glands. At the same time, the ventral portions of the distal ends of the third pouches differentiates into the primordia of the thymus gland (see Plate 2.3C). The ventral portions of the distal ends of the fourth pouches may give rise to thymic primordia, which soon disappear without contributing to the adult thymus.

Usually, two pairs of parathyroid glands are formed. By the end of the sixth gestational week, the primordia of the parathyroids and thymus lose their connection with the pouches. At this time, the lumen of the third and fourth pouches becomes obliterated. Parathyroid tissue from the third pouch and thymic primordia migrate, during the seventh week, in a caudomedial direction. During the eighth week, the lower ends of the thymic primordia enlarge and become superficially fused together in the midline. This bilobated lower end continues to descend, to be located in the superior mediastinum of the thorax, posterior to the manubrium. During this descent, the upper ends of the thymic primordia are drawn out into tail-like extensions that usually disappear. Occasionally, they persist as fragments embedded in the thyroid gland or as isolated thymic nests or cords.

Parathyroid tissue from the third pouch migrates with the thymic primordia and usually comes to rest at the caudal level of the thyroid gland to become the inferior parathyroid glands of the adult. Situated within the cervical fascial sheath of the thyroid, the glands are attached to the back of the proper capsule of each lateral thyroid lobe; however, each has its own proper capsule. Occasionally, parathyroid tissue descends with

the thymic primordia to a lower level, being located in the thorax, close to the thymus.

The parathyroids from the fourth pouch do not shift their position appreciably; therefore parathyroids from the third pouch pass them in their caudal migration to a lower level. Thus parathyroids from the fourth pouch become the superior parathyroid glands of the adult, located within the fascial sheath of the thyroid, attached to the back of the proper capsule of each lateral thyroid lobe at the level of the lower border of the cricoid cartilage. Variations in the number, size, and location of the parathyroids are common. Both the regularly occurring

and accessory glands may be situated at some distance from the thyroid. The parathyroids produce parathyroid hormone, which maintains the normal calcium and phosphorus balance.

The thymus gland is a conspicuous organ in infants. At about 2 years of age, it attains its largest relative size, continuing to grow until puberty. It undergoes a gradual involution after puberty as the thymic tissue is replaced by fat. Therefore in adults, the thymus is of approximately the same form and size as during the earlier years, but it now consists chiefly of adipose tissue.

Source	
1st pharyngeal pouch	Auditory tube Tympanic cavity Eardrum Pharyngeal fistula
1st pharyngeal groove	External acoustic meatus
1st and 2nd branchial arches	Auricle
	Nasopharynx Soft palate (velum) Oropharynx
2nd pharyngeal pouch	Supratonsillar fossa Epithelium of palatine tonsil
Ventral pharyngeal wall	Tongue (cut) Foramen cecum Persistent thyroglossal duct Hyoid bone (cut)
3rd pharyngeal pouch	Aberrant parathyroid gland III
2nd pharyngeal pouch	Pharyngeal fistula
4th pharyngeal pouch	Parathyroid gland IV Ultimobranchial body
Ventral pharyngeal wall	Pyramidal and lateral lobes of thyroid gland
3rd pharyngeal pouch	Parathyroid gland III Persistent cord of thymus
	Common carotid artery
3rd pharyngeal pouch	Pharyngeal fistula
	Manubrium of sternum
3rd pharyngeal pouch	Aberrant parathyroid gland III Thymus gland Heart

Plate 2.5

Endocrine System: VOLUME 2

**Aberrant and normal
locations of thyroid tissue**

Lingual

Intralingual

Thyroglossal tract

Sublingual

Thyroglossal cyst

Prelaryngeal

Normal

Intratracheal

Substernal

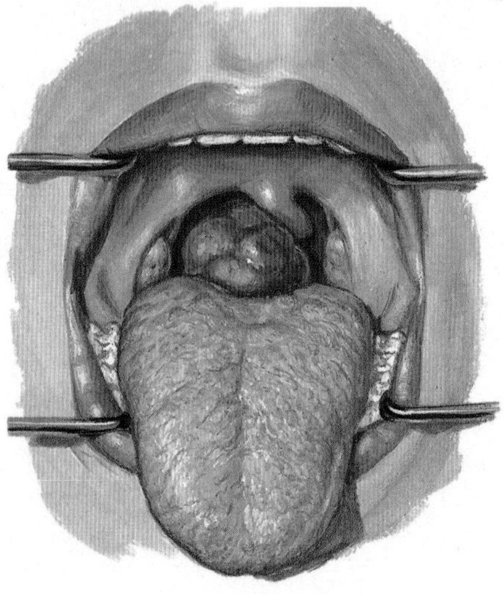

CONGENITAL ANOMALIES OF THE THYROID GLAND

Aberrant, or abnormal, locations of thyroid tissue may be explained on the basis of abnormal embryologic migration of the thyroid and of its close association with lateral thyroid anlagen. These abnormal settings of thyroid tissue can better be understood if one considers the embryology of the thyroid gland, which, in humans, arises about the 17th day of gestation and is derived from the alimentary tract. The median part of the thyroid is formed from the ventral evagination of the floor of the pharynx at the level of the first and second pharyngeal pouches. The lateral thyroid anlage, from the area of the fourth pouch, becomes incorporated into the median thyroid anlage to contribute a small proportion of the final thyroid parenchyma. The thyroid anlage becomes elongated and enlarges laterally, with the pharyngeal region contracting to become a narrow stalk—the thyroglossal tract or duct. This subsequently atrophies, leaving at its point of origin on the tongue a depression known as the *foramen cecum*. Normally, the thyroid continues to grow and simultaneously migrates caudally.

The anatomic sites for the location of anomalously formed thyroid tissue range from the posterior tongue down into the region of the heart, within the mediastinum. Persistence of thyroid tissue on the posterior tongue is a fairly uncommon anomaly known as *lingual thyroid*. This may be the only source of thyroid tissue in the individual. It can often be demonstrated with radioactive iodine scintigraphy, revealing the localization of radioiodine only within the lingual thyroid without any thyroid tissue being demonstrated in the neck.

Intralingual and sublingual rests of thyroid tissue have been described, but these are quite uncommon. The thyroglossal tract that persists usually atrophies completely. However, it may fail to atrophy, remaining as a cystic mass in the midline of the neck, somewhere between the base of the tongue and the hyoid bone. A thyroglossal cyst should therefore be considered in any individual presenting with an enlarging cystic mass immediately beneath the chin in the midline. Occasionally, such cysts may be associated with thyroid tissue capable of concentrating radioactive iodine.

Substernal aberrant thyroid tissue in the mediastinum, is rarely the consequence of abnormal development, representing glandular rests remaining from the time of the caudal descent of the thyroid. However, most often, substernal thyroid tissue is the result of

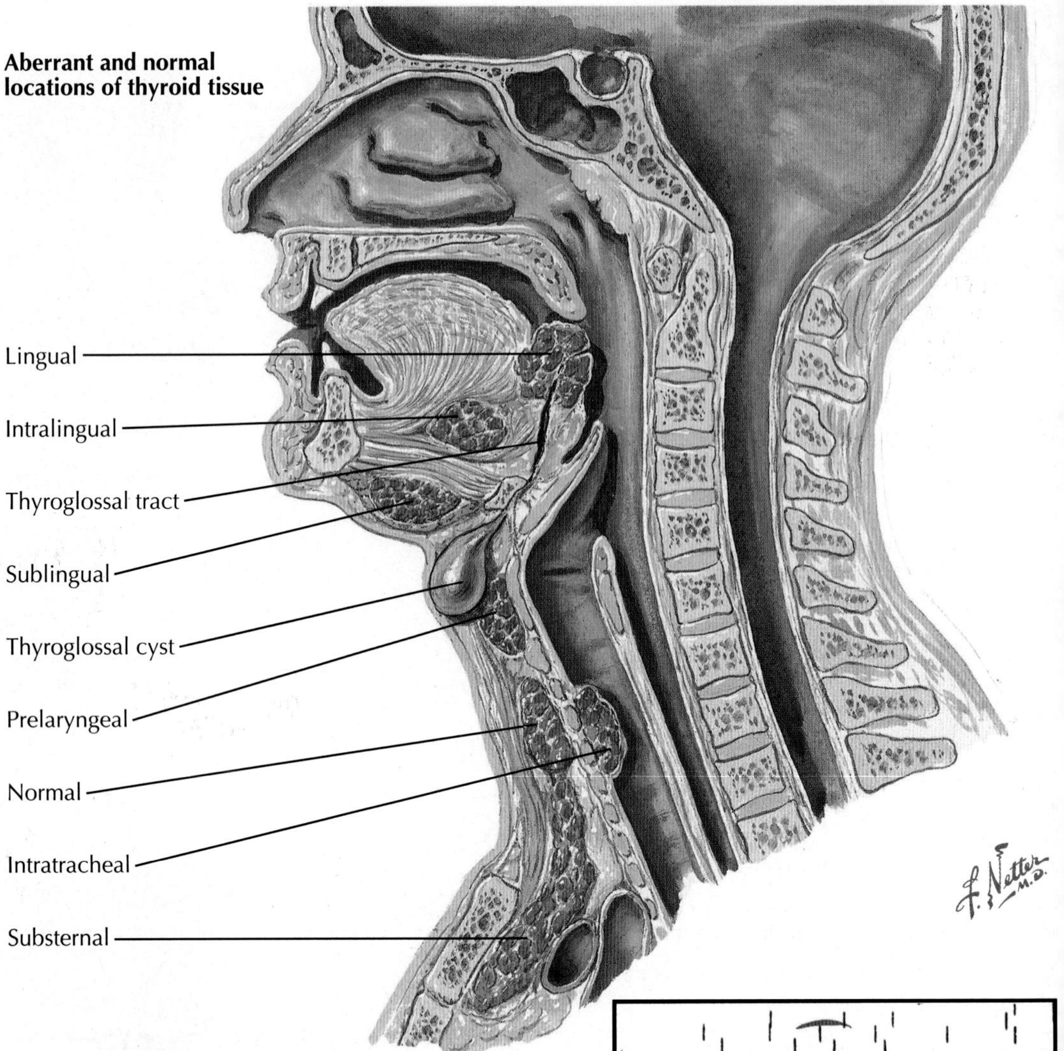

Lingual thyroid

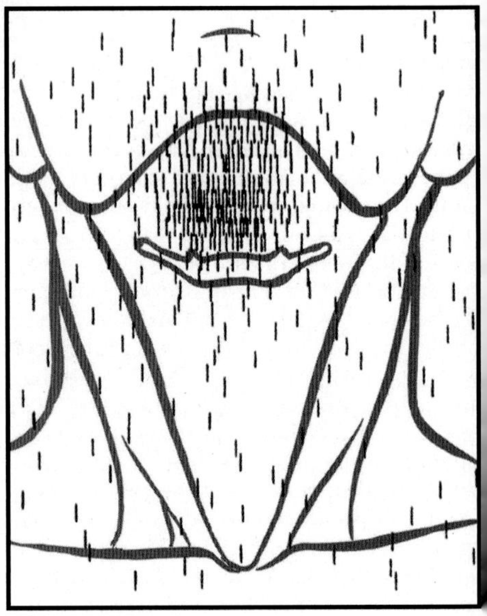

Scintigram; lingual thyroid

downward growth of a nodular goiter. Prelaryngeal thyroid tissue may exist, being attached to a very long pyramidal lobe or to a thyroglossal cyst. Intratracheal thyroid rests have also been reported, although infrequently. The "lateral aberrant thyroid" may represent original branchial tissue that did not fuse with the median thyroid. However, the demonstration of microscopic carcinoma in the thyroids of some patients with so-called lateral aberrant thyroid tissue suggests that, in

most instances, these may actually be metastases from a low-grade, well-differentiated thyroid papillary thyroid carcinoma.

The medical significance of aberrant thyroid tissue is quite limited. Occasionally, an inflammatory change or, rarely, enlargement and consequent thyrotoxicity will call for surgical or radiotherapeutic intervention. The exact interpretation of these lesions necessitates an understanding of their embryologic derivation.

Plate 2.6

Thyroid

EFFECTS OF THYROTROPIN ON THE THYROID GLAND

The hypothalamic-pituitary unit has an indispensable role in the regulation of thyroid function. Hypothalamic dysfunction or anterior pituitary failure leads to diminished thyroid mass and decreased production and secretion of thyroid hormones. The pituitary hormone that targets the thyroid gland is a glycoprotein, thyroid-stimulating hormone (TSH; thyrotropin), which is secreted by pituitary thyrotrophs. TSH is the main regulator of the structure and function of the thyroid gland. TSH is composed of an α subunit and a β subunit. The α subunit consists of 92 amino acids, and it is identical to the α subunit of luteinizing hormone (LH), follicle-stimulating hormone, and human chorionic gonadotropin (hCG). The β subunit of glycoprotein hormones confers specificity. The β subunit synthesized in thyrotrophs is an 112-amino acid protein. Hypothalamic thyrotropin-releasing hormone (TRH) is a modified tripeptide (pyroglutamyl-histidyl-proline-amide) that increases the transcription of both subunits, and thyroid hormones (tetraiodothyronine [T_4; thyroxine] and triiodothyronine [T_3]) suppress the transcription of both subunits. In healthy persons, the serum TSH concentration is between 0.3 and 5.0 mIU/L. TSH concentrations are increased in primary hypothyroidism, increased in secondary hyperthyroidism (e.g., TSH-secreting pituitary tumor), and decreased in primary hyperthyroidism. Blood TSH concentrations vary in both a pulsatile and a circadian manner—a nocturnal surge precedes the onset of sleep.

Both T_4 and T_3 mediate feedback regulation of TRH and TSH secretion. A linear inverse relationship exists between the serum free T_4 concentration and the log of the TSH. Thus the serum TSH concentration is a very sensitive indicator of the thyroid state of patients with intact hypothalamic-pituitary function.

A TSH receptor is expressed on thyroid cells. The TSH receptor is a member of the glycoprotein G protein-coupled receptor family. The TSH receptor couples to Gs and induces a signal via the phospholipase C and intracellular calcium pathways that regulate iodide efflux, H_2O_2 production, and thyroglobulin (Tg) iodination. Signaling by the protein kinase A pathways mediated by cyclic adenosine monophosphate regulates iodine uptake and transcription of Tg, thyroperoxidase, and the sodium-iodide symporter (NIS) mRNAs, leading to thyroid hormone production. In addition to TSH, the TSH receptor also binds thyroid-stimulating antibody (increased in the setting of Graves disease) and thyroid-blocking antibodies (increased in the setting of Hashimoto thyroiditis). At high concentrations, the closely related glycoprotein hormones—LH and hCG—also bind to and activate TSH receptor signaling

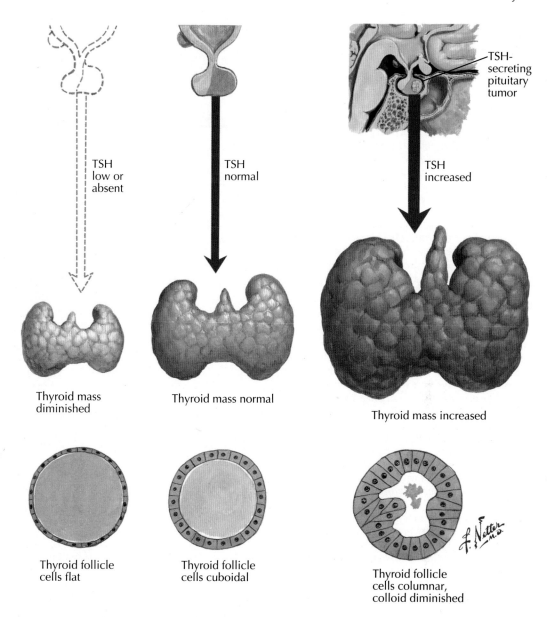

and can cause physiologic hyperthyroidism of early pregnancy.

With an intact hypothalamic-pituitary-thyroid axis, the thyroid gland mass is normal, thyroid follicle cells appear cuboidal, TSH concentration is in the reference range, free T_4 and total T_3 concentrations are in the reference range, and radioactive iodine uptake is normal. In the setting of hypothalamic or pituitary dysfunction, secondary hypothyroidism is manifest by decreased thyroid gland mass (which may not be palpable on physical examination), flat-appearing thyroid follicle cells, low TSH concentration (or inappropriately low for the low thyroid hormone levels), free T_4 and total T_3 concentrations below the reference range, and low radioactive iodine uptake. However, in a patient with a TSH-secreting pituitary tumor, the thyroid gland mass is increased and is usually evident as a firm goiter on physical examination, thyroid follicle cells appear columnar and the colloid is diminished, TSH concentration is inappropriately within or slightly above the reference range, free T_4 and total T_3 concentrations are above the reference range, and radioactive iodine uptake is increased.

TSH low or absent — Thyroid mass diminished — Thyroid follicle cells flat

TSH normal — Thyroid mass normal — Thyroid follicle cells cuboidal

TSH-secreting pituitary tumor — TSH increased — Thyroid mass increased — Thyroid follicle cells columnar, colloid diminished

TSH: low	TSH: normal	TSH: high
Free T_4: low	Free T_4: normal	Free T_4: high
Total T_3: low	Total T_3: normal	Total T_3: high
^{131}I-uptake: low	^{131}I-uptake: normal	^{131}I-uptake: high

Plate 2.7

Endocrine System: VOLUME 2

PHYSIOLOGY OF THYROID HORMONES

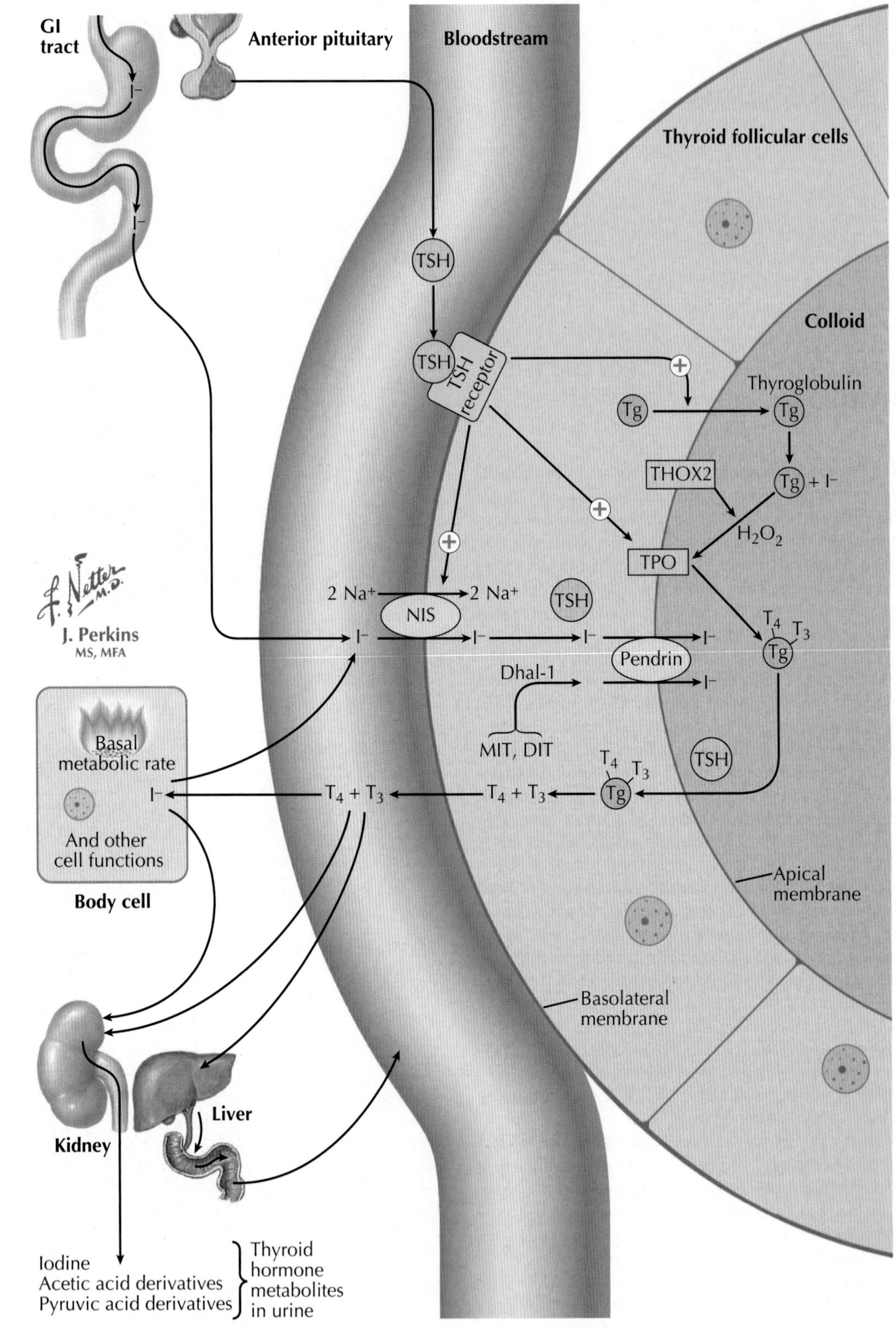

The role of the thyroid gland in the total body economy comprises the synthesis, storage, and secretion of thyroid hormones, which are necessary for growth, development, and normal body metabolism. These thyroid functions can be considered almost synonymous with iodine metabolism. Iodination of the tyrosine molecule leads to synthesis of T_4 and T_3.

Inorganic iodine (I^-) is rapidly absorbed in the gastrointestinal (GI) tract and circulates as iodide, until it is either trapped by the thyroid or salivary glands or excreted by the urinary tract. The thyroid extracts iodine from the plasma, against a 25-fold concentration gradient, by virtue of the NIS. The function of NIS requires a sodium gradient across the basolateral membrane—the transport of two Na^+ ions allows the transport of one iodide atom. NIS also transports TcO_4^-, which is used clinically for thyroid scintigraphy, and potassium perchlorate ($KClO_4^-$), which can block thyroid iodide uptake. NIS gene transcription and protein half-life are enhanced by thyrotropin. Intrafollicular cell iodide is also generated by the action of iodotyrosine dehalogenase 1 isoenzyme (Dhal-1) that deiodinates monoiodotyrosine (MIT) and diiodotyrosine (DIT).

Pendrin is a glycoprotein expressed on the apical border of the thyroid follicular cell, where it facilitates the transfer of iodide into the follicular colloid. After the pendrin-facilitated iodide transfer to the colloid, iodide is oxidized by thyroid peroxidase (TPO) to facilitate the iodination of tyrosine to MIT and DIT. Antithyroid drugs (e.g., propylthiouracil, methimazole, carbimazole) inhibit the function of TPO. TPO requires H_2O_2 that is generated by thyroid oxidase 2 (THOX2), a step that is inhibited by iodide excess. The organic compounds of iodine are stored in the thyroid as part of Tg (molecular weight, 660 kDa). TPO also serves to catalyze the coupling of two molecules of DIT to form T_4 and one molecule of MIT and one molecule of DIT to form T_3. T_4 and T_3 are stored in the colloid as part of the Tg molecule—there are three to four T_4 molecules in each molecule of Tg. TSH stimulates the retrieval of Tg from the colloid by micropinocytosis to form phagolysosomes, where proteases free T_4, T_3, DIT, and MIT within the phagolysosome. T_4 and T_3 are then transported from the phagolysosome across the basolateral cell membrane and into the circulation. This action is inhibited by large amounts of iodine, a finding that can be used therapeutically in the treatment of patients with hyperthyroidism caused by Graves disease. DIT and MIT are deiodinated by Dhal-1, and the iodide is returned to the follicular lumen.

The ratio of T_4 to T_3 in Tg is approximately 15 to 1, and when released from the follicular cell, it is approximately 10 to 1 (the difference reflecting the action of a 5'-deiodination). The deiodination step can be inhibited by propylthiouracil. T_4 is produced only in the thyroid gland. Although T_3 is released from the thyroid, 75% of T_3 in the body is derived from peripheral 5'-deiodination of one of the outer ring iodine atoms in T_4. T_4 and T_3 can be inactivated by inner ring (5-deiodination) to form reverse T_3 and diiodothyronine, respectively. The presence of these deiodinases in various cell types provides for local regulation of thyroid hormone effect.

T_4 and T_3 are poorly water soluble and circulate bound to plasma proteins—thyroxine-binding globulin (TBG), T_4-binding prealbumin (transthyretin), and albumin. TBG has one iodothyronine binding site per molecule. The affinity of TBG for T_3 is 20-fold less than that for T_4.

From the thyroxine-binding proteins, T_4 and T_3 enter the body cells, where they exert their metabolic actions, which are, predominantly, calorigenic (raising the basal metabolic rate). Thyroid hormones act by binding to the thyroid hormone receptor, which, in turn, binds to DNA. T_3 has a 15-fold higher binding affinity for the thyroid hormone receptor than does T_4.

Both T_4 and T_3 are metabolized by kidney and liver tissue to their pyruvic acid and acetic acid derivatives and, eventually, to iodide. These metabolites are concentrated and conjugated in the liver to glucuronic acid, excreted with the bile, hydrolyzed in the small bowel, and reabsorbed.

The thyroid gland is unique with regard to the amount of stored hormone. There is approximately 250 μg of T_4 for every gram of thyroid gland—approximately 5 mg of T_4 in a 20-g thyroid. Thus it is not surprising that thyrotoxicosis is common when the thyroid gland is acutely damaged by inflammation (e.g., subacute thyroiditis).

GI tract

Anterior pituitary

Bloodstream

Thyroid follicular cells

Colloid

TSH

TSH receptor

Thyroglobulin

Tg

THOX2

H_2O_2

TPO

T_4 T_3

2 Na^+ → 2 Na^+

NIS

TSH

Pendrin

Dhal-1

MIT, DIT

T_4 T_3

TSH

Basal metabolic rate

$T_4 + T_3$

$T_4 + T_3$

And other cell functions

Body cell

Apical membrane

Basolateral membrane

Kidney

Liver

Iodine
Acetic acid derivatives
Pyruvic acid derivatives } Thyroid hormone metabolites in urine

J. Netter M.D.

J. Perkins
MS, MFA

Plate 2.8

Thyroid

GRAVES DISEASE

Graves disease is an eponym that describes a thyroid autoimmune syndrome characterized by hyperthyroidism, goiter, ophthalmopathy, and occasionally an infiltrative dermopathy (pretibial or localized myxedema). Graves disease and hyperthyroidism are not synonymous because some patients with Graves disease have ophthalmopathy but not hyperthyroidism. Also, in addition to Graves disease, hyperthyroidism has several other causes. The hyperthyroidism in Graves disease is caused by autoantibodies to the thyrotropin receptor that activate the receptor and stimulate the synthesis and secretion of thyroid hormones (T_4 and T_3) and thyroid gland growth.

Graves disease occurs more commonly in females than in males (4:1) and more frequently during the childbearing years, although it may occur as early as in infancy and in extreme old age. Although this malady's primary signs are an enlarged thyroid gland and prominent eyes, along with cardiovascular symptoms, it actually involves most systems of the body and is thus a systemic disease. The thyroid is diffusely enlarged (goiter) and is anywhere from two to several times its normal size. Some asymmetry may be observed, the right lobe being somewhat larger than the left. The pyramidal lobe is usually enlarged. Rarely in a patient with Graves disease, there is no palpable enlargement of the thyroid gland. The gland has an increased vascularity, as evidenced by a bruit that can be heard with a stethoscope and sometimes by a thrill felt on palpation, which may be demonstrated over the upper poles. Histologically, the gland shows follicular hyperplasia with a marked loss of colloid from the follicles and an increased cell height, with high columnar acinar cells that may demonstrate papillary infolding into the follicles. Late in the disease, there may be multifocal lymphocytic (primarily T cells) infiltration throughout the thyroid gland, and, occasionally, even lymph follicles (primarily B cells) may be seen within the thyroid parenchyma.

The hyperplastic thyroid functions at a markedly accelerated pace, evidenced by an increased uptake and turnover of radioactive iodine and increased levels of T_4 and T_3, which cause an increased rate of oxygen consumption or increased basal metabolic rate and decreased serum total and high-density lipoprotein (HDL) cholesterol concentrations. The increased levels of T_4 and T_3 cause a variety of physical and psychologic manifestations. Patients with this malady are usually nervous, agitated, restless, and experience insomnia, personality changes, and emotional lability. Behavioral findings include difficulty concentrating, confusion, and poor immediate recall.

On physical examination, patients with Graves disease present a fine tremor that may not be obvious but is best demonstrated by placing a paper towel on the extended fingers. The increased levels of T_4 and T_3 and the increased levels of oxygen consumption, with concomitant generalized vasodilation, result in increased cardiac output, presenting with palpitation and sinus tachycardia. The increased stimulus to the heart action may result in atrial fibrillation and heart failure.

The skin of patients with this disease is warm and velvety (because of a decrease in the keratin layer); it may also be flushed and is often associated with marked perspiration caused by increased calorigenesis. Occasionally, vitiligo—another autoimmune manifestation—is observed. Onycholysis (known as *Plummer nails*)—loosening of the nails from the nail bed and softening

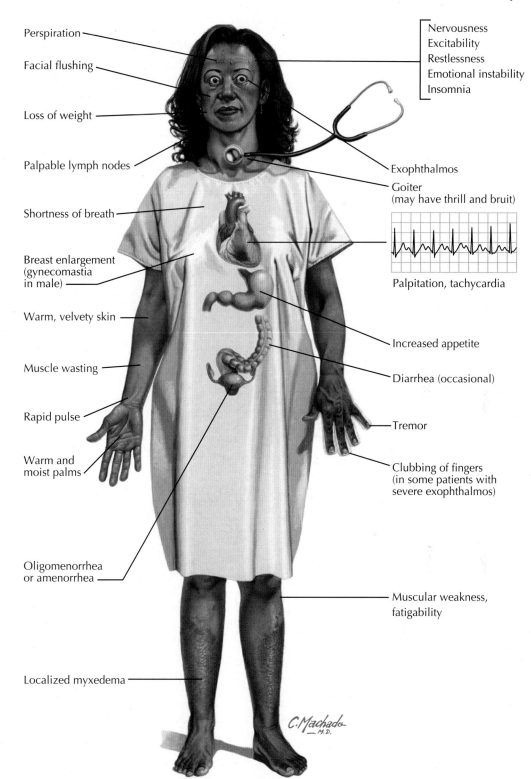

Perspiration

Facial flushing

Loss of weight

Palpable lymph nodes

Shortness of breath

Breast enlargement (gynecomastia in male)

Warm, velvety skin

Muscle wasting

Rapid pulse

Warm and moist palms

Oligomenorrhea or amenorrhea

Localized myxedema

Nervousness
Excitability
Restlessness
Emotional instability
Insomnia

Exophthalmos

Goiter (may have thrill and bruit)

Palpitation, tachycardia

Increased appetite

Diarrhea (occasional)

Tremor

Clubbing of fingers (in some patients with severe exophthalmos)

Muscular weakness, fatigability

C. Machado M.D.

of the nails—occurs in a minority of patients with Graves disease. Infiltrative dermopathy (pretibial myxedema) is the skin change that sometimes occurs in the lower extremities or on the forearms in patients with severe progressive ophthalmopathy. This is associated with a brawny, nonpitting thickening of the skin. It presents as a rubbery, nonpitting swelling of the cutaneous and subcutaneous tissues, with a violaceous discoloration of the skin on the lower third of the legs. Usually, it is predominant in the outer half of the leg. Nodules (as large as 1 cm in diameter) over the tibia,

extending up as high as the knees, may be associated with classic localized pretibial myxedema. This lesion may also occur on the forearms, and it has been known to involve the feet and even the toes. Characteristically, hair does not grow in such myxedematous sites, but the occasional presence of hair follicles, producing hair at the site, does not exclude the diagnosis. When localized myxedema occurs, it is almost always in patients who have severe and progressive ophthalmopathy. Graves disease is also associated with clubbing of the fingers and of the toes (thyroid acropachy).

Plate 2.9

Endocrine System: VOLUME 2

GRAVES DISEASE (Continued)

Sympathetic overactivity results in a stare and eyelid lag in most patients with hyperthyroidism. Eyelid lag is demonstrated by having the patient follow the examiner's finger through a vertical arc—the sclera can usually be seen above the iris as the patient looks down. Unique to Graves disease is ophthalmopathy (see Plate 2.10).

The increased metabolic rate and calorigenesis of these patients leads to a loss of weight despite a good to increased appetite, and to wasting of certain muscles, which is associated with muscular weakness. Hyperthyroidism has mixed effects on glucose metabolism, but patients who are affected typically have fasting hyperglycemia. Severe hyperthyroidism may be associated with hyperdefecation and malabsorption.

In females, the total serum estradiol concentrations are increased because of increased serum sex hormone-binding globulin concentrations. However, free estradiol concentrations are low, and serum LH concentrations are increased—factors that lead to oligomenorrhea or even amenorrhea, which is corrected by restoring the euthyroid state. The increase in serum sex hormone-binding globulin concentrations is also observed in hyperthyroid males, reflected in high serum total testosterone concentrations, low serum free testosterone concentrations, and mild increases in serum LH concentrations. The aromatization of testosterone to estradiol is increased, frequently resulting in gynecomastia, decreased libido, and sexual dysfunction.

Patients with Graves disease manifest the symptoms and signs of profound muscle changes known as *thyroid myopathy*. Atrophy of the temporal muscles, the muscles of the shoulder girdle, and the muscles of the lower extremities—notably the quadriceps femoris group—is typical. Muscular weakness is present, and these patients are often unable to climb steps or to lift their own weight from a chair. The muscular weakness may also contribute to dyspnea. Characteristically, these patients have a tremor, and when asked to extend a leg, they manifest a marked trembling and are usually unable to hold the leg in the extended position for more than 1 minute.

Excess T_4 and T_3 stimulate bone resorption, which reduces trabecular bone volume and increases the porosity of cortical bone. The effect on cortical bone density is usually greater than that on trabecular bone density. The high bone turnover state can be confirmed by measurement of increased blood concentrations of osteocalcin and bone-specific alkaline phosphatase. In some patients, the increased bone resorption leads to hypercalcemia. The hypercalcemia inhibits parathyroid hormone secretion and the genesis of 1,25-dihydroxyvitamin D, which leads to impaired calcium absorption and increased urinary calcium excretion. Thus patients with long-standing hyperthyroidism are at increased risk for bone fracture and osteoporosis.

The earliest descriptions of Graves disease concerned patients who had goiters and some degree of heart failure. Characteristically, patients with hyperthyroidism report a variety of cardiac symptoms and signs. An increased heart rate is usually present. Cardiac output is increased, and those who develop heart failure present the manifestations of high-output failure characterized by a shorter than normal circulation time despite elevated venous pressure. Systolic hypertension is frequently present. Enlargement of the heart is unusual except in a case of frank heart failure or in a patient with

previous heart disease. The heart does not show any characteristic anatomic or microscopic changes that can be attributed to hyperthyroidism. The stimulus to cardiac output has been attributed to the elevated basal metabolic rate and the increased oxygen demands of the body. The usual cardiac effects of the catecholamines are accentuated by thyroid hormones, and all sympathetic activity is exaggerated in hyperthyroidism. Atrial

fibrillation occurs in approximately 15% of patients and is more common in patients older than age 60 years. In most patients, the atrial fibrillation spontaneously converts to normal sinus rhythm when euthyroidism is established. Thus a peripheral β-adrenergic blocker will control most of the circulatory manifestations, reduce sweating, and diminish eyelid retraction—all independent of any effect on circulating levels of T_4 and T_3.

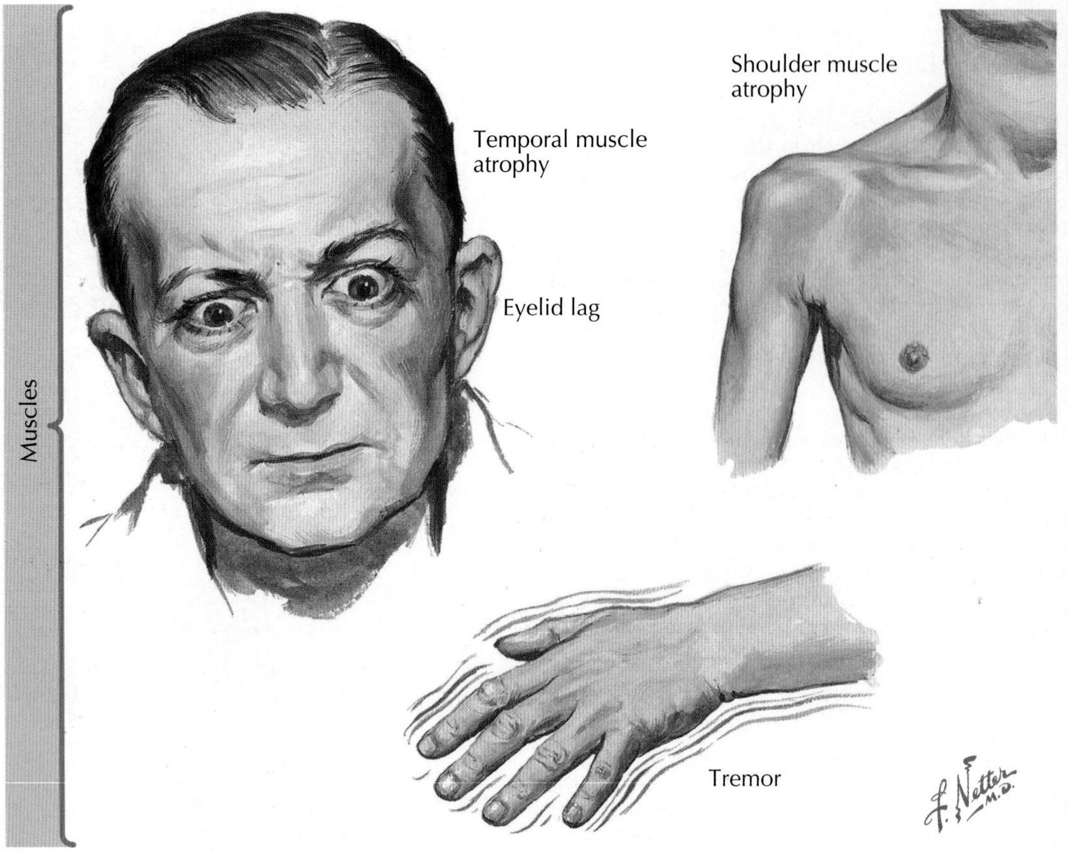

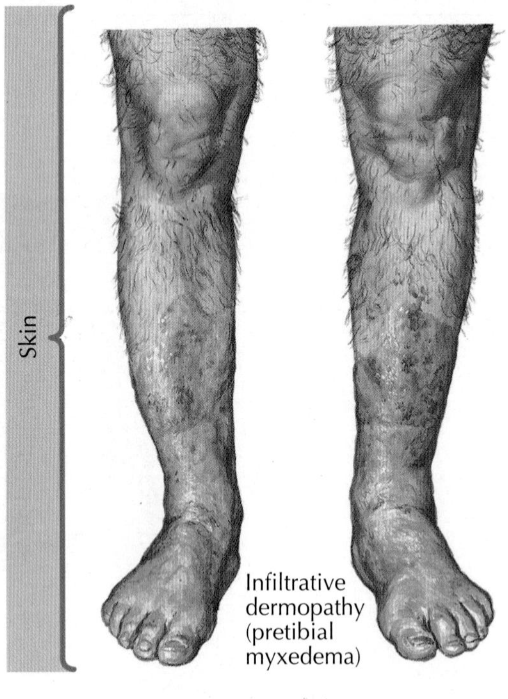

Temporal muscle atrophy

Shoulder muscle atrophy

Eyelid lag

Muscles

Tremor

Skin

Infiltrative dermopathy (pretibial myxedema)

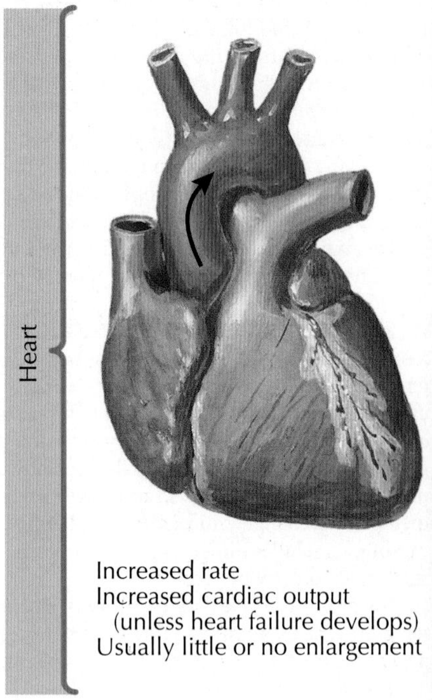

Heart

Increased rate
Increased cardiac output (unless heart failure develops)
Usually little or no enlargement

Plate 2.10

Thyroid

GRAVES OPHTHALMOPATHY

Graves ophthalmopathy (or thyroid eye disease) is an autoimmune disease of the retroorbital tissues, and the eye signs, of which proptosis and periorbital edema are the most common, vary in degree from mild to extremely severe and progressive.

Most patients with hyperthyroidism (regardless of the cause) have retraction of the eyelids (caused by contraction of the eyelid levator palpebrae muscles), which leads to widened palpebral fissures and a stare. Although the stare may give the appearance of proptosis, it must be confirmed with an exophthalmometer (see later text). Frequently, an eyelid lag can be demonstrated. This is a failure of the upper eyelid to maintain its position relative to the globe as the gaze is directed downward. There also may be globe lag—the eyelid moves upward more rapidly than does the globe as the patient looks upward. The eyelid retraction and eyelid lag regress after correction of the hyperthyroidism.

Graves ophthalmopathy includes varying degrees of additional findings such as true proptosis, conjunctival injection, conjunctival edema (chemosis), periorbital edema, weakness of convergence, and palsy of one or more extraocular muscles. Patients often report increased lacrimation (aggravated by bright light, wind, or cold air), a sandy feeling in the eyes, and an uncomfortable sense of fullness in the orbits. When the patient is requested to look in one direction or another, a significant weakness of one or more of the extraocular muscles may be noted. The patient may note blurred vision, or even diplopia on looking either upward or to the side.

If the distance, measured with an exophthalmometer, from the canthus to the front of the cornea exceeds 20 mm in White patients and 22 mm in Black patients, proptosis is present. The proptosis may be asymmetric, and it may be masked by periorbital edema. Testing the eye and the orbital contents for resiliency to pressure is also useful. This is done by applying the fingers to the eyeball over the closed eyelid and attempting to move the eyeball backward. Normally, the eyeball can be pushed back easily and without resistance; in patients with severe ophthalmopathy, however, a significant decrease in resiliency is evident, and in some patients, it is impossible to push the eyeball back at all—a poor prognostic sign of progressive ophthalmopathy. The progression may be so rapid and extensive that the eyelids cannot be closed over the eyes, so that ulcerations of the cornea may result. These ulcerations may become infected and may even lead to loss of the eye. Rarely, the optic nerve may be involved by papilledema, papillitis, or retrobulbar neuritis, causing blindness.

The pathogenesis of Graves ophthalmopathy is related to an increased volume in the retro-orbital space—the extraocular muscles and retroorbital connective and adipose tissues—because of inflammation and the accumulation of hydrophilic glycosaminoglycans (GAGs) (e.g., hyaluronic acid). As GAGs accumulate in these tissues, a change in osmotic pressure and an increase in fluid content displace the globes forward and compromise the function of the extraocular muscles. The extraocular muscles are swollen and infiltrated with T lymphocytes, which appear to be activated by the TSH receptor antigen. There is a positive correlation between the severity of ophthalmopathy and serum TSH receptor antibody concentrations.

In addition to a high titer of TSH receptor antibodies, several other risk factors for the development of ophthalmopathy in patients with Graves disease have been identified. Graves eye disease is more common in

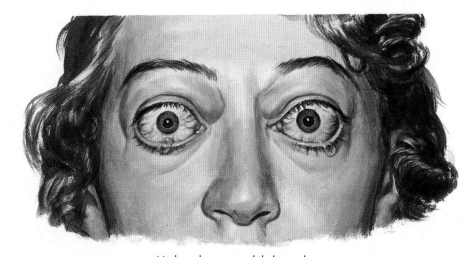

Moderately severe ophthalmopathy

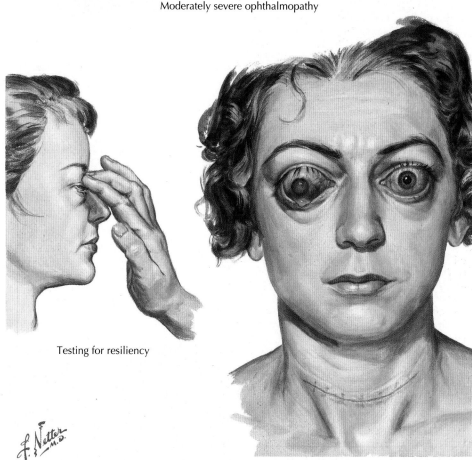

Testing for resiliency

Severe progressive ophthalmopathy

females, as is hyperthyroidism. However, when present, males appear to have more severe ophthalmopathy than females. Cigarette smoking has been clearly shown to increase both the risk for and the severity of ophthalmopathy. Cigarette smoke appears to increase GAG production and adipogenesis. Radioiodine therapy for hyperthyroidism appears to trigger or worsen ophthalmopathy more than subtotal thyroidectomy or antithyroid drug therapy. Although treating hyperthyroidism decreases the eyelid retraction, it does not improve Graves ophthalmopathy. Finally, there is a temporal relationship between the Graves eye disease and the onset of hyperthyroidism. Ophthalmopathy appears before the onset of hyperthyroidism in 20% of patients, concurrently in 40%, when hyperthyroidism is treated in 20%, and in the 6 months after diagnosis in 20%.

Most patients can be successfully treated by raising the head of the bed at night, using saline eye drops frequently through the day, and wearing sunglasses when outside. In patients with more severe symptoms (e.g., chemosis, diplopia), glucocorticoid therapy should be considered. If there is no response to glucocorticoids, additional medical treatment options include insulin-like growth factor 1 receptor inhibitors (e.g., teprotumumab), immunosuppressive agents (e.g., mycophenolate mofetil), anti-interleukin-6 receptor monoclonal antibody (e.g., tocilizumab), and chimeric monoclonal antibody targeted against the CD20 surface antigen on B cells (e.g., rituximab). Orbital decompression surgery should be considered if the ophthalmopathy progresses despite the treatment options listed above, if vision is threatened, or if there is a cosmetic reason in patients with severe proptosis.

Plate 2.11

Endocrine System: VOLUME 2

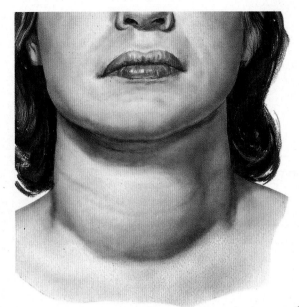

Diffuse goiter of moderate size

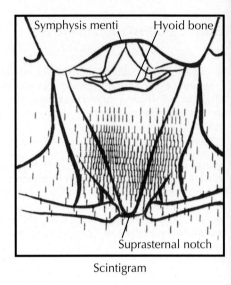

Scintigram

THYROID PATHOLOGY IN GRAVES DISEASE

In patients with Graves disease, the most dramatic anatomic changes are those found in the thyroid gland, although characteristic changes in organs other than the thyroid also occur. The thyroid, which in healthy adults weighs between 15 and 20 g, is usually two to four times its normal size in patients with Graves disease. In extreme situations, it may be as large as 10 times the normal size. Rarely, patients with Graves disease do not have any significant enlargement of the thyroid gland. Diffuse enlargement and engorgement of the thyroid occurs in a more or less symmetric fashion. These features can very well be demonstrated by scintigraphy of the thyroid after the administration of a test dose of radioactive iodine. As shown here, the thyroid gland of such patients concentrate radioactive iodine very diffusely and evenly. Characteristically, the pyramidal lobe, which extends above the isthmus on one or the other side of the trachea, is enlarged enough to be easily palpable. The enlarged thyroid gland is firm, smooth, and rubbery to palpation. Typically, it is very vascular, as evidenced by an audible bruit (which may be heard usually over the superior poles of either lobe) and in some instances by a palpable thrill over the lateral lobes. The untreated thyroid gland, being vascular and friable in this disease, can be a source of serious bleeding during surgery.

Histologic examination of the untreated thyroid reveals a very characteristic microscopic picture of diffuse hyperplasia. Usually, the colloid is completely lost from within the follicle. Any colloid that remains is pale staining and demonstrates marginal scalloping and vacuolization. The thyroid cells are hypertrophied and hyperplastic. The acinar cells, which are normally low cuboidal, become high cuboidal or columnar and, by measurement, may be more than twice as high as those in the normal thyroid gland. In some instances, the hyperplasia of the acinar cells is so great that an intraacinar papillary infolding takes place.

Along with the marked hyperplasia, there is a pronounced increase in avidity for radioactive iodine. Whereas the normal iodine uptake is 3% to 16% at 6 hours and 8% to 25% at 24 hours, in patients with Graves disease, it is nearly always more than 50% and may be as great as 80% or 90%.

In a small number of patients with long-standing Graves disease, hyperplasia is accompanied by significant to extensive lymphocytic infiltration (most are T lymphocytes) of the thyroid parenchyma, occasionally with large lymph follicles being present. The degree of lymphocytic infiltration may be decreased by antithyroid drug therapy. The size of the follicular epithelial cells correlates with the intensity of the local lymphocytic infiltrate, implicating local thyroid cell stimulation by thyrotropin receptor antibodies.

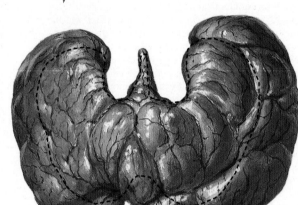

Diffuse enlargement and engorgement of thyroid gland (*broken line* indicates normal size of gland).

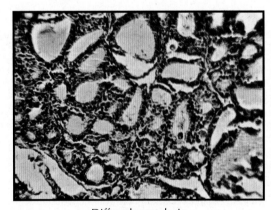

Diffuse hyperplasia

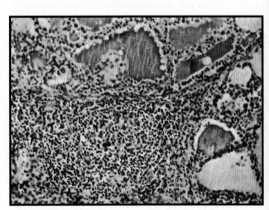

Hyperplasia with lymphocytic infiltration

Other anatomic and functional changes include those in the eyes, skin, skeletal muscles, nervous system, heart, liver, thymus, and lymphoid tissues. The eyes are frequently proptosed; associated with this condition are enlarged, edematous extraocular muscles with increased fluid and fat in the retroorbital space (see Plate 2.10). These muscles and the skeletal muscles show edema, round cell infiltration, hyalinization, fragmentation, and destruction.

Hyperthyroidism can affect the central and peripheral nervous systems—most of these represent direct or indirect effects of thyrotoxicosis. Other nervous system effects are related to the autoimmune nature of Graves disease (e.g., myasthenia gravis). The heart may be somewhat enlarged, but it does not present any characteristic or classic pathologic changes. Characteristically, the thymus and lymphoid tissues are enlarged, displaying simple hypertrophy.

Plate 2.12

Thyroid

CLINICAL MANIFESTATIONS OF TOXIC ADENOMA AND TOXIC MULTINODULAR GOITER

The hyperthyroidism associated with toxic adenomas and toxic multinodular goiters is caused by hyperfunctioning adenoma(s), which are the most common cause of hyperthyroidism after Graves disease. Hyperthyroidism is caused by nodular hyperplasia of thyroid follicular cells that is independent of thyrotropin regulation. The clinical picture of this type of hyperthyroidism differs in important ways from that observed in patients with Graves disease. Patients with adenomatous goiters with hyperthyroidism are usually older than 40 years. They often give a history of having had either a multinodular thyroid or a single nodule in the thyroid for a long time. As a rule, they have cardiovascular symptoms, and frequently they have been referred to a cardiologist before being sent to an endocrinologist. They describe marked shortness of breath and have tachycardia, frequently with atrial fibrillation. When in heart failure, they may manifest all the signs and symptoms of this disease except that they usually do not have an increased circulation time, as in Graves disease. Characteristically, these patients do not have ophthalmopathy. Rarely, one may observe a minimal eyelid retraction or even a minimal eyelid lag. There is no thyroid acropachy or pretibial myxedema. Patients with this type of hyperthyroidism have less of the muscular weakness so characteristic of Graves disease. The basal metabolic rate is not as markedly elevated as it is in Graves disease, and these patients are not especially nervous or excitable. Typically, they do not show signs of marked weight loss or of muscle wasting, both of which are striking in Graves disease. Because a large percentage of female patients who are affected are postmenopausal, changes in the menstrual cycle, often seen in Graves disease, are not present.

The pathogenesis of a toxic adenoma and toxic multinodular goiter is frequently associated with activating somatic mutations in the gene encoding the thyrotropin receptor. Toxic multinodular goiter tends to be more common in geographic areas where iodine intake is relatively low, but the incidence of solitary toxic thyroid adenomas does not seem to be affected by iodine intake.

Patients with this malady have a moderate elevation in serum free T_4 and total T_3 concentrations. The serum total and HDL cholesterol concentrations are slightly decreased.

Studies with radioactive iodine are highly useful in examining these patients, especially if the site of radioactive iodine concentration is localized. Although the uptake of radioactive iodine may not be as great as is observed in classic Graves disease, in this malady, the radioactive iodine is usually concentrated primarily in the hyperfunctioning adenoma, with practically none in the remainder of the thyroid gland. However, in patients with toxic multinodular goiter, typically one or more focal areas of increased radioiodine uptake are found; nonfunctioning (or "cold") nodules are also evident in some of these patients.

Effective treatment of hyperthyroidism is aimed at both symptomatic relief and decreasing the excess production of thyroid hormone. β-Adrenergic blockers control many of the hypermetabolic-type symptoms of hyperthyroidism. The treatment options to normalize T_4 and T_3 excess include thionamide administration, radioiodine administration, or surgery.

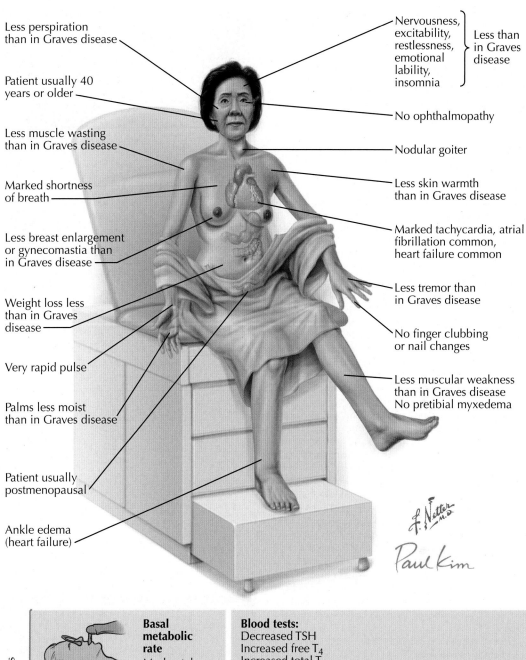

Less perspiration than in Graves disease

Patient usually 40 years or older

Less muscle wasting than in Graves disease

Marked shortness of breath

Less breast enlargement or gynecomastia than in Graves disease

Weight loss less than in Graves disease

Very rapid pulse

Palms less moist than in Graves disease

Patient usually postmenopausal

Ankle edema (heart failure)

Nervousness, excitability, restlessness, emotional lability, insomnia — Less than in Graves disease

No ophthalmopathy

Nodular goiter

Less skin warmth than in Graves disease

Marked tachycardia, atrial fibrillation common, heart failure common

Less tremor than in Graves disease

No finger clubbing or nail changes

Less muscular weakness than in Graves disease
No pretibial myxedema

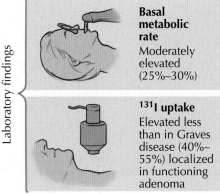

Laboratory findings

Basal metabolic rate
Moderately elevated (25%–30%)

^{131}I uptake
Elevated less than in Graves disease (40%–55%) localized in functioning adenoma

Blood tests:
Decreased TSH
Increased free T_4
Increased total T_3
Undetectable TSH-receptor antibodies
Decreased total and HDL cholesterol
Increased sex hormone–binding globulin
Increased estradiol (in both males and females)
Increased osteocalcin and bone-specific alkaline phosphatase

Thionamides (methimazole and propylthiouracil) are frequently used as the initial treatment of choice in patients who are elderly and have underlying cardiovascular disease. However, unlike Graves hyperthyroidism, which may go into long-term remission after the thionamide is discontinued, hyperthyroidism associated with toxic nodules and toxic multinodular goiters recurs when thionamide therapy is discontinued. The goal of thionamide therapy is to achieve a euthyroid state before definitive therapy (e.g., radioiodine or surgery). Patients who are young and healthy usually do not need thionamide treatment before definitive therapy. A permanent cure can be achieved with radioiodine; it causes extensive tissue damage and destroys the adenoma or autonomous foci within 2 to 4 months after treatment. However, because the radioiodine is taken up primarily by the hyperfunctioning nodules and intervening normal thyroid tissue is quiescent, most patients are euthyroid after radioiodine therapy. Because the cure rate of radioiodine therapy decreases with very large toxic multinodular goiters, surgery is the treatment of choice for this subset of patients.

Plate 2.13

Endocrine System: VOLUME 2

PATHOPHYSIOLOGY OF TOXIC ADENOMA AND TOXIC MULTINODULAR GOITER

Hyperthyroidism arising in a hyperfunctioning adenoma(s) of the thyroid is the second most common cause of hyperthyroidism. This syndrome usually occurs in patients who previously had nontoxic nodular goiters. In the most clear-cut and classic setting, the patient, usually a middle-aged woman, presents with cardiovascular symptoms varying from complaints of palpitation and dyspnea to the picture of chronic atrial fibrillation and frank heart failure. The heart failure of hyperthyroidism exhibits a few characteristic features that should direct the physician to an investigation of the thyroid. Such patients have high-output failure with a decreased circulation time despite an elevated venous pressure. Other extrathyroidal pathology in patients with hyperthyroidism arising from hyperfunctioning adenomas of the thyroid is uncommon. Patients do not develop the typical eye signs, thyroid acropachy, or pretibial myxedema of Graves disease. These patients do not have the muscle weakness so characteristic of Graves disease.

Pathologically, the most classic feature of this disease is that found in the patient with a rare "single" hyperfunctioning adenoma of the thyroid, which may be significantly enlarged, whereas the rest of the thyroid gland remains uninvolved. No palpable nodules are present in the remainder of the gland, which may actually be smaller than normal. In such unique situations, the examiner may be impressed by the small size or the impalpability of the unaffected lobe, as contrasted with the large, single nodule in the opposite lobe. It is extremely uncommon to hear a bruit or to detect a thrill over a hyperfunctioning adenoma of the thyroid. If a test dose of radioactive iodine is administered to the patient and a scintigram is made over the neck at 24 hours, all the radioactive iodine will be found in the nodule, the remainder of the gland having concentrated none.

Grossly, whereas the nodule may be red, the rest of the gland is pale in color.

Histologic examination of the hyperfunctioning adenoma demonstrates a uniform hypertrophy and hyperplasia of the acinar cells. Some papillary infolding may be present, although this is much less common than in the diffusely hyperplastic gland of Graves disease. Lymphocytic infiltration is not found in this type of hyperplastic thyroid lesion. The remainder of the gland shows involution. If the acinar cells are measured, the cell height will be uniformly increased, averaging around 12 to 14 μm, whereas the cell height of the uninvolved tissue may be less than that of a normal thyroid, averaging around 5 to 6 μm.

The toxic adenoma is a true follicular adenoma that has one of several somatic point mutations in the gene encoding the TSH receptor, which lead to constitutive activation of the TSH receptor in the absence of TSH.

The more common type of hyperfunctioning adenomatous goiter, the "multinodular" type, occurs in patients who had a long-standing multinodular goiter before developing hyperthyroidism, with a number of adenomas within the gland. Some of these nodules may be highly undifferentiated adenomas, and, rarely, even a cancerous lesion may be found within one of the

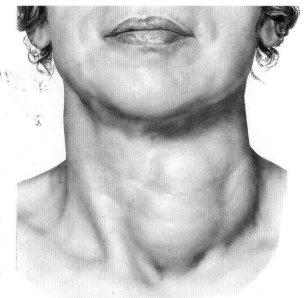

Hyperfunctioning adenoma

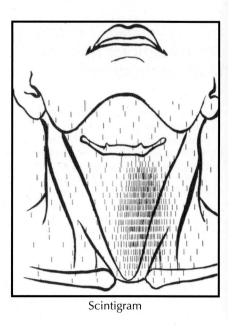

Scintigram

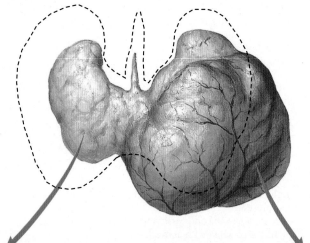

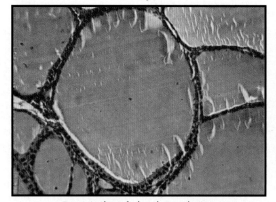

Remainder of gland: involution

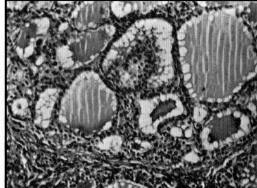

Adenoma: hyperplasia

nodules. If all multinodular thyroids could be examined, it is quite possible that in many of them, the structure of undifferentiated adenomas would be present; others would show varying degrees of differentiation; and a few would exhibit the structure of a well-differentiated, functional adenoma.

The somatic mutations in the TSH receptor gene found in solitary toxic nodules may also be seen in some cases of toxic multinodular goiter but may differ from one nodule to another. Radioiodine scans show localization of isotope in more than one of the nodules; iodine uptake in the rest of the gland is usually suppressed. Histopathologic examination shows that the functioning areas resemble adenomas and are distinct from the surrounding tissue. These multinodular thyroid glands contain multiple solitary hyperfunctioning and hypofunctioning adenomas in the midst of suppressed normal thyroid tissue.

Plate 2.14

Thyroid

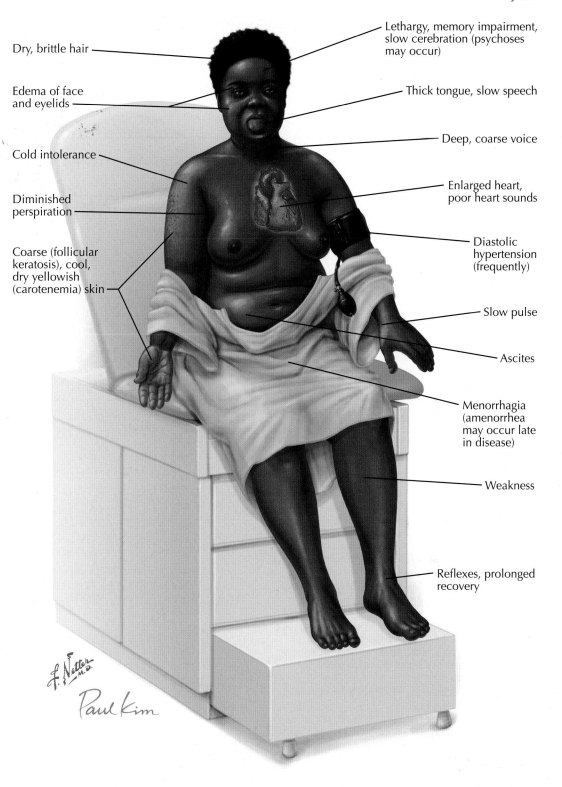

Dry, brittle hair

Edema of face and eyelids

Cold intolerance

Diminished perspiration

Coarse (follicular keratosis), cool, dry yellowish (carotenemia) skin

Lethargy, memory impairment, slow cerebration (psychoses may occur)

Thick tongue, slow speech

Deep, coarse voice

Enlarged heart, poor heart sounds

Diastolic hypertension (frequently)

Slow pulse

Ascites

Menorrhagia (amenorrhea may occur late in disease)

Weakness

Reflexes, prolonged recovery

CLINICAL MANIFESTATIONS OF HYPOTHYROIDISM IN ADULTS

SYMPTOMS AND SIGNS

Primary hypothyroidism, although not described until 1874, is a common endocrine disorder that occurs about seven or eight times more often in females than in males. The clinical presentation of hypothyroidism depends on the degree of thyroid hormone deficiency and the rapidity of the loss of the thyroid hormones, T_4 and T_3. Patients with gradual onset of hypothyroidism may not be diagnosed for many years—patients often attribute the signs and symptoms to aging. In addition, the clinical presentation of hypothyroidism may be affected by coexisting morbidities. For example, in patients with hypothyroidism caused by hypothalamic or pituitary disease, the presentation may be dominated by the signs and symptoms of secondary adrenal failure, hypogonadism, or diabetes insipidus.

The basis of the pathophysiology of hypothyroidism can be thought of as the "slowing down" of most metabolic processes. Patients may be lethargic with slow cerebration, slow speech patterns, cold intolerance, constipation, and bradycardia. These patients typically have dry, brittle hair, which, if previously curly, loses its curl. Individuals with profound hypothyroidism may actually manifest many psychotic features, which have been labeled "myxedema madness." The edema of the face and eyelids (periorbital edema) is associated with the subcutaneous accumulation of GAGs. The tongue is thick, and the voice is deep and coarse, with a relative lack of inflection.

The skin is cool and dry because of diminished perspiration and may be coarse. Often, a sandpapery follicular hyperkeratosis occurs over the extensor surfaces of the arms and elbows, frequently on the lateral thoracic wall and over the lateral thighs, and occasionally over the shoulders. The skin of the hands or face frequently acquires a yellowish color, suggesting carotenemia. The fingernails may be brittle and chip easily. Loss of hair of the lateral third of the eyebrows is frequently observed. Vitiligo and alopecia may be present in patients with autoimmune polyglandular failure.

Patients with hypothyroidism generally have a slow pulse and diastolic hypertension; the latter is associated with increased peripheral vascular resistance. Cardiac output is decreased, and patients may note dyspnea on exertion. A typical feature in patients with marked and long-standing primary hypothyroidism is diffuse cardiac enlargement owing to myxedematous fluid in the myocardium and to pericardial effusions, which may also be associated with pleural effusions and even with ascites. Heart sounds are distant. There is a decreased rate of cholesterol metabolism that leads to hypercholesterolemia.

Respiratory muscle weakness may contribute to dyspnea on exertion. Some of these patients may have hypoxia and hypercapnia. Macroglossia may contribute to obstructive sleep apnea.

Younger female patients may have menorrhagia severe enough to require surgical curettage. Later in the disease, reversible secondary amenorrhea may occur. Hyperprolactinemia and galactorrhea may be seen in females with primary hypothyroidism, in whom increased hypothalamic TRH secretion can stimulate prolactin release from pituitary lactotrophs.

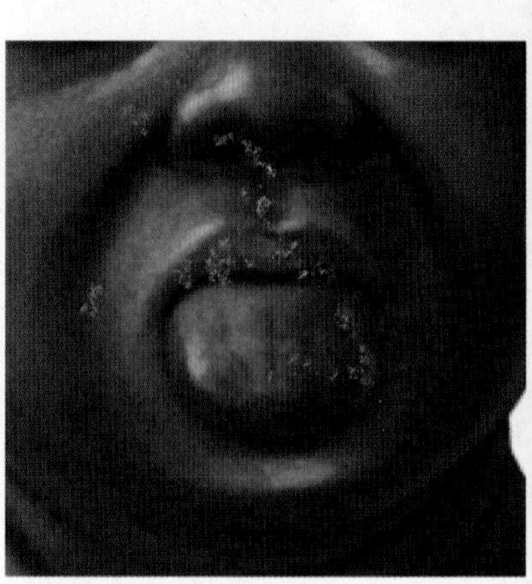

Plate 2.15

Endocrine System: VOLUME 2

Macroglossia, showing dental impressions

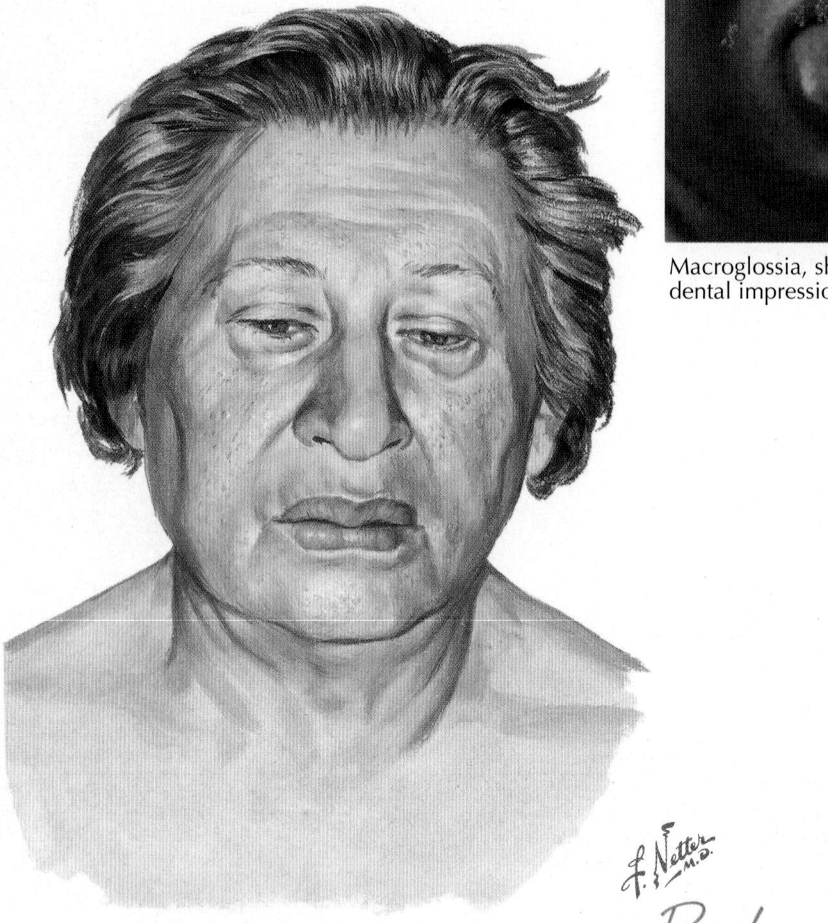

CLINICAL MANIFESTATIONS OF HYPOTHYROIDISM IN ADULTS (Continued)

Neurologic findings include a prolonged relaxation phase of the ankle jerk reflex and generalized weakness. Carpal tunnel syndrome is fairly common in these patients. Myxedema coma—a rare complication—should be considered in patients who have hyponatremia, hypercapnia, and hypothermia. Myxedema coma may be triggered in patients with severe hypothyroidism by the administration of opiates or by infection or trauma.

Hypochromic anemia, if present, may be of any type—microcytic or normocytic. Occasionally, normochromic macrocytic anemia is found. If the patient has polyglandular failure, pernicious anemia may be present. The menorrhagia seen in hypothyroid premenopausal females may lead to iron-deficiency anemia. Decreased free water clearance may result in hyponatremia.

Primary hypothyroidism (resulting from disease of the thyroid gland itself) must be distinguished from central hypothyroidism (resulting from disease of the pituitary gland or hypothalamus). Some signs and symptoms may provide clues as to the cause of hypothyroidism. The history of patients with the latter disease often includes severe postpartum hemorrhage followed by absence of lactation and failure of the menstrual cycle to return after recovery from the postpartum period. Usually, the picture of myxedema does not develop until some time after the first sign of pituitary insufficiency (e.g., amenorrhea without hot flushes). These individuals usually describe extreme weakness, somnolence, intolerance to the cold, impaired memory, and slow cerebration. On physical examination, they differ from patients with primary hypothyroidism if they lack other pituitary hormones. Thus patients with central hypothyroidism may also have finer, softer hair; loss of axillary and pubic hair; a small heart (in contrast to the enlarged heart of patients with primary myxedema); some degree of hypotension; and skin that is less dry and not scaly.

Characteristic facies in hypothyroidism: coarse features; thick lips; dry skin; puffy eyelids; dull, lethargic expression; coarse hair

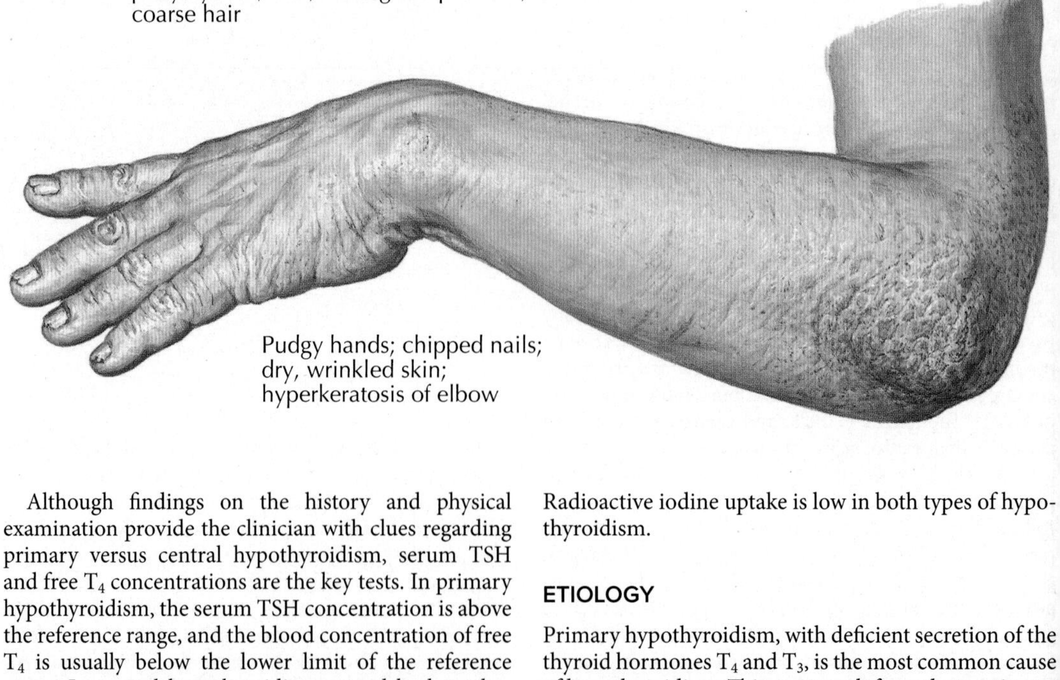

Pudgy hands; chipped nails; dry, wrinkled skin; hyperkeratosis of elbow

Although findings on the history and physical examination provide the clinician with clues regarding primary versus central hypothyroidism, serum TSH and free T_4 concentrations are the key tests. In primary hypothyroidism, the serum TSH concentration is above the reference range, and the blood concentration of free T_4 is usually below the lower limit of the reference range. In central hypothyroidism caused by hypothalamic or pituitary dysfunction, the serum TSH concentration is inappropriately low for the low level of free T_4.

Radioactive iodine uptake is low in both types of hypothyroidism.

ETIOLOGY

Primary hypothyroidism, with deficient secretion of the thyroid hormones T_4 and T_3, is the most common cause of hypothyroidism. This may result from destruction or removal of the thyroid gland or from thyroid gland atrophy and subsequent replacement by fibrous tissue.

Plate 2.16

Thyroid

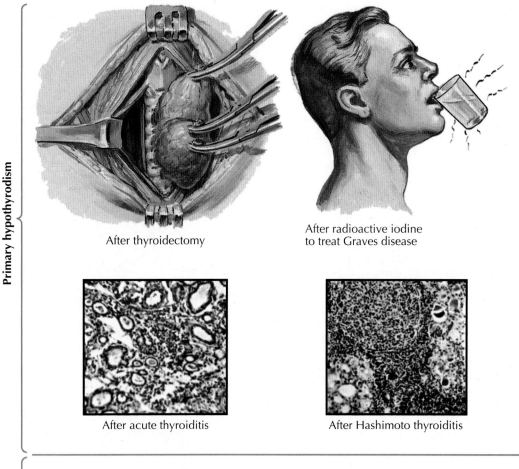

Primary hypothyroidism

After thyroidectomy

After radioactive iodine
to treat Graves disease

After acute thyroiditis

After Hashimoto thyroiditis

CLINICAL MANIFESTATIONS OF HYPOTHYROIDISM IN ADULTS (Continued)

Primary hypothyroidism may also develop with goiters, which are incapable of synthesizing thyroid hormone either because of the administration of some agent that inhibits the organification of iodine or because of some defect in the enzymes necessary for the synthesis of thyroid hormone. It may also result from autoimmune chronic thyroiditis, such as Hashimoto thyroiditis. Central hypothyroidism is caused by a process that inhibits release of TSH-releasing hormone from the hypothalamus or TSH release from the pituitary.

The most common cause of primary hypothyroidism is Hashimoto thyroiditis. The second most common cause is iatrogenic. For example, most patients who have undergone thyroidectomy in the treatment of nontoxic goiter or of Graves disease develop primary hypothyroidism. The most common treatment of Graves disease is radioactive iodine with the goals of total thyroid gland destruction and primary hypothyroidism.

Hashimoto thyroiditis is the most common spontaneous cause of primary hypothyroidism. Transient primary hypothyroidism may develop after subacute and acute thyroiditis (see Plate 2.22). A high serum TPO antibody concentration is consistent with Hashimoto thyroiditis.

Central hypothyroidism is the result of a variety of processes that affect the anterior pituitary gland, resulting in loss of TSH secretion. TSH deficiency may occur in isolation (e.g., with lymphocytic hypophysitis) or, more commonly, as part of complete anterior pituitary failure. Complete anterior pituitary failure may be the result of inflammation, infarction (e.g., postpartum apoplexy), primary neoplasms, metastatic disease, infiltrative disorders (e.g., sarcoidosis, Langerhans cell histiocytosis, hemochromatosis); surgery, head trauma, or radiation therapy (see Plates 1.12–1.18). Pituitary-directed head magnetic resonance imaging (MRI) is indicated in these patients to assist in differentiating among these multiple causes.

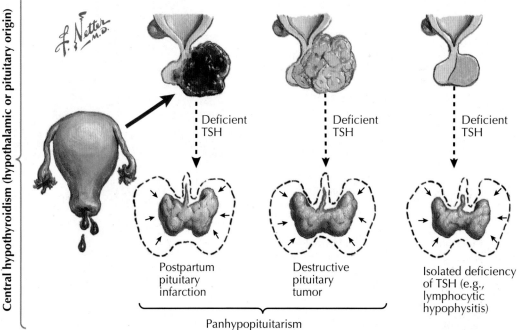

Central hypothyroidism (hypothalamic or pituitary origin)

Deficient TSH

Deficient TSH

Deficient TSH

Postpartum pituitary infarction

Destructive pituitary tumor

Isolated deficiency of TSH (e.g., lymphocytic hypophysitis)

Panhypopituitarism

TREATMENT

Whether primary or secondary in etiology, the treatment of hypothyroidism is daily levothyroxine administered orally. In patients with primary hypothyroidism, the serum TSH concentration is measured to guide the adjustment of the levothyroxine dosage; the goal is a TSH concentration in the middle of the reference range. In patients with central hypothyroidism, blood TSH measurement is useless, and the levothyroxine dosage is adjusted to a free T_4 concentration in the middle of the reference range. However, before starting levothyroxine therapy in patients with central hypothyroidism, it is essential to assess the hypothalamic-pituitary-adrenal axis. If levothyroxine, which can accelerate cortisol metabolism, is administered to a patient with concomitant untreated adrenal insufficiency, it may precipitate an adrenal crisis.

Plate 2.17

Endocrine System: VOLUME 2

CONGENITAL HYPOTHYROIDISM

Congenital hypothyroidism is the most common cause of intellectual disability that can be prevented and treated. The intelligence quotient later in life is inversely related to the age at the time of diagnosis; thus identifying congenital hypothyroidism as soon as possible after birth is critical. The most common cause is thyroid dysgenesis, including congenital absence (agenesis) of the thyroid gland itself, thyroid hypoplasia, or thyroid gland ectopy. Less commonly, congenital hypothyroidism is associated with nonfunctioning goiters or with goiters that have inborn errors of thyroid hormone biosynthesis (goitrous hypothyroidism). The synthetic defects are usually inherited in an autosomal recessive pattern and include deficits in impaired TPO activity, abnormal iodide transport, iodotyrosine deiodinase deficiency, and abnormal Tg molecules. This malady occurs most frequently in endemic goiter regions, but goitrous congenital hypothyroidism has been observed in areas where goiters are quite uncommon.

Central (hypothalamic or pituitary) hypothyroidism is a much less common cause of congenital hypothyroidism (1 in 100,000 infants) and can be detected only by measuring the serum T_4 concentration. When present, it may occur in the setting of other midline developmental disorders (e.g., cleft lip and palate, septooptic dysplasia) and be associated with other anterior pituitary gland hormone deficiencies.

The physical stigmata of congenital hypothyroidism may be mild or absent at the time of birth because some maternal T_4 crosses the placenta. Congenital hypothyroidism is sporadic more than 85% of the time and is thus unsuspected. In the mid-1970s, statewide newborn screening programs in the United States were developed. These programs measure either TSH, T_4, or both in blood samples collected by heel stick on filter paper cards 24 to 48 hours after delivery. On the basis of these data, the incidence of elevated TSH levels varies from 1 in 2000 to 1 in 32,000 infants; the variance depends on geographic location and ethnicity. The frequency of congenital hypothyroidism is approximately twofold higher in baby girls. Rapid institution of thyroid hormone replacement therapy can prevent subsequent irreversible disabilities.

When untreated, congenital hypothyroidism in infants has similar features to those seen in adults with hypothyroidism, but there are some important differences. There is a failure of skeletal growth and maturation and a marked disability and deficiency in intellect. The development of centers of ossification is markedly delayed, and the epiphyses show a characteristic stippling. Delayed ossification of bone, of epiphysial union, and of dentition is observed. The skull base is usually short; there may be persistence of the cartilaginous junctions between the presphenoid and postsphenoid bones, which normally ossify in the eighth month of fetal life. Furthermore, because of a delay in ossification of the membranous bones, the frontal suture is usually wide, and the anterior fontanels are exceptionally large.

The face of a child with untreated congenital hypothyroidism is round, with a dull expression and yellowish color. The eyelids are puffy, and the palpebral fissures are generally narrowed but horizontal. The nose is frequently flat and thick, the lips are thick, the mouth remains open, and a large, thick tongue protrudes. The voice is flat and harsh. The neck is usually short and thick. The skin is dry and cool and presents a picture of nonpitting edema. There is usually marked hyperkeratosis in the skin over the anterior abdominal wall. The hair is fine, lifeless, dry, and often quite sparse. Juvenile patients with untreated congenital hypothyroidism may also have a marked growth of fine, short hair, of a lanugo type, over the shoulders, upper arms, and face.

The physical features of children with congenital hypothyroidism may be confused with the features observed in trisomy 21. Persons with trisomy 21 have finer features, absent coarse skin, slanted eyes, a palmar crease, and excessive extensor flexibility of the fingers arc. On laboratory evaluation, infants with trisomy 21 have normal blood concentrations of TSH and T_4.

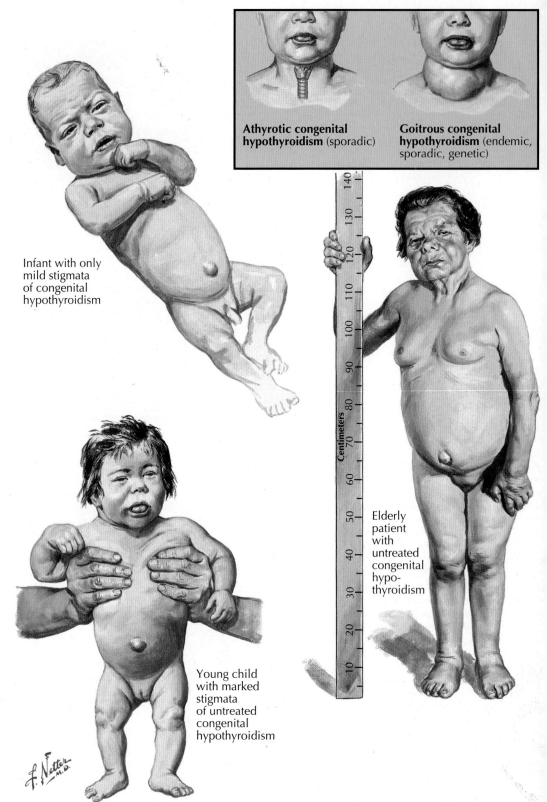

Athyrotic congenital hypothyroidism (sporadic)

Goitrous congenital hypothyroidism (endemic, sporadic, genetic)

Infant with only mild stigmata of congenital hypothyroidism

Young child with marked stigmata of untreated congenital hypothyroidism

Elderly patient with untreated congenital hypothyroidism

Plate 2.18

Thyroid

EUTHYROID GOITER

Euthyroid (nontoxic) goiters occur throughout the world, although they are more common in areas where the iodine content in the water and soil is low. In iodine-deficient goiters, there is characteristic enlargement of the thyroid with a moderate-sized, nontoxic, diffuse goiter that occurs in both boys and girls at about the time of puberty. Such goiters are diffuse in the early stage; later, they may become nodular, feeling hard in one area or cystic in another. Nodular goiters may be more or less symmetric or quite asymmetric. Such a goiter, if allowed to progress, may descend beneath the sternum and produce the picture of an intrathoracic goiter. With the increase in goiter size, especially if some of it is lodged beneath the sternum, obstructive symptoms may result from distortion of the trachea, esophagus, nerves, or jugular veins. This may occur because the thoracic inlet is a small area (~5 × 10 cm) that has bony boundaries—first ribs laterally, first thoracic vertebral body posteriorly, and manubrial and sternal bones anteriorly. Typically, these multinodular goiters grow very slowly, and the development of early obstructive symptoms can be quite insidious. Dyspnea on exertion may be the first symptom related to a substernal goiter. With advancing tracheal compression, stridor may become evident. Other thoracic inset compressive symptoms include dysphagia, vocal cord palsy from recurrent laryngeal nerve compression, and Horner syndrome from compression of the cervical sympathetic chain. On physical examination, the Pemberton maneuver may be used to detect thoracic inlet obstruction. The patient is asked to hold the arms straight up vertically for 1 minute; if the patient develops marked facial plethora, cyanosis, or stridor, the result is considered positive for thoracic inlet obstruction.

Occasionally, a nodular goiter may enlarge in one area very suddenly, producing pain that may be referred to the ear, neck structures, or shoulder. This is frequently explained on the basis of a hemorrhage into a follicle or into an adenoma or a large cyst in the thyroid.

In such multinodular goiters, adenomas of various types may be observed, and these may present various kinds of histologic structures. Some may be capable of function and may develop hyperfunction, resulting in a clinical picture of hyperthyroidism in an adenomatous goiter, a so-called hot nodule (see Plates 2.12 and 2.13). Cancer is much less common in these multinodular goiters than in thyroids with a single nodule. However, the fact that the goiter is multinodular does not rule out the possibility of cancer developing or being found in it.

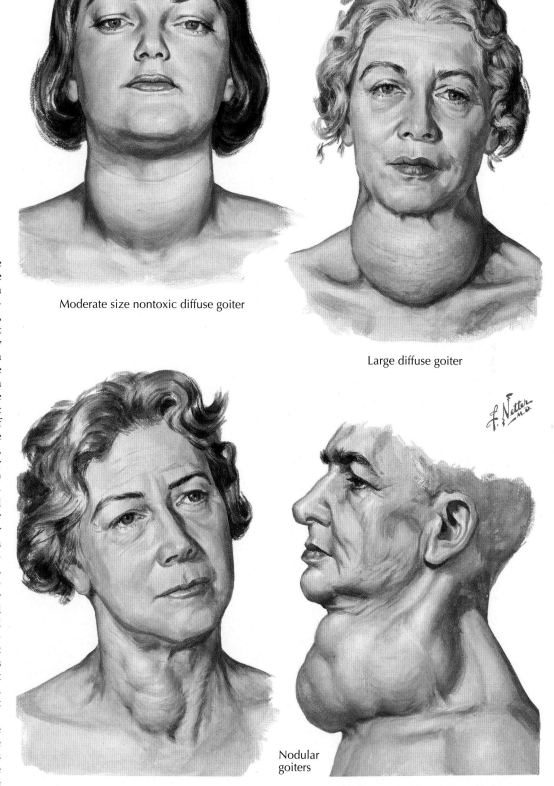

Moderate size nontoxic diffuse goiter

Large diffuse goiter

Nodular goiters

Hyperthyroidism should be excluded by measuring the serum thyrotropin concentration. Thyroid ultrasonography is helpful in assessing the structure of the suprasternal component of a multinodular goiter. If needed, the extent of substernal goiters can be determined with either computed tomography (CT) or MRI. If prominent nodules are present, the underlying pathophysiology can be assessed with ultrasound-guided fine-needle aspiration (FNA) biopsy.

The indications for surgical removal of such thyroids may fall into several categories: (1) cosmetic reasons that may impel the patient to seek surgical removal of the gland; (2) sudden enlargement of the gland, especially if the site of rapid growth is hard, suggesting a neoplastic change; and (3) most importantly, to correct any obstructive symptoms produced by the impingement of such a large mass on either the trachea or the esophagus.

Plate 2.19

Endocrine System: VOLUME 2

GROSS PATHOLOGY OF GOITER

The term *goiter* refers to an enlargement of the thyroid gland. In general, the prevalence of goiter depends on the dietary iodine intake. Thus goiters may be endemic in geographic areas of iodine deficiency. Early in the development of a nontoxic goiter, the gland is usually diffusely and uniformly enlarged, with an increase in the size of the pyramidal lobe. This is known as a *diffuse nontoxic*, or *colloid*, *goiter*. Nontoxic goiters are eight-fold more common in females and frequently become evident in adolescence or pregnancy. Such glands may be two to three times the normal size or even larger. The patient may become aware of the condition because others have commented on the fullness of the neck, because shirt collars may feel too tight, or because it may become difficult to swallow. Large goiters may compress the trachea and result in stridor. Venous engorgement from narrowing of the thoracic inlet may occur. Most simple and multinodular goiters are associated with a euthyroid state.

On physical examination, the gland feels firm but not hard. As the process progresses, with the advancing age of the patient the thyroid may become asymmetric and multinodular, which is evident on gross examination of the gland. Significant variations in the size and structure of the nodules become apparent. In very long-standing nodular goiters, hemorrhages into various sites in the gland, cyst formation, fibrosis, and even calcification are likely to be observed. On chest radiographs, asymmetric goiters typically cause lateral displacement of the trachea; in addition, any retrosternal extension of such a goiter may, if calcified, initially simulate intrapulmonary calcifications.

The cut surface of a colloid goiter shows a uniform amber color with a translucent appearance. Colloid goiters may weigh anywhere from 40 to 1000 g or more. The thyroid gland is distorted in shape and nodular, with some nodules partially or completely separated from the gland. The gross pathology appearance on cut section typically shows areas of nodularity, fibrosis, hemorrhage, and calcification. Some nodules may show cystic change, and some may have a thickened fibrous connective tissue capsule and have the general appearance of a follicular neoplasm.

Cytologic examination from FNA biopsy of colloid nodules typically shows colloid and mixed cell populations with relatively few cells in the aspirate. The types of cells usually seen on cytologic examination include follicular cells with uniform nuclei, inflammatory cells, and Hürthle cells. Hypercellular foci within a multinodular goiter may simulate a follicular neoplasm.

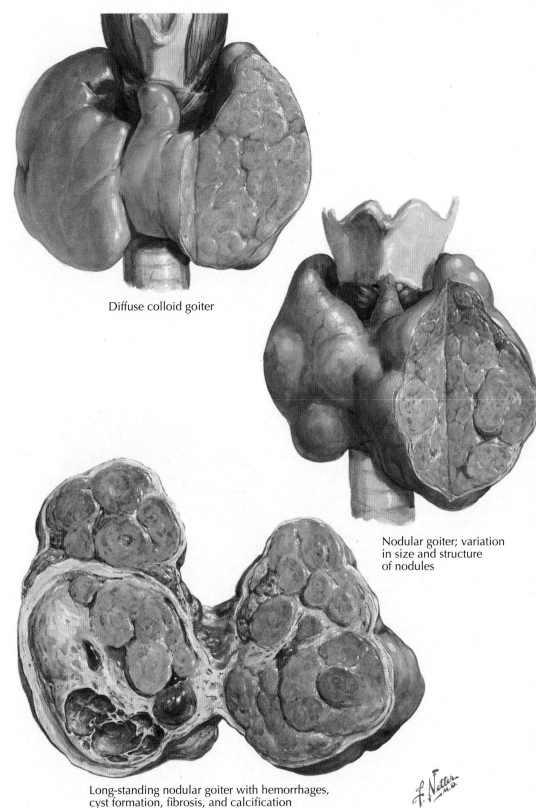

Diffuse colloid goiter

Nodular goiter; variation in size and structure of nodules

Long-standing nodular goiter with hemorrhages, cyst formation, fibrosis, and calcification

Microscopic examination of the colloid nodular goiter may reveal every conceivable type of benign adenoma, including a highly undifferentiated trabecular pattern or the earliest stage of differentiation of tubular structure, the structure of microfollicles, or the picture of a hyperplastic adenoma. The follicles—usually lined by flattened epithelium with involutional changes—can be of varying size and as large as 2 mm in diameter. Large, distended follicles may coalesce to create cystic areas.

Rarely, within these nodules may be seen various types of cancerous growths, such as differentiated thyroid carcinomas (papillary and follicular). However, the cancerous changes in such thyroids are much less common than they are in those of patients presenting with a single nodule in the thyroid. Thoracic inlet obstructive symptoms represent the most important indication for therapeutic intervention, but the rare occurrence of a small malignancy must always be kept in mind.

Plate 2.20

Thyroid

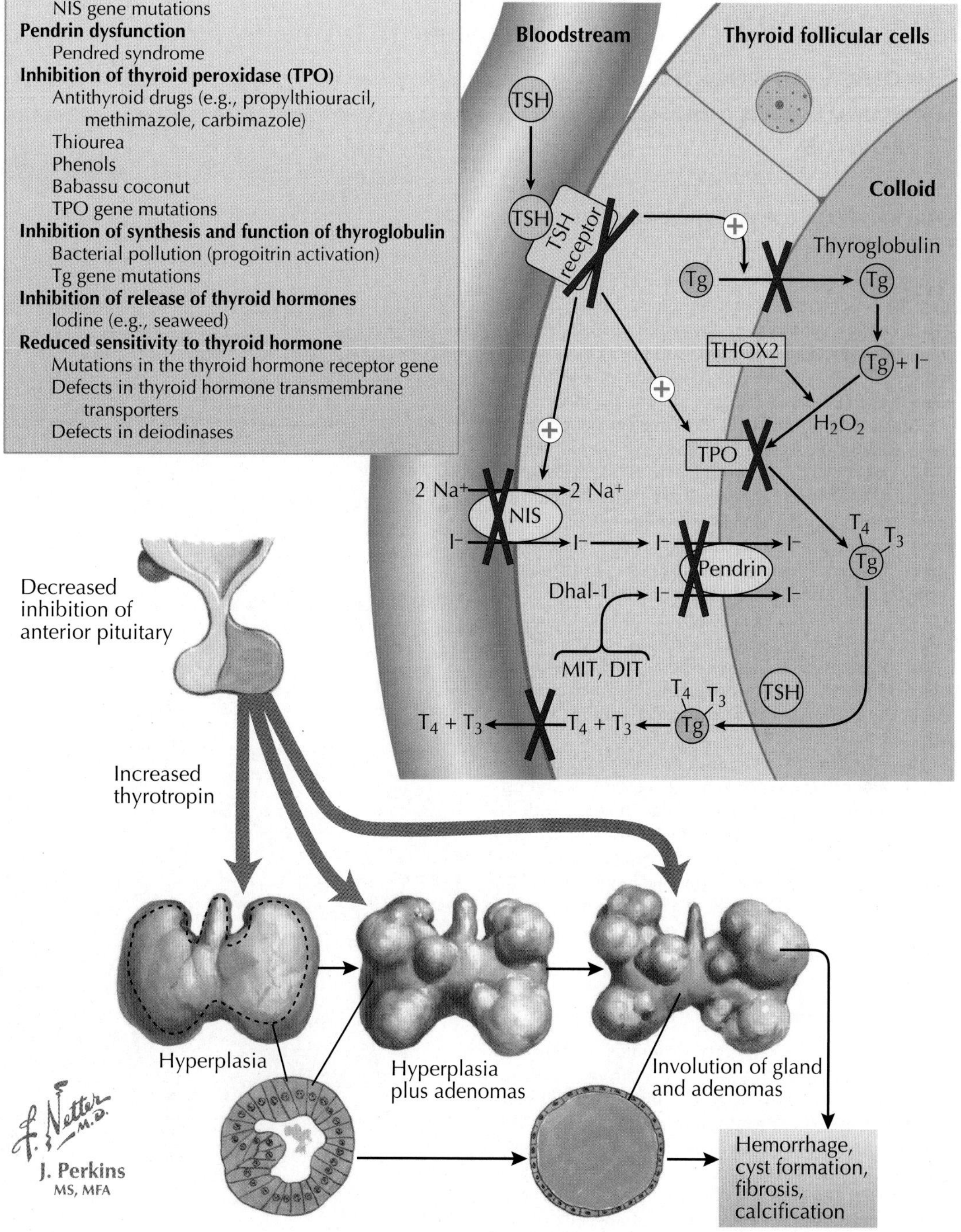

ETIOLOGY OF NONTOXIC GOITER

The development of nontoxic goiter—thyroid enlargement (diffuse or nodular) that is not associated with overt hyperthyroidism or hypothyroidism or caused by neoplasia or inflammation—can usually be attributed to a genetic or environmental factor that leads to deficiency in thyroid hormone secretion, to which the pituitary responds with an increased output of TSH. For example, iodine deficiency may result in decreased thyroid gland production of T_4 and T_3, resulting in increased TSH secretion that in turn promotes thyroid gland growth. Iodine deficiencies are usually related to geographic areas where the soil and water lack iodine, especially in mountainous and formerly glaciated regions. Approximately 1 billion people live in iodine-deficient regions of the world and are at risk for endemic goiter. Plasma iodide is replenished in part by iodide liberated through deiodination of iodothyronines in peripheral tissues. Ultimately, however, the diet is the most important source. The thyroid requires 75 μg of iodine daily; in North America, the daily dietary intake of iodine ranges between 150 and 300 μg. The use of iodized table salt in North America has markedly reduced the incidence of iodine deficiency goiter. Thus the impairment of, or interference with, the synthesis of thyroid hormone is the most common cause of goiter in the United States.

A growing number of clinical entities are recognized in which congenital deficiencies of a step necessary to the intrathyroidal metabolism of iodine or to the synthesis of thyroid hormone explain the congenital hypothyroidism and the development of nontoxic goiters. For example, a number of families that have goiter with congenital hypothyroidism have now been identified in which various mutations in the NIS gene and an iodide transport defect are evident. Mutations in the genes responsible for the synthesis of Tg, TPO, and the TSH receptor may all lead to nontoxic goiters. However, predisposing gene mutations are not found in most patients with nontoxic goiter.

Pendred syndrome is the association of impaired thyroid hormone synthesis and sensorineural hearing loss. Pendrin, the protein critical to iodide transport into the lumen of the thyroid follicular cell, is also required for ion and fluid transport in the cochlear apparatus.

Congenital defects in organification of thyroid hormone lead to goiter. For example, congenital absence of TPO or inadequate production of hydrogen peroxide by THOX2 is goitrogenic.

Patients with reduced sensitivity to thyroid hormone may have mutations in the gene encoding the thyroid

hormone receptor (thyroid hormone resistance, which is usually caused by mutations in the T_3-binding domain in the thyroid receptor β gene), or defects in thyroid hormone transmembrane transporters, or deiodinases responsible for intracellular activation of T_4 to T_3. Patients with thyroid hormone resistance typically present with a nontoxic goiter, are clinically euthyroid, and have serum T_4 to T_3 concentrations above the reference range.

After a prolonged period of thyroid hyperplasia, incompletely encapsulated nodules of various types develop within the hyperplastic thyroid. Finally, after a period of extreme hyperplasia, exhaustion or involution occurs. The epithelium becomes flat, the follicles fill with a viscous colloid, and, eventually, hemorrhagic cysts may occur, some becoming calcified or fibrosed. Rarely, carcinoma may form within such a hyperplastic gland.

Etiologic factors of nontoxic goiter:
Iodine deficiency
  Nutritional
Thyrotropin (TSH) receptor dysfunction
  TSH receptor mutations
Block of sodium-iodide symporter (NIS)
  Iodine
  Thiocyanate (e.g., millet, cassava)
  Perchlorate
  NIS gene mutations
Pendrin dysfunction
  Pendred syndrome
Inhibition of thyroid peroxidase (TPO)
  Antithyroid drugs (e.g., propylthiouracil,
    methimazole, carbimazole)
  Thiourea
  Phenols
  Babassu coconut
  TPO gene mutations
Inhibition of synthesis and function of thyroglobulin
  Bacterial pollution (progoitrin activation)
  Tg gene mutations
Inhibition of release of thyroid hormones
  Iodine (e.g., seaweed)
Reduced sensitivity to thyroid hormone
  Mutations in the thyroid hormone receptor gene
  Defects in thyroid hormone transmembrane
    transporters
  Defects in deiodinases

Plate 2.21

Endocrine System: VOLUME 2

CHRONIC LYMPHOCYTIC THYROIDITIS AND FIBROUS THYROIDITIS

CHRONIC LYMPHOCYTIC (HASHIMOTO) THYROIDITIS

In iodine-replete regions of the world, Hashimoto thyroiditis is the most common cause of primary hypothyroidism. It is a chronic autoimmune thyroiditis characterized by circulating antibodies to thyroid antigens (TPO and Tg) and by diffuse lymphocytic infiltration of the thyroid gland. As with other endocrine autoimmune disorders, it is more common in females (8:1 female:male ratio) and has a genetic predisposition. Although thyroid reserve allows for normal thyroid hormone levels for many years, gradual loss of function occurs, and patients eventually progress from subclinical to overt hypothyroidism. Hashimoto thyroiditis becomes clinically evident most commonly between 20 and 40 years of age. On pathology, these thyroid glands demonstrate marked lymphocytic infiltration (both T and B cells), destruction of thyroid follicles, and lymphoid germinal centers.

On physical examination, most patients who are affected have an asymptomatic, firm, symmetric goiter; the borders are scalloped with pseudopodia, and the surface is bosselated.

After Hashimoto thyroiditis has been documented with increased serum TPO and Tg antibodies, and primary hypothyroidism has been documented with an increased serum thyrotropin concentration, patients with Hashimoto thyroiditis are simply treated with levothyroxine replacement. Thyroid biopsy is usually not needed to confirm the diagnosis of Hashimoto thyroiditis. Surgery is rarely needed except, for example, in patients with symptomatic large goiters.

FIBROUS (RIEDEL) THYROIDITIS

Riedel thyroiditis, or fibrous thyroiditis, is rare and occurs predominantly in males. It is a chronic, proliferative, invasive, and fibrosing process involving the thyroid gland. It may extend to displace and/or compress the trachea and esophagus and the overlying fasciae and muscles. Although the cause of Riedel thyroiditis is unknown, it is a primary fibrosing disorder, and some patients may also have retroperitoneal and mediastinal fibrosis. Riedel thyroiditis may occur within the spectrum of immunoglobulin G4-related systemic disease.

Microscopically, this disease is characterized by a marked diffuse fibrosis, with macrophage and eosinophilic infiltration of the thyroid gland. A woodlike, hard texture is characteristic. The unaffected portions of the gland reveal varying numbers of persistent acini, which appear to be compressed by the surrounding dense, fibrous stroma.

On physical examination, Riedel thyroiditis is characterized by a stony-hard, enlarged thyroid gland, which is firmly adherent to adjacent structures but not

Hashimoto thyroiditis

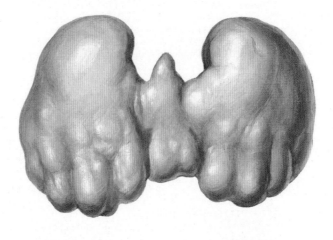

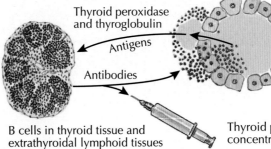

Thyroid peroxidase and thyroglobulin

Antigens

Antibodies

B cells in thyroid tissue and extrathyroidal lymphoid tissues

Thyroid peroxidase and thyroglobulin antibody concentrations can be measured in serum.

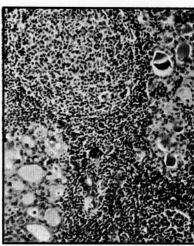

Microscopy of Hashimoto thyroiditis. Mixture of hyperplastic and atrophic follicles with diffuse lymphocytic infiltration.

Riedel thyroiditis

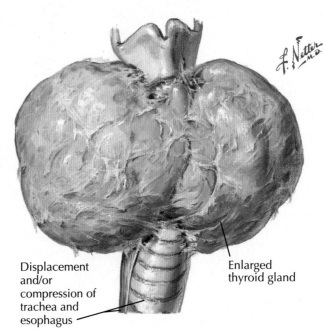

Displacement and/or compression of trachea and esophagus

Enlarged thyroid gland

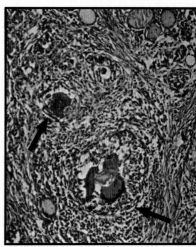

Microscopy of Riedel thyroiditis. Macrophage and eosinophilic infiltration with atrophy of follicles (*arrows*) and marked diffuse fibrosis.

to the skin. Often, the gland may be asymmetric, with greater enlargement of one side.

Subjectively, patients with Riedel thyroiditis may describe neck pressure and tightness, dysphagia, and hoarseness. Just as with Hashimoto thyroiditis, antibodies to TPO and Tg may be increased. However, frequently these patients are clinically euthyroid, and the serum TSH concentration may be normal. When

suspected on physical examination, the diagnosis of Riedel thyroiditis is confirmed by thyroid biopsy.

Treatment with glucocorticoids or tamoxifen may stop the progression or help resolve the advancing fibrotic process. Rituximab and mycophenolate mofetil are additional agents that may be tried if glucocorticoids and tamoxifen are ineffective. Surgery may be required for advancing symptomatic tracheal compression.

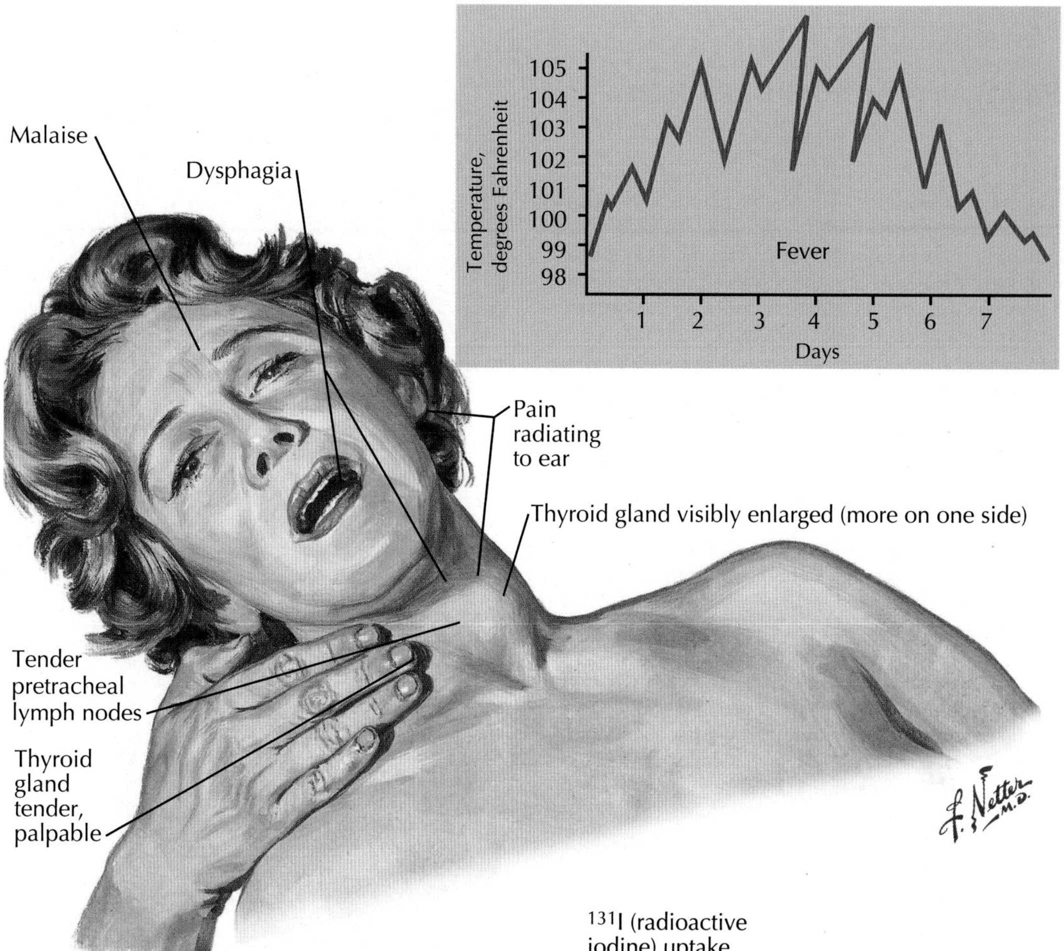

Plate 2.22

Thyroid

Malaise

Dysphagia

Pain radiating to ear

Thyroid gland visibly enlarged (more on one side)

Tender pretracheal lymph nodes

Thyroid gland tender, palpable

Temperature, degrees Fahrenheit

105 104 103 102 101 100 99 98

Fever

1 2 3 4 5 6 7

Days

SUBACUTE THYROIDITIS

Subacute thyroiditis—also known as *subacute granulomatous thyroiditis*, *acute nonsuppurative thyroiditis*, or *de Quervain thyroiditis*—is characterized by an abrupt onset of hyperthyroid-related symptoms: fever, fatigue, myalgias, and a very tender enlargement of the thyroid gland. It is an uncommon disorder that is five times more frequent in females than in males. The thyroid gland enlargement is usually asymmetric, and it may be 1.5- to 2-fold times its normal size. The thyroid gland pain may be referred to the mandibular joints or to the ears. A marked tenderness in the thyroid, even in lymph nodes near the gland, is evident, and the patient may report dysphagia.

The cause of this disease appears to be related to viral infections; most patients have a recent history of an upper respiratory infection. The insult results in thyroid gland inflammation, follicular damage, and the release of stored T_4 and T_3, causing symptomatic hyperthyroidism followed by a hypothyroid phase. The hyperthyroidism persists until the thyroid gland stores are exhausted; the typical duration is 2 to 8 weeks. As the thyroid gland inflammation resolves, the thyroid follicles regenerate, and eventually normal thyroid function returns.

On physical examination, the thyroid gland is symmetrically enlarged and is exquisitely tender to palpation. Some patients refuse to have their neck palpated.

If a thyroid biopsy is performed, an inflammatory reaction is seen with infiltration with lymphocytes and neutrophils. Necrosis of thyroid follicular cells and disruption of thyroid follicles are seen within various parts of the specimen.

Laboratory studies demonstrate increased serum concentrations of free T_4, total T_3, and Tg and low levels of TSH. The erythrocyte sedimentation rate (ESR) is usually greater than 50 mm/h, and leukocytosis may also be present. If an ^{131}I uptake scan is performed, these inflamed thyroid glands do not concentrate significant amounts of iodine—the 24-hour uptake is usually only 1% to 2%. The combination of a low ^{131}I

$\uparrow T_4$
$\uparrow T_3$
$\uparrow$ Thyroglobulin

^{131}I (radioactive iodine) uptake very low

Block by inflammation

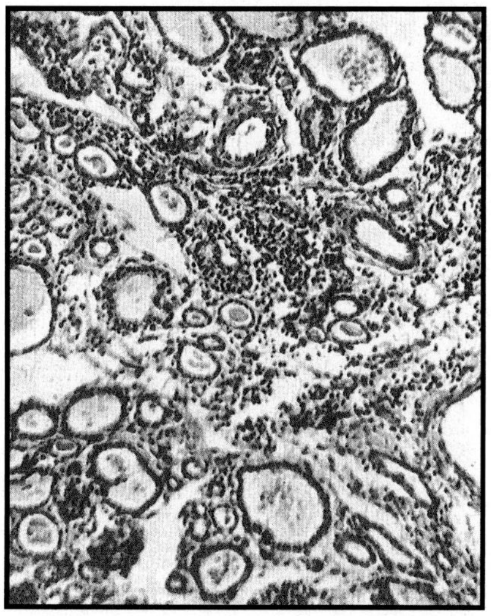

Diffuse infiltration of thyroid stroma

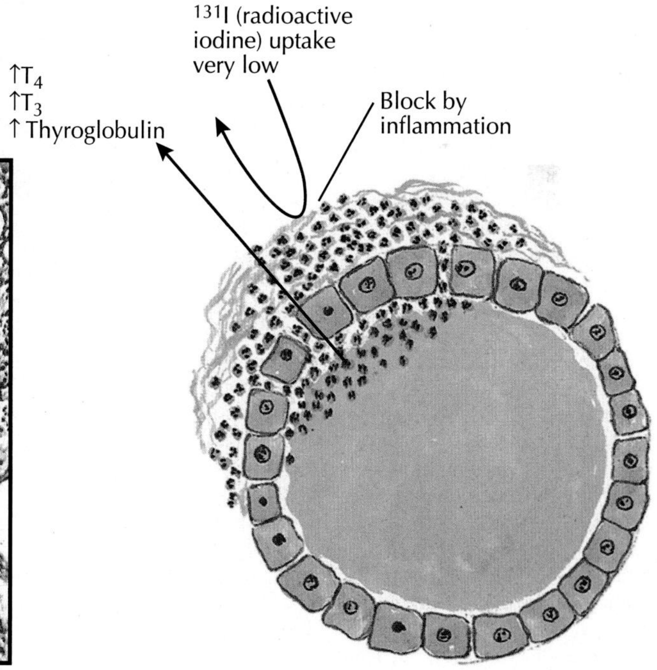

uptake, normal or increased blood T_4 and T_3 concentrations, increased blood Tg concentration, suppressed TSH, and increased ESR are diagnostic of subacute thyroiditis. Silent and postpartum thyroiditis have similar findings, except that neck pain and an increased ESR are absent.

Treatment should focus on pain control and treatment of hyperthyroid symptomatology. Typically, management includes a 2- to 8-week course of either a

nonsteroidal antiinflammatory drug or glucocorticoids. The hyperthyroid symptoms (e.g., tremor, anxiety, palpitations) can be treated with a β-adrenergic blocker.

After the hyperthyroid phase resolves, the hypothyroid phase may be subclinical, or patients may have hypothyroid symptoms. For patients who are symptomatic, treatment with levothyroxine may be prescribed for 6 to 8 weeks. Thyroid function eventually returns to normal.

Plate 2.23

Endocrine System: VOLUME 2

Papillary Thyroid Carcinoma

Papillary thyroid carcinoma (PTC) is one of the four thyroid epithelial-derived thyroid cancers (follicular thyroid carcinoma [FTC], oncocytic thyroid carcinoma, and anaplastic thyroid carcinoma [ATC] being the other three). PTC is the most common malignant tumor of the thyroid gland, accounting for approximately 75% of cases. PTC incidence is greatest in the fourth and fifth decades of life and is 2.5 times more common in females than in males. PTCs may be very small or may be readily palpable. The most frequent presentation is that of a solitary thyroid nodule. However, with the advent of widespread use of CT imaging and ultrasonography, such a tumor may also present as an incidentally discovered thyroid nodule.

PTCs frequently have multiple foci within the thyroid gland. It is common to find two or more lesions in the thyroid gland of a patient who presents with a lymph node in the neck, which, on FNA biopsy, proves to be a papillary lesion of thyroid origin. Although some of these sites represent intraglandular metastases, at least half have different clonal origins.

Histologically, PTC is usually unencapsulated and is composed of papillary cords, with a delicately vascularized connective tissue that is lined by one to many layers of cuboidal and columnar cells. Thyroid colloid and follicles are absent from a pure PTC. The nuclei are quite characteristic in their large size and oval shape with hypodense chromatin; they show cytoplasmic "pseudoinclusions" (redundant nuclear membrane). In approximately 50% of PTCs, calcified, scarred remains of tumor papillae (psammoma bodies) are found. Approximately 10% of all PTCs are of the follicular variant type, characterized by the presence of follicles in addition to the characteristic microscopic findings of PTC. Although follicular variant PTC is usually smaller in diameter at the time of diagnosis, the overall prognosis is the same as the prognosis of common PTC. However, the tall-cell variant of PTC (1% of all PTCs) is a more aggressive tumor; they are larger at the time of diagnosis and are more likely to be invasive than the common type of PTC. Other less common PTC variants that are associated with increased aggressive tumor behavior include the clear-cell, insular, columnar, trabecular, oxyphilic, and diffuse sclerosing variants.

PTC metastasizes frequently to the cervical and upper-mediastinal lymph nodes. At the time of initial diagnosis, PTC is found beyond the confines of the neck in only 2% of patients, usually in the lung and less commonly in bone. (Other less common sites of metastatic disease include the brain, liver, kidneys, and adrenal glands.) In the setting of metastatic disease to the lungs, chest radiography or chest CT typically shows miliary nodules fanning out from the hilum. Skeletal metastases occur infrequently. When the bones are involved, the patient is usually older.

PTC is one of the least aggressive and least malignant of the cancers occurring in the human body; most patients with PTC do not die of this tumor. However, it is capable of causing death. The highest risk of dying from thyroid cancer is associated with older patients (>55 years of age at diagnosis) who present with distant metastases or soft tissue invasion (e.g., trachea, esophagus). Additional factors that increase the risk of recurrent disease include male gender, multicentric thyroidal PTC, large number of lymph node metastases (>10), and age younger than 7 years.

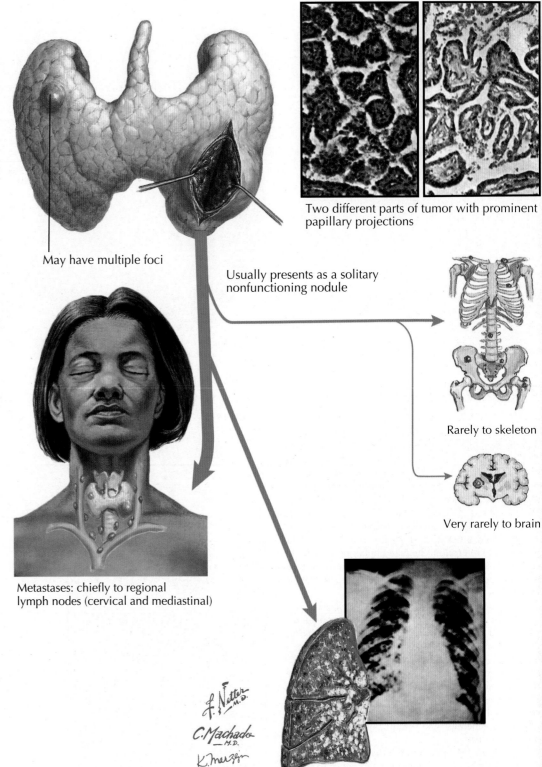

Two different parts of tumor with prominent papillary projections

May have multiple foci

Usually presents as a solitary nonfunctioning nodule

Rarely to skeleton

Very rarely to brain

Metastases: chiefly to regional lymph nodes (cervical and mediastinal)

Secondary to lungs (miliary spread)

For PTCs larger than 1 cm in diameter or for PTCs with known lymph node metastases, total thyroidectomy with central compartment lymphadenectomy is the treatment of choice. More extensive surgery is indicated for patients with invasion of other neck tissues (e.g., trachea, esophagus), but less aggressive surgery (e.g., lobectomy and isthmusectomy) may be considered in patients with solitary PTCs smaller than 1 cm in diameter. ^{133}I treatment serves as an adjuvant therapy for PTC, but it is not universally administered and should be considered individually. External-beam radiotherapy may be considered in patients who have metastatic disease that cannot be resected and that is refractory to ^{131}I therapy. Systemic therapies may be beneficial in patients with aggressive and symptomatic PTC that is refractory to all other treatment options. All patients should be treated with levothyroxine after surgery to prevent pituitary thyrotropin secretion from stimulating PTC growth.

Plate 2.24

Thyroid

FOLLICULAR THYROID CARCINOMA

FTC is one of the four thyroid epithelial-derived thyroid cancers (PTC, oncocytic thyroid carcinoma, and ATC being the other three). After PTC, FTC is the second most common type of thyroid cancer, accounting for 10% of cases. Compared with PTC, FTC occurs more commonly in older persons; the peak incidence is between 40 and 60 years of age and is threefold more common in females than in males. FTC is more common in iodine-deficient regions of the world.

FTC may present as a small nodule or as a large mass within the thyroid. Unlike PTC, FTC usually has a solitary intrathyroidal focus. Cytologic examination of a thyroid FNA biopsy specimen cannot be used to distinguish between FTC and a benign follicular adenoma. On FNA specimens from FTC are typically categorized as follicular neoplasms or follicular lesions of undetermined significance (FLUS). FTC can be diagnosed only on the basis of en bloc thyroid tissue removed at surgery and documentation of tumor capsule or vascular invasion.

Histologically, FTC shows a fairly well-organized follicular pattern, with small but frequently irregular follicles lined by high cuboidal epithelium. The follicles with a more orderly arrangement commonly contain colloid. Findings consistent with PTC (e.g., psammoma bodies) are absent. FTC is classified based on the type and extent of invasion into three groups: (1) minimally invasive FTC (i.e., invasion only of the capsule of the tumor without vascular invasion); (2) encapsulated angioinvasive FTC (i.e., encapsulated tumors with any evidence of vascular invasion); and (3) widely invasive FTC (i.e., tumors with clinically obvious gross invasion of the thyroid gland and extrathyroidal soft tissues).

Most FTCs appear to be monoclonal, and approximately 40% are associated with somatic point mutations in the *RAS* oncogenes, a finding associated with a more aggressive tumor.

FTC frequently metastasizes early via hematogenous dissemination; distant metastases are evident at the time of primary tumor detection in 15% of patients with FTC. The most common sites of metastatic disease are bone and lung (less common sites of involvement include the liver, brain, urinary bladder, and skin). Neck lymph node involvement is much less common in FTC than in PTC. Skeletal metastases, when biopsied, may look like normal thyroid tissue.

FTC tends to have a more aggressive clinical course than PTC. A worse prognosis is associated with larger tumor size, distant metastasis, and vascular invasion. Insular carcinoma is a poorly differentiated form of FTC that is associated with a poor prognosis.

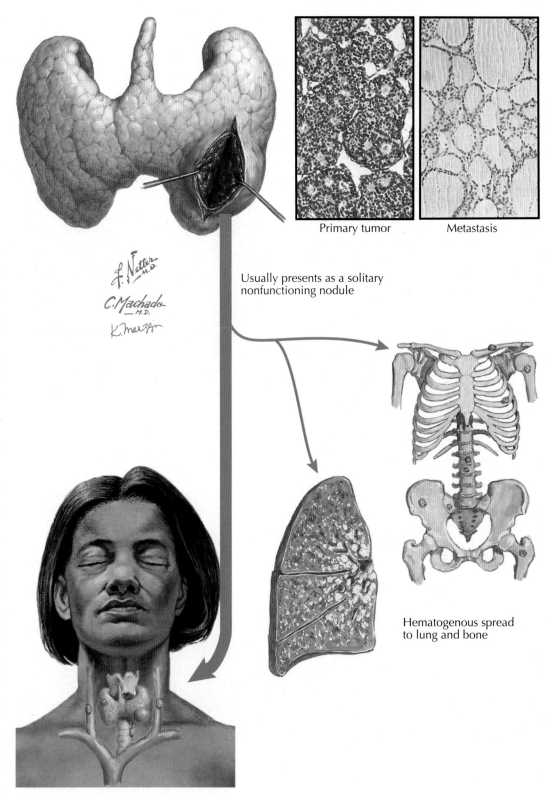

Primary tumor   Metastasis

Usually presents as a solitary nonfunctioning nodule

Hematogenous spread to lung and bone

Rare neck lymph node involvement

The treatment of patients with FTC is similar to that for those with PTC. Total thyroidectomy with central compartment lymph node dissection is the treatment of choice. Preoperative neck ultrasonography with lymph node mapping is essential in planning a successful operation. FTC cells are able to retain ^{131}I but not as well as normal thyroid follicular cells. Iodine-131 may be administered after surgery to destroy thyroid remnant tissue in the thyroid bed and microscopic metastatic disease. After treatment, levothyroxine replacement therapy is initiated to suppress pituitary thyrotropin, with the intent to prevent thyrotropin-driven growth of any residual FTC cells. External-beam radiation therapy may be used when primary or metastatic disease cannot be resected. Systemic therapies may be needed in the small subset of patients whose disease is refractory to all other treatment options.

Plate 2.25

Endocrine System: VOLUME 2

MEDULLARY THYROID CARCINOMA

Medullary thyroid carcinoma (MTC) is a neoplasm of the thyroid parafollicular or "C cells." Approximately 3% of all thyroid malignancies prove to be MTC. The C cells are located in the upper portion of each thyroid lobe and originate from the embryonic neural crest; thus from the clinical and histologic perspectives, MTC is more of a neuroendocrine tumor than a thyroid neoplasm.

In approximately 80% of patients, MTC is sporadic, but it may be familial either as part of multiple endocrine neoplasia type 2 (MEN 2) syndrome or familial MTC (FMTC). Sporadic MTC typically presents as a solitary thyroid nodule at age 40 to 60 years, with a slight female preponderance. MTC is easily diagnosed by FNA biopsy of a thyroid nodule. At the time of diagnosis, more than half of patients with sporadic MTC have metastatic disease, typically involving regional lymph nodes.

MTC secretes the hormone calcitonin. Markedly elevated levels of calcitonin may be found in patients with MTC and may result in severe diarrhea. Also, because of its neuroendocrine embryology, MTC has the potential to secrete other hormones that may cause additional clinical symptomatology. For example, MTC may hypersecrete corticotropin and cause Cushing syndrome.

On histology, MTC shows a solid trabecular pattern with closely packed cells, with considerable variation in hyperchromatism and the size of the nuclei. The cells usually immunostain for calcitonin, galectin-3, and carcinoembryonic antigen.

Inherited MTC is associated with mutations in the *RET* protooncogene and presents as MEN 2A, MEN 2B, or FMTC. The penetrance of MTC in patients with MEN 2 is 100%. Males and females are affected with equal frequency. Patients with MEN 2B have a more aggressive form of MTC, and they should have prophylactic thyroidectomy in the first year of life. Patients with inherited MTC that is not recognized earlier in life typically present between the ages of 20 and 30 years. However, when the risk of familial MTC is known, MTC can be diagnosed before it is palpable or clinically evident. After the specific *RET* protooncogene mutation has been identified in the proband, at-risk family members can have genetic testing for the specific mutation to determine their risk for MTC.

Even patients with apparently sporadic MTC should have genetic testing for mutations in the *RET* protooncogene because approximately 7% have a mutation. This finding can facilitate genetic testing of at-risk family members to identify individuals with MTC and treat them surgically before metastases develop.

All patients with MTC should have biochemical testing to exclude primary hyperparathyroidism and pheochromocytoma (components of MEN 2). Serum calcitonin concentration should be measured

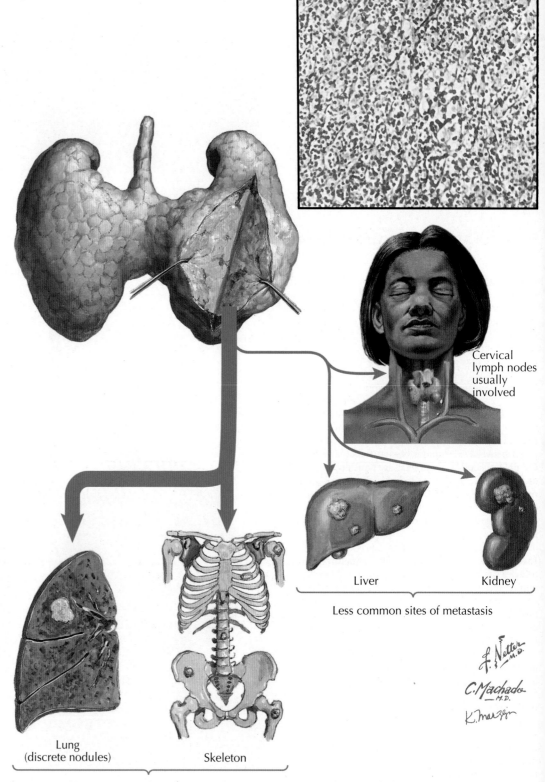

Cervical lymph nodes usually involved

Liver

Kidney

Less common sites of metastasis

Lung (discrete nodules)

Skeleton

Most common sites of metastasis

preoperatively in all patients with MTC. The higher the serum calcitonin concentration, the more likely it is that the patient has metastatic disease and will not be cured with thyroidectomy.

The treatment of choice is total thyroidectomy. Prognosis is determined in part by the age at the time of diagnosis (the older the patient, the poorer the prognosis). For patients with familial disease, the prognosis is determined by the age at which thyroidectomy is

performed; cure rates are higher when thyroidectomy is performed at a younger age. Serum calcitonin concentration should be measured postoperatively to determine whether a surgical cure has been achieved. Metastatic disease may involve the neck, mediastinum, lungs, liver, bone, and kidneys. Persistent metastatic disease that cannot be surgically resected may be treated with molecular pathway-blocking drugs (e.g., tyrosine kinase inhibitors).

Plate 2.26

Thyroid

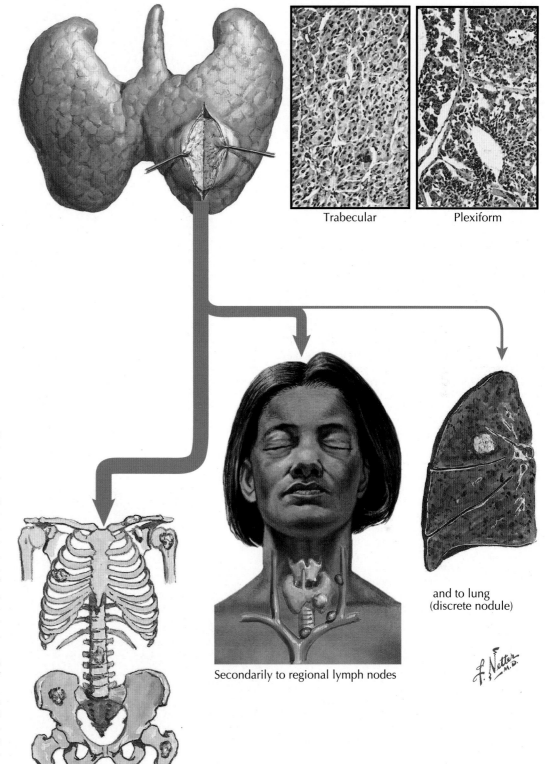

Trabecular

Plexiform

and to lung
(discrete nodule)

Secondarily to regional lymph nodes

Metastases: chiefly to skeleton

ONCOCYTIC (HÜRTHLE CELL) THYROID CARCINOMA

Oncocytic thyroid carcinoma, previously referred to as Hürthle cell thyroid carcinoma, was previously considered to be a variant of follicular thyroid cancer. However, recent clinical and molecular studies have shown that it is a distinct tumor type. Oncocytic thyroid carcinoma represents 3% to 4% of all thyroid malignancies and is distinctive because of a cell population of oncocytes that form at least 75% of the neoplasm. Eosinophilic oxyphilic cells are distinguished by their abundant cytoplasm, oval nuclei with prominent nucleoli, and closely packed mitochondria. Compared with FTC, oncocytic thyroid carcinoma is associated with a poorer prognosis, and it has an increased recurrence rate in local lymph nodes. Peak age range at the time of diagnosis is 40 to 70 years (median age, 61 years). Oncocytic thyroid carcinoma is twofold more common in females than in males.

Oncocytic thyroid carcinoma typically presents as a painless single nodule; it may be barely palpable, or it may be large enough to involve an entire lobe of the thyroid.

Gross pathology usually shows a mahogany brown tumor. Histologically, oncocytic thyroid carcinoma is characterized by the appearance of bright, opaque, eosinophilic, and granular cells that are high cuboidal to low columnar and that may occur in an orderly trabecular arrangement, with each column being separated by a rich, thin-walled capillary blood supply, or they may be stratified in plexiform groups, which are also separated by the capillaries of the rich blood supply. Colloid is scant or absent. The nuclei are hyperchromatic and pleomorphic with prominent eosinophilic nucleoli. Ultrastructurally, oncocytic thyroid carcinoma cells are filled with mitochondria. The diagnosis of carcinoma rests on the demonstration of capsular invasion, vascular invasion, or metastatic spread.

About 5% of patients with oncocytic thyroid carcinoma have distant metastases to lung or bone at the time of diagnosis. Regional lymph node metastases are evident in approximately 25% of cases. Fewer than 10% of oncocytic thyroid carcinomas take up radioiodine.

The prognosis for patients with oncocytic thyroid carcinoma can be predicted on the basis of the presence of distant metastases at presentation, increasing patient age, large primary tumor size, gender, and local extrathyroidal invasion. In general, oncocytic thyroid carcinoma is a more aggressive cancer than papillary or follicular thyroid cancers. The recurrence rate after surgery is approximately 35%. The presence of distant metastases is the strongest predictor of poor outcome. In addition, oncocytic thyroid carcinoma is more aggressive in males than in females.

The treatment of patients with oncocytic thyroid carcinoma is identical to that of patients with FTC. Total thyroidectomy with ipsilateral central neck lymph node dissection is the most common treatment approach. Treatment with radioiodine does not appear to improve outcomes in patients with oncocytic thyroid carcinoma. External-beam radiotherapy may be considered in patients with unresectable oncocytic thyroid carcinoma. In addition, systemic therapies may be beneficial in some patients with refractory disease.

Plate 2.27

Endocrine System: VOLUME 2

ANAPLASTIC THYROID CARCINOMA

ATC is one of four thyroid epithelial-derived thyroid cancers (PTC, FTC, and oncocytic thyroid carcinoma being the other three). Whereas PTC, FTC, and oncocytic thyroid carcinoma are considered differentiated thyroid cancers, ATC is an undifferentiated thyroid cancer. ATC is one of the most malignant and deadly of all carcinomas occurring in humans and accounts for approximately 2% of all thyroid cancers. It usually occurs after age 50 years (mean age, 65 years), and approximately two-thirds of ATCs occur in females.

ATC develops as a rapidly growing, tender tumor of the neck, and it never shows any sign of hormonal function. The patient can often give the exact date of onset (usually a very recent one) and describes rapid growth causing pressure symptoms, dyspnea, dysphagia, hoarseness, cough, and even tenderness or pain in the mass. Systemic symptoms of weight loss, anorexia, fatigue, and fever may also be present. Examination of the nodule reveals a large (frequently larger than 5 cm in diameter), hard mass, which may be fixed. It is usually tender. Heat and even redness in the skin over the nodule may be present. Cervical adenopathy is frequently present. The trachea may be deviated, and the patient may have vocal cord paralysis. In addition, superior vena cava syndrome may be evident in patients whose tumor occupies most of the thoracic inlet.

Approximately 20% of patients with ATC have a history of differentiated thyroid carcinoma (either PTC or FTC), and approximately 50% have a history of goiter. Thus it appears that ATC arises from differentiated thyroid neoplasms, probably caused by a dedifferentiating step (e.g., loss of a tumor suppressor protein or an acquired activating mutation).

The diagnosis of ATC can be confirmed on FNA biopsy or surgical biopsy. Histologically, this tumor is a solid, highly anaplastic growth, with spindle cells predominating but with many large giant cells occurring throughout the tumor. Immunohistochemical staining for the *BRAF V600E*-mutated protein on the fine needle aspiration or core biopsy samples should be obtained. Also, next-generation molecular sequencing should be performed to evaluate for the presence of other treatment-targetable mutations.

This cancer, which is so highly malignant, seldom metastasizes widely. Its rapid growth is local and invasive into the surrounding neck structures (e.g., muscle, lymph nodes, larynx, trachea, esophagus, and great vessels of the neck), usually causing death by direct invasion of the trachea, resulting in compression and asphyxiation. The lungs are the most frequent site of distant spread. ATC may also metastasize to bone, skin over the chest wall, liver, heart, kidneys, and adrenal glands.

CT imaging of the neck, brain, and chest is helpful in planning therapy and monitoring the response to treatment interventions. Positron emission tomography (PET)-CT using 18F-fluorodeoxyglucose is also indicated to determine the extent and sites of metastatic disease. All ATCs are considered stage IV cancers with the following subdivisions: stage IVA for intrathyroidal

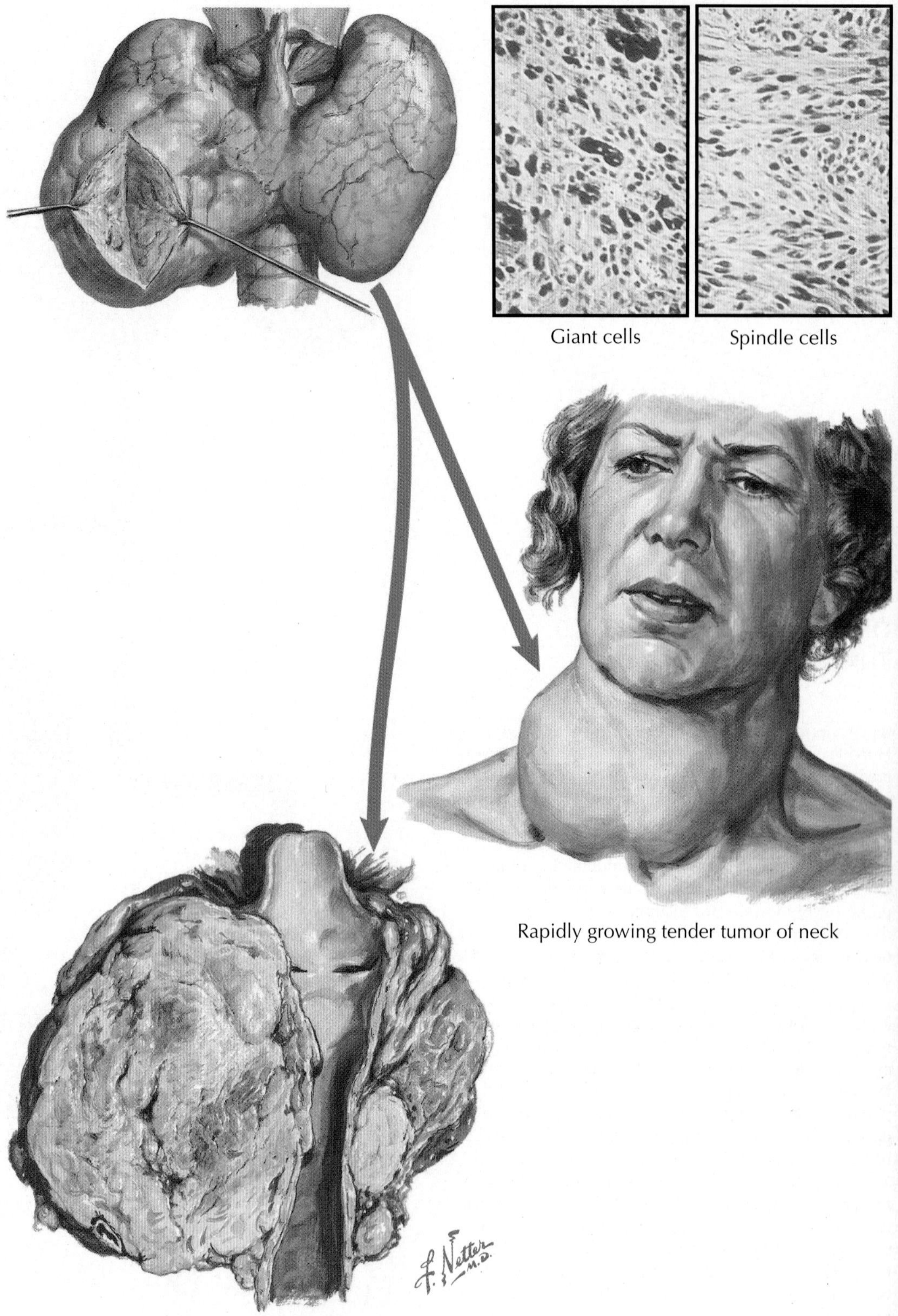

Giant cells

Spindle cells

Rapidly growing tender tumor of neck

Compression and invasion of trachea

ATCs; stage IVB for ATCs with gross extrathyroidal extension or cervical lymph node metastases; and stage IVC when distant metastases are present. ATC has a disease-specific mortality that approaches 100%—the rare exceptions are the patients with small stage IVA ATCs who are treated very aggressively.

For stage IVA ATCs, complete resection should be attempted. However, ATC usually recurs within months after surgical removal even though the lesion appeared

at operation to have been completely eradicated. Thus adjuvant external-beam radiotherapy after surgery should be considered.

For patients with IVB ATCs, if a *BRAF V600E* mutation is present, neoadjuvant treatment (e.g., with dabrafenib and trametinib) might improve the chance of complete tumor resection. For patients with stage IVC disease, there is no curative therapy, and it is uniformly fatal with a median survival of 4 months.

Plate 2.28

Thyroid

THYROID BIOPSY

Thyroid nodules are found in approximately 60% of adults, but only 5% are malignant. Risk factors for thyroid nodules include female sex, older age, iodine deficiency, and history of radiation involving the head and neck before 18 years of age. Imaging characteristics on ultrasound are more useful than nodule size for identifying nodules that are likely to be malignant. For example, spongiform nodules (defined as an aggregate of microcystic areas in >50% of an isoechoic nodule) are at very low risk for cancer (<3%), whereas features of solid hypoechoic nodules that are associated with a much higher risk of malignancy include irregular margins, a taller than wide nodule shape as measured on a transverse image, and punctate echogenic foci, which may sometimes represent psammomatous calcifications of papillary thyroid cancer. Based on thyroid ultrasound findings, the American College of Radiology's Thyroid Imaging, Reporting, and Data System recommends biopsy of all mildly suspicious nodules 1.5 cm or larger, suspicious nodules that are 1 cm or larger, and highly suspicious nodules 0.5 cm or larger.

Fine-needle aspiration (FNA) biopsy of thyroid nodules is a minimally invasive and safe outpatient procedure. Either palpation or ultrasonography may be used to guide needle placement. Ultrasound has the advantage of providing visualization of the needle within the nodule. Thyroid FNA biopsy is performed with the patient in the supine position with the neck extended using a rolled towel. Local anesthesia, if needed, can be achieved with 1% to 2% lidocaine. Sterile technique is achieved with iodine swabs or chlorohexidine and the area draped. A high-resolution linear-array ultrasound transducer with a sterile cover is used. A 22- to 27-gauge needle is attached to a 2- to 20-mL syringe that is placed either in the operator's hand or in a syringe holder. Ultrasonography is performed in the transverse plane for lesion localization. Color Doppler should be used along the planned needle trajectory to ensure there are no large blood vessels. The patient is advised to hold still and avoid swallowing or speaking during the biopsy. When the needle reaches the nodule the biopsy is performed by either aspiration or nonaspiration techniques. With the aspiration technique, the needle tip is advanced into various positions in the nodule and the needle should be gently rotated while moving back and forth in the nodule to allow for sheering of the cells while suction is applied (negative suction is created by pulling back to 1–2 mL on the syringe plunger). Suction is stopped before the needle is removed from the lesion. With the nonaspiration technique, the needle is advanced into the nodule and vigorously moved back and forth while being rotated on its axis until a small amount of cellular material collects inside the needle hub. No suction is performed. This technique is useful in very hypervascular nodules. Two or three FNA needles should be used to ensure a sufficient number of cells for examination by the pathologist. The collected material is placed on glass slides, smeared, and fixed in 95% ethyl alcohol.

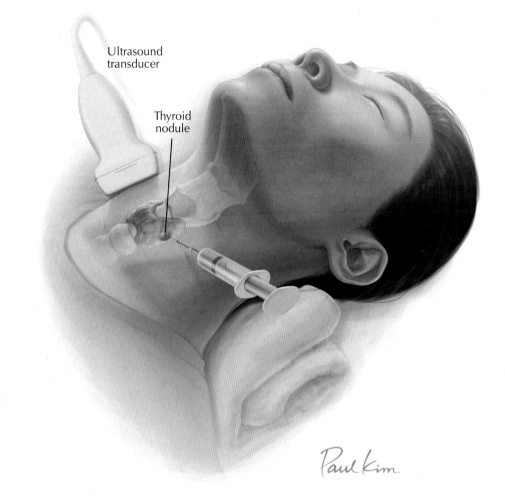

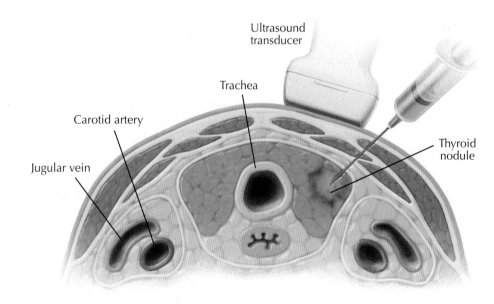

Limited intrathyroidal bleeding and mild local pain radiating to the ear may occur. Neck hematoma is a very rare complication.

The National Cancer Institute Thyroid FNA State of the Science Conference (Bethesda Conference) suggests the following six major cytologic classes: I, nondiagnostic; II, benign; III, follicular lesion or atypia of undetermined significance (FLUS or AUS); IV, follicular neoplasm; V, suspicious for malignancy; and VI, malignant.

Molecular analysis on indeterminate FNA biopsy aspirates (follicular neoplasm, AUS, FLUS) can reduce the number of patients who require diagnostic thyroid surgery. Molecular studies are designed to identify molecular markers of malignancy and high-density genomic data for molecular classification.

Plate 2.29

Endocrine System: VOLUME 2

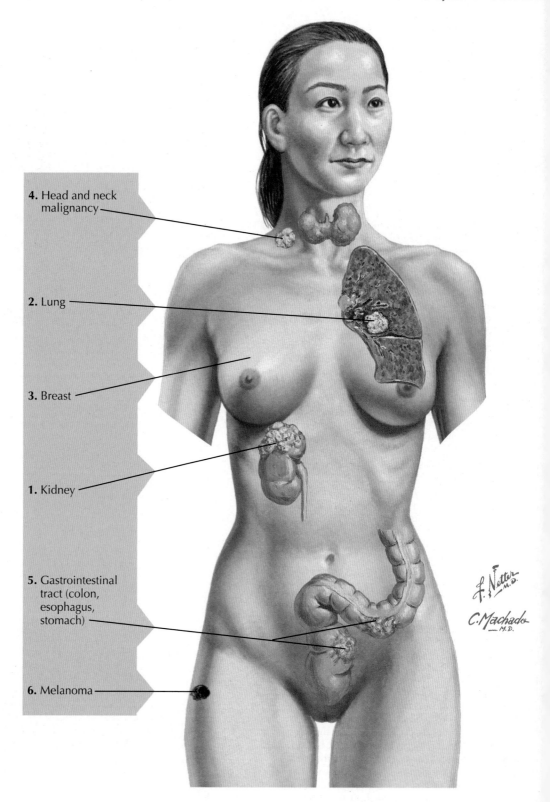

4. Head and neck malignancy

2. Lung

3. Breast

1. Kidney

5. Gastrointestinal tract (colon, esophagus, stomach)

6. Melanoma

TUMORS METASTATIC TO THE THYROID

Metastatic disease to the thyroid is common; it likely relates to its rich blood supply of approximately 560 mL/100 g tissue/min (a flow rate per gram of tissue that is second only to the adrenal glands). The prevalence of metastases to the thyroid gland in autopsy series varies from 1.25% in unselected autopsy studies to 24% in those that died with widespread malignant neoplasms. When preoperative FNA biopsies are performed, the frequency of clinically important metastases to the thyroid gland is approximately 5%. In a patient with a thyroid nodule and a history of cancer, metastatic disease should be the prime consideration.

Although patients with metastatic disease to the thyroid may present with mass-effect symptoms (e.g., hoarseness, dysphagia, stridor, or neck mass), most have asymptomatic disease, and the thyroid nodule is found on physical examination or it is an incidental finding on radiologic imaging (e.g., PET) obtained for tumor staging. The diagnostic procedure of choice in these patients is thyroid FNA biopsy, a highly sensitive and specific procedure.

The most common organ locations for the primary malignancy (in order of frequency) are the kidney (clear cell), lung, breast, head and neck, gastrointestinal tract (colon, esophagus, stomach), and skin (melanoma). Other organ locations and cell types that have

been reported to metastasize to the thyroid include the uterus, ovary, prostate, pancreas, parathyroid, and sarcoma. Most metastases to the thyroid present within 3 years of the primary tumor resection, although intervals as long as 26 years (in a patient with renal cell carcinoma) have been reported.

The metastatic site in the thyroid may be the only apparent location of metastatic involvement. Although there is no consensus on the role for surgery in these patients, most endocrinologists and endocrine

surgeons recommend thyroid lobectomy. If the metastasis is large or if it involves both lobes, a near-total thyroidectomy may be needed. Although it is usually a palliative procedure, aggressive surgical treatment of thyroid metastases in the patients with isolated metastatic renal cell carcinoma have been curative. Radiotherapy may be considered for treatment of metastases that cannot be completely resected. Systemic chemotherapy may be indicated when there are multiple other sites of metastatic disease.

ADRENAL

Plate 3.1   Endocrine System: VOLUME 2

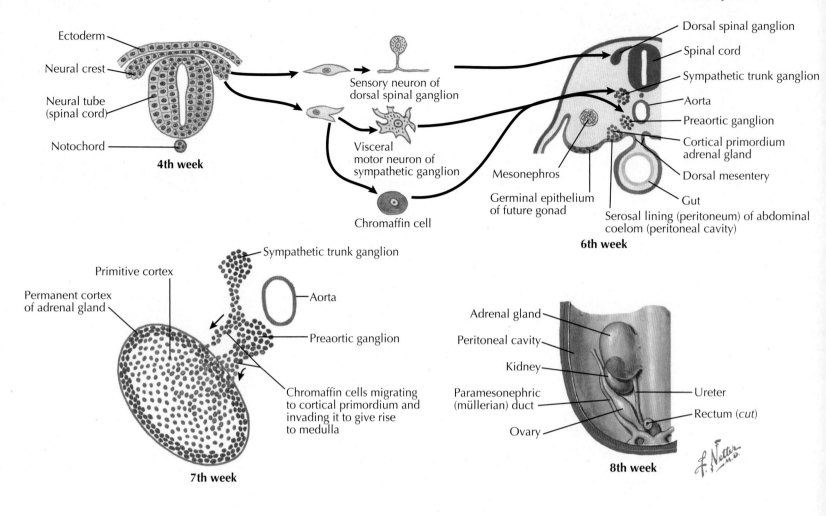

DEVELOPMENT OF THE ADRENAL GLANDS

The detailed anatomy of the adrenal glands was first described by Bartholomeo Eustacius in 1563. Each adrenal gland consists of two parts—the cortex and medulla—that are enveloped in a common capsule. The cortex is derived from mesenchymal tissue and the medulla from ectodermal tissue. From the fifth to sixth week of embryogenesis, the cortical portion of each adrenal gland begins as a proliferation of cells, which originate from the coelomic cavity lining adjacent to the urogenital ridge. The cells proliferate rapidly and penetrate the retroperitoneal mesenchyme to form the primitive cortex. The primitive cortex soon becomes enveloped by a thin layer of more compactly arranged cells that become the permanent cortex, the cells being derived from the same source as those of the primitive cortex. By the eighth week, the cortical tissue has an intimate relationship with the cranial pole of the kidney. Toward the end of the eighth week, the cortical mass attains a considerable size, separates from its peritoneal mesothelial cell layer of origin, and becomes invested in the capsule of connective tissue. At this time, the developing adrenal gland is much larger than the developing kidney.

The primitive, or fetal, cortex constitutes the chief bulk of the adrenal glands at birth. By the second week after birth, the adrenal glands lose one third of their weight; this is a result of the degeneration of the bulky primitive cortex, which disappears by the end of the first year of life. The outer permanent cortex, which is thin at birth, begins to differentiate as the inner primitive cortex undergoes involution. However, full differentiation of the permanent cortex into the three zones of the adult gland (glomerulosa, fasciculata, and reticularis) is not completed until about the third year after birth. The differentiation of the adrenal cortex is dependent on the temporal expression of transcription factors (e.g., steroidogenic factor 1, zona glomerulosa-specific protein, and inner zone antigen).

Certain ectodermal cells arise from the neural crest and migrate from their source of origin to differentiate into sympathetic neurons of the autonomic nervous system. However, not all of the cells of the primitive autonomic ganglia differentiate into neurons. Some become endocrine cells, designated as chromaffin cells because they stain brown with chromium salts. Cytoplasmic granules turn dark when stained with chromic acid because of the oxidation of epinephrine and norepinephrine to melanin. Certain chromaffin cells migrate from the primitive autonomic ganglia adjacent to the developing cortex to give rise eventually to the medulla of the adrenal glands. When the cortex of the adrenal gland has become a prominent structure (during the seventh week of embryogenesis), masses of these migrating chromaffin cells come into contact with the cortex and begin to invade it on its medial side. By the middle of fetal life, some of the chromaffin cells have migrated to the central position within the cortex. Some chromaffin cells also migrate to form paraganglia, collections of chromaffin cells on both sides of the aorta. The largest cluster of chromaffin cells outside the adrenal medulla is near the level of the inferior mesenteric artery and is referred to as the *organ of Zuckerkandl*, which is quite prominent in fetuses and is a major source of catecholamines in the first year of life.

True accessory adrenal glands, consisting of both cortex and medulla, are rarely found in adults. When they are present, they may be within the celiac plexus or embedded in the cortex of the kidney. Adrenal rests, composed of only cortical tissue, occur frequently and are usually located near the adrenal glands. In adults, accessory separate cortical or medullary tissue may be present in the spleen, in the retroperitoneal area below the kidneys, along the aorta, or in the pelvis. Because the adrenal glands are situated close to the gonads during their early development, accessory tissue may also be present in the spermatic cord, attached to the testis in the scrotum, attached to the ovary, or in the broad ligament of the uterus. Although one adrenal gland may be absent occasionally, complete absence of the adrenal glands is extremely rare.

Plate 3.2   Adrenal

ANATOMY AND BLOOD SUPPLY
OF THE ADRENAL GLANDS

The adrenal glands are two small triangular structures located retroperitoneally at the upper poles of the kidneys. They are found on the posterior parietal wall, on each side of the vertebral column, at the level of the 11th thoracic rib and lateral to the first lumbar vertebra. The typical weight of each adrenal gland is 3.5 to 6.0 g. The surface of the gland is corrugated or nodular to a variable extent. Each gland measures 2 to 3 cm in width, 4 to 6 cm in length, and 0.3 to 0.6 cm in thickness. They are surrounded by areolar tissue, containing much fat and are covered by a thin, fibrous capsule attached to the gland by many fibrous bands. The adrenal glands have their own fascial supports so they do not descend with the kidneys when these are displaced. The glands appear golden-yellow, distinct from the paler surrounding fat. The cut section demonstrates a golden cortical layer and a flattened mass of darker (reddish-brown) medullary tissue.

The right adrenal gland is pyramidal or triangular in shape. It occupies a somewhat higher and more lateral position than does the left one. Its posterior surface is in close apposition to the right diaphragmatic crus. The gland is located retroperitoneally in the recess, bounded superiorly by the posteroinferior border of the right lobe of the liver and medially by the right border of the inferior vena cava (IVC). The base of the pyramid is in close apposition to the anteromedial aspect of the upper pole of the right kidney.

The left adrenal gland is generally elongated or semilunar in shape and is a little larger than the right one. It is more centrally located, its medial border frequently overlapping the lateral border of the abdominal aorta. Its posterior surface is in close relationship to the diaphragm and to the splanchnic nerves. The upper two-thirds of the gland lie behind the posterior peritoneal wall of the lesser sac. The lower third is in close relationship to the posterior surface of the body of the pancreas and to the splenic vessels.

The adrenal glands have a very rich vascular supply, characterized by the following features:

1. Unlike those in other organs, the arteries and veins do not usually run together.
2. The arterial supply is abundant, with as many as 12 small arteries.
3. The venous blood is channeled almost completely through a large, single venous trunk that is easily identified.

Arterial blood reaches the adrenal glands through a variable number of slender, short, twiglike arteries, encompassing the gland in an arterial circle (see Plate 3.5). Three types must be distinguished: short capsular arterioles, intermediate cortical ones, and long branches that go through the cortex to the medulla and its sinusoids. These small arteries are terminal branches of the inferior phrenic artery superiorly forming the superior adrenal artery (located along the superior medial margin of the gland). The middle adrenal artery arises from the aorta; the inferior adrenal artery on the inferomedial margin of the adrenal gland arises from the renal artery. This general pattern is occasionally supplemented by additional branches from vessels adjacent to

the gland, such as the ovarian artery in females or the internal spermatic artery in males (on the left side).

Venous blood from the right adrenal gland empties into the vena cava through the right adrenal vein. This vein is short, generally measuring only 4 to 5 mm, and is located in an indentation on the anteromedial aspect of the right adrenal gland at the junction of the upper and middle thirds. On the left side, the left adrenal vein

is situated inferomedially and empties directly into the left renal vein. The left adrenal vein is often joined by the left inferior phrenic vein to become the short common phrenic trunk before it empties into the left renal vein.

Arterial and venous capillaries within the adrenal gland help integrate the function of the cortex and medulla. For example, cortisol-enriched blood flows from the cortex to the medulla, where cortisol

Abdominal exposure of right adrenal gland

Liver (*retracted superiorly*)
Superior adrenal arteries (from inferior phrenic artery)
Inferior vena cava (*retracted medially*)
Adrenal vein
Adrenal gland
Peritoneum (*cut edge*)
Branches of middle adrenal arteries (from abdominal aorta)
Duodenum (*pulled down*)
Inferior adrenal artery (from renal artery)
Renal (Gerota) fascia
Right kidney (*pulled down*)

Abdominal exposure of left adrenal gland

Left inferior phrenic artery
Superior adrenal arteries
Pancreas and spleen (*retracted superiorly*)
Splenic vein
Middle adrenal artery
Aorta
Duodenojejunal flexure
Inferior adrenal artery
Adrenal vein
Left colic (splenic) flexure (*pulled medially*)
Left renal artery and vein
Renal (Gerota) fascia
Adrenal gland
Left kidney
Peritoneum (*cut edges*)

Plate 3.3

Endocrine System: VOLUME 2

ANATOMY AND BLOOD SUPPLY OF THE ADRENAL GLANDS (Continued)

enhances the activity of phenylethanolamine-*N*-methyltransferase that converts norepinephrine to epinephrine. Extraadrenal chromaffin tissues lack these high levels of cortisol and produce norepinephrine almost exclusively.

SURGICAL APPROACHES TO THE ADRENAL GLANDS

The pathologic process, tumor size, patient size, and previous operations are all factors that help determine the surgical approach to the adrenal glands. No one particular approach can be considered suitable for all cases, and the removal of a diseased gland or an adrenal tumor may, at times, present formidable difficulties.

Open Transabdominal Adrenalectomy

The patient is in the supine position, and the incision is typically in an extended subcostal location. A midline incision may be used if the patient has a narrow costal angle or bilateral adrenal disease is present. The approach to the left adrenal gland is typically through the gastrocolic ligament into the lesser sac. The left adrenal is exposed by lifting the inferior surface of the pancreas upward, Gerota fascia is opened, and the upper pole of the kidney is retracted inferiorly. The approach to the right adrenal gland involves mobilizing the hepatic flexure of the colon inferiorly and retracting the right lobe of the liver upward.

Open Posterior Adrenalectomy

Compared with the open anterior approach, the open posterior approach causes less pain, ileus, and other complications. The patient is in the prone position and the incision is either curvilinear extending from the 10th rib (4 cm from the midvertebral line) to the iliac crest (8 cm from the midvertebral line) or a single straight incision over the 12th rib with a small vertical paravertebral upward extension. The 12th rib is resected, the pleura is reflected upward, and Gerota fascia is incised.

Laparoscopic Transabdominal Adrenalectomy

Since its description in 1992, laparoscopic adrenalectomy has rapidly become the procedure of choice for unilateral adrenalectomy when the adrenal mass is smaller than 8 cm and there are no frank signs of malignancy (e.g., invasion of contiguous structures). The postoperative recovery time and long-term morbidity associated with laparoscopic adrenalectomy are significantly reduced compared with open adrenalectomy. The patient is placed in the lateral decubitus position with the side to be operated facing upward. Four trocars are placed in a straight line, 1 to 2 cm below the subcostal margin. On the right side, the liver with the gallbladder is retracted upward, and the retroperitoneum is incised. On the left side, the left colonic flexure and the descending colon are mobilized inferiorly and medially to expose the upper pole of the left kidney, and the retroperitoneum is incised.

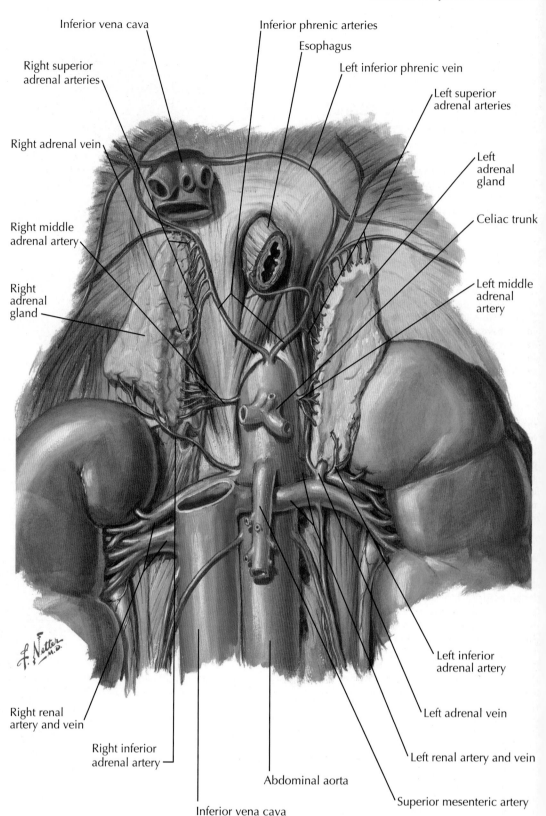

Posterior Retroperitoneoscopic Adrenalectomy

A minimally invasive posterior approach to the adrenal is favored by some endocrine surgeons and is advantageous in patients who have had previous anterior upper abdominal operations. The patient is in the prone position, and three trocars are used. A gas pressure of 20 to 25 mm Hg allows the creation of sufficient space in the retroperitoneum to facilitate the operation.

Keys to Successful Adrenal Surgery

The keys to successful adrenal surgery are appropriate patient selection, knowledge of anatomy, delicate tissue handling, meticulous hemostasis, and experience with the approach used. Familiarity with the vascular anomalies of the blood supply of the adrenal glands is indispensable. Finally, the gland should be handled gently because it fractures easily when traumatized, jeopardizing its complete removal.

Plate 3.4

Adrenal

INNERVATION OF THE ADRENAL GLANDS

Relative to their size, the adrenal glands have a richer innervation than other viscera. The sympathetic preganglionic fibers for these glands are the axons of cells located in the intermediolateral columns of the lowest two or three thoracic and highest one or two lumbar segments of the spinal cord. They emerge in the anterior rootlets of the corresponding spinal nerves; pass in the white rami communicantes to the homolateral sympathetic trunks; and leave them in the greater, lesser, and least thoracic and first lumbar splanchnic nerves, which run to the celiac, aorticorenal, and renal ganglia. Some fibers end in these ganglia, but most pass through them without relaying and enter numerous small nerves that run outward on each side from the celiac plexus to the adrenal glands. These nerves are joined by direct contributions from the terminal parts of the greater and lesser thoracic splanchnic nerves, and they communicate with the homolateral phrenic nerve and renal plexus. Small ganglia exist on the adrenal nerves and within the actual adrenal medulla; a proportion of sympathetic fibers may relay in these ganglia.

Parasympathetic fibers are conveyed to the celiac plexus in the celiac branch of the posterior vagal trunk, and some of these are involved with adrenal innervation and may relay in ganglia in or near the gland.

On each side, the adrenal nerves form an adrenal plexus along the medial border of the adrenal gland. Filaments associated with occasional ganglion cells spread out over the gland to form a delicate subcapsular plexus, from which fascicles or solitary fibers penetrate the cortex to reach the medulla, apparently without supplying cortical cells en route, although they do supply cortical vessels. Most of the branches of the adrenal plexus, however, enter the gland through or near its hilum as compact bundles, some of which accompany the adrenal arteries. These bundles run through the cortex to the medulla, where they ramify profusely and mostly terminate in synaptic-type endings around the medullary chromaffin cells; some fibers invaginate but do not penetrate the plasma membranes of these cells. The preganglionic sympathetic fibers end directly around the medullary cells because these cells are derived from the sympathetic anlage and are the homologues of sympathetic ganglion cells. Other fibers innervate the adrenal vessels, including the central vein.

Catecholamines are released from the adrenal medullary and sympathoneuronal systems—both are key components of the fight-or-flight reaction. The signs and symptoms of the fight-or-flight reaction include cutaneous and systemic vasoconstriction with cold and clammy skin, anxiety, agitation, piloerection, tachycardia, dilated pupils, hyperventilation, hyperglycemia, decreased gastrointestinal motility, and decreased urinary output. This reaction is triggered by neural signals from several sites in the brain (e.g., the hypothalamus, pons, and medulla), leading to synapses on cell bodies in the intermediolateral cell columns of the thoracolumbar spinal cord. The preganglionic sympathetic nerves leave the spinal cord and synapse in paravertebral and preaortic ganglia of the sympathetic chain. Preganglionic axons from the lower thoracic and lumbar ganglia innervate the adrenal medulla via the splanchnic nerve and ramify about cells of the medulla. Acetylcholine is the neurotransmitter in the ganglia, and the postganglionic fiber releases norepinephrine. The chromaffin cell of the adrenal medulla is a "postganglionic fiber equivalent," and its chemical transmitters are epinephrine and norepinephrine.

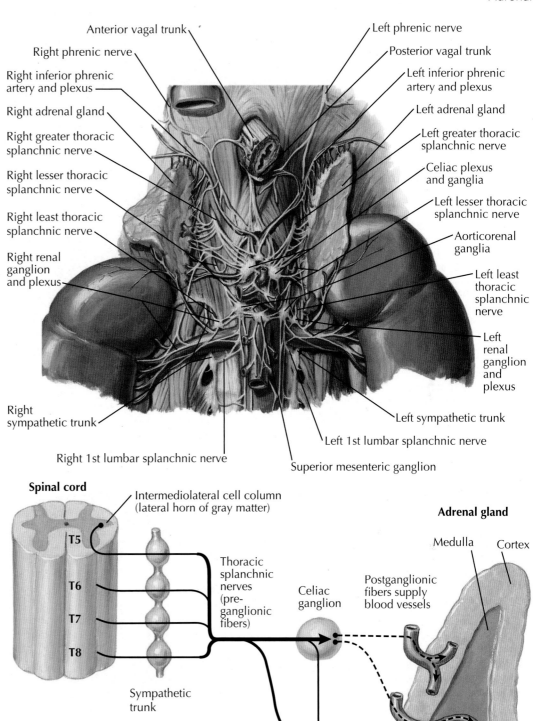

Plate 3.5

Endocrine System: VOLUME 2

HISTOLOGY OF THE ADRENAL GLANDS

The adrenal glands are composed of two separate and distinct endocrine tissues—the adrenal cortex and the adrenal medulla—and each is entirely different in embryologic origin, structure, and function. In adults, the cortex constitutes about 90% of the adrenal gland and completely surrounds the thin layer of centrally located medulla. In histologic sections, the cortex is seen to be composed mainly of radially oriented cords of cells. During embryogenesis, cells destined to form the medulla migrate through the cortex. At birth, in addition to a thin outer layer of permanent cortex, there is a thick band of fetal cortex, which soon involutes.

The cells of the adrenal cortex are typically epithelioid in appearance, with centrally placed nuclei having two or more prominent nucleoli. The cytoplasm features a variable abundance of lipid-containing vacuoles in addition to mitochondria and the Golgi apparatus.

In the adrenal cortex, three concentrically arranged cell layers, or zones, can be identified on the basis of the grouping of cells and the disposition of cell cords. In the thin outermost layer, the zona glomerulosa, the cells occur in arched loops or round balls. The middle layer, the zona fasciculata, is the widest of the three zones and is composed of cells arranged in long straight cords, or fascicles. The innermost layer, the zona reticularis, is contiguous with the medulla, and the cell cords are entwined, forming a reticulum. The two inner zones are entirely dependent on pituitary adrenocorticotropic hormone (ACTH; corticotropin) secretion for the maintenance of their structure and function. However, the zona glomerulosa remains structurally and functionally normal in the absence of ACTH. Under normal conditions, the cortical cells at the inner border of the cortex have few lipid vacuoles and are referred to as *compact cells*, in contrast to the lipid-laden light cells that occupy the midportion of the cortex. Under ACTH stimulation, the layer of compact cells increases in width at the expense of the layer of light cells.

The zona glomerulosa is primarily responsible for the secretion of aldosterone, a mineralocorticoid having the prime function of regulating sodium and potassium balance. The function of the zona glomerulosa is essentially independent of that of the remainder of the cortex. The control of aldosterone secretion involves the renal juxtaglomerular apparatus and the renin-angiotensin system. The zona fasciculata and reticularis can best be regarded as a functional unit, having as its primary purpose the secretion of the glucocorticoid cortisol and some adrenal androgens. Cortisol has a prominent role in regulating the catabolism of protein, facilitating gluconeogenesis, and suppressing inflammation.

The adrenal gland receives blood from 30 to 50 small arteries that penetrate the capsule at different points and form the capsular plexus of arterioles. These supply the capillaries that extend radially through the cortex

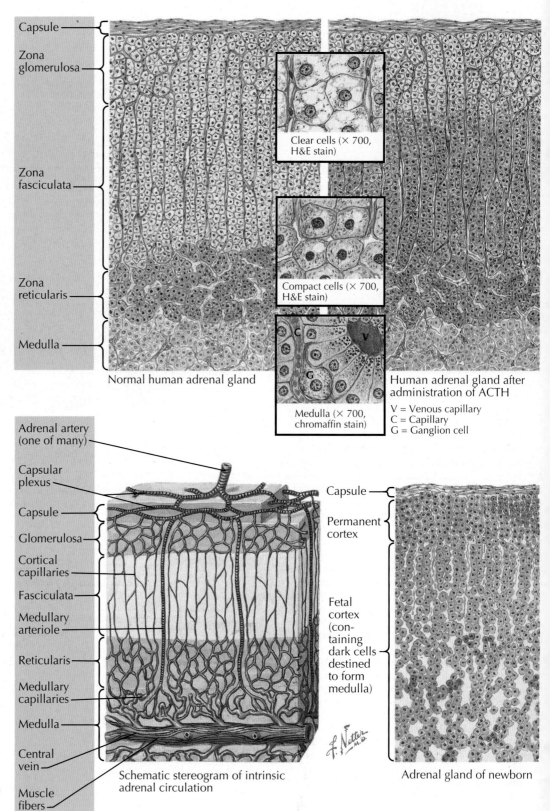

Capsule

Zona glomerulosa

Zona fasciculata

Zona reticularis

Medulla

Normal human adrenal gland

Clear cells (× 700, H&E stain)

Compact cells (× 700, H&E stain)

Medulla (× 700, chromaffin stain)

Human adrenal gland after administration of ACTH

V = Venous capillary
C = Capillary
G = Ganglion cell

Adrenal artery (one of many)

Capsular plexus

Capsule

Glomerulosa

Cortical capillaries

Fasciculata

Medullary arteriole

Reticularis

Medullary capillaries

Medulla

Central vein

Muscle fibers

Capsule

Permanent cortex

Fetal cortex (containing dark cells destined to form medulla)

Schematic stereogram of intrinsic adrenal circulation

Adrenal gland of newborn

and separate the cords of cells. The adrenal medulla has both a venous and an arterial blood supply. Capillaries from the cortex extend into the medulla as venous capillaries; a few medullary arterioles extend through the cortex to form arterial capillaries in the medulla. Both categories of vessels join to form veins that drain through the single large central adrenal vein. The venous tributaries enter the latter between thick bands of smooth muscle, longitudinally disposed in its wall.

The adrenal medulla is composed of columnar cells that secrete the catecholamines epinephrine, norepinephrine, and dopamine (DA). Because the catecholamines are readily darkened by the oxidizing agent potassium dichromate, the medulla is often referred to as *chromaffin tissue*. Preganglionic sympathetic fibers enter the medulla and terminate directly on the parenchymal cells or scattered sympathetic ganglion cells.

Plate 3.6

Adrenal

Biosynthesis and Metabolism of Adrenal Cortical Hormones

The steroids produced by the adrenal cortex include glucocorticoids, mineralocorticoids, adrenal androgens (17-ketosteroids), estrogens, and progestogens. Although some steroids are highly potent biologically, others are relatively inactive. Whereas the secretory activity and growth of the zona fasciculata and zona reticularis of the adrenal cortex are regulated by the pituitary secretion of ACTH, the secretion of aldosterone from the zona glomerulosa of the adrenal cortex is regulated by angiotensin II, potassium, and (to a lesser extent) ACTH. ACTH is released from pituitary corticotrophs on the basis of feedback regulation—if there is a decrease in the blood cortisol concentration, pulsatile corticotropin-releasing hormone (CRH) and ACTH secretion increase and raise the cortisol level again, which in turn inhibits further CRH and ACTH release. The hypothalamic-pituitary-adrenal axis feedback control is accompanied by a diurnal variation in ACTH secretion. The ACTH pulse frequency and amplitude are maximal between 2 and 8 AM. After 8 AM, there is a gradual daytime decrease in ACTH and cortisol secretion, reaching a nadir in the late evening hours. The circadian rhythm is dependent on both sleep-wake and day-night patterns. With overseas travel, it may take 10 to 14 days for the circadian rhythm to reset to the new time zone.

The diurnal rhythm in cortisol secretion is abolished in individuals with Cushing syndrome, whether the syndrome is caused by a primary adrenal tumor, eutopic ACTH, or ectopic ACTH hypersecretion. The feedback inhibition of ACTH by cortisol may be interrupted at any time by an overriding mechanism (e.g., stress). Stressful stimuli (e.g., fever, trauma, hypoglycemia, hypotension) reaching the cerebral cortex release the inhibition of the reticular formation or of the limbic system on hypothalamic centers in and around the tuberoinfundibular nucleus and the median eminence. Large neurons then secrete hypothalamic CRH. Vasopressin also has an ACTH-releasing effect. The proinflammatory

cytokines (e.g., interleukins) increase ACTH secretion either directly or by augmenting CRH secretion. The greater the stress, the more ACTH is secreted. The upper secretory limit of endogenous cortisol is approximately 250 mg/day.

Cholesterol derived from acetate is stored in the adrenal cortex. Its cyclopentanophenanthrene four-ring hydrocarbon nucleus (three cyclohexane rings and a single cyclopentane ring) is modified by enzymes that induce hydroxyl groups into the ring (hydroxylases), but other enzymes (dehydrogenases) may remove hydrogen from a hydroxyl group, and others (oxidases) remove hydrogen from a CH group. Chemical structure determines function; for example, glucocorticoids are distinguished by an α-ketol group and an 11-hydroxyl group. Cleaving cholesterol into pregnenolone (the C21 precursor of all active steroid hormones) and isocaproaldehyde is the critical first step and occurs in a limited number of sites in the body (e.g., adrenal cortex, testicular Leydig cells, ovarian theca cells, trophoblast cells of the placenta, and certain glial and neuronal cells of the brain). The roles of different steroidogenic tissues are determined by how this process is regulated and in how pregnenolone is subsequently metabolized. Most of the steroidogenic enzymes are unidirectional, so the accumulation of product does not drive flux back to the substrate. In addition, whereas the P450-mediated hydroxylations and carbon-carbon bond cleavage reactions are irreversible, the hydroxysteroid dehydrogenase reactions are reversible. Glucocorticoids and progestogens have 21 carbon atoms (C21 steroids), androgens have 19 carbon atoms (C19 steroids), and estrogens have 18 carbon atoms (C18 steroids).

The steroidogenic acute regulatory protein (StAR) mobilizes cholesterol from the outer mitochondrial membrane to the inner mitochondrial membrane, where the rate-limiting steroid side-chain cleavage enzyme (P450scc) cleaves cholesterol to pregnenolone. StAR is induced by an increase in intracellular cyclic adenosine monophosphate (cAMP) after receptor activation by ACTH. P450scc and the CYP11B enzymes (11β-hydroxylase and aldosterone synthase) are mitochondrial enzymes and require an electron shuttle system (adrenodoxin/adrenodoxin reductase) to oxidize

steroids, whereas 17α-hydroxylase and 21-hydroxylase are located in the endoplasmic reticulum, and electron transfer is accomplished from nicotinamide adenine dinucleotide phosphate by the enzyme P450 oxidoreductase (P450 OR). Finally, the 17,20-lyase activity of P450 CYP17 requires flavoprotein b5 that functions as an allosteric facilitator of the CYP17 and P450 OR interaction.

In the cytoplasm, pregnenolone is converted to progesterone by 3β-hydroxysteroid dehydrogenase (3β-HSD) by a reaction involving dehydrogenation of the 3-hydroxyl group and isomerization of the double bond at C5. Progesterone is hydroxylated to 17-hydroxyprogesterone through the activity of 17α-hydroxylase (P450c17). 17-Hydroxylation is a prerequisite for glucocorticoid synthesis (the zona glomerulosa does not express P450c17). P450c17 also possesses 17,20-lyase activity, which results in the production of the C19 adrenal androgens (dehydroepiandrosterone [DHEA] and androstenedione). Most of the adrenal androstenedione production is dependent on the conversion of DHEA to androstenedione by 3β-HSD. 21-Hydroxylation of either progesterone in the zona glomerulosa or 17-hydroxyprogesterone (zona fasciculata) is performed by 21-hydroxylase (P450c21) to yield deoxycorticosterone (DOC) or 11-deoxycortisol, respectively. The final step in cortisol biosynthesis—the conversion of 11-deoxycortisol to cortisol by 11β-hydroxylase (P450c11β)—takes place in the mitochondria. In the zona glomerulosa, P450c11β and aldosterone synthase (P450c11AS) convert DOC to corticosterone. P450c11AS is also required for the 18-hydroxylation and 18-methyloxidation steps to convert corticosterone to aldosterone via the intermediate 18-hydroxycorticosterone. Whereas aldosterone secretion is confined to the zona glomerulosa through the restricted expression of *CYP11B2*, the zona glomerulosa cannot synthesize cortisol because it does not express *CYP17*. In the zona reticularis, high levels of cytochrome b5 facilitate 17,20-lyase activity on P450c17, and the production of DHEA. DHEA is either converted to androstenedione by 3β-HSD or sulfated in the zona reticularis by the DHEA sulfotransferase (*SULT2A1*) to form DHEA sulfate (DHEA-S). Androstenedione may be converted to testosterone by

Plate 3.6

Endocrine System: VOLUME 2

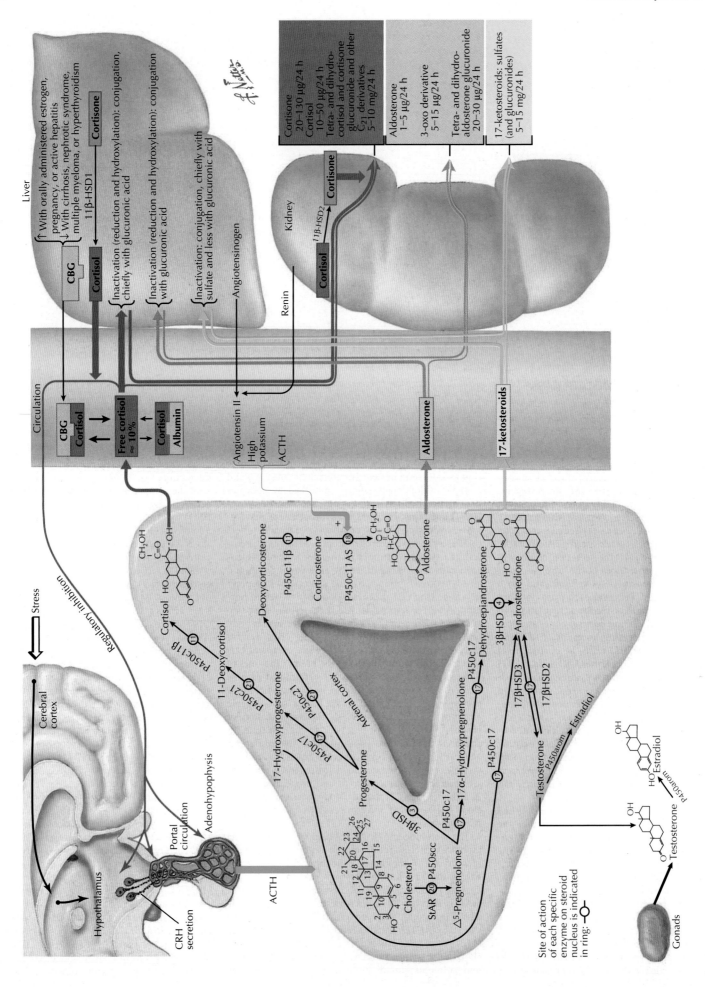

Liver

↑ With orally administered estrogen, pregnancy, or active hepatitis
↓ With cirrhosis, nephrotic syndrome, multiple myeloma, or hyperthyroidism

Cortisone

11β-HSD1

Cortisol

CBG

Inactivation (reduction and hydroxylation): conjugation, chiefly with glucuronic acid

Inactivation (reduction and hydroxylation): conjugation with glucuronic acid

Inactivation: conjugation, chiefly with sulfate and less with glucuronic acid

Angiotensinogen

Kidney

Cortisone

11β-HSD2

Cortisol

Cortisone 20–130 μg/24 h
Cortisol 10–50 μg/24 h
Tetra- and dihydro-cortisol and cortisone glucuronide and other C₂₁ derivatives 5–10 mg/24 h

Aldosterone 1–5 μg/24 h
3-oxo derivative 5–15 μg/24 h
Tetra- and dihydro-aldosterone glucuronide 20–30 μg/24 h

17-ketosteroids: sulfates (and glucuronides) 5–15 mg/24 h

Renin

Circulation

CBG Cortisol

Free cortisol ≈ 10%

Cortisol Albumin

Angiotensin II

High potassium

ACTH

Aldosterone

17-ketosteroids

Stress

Regulatory inhibition

Cerebral cortex

Deoxycorticosterone

P450c11β

Corticosterone

P450c11AS

Aldosterone

Dehydroepiandrosterone

3βHSD

Androstenedione

P450c17

Cortisol

P450c11β

11-Deoxycortisol

P450c21

P450c21

17-Hydroxyprogesterone

P450c17

Adrenal cortex

Progesterone

3βHSD

P450c17

17α-Hydroxypregnenolone

P450c17

17βHSD3

17βHSD2

Testosterone

P450arom

Estradiol

Adenohypophysis

Portal circulation

Hypothalamus

CRH secretion

ACTH

StAR P450scc

Cholesterol

Δ5-Pregnenolone

Estradiol

Testosterone

Gonads

Site of action of each specific enzyme on steroid nucleus is indicated in ring: ◯

Plate 3.7

Adrenal

Adrenal Steroidogenic Enzymes, Their Genes, Locations, and Substrates

Enzyme name	Abbreviation	Gene	Location	Substrate
Cholesterol side-chain cleavage (desmolase)	P-450scc	CYP11A1	ZG, ZF, ZR, gonads, placenta, brain	Cholesterol
3β-Hydroxysteroid dehydrogenase (3β-HSD1) (type I isozyme)	3β-HSD1	HSD3B1	Placenta, liver, brain	Pregnenolone, 17α-OH-pregnenolone
3β-Hydroxysteroid dehydrogenase (3β-HSD2) (type II isozyme)	3β-HSD2	HSD3B2	ZG, ZF, ZR, gonads	DHEA, pregnenolone, 17α-OH-pregnenolone
17α-Hydroxylase/ 17,20 lyase	P-450c17	CYP17	ZF, ZR, gonads, brain	Pregnenolone, 17α-OH-pregnenolone, progesterone, 17α-OH-progesterone
21-Hydroxylase	P-450c21	CYP21A2	ZG, ZF, ZR	Progesterone, 17α-OH-progesterone
11β-Hydroxylase	P-450c11β	CYP11B1	ZG, ZR, brain	11-deoxycortisol, 11-deoxycorticosterone
Aldosterone synthase	P-450c11AS	CYP11B2	ZG, brain, heart	Deoxycorticosterone, 18-OH-corticosterone
Aromatase	P-450arom	CYP19A1	Gonads, placenta, brain, bone, fat	Testosterone, androstenedione
17β-Ketosteroid reductase	17β-HSD1	HSD17B1	Gonads, placenta, breast	Estrone
17β-Hydroxysteroid dehydrogenase	17β-HSD2	HSD17B2	Broadly	Estradiol, testosterone
17β-Ketosteroid reductase	17β-HSD3	HSD17B3	Gonads	Androstenedione
11β-Hydroxysteroid dehydrogenase 1	11β-HSD1	HSD11B1	Liver, brain, placenta, fat	Cortisone
11β-Hydroxysteroid dehydrogenase 2	11β-HSD2	HSD11B2	Kidney, colon, salivary glands, placenta	Cortisol

DHEA, Dehydroepiandrosterone; *ZF*, adrenal zona fasciculata; *ZG*, adrenal zona glomerulosa; *ZR*, adrenal zona reticularis.

BIOSYNTHESIS AND METABOLISM OF ADRENAL CORTICAL HORMONES (Continued)

17β-ketosteroid reductase (17β-HSD3) in the adrenal glands or gonads.

Under normal conditions, 10 to 20 mg of cortisol and 0.1 to 0.15 mg of aldosterone are secreted over 24 hours. The adult adrenal gland secretes approximately 4 mg of DHEA, 10 mg of DHEA-S, 1.5 mg of androstenedione, and 0.05 mg of testosterone over 24 hours. However, testosterone has 60 times the androgenic potency of even the most potent 17-ketosteroid (characterized by an oxygen atom in the 17 position). The adrenal androgens supply approximately 50% of circulating androgens in premenopausal women. The adrenal glands secrete small amounts of estradiol (derived from testosterone) and estrone (derived from androstenedione); both become important after menopause when the adrenal glands are the only source of estrogens in females.

Approximately 90% of cortisol in the plasma is bound, primarily by cortisol-binding globulin (CBG) and to a lesser extent by albumin. The hepatic production of CBG is increased in patients taking orally administered estrogen (e.g., oral contraceptive pill or postmenopausal estrogen replacement therapy), in pregnant females, and in patients with active hepatitis. Blood CBG concentrations are decreased in patients with cirrhosis, nephrotic syndrome, multiple myeloma, or hyperthyroidism. When cortisol is measured in the blood, it is the sum of the bound and free forms; thus the CBG concentration has a substantial effect on the measured level of cortisol, appearing high in patients taking oral estrogen and low in patients with low CBG concentrations. In these settings, the clinician can measure the unbound or free cortisol concentration in the blood or the excretion of free cortisol through the kidneys, termed *urinary free cortisol* (UFC) (which represents approximately 1% of the total cortisol secretion rate).

The circulating half-life of cortisol varies between 60 and 120 minutes. The interconversion of cortisol and cortisone via 11β-hydroxysteroid dehydrogenase (11β-HSD) regulates local corticosteroid hormone action. There are 2 distinct 11β-HSD isozymes: type 1 (11β-HSD1) is expressed primarily in the liver and converts cortisone to cortisol; type 2 (11β-HSD2) is found near the mineralocorticoid receptor (MR) in the kidney, colon, and salivary glands and inactivates cortisol to cortisone. Apparent mineralocorticoid excess is the result of impaired 11β-HSD2 activity. Cortisol can be a potent mineralocorticoid, and as a result of the enzyme deficiency, high levels of cortisol accumulate in the kidney. Thus 11β-HSD2 normally excludes physiologic glucocorticoids from the nonselective MR by converting them to the inactive 11-keto compound, cortisone. Decreased 11β-HSD2 activity may be hereditary or secondary to pharmacologic inhibition of enzyme activity by glycyrrhizic acid, the active principle of licorice root (*Glycyrrhiza glabra*). The clinical phenotype of patients with apparent mineralocorticoid excess includes hypertension, hypokalemia, metabolic alkalosis, low plasma renin activity (PRA), low plasma aldosterone concentration (PAC), and normal plasma cortisol levels. The diagnosis is confirmed by demonstrating an abnormal ratio of cortisol to cortisone (e.g., >10:1) in a 24-hour urine collection. The apparent mineralocorticoid excess state caused by ectopic ACTH secretion, commonly seen in patients with Cushing syndrome, is related to the high rates of cortisol production that overwhelm 11β-HSD2 activity.

The usual level of cortisone in the urine is approximately two- to threefold higher than the level of cortisol. The subsequent metabolism of cortisol and cortisone then follows similar pathways with reduction of the C4–5 double bond to form dihydrocortisol or dihydrocortisone followed by a hydroxylation step to form tetrahydrocortisol and tetrahydrocortisone, which are rapidly conjugated with glucuronic acid and excreted in the urine. Thus primary sites of cortisol metabolism are the liver and kidney.

Aldosterone is also metabolized in the liver, where it undergoes tetrahydro reduction and is excreted by the kidneys as 3-glucuronide tetrahydroaldosterone; 20 to 30 μg of this conjugate is excreted daily in the urine. In addition, 5 to 15 μg per day of the aldosterone 3-oxoglucuronic acid conjugate is found in the urine as hydrolyzable aldosterone. A much smaller fraction of aldosterone (1–5 μg) appears in the urine in the free form.

Plate 3.8

Endocrine System: VOLUME 2

BIOLOGIC ACTIONS OF CORTISOL

CARBOHYDRATE, PROTEIN, AND LIPID METABOLISM

Because of their actions on glycogen, protein, and lipid metabolism, glucocorticoids increase blood glucose concentrations. Glucocorticoids stimulate glycogen deposition in the liver by inhibiting the glycogen-mobilizing enzyme (glycogen phosphorylase) and by increasing glycogen synthase. They increase hepatic glucose output by activation of the gluconeogenic enzymes (glucose-6-phosphatase and phosphoenolpyruvate kinase). Lipolysis is activated in adipose tissue, increasing blood free fatty acid concentrations. Because of their enhancing and synergistic effects on the actions of other hormones (e.g., glucagon and catecholamines), increased glucocorticoid concentrations cause insulin resistance and an increased blood glucose concentration. Thus over the short term, glucocorticoids support stress responses that require glucose for rapid and intense exertion. With long-term excess, glucocorticoids are diabetogenic. In addition, there is enhanced adipogenesis, especially in the visceral or central adipose tissue depots (centripetal distribution).

SKIN, MUSCLE, AND CONNECTIVE TISSUES

Excess glucocorticoids are catabolic and divert amino acids from muscle to the liver for deamination, resulting in muscle wasting and proximal muscle weakness. There is decreased protein synthesis and increased resorption of bone matrix, resulting in growth arrest in children. Glucocorticoids decrease collagen synthesis and production and inhibit epidermal cell division and DNA synthesis.

BONE AND CALCIUM METABOLISM

Excess glucocorticoids cause osteopenia and osteoporosis by inhibiting osteoblast function and enhancing resorption of bone matrix. The most serious bone-related complication from excess glucocorticoids is osteonecrosis (avascular necrosis); it is caused by osteocyte apoptosis, resulting in focal deterioration and collapse of bone that primarily affects the femoral head. Excess glucocorticoids inhibit intestinal calcium absorption and increase renal calcium excretion, resulting in a negative calcium balance.

BLOOD PRESSURE CONTROL

Glucocorticoids increase glomerular filtration rate, proximal tubular epithelial sodium transport, and free water clearance. Excess glucocorticoids can overwhelm renal 11β-HSD2, allowing access of cortisol to the MR (see Plates 3.6 and 3.7) and resulting in renal sodium retention and potassium loss. Under normal physiologic conditions, glucocorticoids increase sensitivity to pressor agents such as catecholamines and angiotensin II in vascular smooth muscle. In addition, the synthesis of angiotensinogen is increased by glucocorticoids.

ANTIINFLAMMATORY ACTIONS

Glucocorticoids suppress the immunologic responses of autoimmune and inflammatory conditions. They reduce blood lymphocyte counts (by redistributing them from the intravascular compartment to spleen, lymph

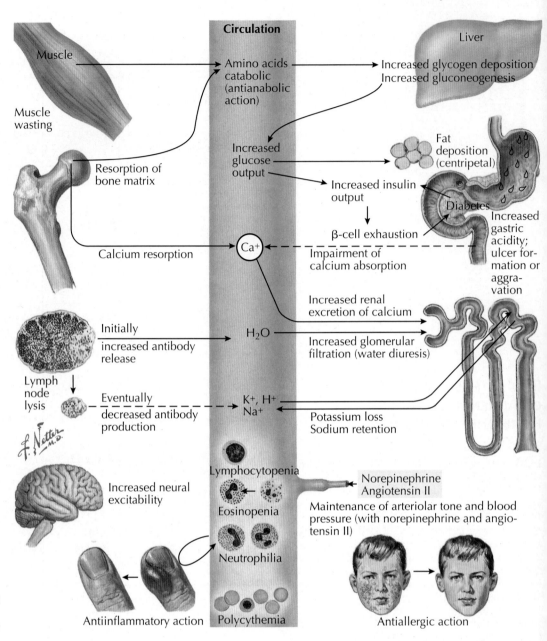

nodes, and bone marrow), inhibit immunoglobulin synthesis, stimulate lymphocyte apoptosis, and inhibit proinflammatory cytokine production. Glucocorticoid administration also increases blood neutrophil counts and decreases eosinophil counts. Another mechanism underlying the antiinflammatory effects of glucocorticoids involves inhibition of monocyte differentiation into macrophages and subsequent macrophage phagocytosis and cytotoxic activity. They reduce the local inflammatory response by preventing the action of histamine and plasminogen activators and by impairing prostaglandin synthesis. A mild polycythemia may be present in patients treated with pharmacologic dosages of glucocorticoids.

CENTRAL NERVOUS SYSTEM AND EYES

Behavioral changes are frequently observed with both excess and deficient glucocorticoids. Depression, euphoria, psychosis, apathy, or lethargy may be observed in patients treated with pharmacologic dosages of glucocorticoids. The increased neuroexcitability frequently

results in insomnia. Depression and lassitude may be seen in individuals with glucocorticoid deficiency. Glucocorticoids may also cause glaucoma by raising intraocular pressure via increased aqueous humor production and prevention of aqueous drainage by matrix deposition in the trabecular meshwork.

GASTROINTESTINAL TRACT

Administration of supraphysiologic dosages of glucocorticoids increases the risk of developing peptic ulcer disease because of increased secretion of hydrochloric acid and pepsin and mucus thinning in the stomach.

ENDOCRINE EFFECTS

Glucocorticoids directly decrease thyrotropin secretion and inhibit 5′ deiodinase activity that converts thyroxine to triiodothyronine. They also inhibit hypothalamic gonadotropin-releasing hormone pulsatility and release of pituitary gonadotropins.

Plate 3.9

Adrenal

CUSHING SYNDROME: CLINICAL FINDINGS

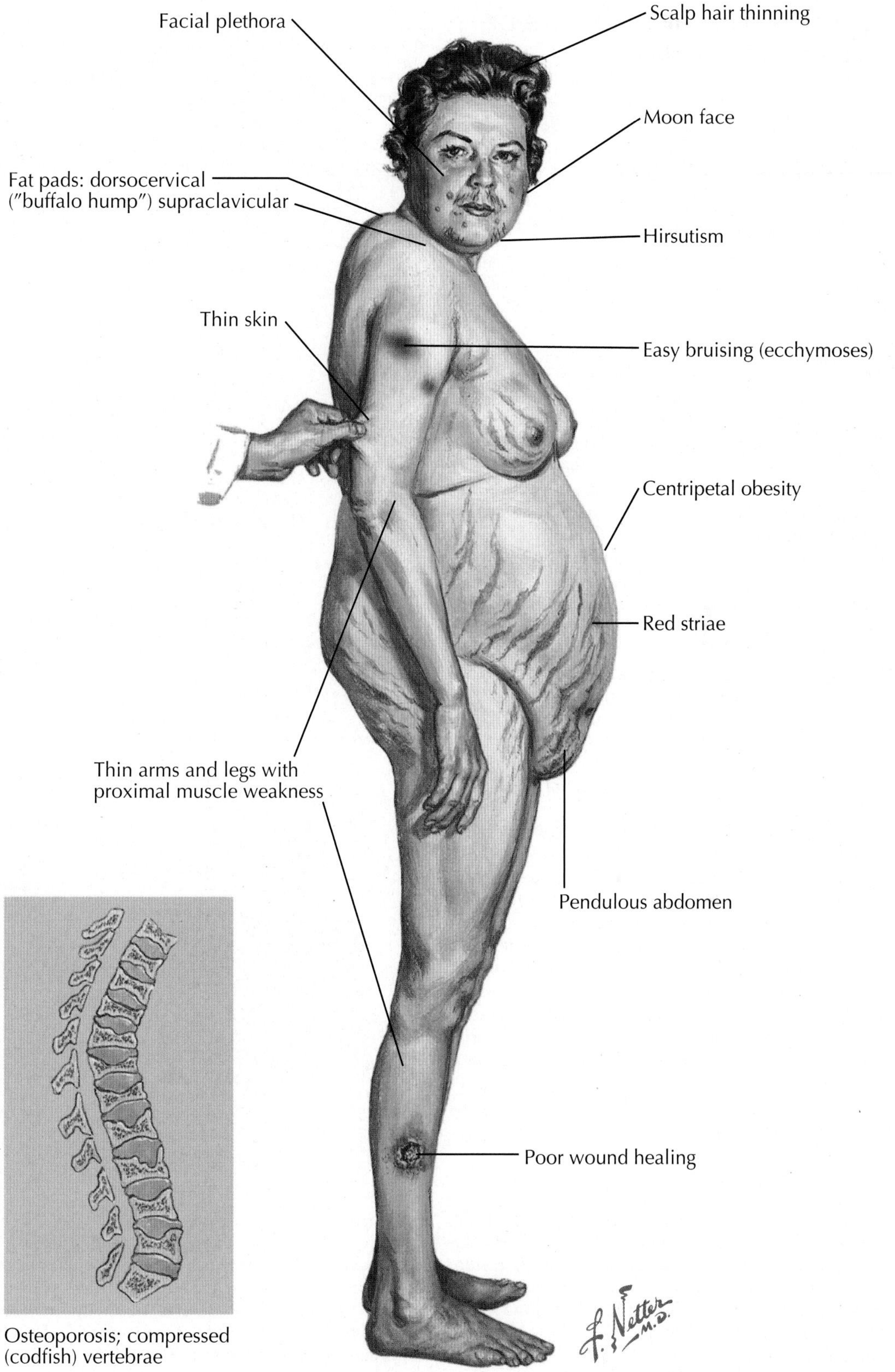

Cushing syndrome is a symptom complex that results from prolonged exposure to supraphysiologic concentrations of glucocorticoids. The most common cause of Cushing syndrome is the use of synthetic glucocorticoids to treat an inflammatory condition, termed *exogenous* or *iatrogenic Cushing syndrome*. Endogenous or spontaneous Cushing syndrome is rare and is caused by hypersecretion of corticotropin (ACTH-dependent Cushing syndrome) or by primary adrenal hypersecretion of glucocorticoids (ACTH-independent Cushing syndrome).

Although Cushing syndrome is not common, the clinical features of hypercortisolism are common. The clinician's role is to (1) recognize Cushing syndrome, (2) confirm endogenous Cushing syndrome with biochemical tests, (3) determine the cause of Cushing syndrome, and (4) provide a definitive cure.

Typical signs and symptoms of Cushing syndrome include weight gain with central (centripetal) obesity; facial rounding with fat deposition in the temporal fossae and cheeks ("moon face") and plethora; supraclavicular fat pads; dorsocervical fat pad ("buffalo hump"); easy ("spontaneous") bruising (ecchymoses); fine "cigarette paper-thin skin" (subcutaneous blood vessels can be seen) that tears easily; poor wound healing; red-purple striae (usually >1 cm in diameter located over the abdomen, flanks, axilla, breasts, hips, and inner thighs); hyperpigmentation over the extensor surfaces and palmar creases (typically only apparent with markedly increased levels of ACTH); scalp hair thinning; proximal muscle weakness associated with muscle loss and resulting in thin extremities; emotional and cognitive changes (e.g., irritability, crying, depression, insomnia, restlessness); hirsutism and hyperandrogenism (e.g., acne); hypertension; osteopenia and osteoporosis with vertebral compression fractures; low back pain (associated with vertebral compression fractures, muscle wasting, and lordotic posture from abdominal weight gain); renal lithiasis; glucose intolerance and diabetes mellitus (caused by glucocorticoid-induced gluconeogenesis and peripheral insulin resistance from increased body fat); polyuria; hyperlipidemia; opportunistic and fungal infections (e.g., mucocutaneous candidiasis, tinea versicolor, pityriasis); menstrual dysfunction (oligomenorrhea or amenorrhea); and infertility. In addition to the preceding features, children with Cushing syndrome may present with generalized obesity and growth retardation.

The clinical features of Cushing syndrome may occur slowly over time; thus comparison of the patient's current appearance with their appearance in old photographs is invaluable. Many of the signs and symptoms in the preceding text are common and are not distinguishing features (e.g., obesity, hypertension, abnormal glucose tolerance, menstrual dysfunction). Clinical suspicion for Cushing syndrome should increase with the simultaneous development of some of the more specific features (e.g., supraclavicular fat pads, wide red-purple striae, proximal muscle weakness). Because of the catabolic effect of glucocorticoids on skeletal muscle, most patients describe difficulty climbing stairs and an inability to rise from a seated position without using their arms. Cortisol has no androgenic activity, and the presence of hirsutism and acne depends on androgen excess, a finding more common in females with ACTH-dependent Cushing syndrome or adrenocortical carcinoma (ACC). The most common form of facial hair associated with Cushing syndrome in

females is thin vellus hair over the sideburn area, cheeks, and upper lip. When Cushing syndrome is caused by an adrenal adenoma, it typically secretes only cortisol.

Standard laboratory studies may reveal fasting hyperglycemia, hyperlipidemia, hypokalemia (from glucocorticoid activity at the mineralocorticoid receptor), leukocytosis with relative lymphopenia, and albuminuria. Marked hypokalemia and severe hypertension are more common in persons with the more severe

hypercortisolism of ectopic ACTH syndrome or ACC. When bone mineral density is measured, most patients with Cushing syndrome have osteoporosis. Causation is multifactorial and includes decreased intestinal calcium absorption, increased bone resorption, decreased bone formation, and decreased renal calcium reabsorption. These patients are also at increased risk for thrombophlebitis and thromboembolic events. Untreated Cushing syndrome can be lethal.

Facial plethora · Scalp hair thinning · Moon face · Fat pads: dorsocervical ("buffalo hump") supraclavicular · Hirsutism · Thin skin · Easy bruising (ecchymoses) · Centripetal obesity · Red striae · Thin arms and legs with proximal muscle weakness · Pendulous abdomen · Poor wound healing

Osteoporosis; compressed (codfish) vertebrae

Plate 3.10

Endocrine System: VOLUME 2

TESTS USED IN THE DIAGNOSIS OF CUSHING SYNDROME

The evaluation of Cushing syndrome can be considered in three steps: (1) case-detection testing, (2) confirmatory testing, and (3) subtype testing.

CASE-DETECTION TESTING

Case detection testing should start with measurements of 24-hour UFC, 11 PM salivary cortisol, and serum cortisol concentrations measured at 8 AM and 4 PM. Unfortunately, the diagnosis of the Cushing syndrome is usually not straightforward. For example, a normal 24-hour UFC value does not exclude Cushing syndrome—10% to 15% of patients with Cushing syndrome have normal 24-hour UFC excretion in one of four measurements. In addition, all forms of endogenous Cushing syndrome can produce cortisol in a cyclical fashion that confounds the biochemical documentation and interpretation of suppression testing. If the clinical suspicion for Cushing syndrome is high and the 24-hour UFC excretion results are normal, obtaining multiple 24-hour UFC measurements is indicated (e.g., every month for 4 months). The baseline 24-hour UFC measurements may also be increased by alcoholism, depression, severe illness, or high urine volume (>4 L). When measured by tandem mass spectrometry, the upper limit of the reference range for 24-hour UFC is 45 µg (124 nmol).

Salivary cortisol concentrations, obtained at 11 PM, are 92% sensitive for Cushing syndrome. Lack of diurnal variation in serum cortisol concentrations is a finding that is also supportive evidence for glucocorticoid secretory autonomy.

The 1-mg overnight dexamethasone suppression test (DST) is an additional case-detection test. At 11 PM, 1 mg of dexamethasone is administered, and serum cortisol is measured the next morning at 8 AM. The serum cortisol concentration in healthy persons suppresses to below 1.8 µg/dL (50 nmol/L). In addition to Cushing syndrome, causes for cortisol nonsuppression with the overnight 1-mg DST include patient error in taking dexamethasone, increased CBG (e.g., with estrogen therapy or pregnancy), obesity, ingestion of a drug that accelerates dexamethasone metabolism (e.g., anticonvulsants, phenobarbital, primidone, rifampin), renal failure, alcoholism, psychiatric disorder (e.g., depression), stress, or laboratory error.

CONFIRMATORY TESTING

Additional confirmatory studies are not needed if the baseline 24-hour UFC excretion is more than 200 µg/24 h (>552 nmol/24 h) and the clinical picture is consistent with Cushing syndrome. However, when the clinical findings are "soft" and when the 24-hour UFC excretion is less than 200 µg/24 h (<552 nmol/24 h), autonomous hypercortisolism should be confirmed with the 2-day low-dose DST (dexamethasone, 0.5 mg orally every 6 hours for 48 hours). A 24-hour UFC excretion more than 10 µg/24 h (28 nmol/24 h) confirms the diagnosis. However, the 2-day low-dose DST is far from perfect (79% sensitivity, 74% specificity, and 71% accuracy). The 2-day low-dose DST works best when the clinician has a low index of suspicion for Cushing syndrome. If clinical suspicion is high, normal suppression with the 2-day low-dose DST does not exclude ACTH-dependent Cushing syndrome; patients with mild pituitary-dependent disease can demonstrate suppression with low-dose DST.

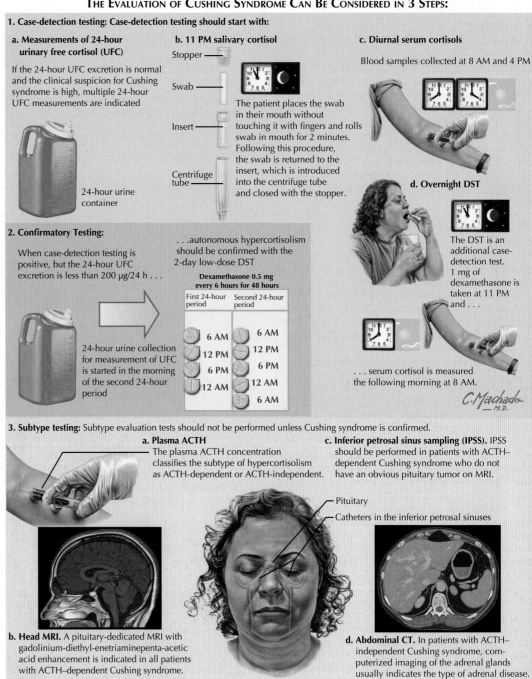

THE EVALUATION OF CUSHING SYNDROME CAN BE CONSIDERED IN 3 STEPS:

1. Case-detection testing: Case-detection testing should start with:

a. Measurements of 24-hour urinary free cortisol (UFC)

If the 24-hour UFC excretion is normal and the clinical suspicion for Cushing syndrome is high, multiple 24-hour UFC measurements are indicated

24-hour urine container

b. 11 PM salivary cortisol

Stopper

Swab

Insert

Centrifuge tube

The patient places the swab in their mouth without touching it with fingers and rolls swab in mouth for 2 minutes. Following this procedure, the swab is returned to the insert, which is introduced into the centrifuge tube and closed with the stopper.

c. Diurnal serum cortisols

Blood samples collected at 8 AM and 4 PM

d. Overnight DST

The DST is an additional case-detection test. 1 mg of dexamethasone is taken at 11 PM and . . .

. . . serum cortisol is measured the following morning at 8 AM.

2. Confirmatory Testing:

When case-detection testing is positive, but the 24-hour UFC excretion is less than 200 µg/24 h . . .

. . . autonomous hypercortisolism should be confirmed with the 2-day low-dose DST

24-hour urine collection for measurement of UFC is started in the morning of the second 24-hour period

Dexamethasone 0.5 mg every 6 hours for 48 hours

First 24-hour period	Second 24-hour period
6 AM	6 AM
12 PM	12 PM
6 PM	6 PM
12 AM	12 AM
	6 AM

3. Subtype testing: Subtype evaluation tests should not be performed unless Cushing syndrome is confirmed.

a. Plasma ACTH The plasma ACTH concentration classifies the subtype of hypercortisolism as ACTH-dependent or ACTH-independent.

c. Inferior petrosal sinus sampling (IPSS). IPSS should be performed in patients with ACTH–dependent Cushing syndrome who do not have an obvious pituitary tumor on MRI.

Pituitary

Catheters in the inferior petrosal sinuses

b. Head MRI. A pituitary-dedicated MRI with gadolinium-diethyl-enetriaminepenta-acetic acid enhancement is indicated in all patients with ACTH–dependent Cushing syndrome.

d. Abdominal CT. In patients with ACTH–independent Cushing syndrome, computerized imaging of the adrenal glands usually indicates the type of adrenal disease.

C. Machado —M.D.

SUBTYPE TESTING

Subtype evaluation tests should not be performed unless Cushing syndrome is confirmed. The application of these tests should be personalized; there is no algorithm that can be applied to all patients with Cushing syndrome. Many of these tests may be superfluous and would delay lifesaving therapy in patients with severe clinical Cushing syndrome.

The plasma ACTH concentration classifies the subtype of hypercortisolism as ACTH dependent (normal to high levels of ACTH) or ACTH independent (undetectable ACTH). Pituitary-dedicated magnetic resonance imaging (MRI) with gadolinium-diethylenetriamine pentaacetic acid enhancement is indicated in all patients with ACTH-dependent Cushing syndrome. If a definite pituitary tumor is found (≥4 mm or larger) and the clinical scenario is consistent with pituitary disease (e.g., female gender, slow onset of disease, and baseline 24-hour UFC < fivefold increase above the reference range), then additional studies are usually not required before definitive treatment. Smaller apparent pituitary lesions (<4 mm) are common in healthy persons and should be considered nonspecific; inferior petrosal sinus sampling (IPSS) should be performed. Also, if the pituitary MRI findings are normal (seen in ~50% of patients with pituitary-dependent Cushing syndrome), performing IPSS should be considered.

In patients with ACTH-independent Cushing syndrome, computed tomography (CT) imaging of the adrenal glands usually indicates the type of adrenal disease—adrenal adenoma (usually 3–6 cm in diameter), ACC (usually 5–20 cm in diameter), bilateral macronodular hyperplasia (massive nodular bilateral adrenal enlargement), or primary pigmented nodular adrenocortical disease (PPNAD) (on CT, the adrenal glands may appear normal or micronodular).

Plate 3.11

Adrenal

CUSHING SYNDROME: PATHOPHYSIOLOGY

The underlying pathophysiology of endogenous Cushing syndrome is either ACTH dependent or ACTH independent.

ACTH-dependent Cushing syndrome results in bilateral adrenocortical hyperplasia. An ACTH-secreting pituitary adenoma (Cushing disease) is the most common cause of endogenous hypercortisolism. Tumorous ectopic hypersecretion of ACTH (ectopic ACTH syndrome) or CRH are less common causes. Eutopic CRH hypersecretion is a very rare cause.

ACTH-independent Cushing syndrome may be caused by adrenocortical adenoma, ACC, primary bilateral macronodular adrenal hyperplasia (PBMAH), or PPNAD (see Plate 3.12).

The clinical presentation of Cushing syndrome is determined by the underlying pathophysiology. When there are markedly excessive adrenal androgens (e.g., with ectopic ACTH syndrome or ACC), hirsutism, acne, and scalp hair recession may be prominent. When the cortisol levels are markedly increased (e.g., with ectopic ACTH syndrome), severe hypertension and hypokalemia may be prominent. When the hypercortisolism develops slowly over years (e.g., pituitary-dependent Cushing syndrome, PBMAH, or PPNAD), central obesity, osteoporosis, and proximal muscle weakness may be the most prominent features. With markedly increased levels of ACTH (e.g., with ectopic ACTH syndrome or pituitary macroadenoma-dependent Cushing syndrome), skin hyperpigmentation may be a prominent feature.

ACTH-DEPENDENT CUSHING SYNDROME

Most patients with Cushing syndrome have pituitary-dependent disease. Approximately 95% of pituitary corticotroph tumors are microadenomas ($\leq$10 mm), and 50% of the time they are not visible on pituitary-dedicated MRI. The serum ACTH concentrations in patients with ACTH-secreting microadenomas are typically in the reference range but are inappropriate for the prevailing hypercortisolism. In contrast, the serum ACTH concentrations in patients with ACTH-secreting macroadenomas are usually above the reference range and may result in hyperpigmentation. The increased blood concentrations of ACTH result in bilateral adrenocortical hyperplasia and hypersecretion of cortisol. The adrenal cortices are typically mildly hyperplastic and typically weigh 6 to 12 g each (the normal adrenal gland weight is 4–6 g each). With ectopic ACTH syndrome, the adrenal glands usually weigh more than 12 g each.

The signs and symptoms, as well as the pathology, of Cushing syndrome are primarily caused by excess cortisol, but adrenal androgens may be elevated, and there may be excess mineralocorticoid effect. When a

corticotroph adenoma of the pituitary is the source of excess ACTH, histologic sections of the pituitary gland typically demonstrate a pituitary microadenoma that stains for ACTH on immunohistochemistry, and the surrounding nontumorous corticotrophs are hyalinized—known as *Crooke hyaline change*. The latter is also seen in all forms of hypercortisolism (e.g., ectopic ACTH, adrenal dependent, and exogenous). It is atrophy of the normally ACTH-producing basophilic corticotrophs because of negative feedback by cortisol. The corticotroph adenoma cells are relatively resistant to negative feedback inhibition by cortisol. The blood concentration of DHEA-S—an ACTH-dependent adrenal androgen—is mildly increased in patients with pituitary-dependent Cushing syndrome. Selective transnasal endoscopic adenectomy is the treatment of choice for patients with ACTH-secreting pituitary tumors.

The nonpituitary tumor hypersecretion of ACTH in the ectopic ACTH syndrome results in marked bilateral adrenocortical hyperplasia and hypercortisolism. The increased serum cortisol concentrations inhibit hypothalamic CRH and pituitary ACTH secretion. The most common cause of ectopic ACTH syndrome is a bronchial carcinoid tumor. Other tumors that can produce ACTH include small cell lung cancer, medullary thyroid carcinoma, thymic carcinoid, pancreatic neuroendocrine tumors, and pheochromocytoma. The mineralocorticoid excess state caused by ectopic ACTH secretion is related to the high rates of cortisol production that overwhelm 11β-hydroxysteroid dehydrogenase activity, allowing free access of cortisol to the mineralocorticoid receptor. DOC levels may also be increased in severe ACTH-dependent Cushing syndrome and contribute to the hypertension and hypokalemia in this disorder. Complete resection of the ectopic ACTH-secreting tumor is the treatment of choice to cure Cushing syndrome. If the tumor cannot be resected, bilateral laparoscopic adrenalectomy should be considered.

In the rare case of ectopic CRH syndrome, the CRH secretion by the ectopic neoplasm (e.g., bronchial carcinoid tumor, pheochromocytoma) causes pituitary corticotroph hyperplasia and hypersecretion of ACTH.

ACTH-INDEPENDENT CUSHING SYNDROME

In the presence of a cortisol-secreting benign cortical adenoma of the adrenal cortex, there is a complete inhibition of hypothalamic CRH and pituitary ACTH production through the negative feedback mechanism by excess cortisol. Thus the adrenal cortex from the contralateral adrenal and the ipsilateral cortex adjacent to a cortisol-secreting adrenal adenoma become atrophic. Adrenal adenomas typically secrete only cortisol, so that the ACTH-dependent adrenal androgens (measured as DHEA-S in the blood and 17-ketosteroids in the urine) are very low (frequently below the assay limit of detection). To generate enough cortisol secretion to cause clinical Cushing syndrome, cortisol-secreting adrenal adenomas are typically at least 2.5 cm in diameter. Unilateral laparoscopic adrenalectomy is the

treatment of choice to cure Cushing syndrome associated with solitary adrenocortical adenoma.

A carcinoma of the adrenal cortex may be limited to the adrenal gland or may be metastatic (regional lymph nodes or distant to liver and lungs). Here, too, the adjacent cortex and the contralateral adrenal gland cortex become atrophic. Approximately half of ACCs are hormone producing; they may hypersecrete a single hormone or multiple hormones (e.g., glucocorticoids, mineralocorticoids, adrenal androgens). With hormonally active ACCs, the blood concentration of DHEA-S is typically increased. In addition, DOC and aldosterone may be hypersecreted, resulting in hypokalemic hypertension. Open laparotomy with en bloc tumor resection, if possible, is the treatment of choice for ACCs. However, even with apparent curative surgery, the recurrence rate is high, and the overall 5-year survival is 30%.

PBMAH is bilateral massive macronodular cortical hyperplasia (the adrenal glands typically weigh 100–500 g each). The bilateral macronodular appearance on cross-sectional computed imaging is usually diagnostic. In some cases, the pathogenesis of PBMAH involves inappropriate expression of ectopic receptors (e.g., gastric inhibitory polypeptide, β-adrenergic, vasopressin, serotonin, or luteinizing hormone/human chorionic gonadotropin [LH/hCG]) or overexpression of eutopic receptors. The mechanism underlying the promiscuous expression of the ectopic receptors is unknown. It has been shown that cortisol secretion in PBMAH is at least partially regulated by intraadrenal paracrine secretion of ACTH. Another cause of PBMAH is germline pathogenic variants in the armadillo repeat-containing 5 gene (*ARMC5*), which have been found in approximately 25% of patients with apparent sporadic PBMAH and is the major cause of familial PBMAH. Another rare variant of PBMAH is Cushing syndrome associated with McCune-Albright syndrome (see Plate 8.8). McCune-Albright syndrome is caused by an activating somatic pathogenic variant of the alpha-subunit stimulatory guanine nucleotide-binding protein, Gs. Finally, PBMAH can rarely be seen in patients with multiple endocrine neoplasia type 1 (see Plate 8.1). Thus the etiology of PBMAH is heterogeneous. In addition, the presentation is variable and ranges from subclinical glucocorticoid secretory autonomy (subclinical Cushing syndrome) to overt and severe Cushing syndrome.

Patients with PBMAH typically have subclinical Cushing syndrome or mild and slowly progressive Cushing syndrome. For patients with overt Cushing syndrome, bilateral laparoscopic adrenalectomy is the treatment of choice, whereas unilateral adrenalectomy of the larger adrenal can be considered in patients with subclinical or mild Cushing syndrome.

PPNAD may occur in sporadic or familial forms (as part of the Carney complex) (see Plate 3.12). The hypercortisolism in individuals with PPNAD is caused by multiple, small, pigmented, autonomously functioning adrenocortical nodules. Bilateral laparoscopic adrenalectomy is the treatment of choice to cure Cushing syndrome associated with PPNAD.

Plate 3.11

Endocrine System: VOLUME 2

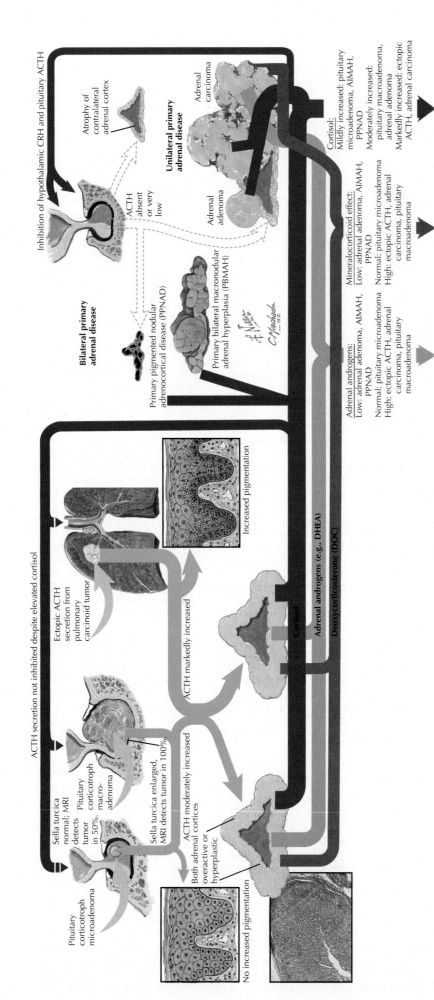

Inhibition of hypothalamic CRH and pituitary ACTH

Atrophy of contralateral adrenal cortex

Unilateral primary adrenal disease

Adrenal carcinoma

ACTH absent or very low

Adrenal adenoma

Bilateral primary adrenal disease

Primary pigmented nodular adrenocortical disease (PPNAD)

Primary bilateral macronodular adrenal hyperplasia (PBMAH)

Cortisol:
Mildly increased: pituitary microadenoma, AIMAH, PPNAD
Moderately increased: pituitary macroadenoma, adrenal adenoma
Markedly increased: ectopic ACTH, adrenal carcinoma

Mineralocorticoid effect:
Low: adrenal adenoma, AIMAH, PPNAD
Normal: pituitary microadenoma
High: ectopic ACTH, adrenal carcinoma, pituitary macroadenoma

Adrenal androgens:
Low: adrenal adenoma, AIMAH, PPNAD
Normal: pituitary microadenoma
High: ectopic ACTH, adrenal carcinoma, pituitary macroadenoma

ACTH secretion not inhibited despite elevated cortisol

Ectopic ACTH secretion from pulmonary carcinoid tumor

Increased pigmentation

Pituitary corticotroph macroadenoma

Sella turcica enlarged, MRI detects tumor in 100%.

ACTH markedly increased

Sella turcica normal; MRI detects tumor in 50%.

Pituitary corticotroph microadenoma

ACTH moderately increased

Both adrenal cortices overactive or hyperplastic

No increased pigmentation

Cortisol

Adrenal androgens (e.g., DHEA)

Deoxycorticosterone (DOC)

Clinical features	Weight gain with central obesity			
	Facial rounding and plethora			
	Supraclavicular and dorsocervical fat pads		Moderate hypertension	
	Easy bruising and poor wound healing			Acne
	Red-purple striae			Hirsutism
	Proximal muscle weakness			Recess of scalp hair
				Clitoral enlargement (rarely)
				Breast atrophy
				Increased libido
Blood	Neutrophilia			
	Relative lymphopenia (less than 20%)		Na+: slightly elevated	DHEA-S: increased
	Relative eosinopenia		K+: normal or low	Androstenedione: increased
	Hyperglycemia		Plasma renin activity: low	Testosterone: increased
	Cortisol: increased and lack of diurnal variation		DOC or aldosterone: high	
Saliva	Midnight salivary cortisol: increased			
Urine	24-hour urinary cortisol: increased		24-hour urinary aldosterone: increased	17–ketosteroids: increased
	Hypercalciuria			

Plate 3.12   Adrenal

CUSHING SYNDROME IN A PATIENT WITH THE CARNEY COMPLEX

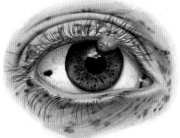

The Carney complex is characterized by spotty skin pigmentation. Pigmented lentigines and blue nevi can be seen on the face—including the eyelids, vermilion borders of the lips, the conjunctivae, the sclera—and the labia and scrotum.

CARNEY COMPLEX: CUSHING SYNDROME CAUSED BY PRIMARY PIGMENTED NODULAR ADRENOCORTICAL DISEASE

A rare form of Cushing syndrome is ACTH-independent PPNAD, which may be sporadic or familial (as part of the Carney complex; MIM #160980). The hypercortisolism in individuals with PPNAD is caused by multiple, pigmented, autonomously functioning adrenocortical nodules. Patients with PPNAD may present with the typical signs and symptoms of hypercortisolism, including central weight gain, hyperglycemia, proximal muscle weakness, purple-red abdominal striae, hypertension, and menstrual cycle disturbance. However, patients with PPNAD tend to be young (i.e., younger than 30 years), have mild signs and symptoms related to hypercortisolism, have marked osteoporosis (presumably because of long-standing mild hypercortisolism before clinical detection), and may have cyclic disease. Baseline hormonal evaluation documents increased levels of cortisol in the blood and urine, suppressed ACTH, suppressed serum DHEA-S, and a paradoxical increase in UFC with DST.

In patients with this disease, the adrenal glands are usually of normal size, and most are studded with black, brown, or red nodules ranging in size from 1 mm to 3 cm. Most of the pigmented nodules are smaller than 4 mm in diameter and are interspersed in the adjacent atrophic cortex. The weight of a PPNAD adrenal gland is either normal (e.g., 4 g) or mildly enlarged (e.g., 5–15 g). The cells in the PPNAD nodules contain granular brown pigment (lipofuscin) and are globular with clear or eosinophilic cytoplasm.

In 66% of cases, PPNAD occurs as part of the Carney complex. Carney complex is characterized by spotty skin pigmentation (pigmented lentigines and blue nevi on the face—including the eyelids, vermilion borders of the lips, the conjunctivae, and the sclera—and the labia and scrotum) in 80% of patients; myxomas (cardiac atrium, cutaneous, and mammary) in 50% of patients; Cushing syndrome due to PPNAD in 40% of patients; testicular large-cell calcifying Sertoli cell tumors in 75% of male patients; growth hormone-secreting pituitary adenomas in 10% of patients; and psammomatous melanotic schwannomas in 10% of patients.

Heterozygous inactivating pathogenic variants in *PRKAR1A*—an apparent tumor suppressor gene that

Additional features of the Carney complex can include:

▶ Myxomas: cardiac atrium, cutaneous (e.g., eyelid), and mammary

▶ Testicular large-cell calcifying Sertoli cell tumors

▶ Growth hormone–secreting pituitary adenomas

▶ Psammomatous melanotic schwannomas

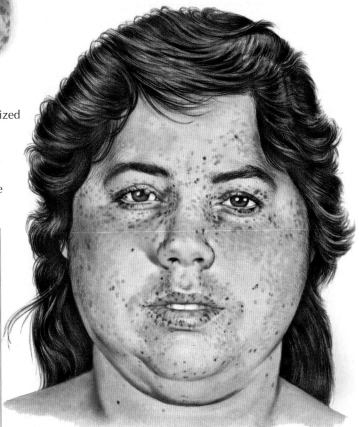

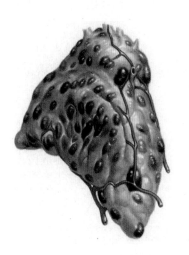

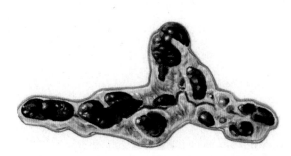

PPNAD adrenal glands are usually of normal size, and most are studded with black, brown, or red nodules. Most of the pigmented nodules are less than 4 mm in diameter and interspersed in the adjacent atrophic cortex.

encodes the protein kinase A regulatory 1α subunit—are found in approximately 70% of patients with the Carney complex. In most familial cases, the Carney complex appears to be autosomal dominant in inheritance with high penetrance but heterogeneous expression. Germline pathogenic variants in *PRKAR1A* may also be present in patients with isolated PPNAD. Approximately 75% of the cases of the Carney complex are familial; 25% of cases occur sporadically, as a result of a de novo mutation.

Even more rare forms of micronodular bilateral hyperplasia that cause Cushing syndrome are associated with nonpigmented nodules and due to pathogenic variants in the phosphodiesterase 11A isoform 4 (*PDE11A* gene) or phosphodiesterase 8B (*PDE8B* gene).

Bilateral laparoscopic adrenalectomy is the treatment of choice to cure Cushing syndrome associated with PPNAD.

Plate 3.13

Endocrine System: VOLUME 2

MAJOR BLOCKS IN ABNORMAL STEROIDOGENESIS

Genetically determined deficiencies in the enzymes responsible for the biosynthesis of cortisol are referred to as *blocks in adrenal steroidogenesis*. Congenital adrenal hyperplasia (CAH) refers to clinical disorders associated with the decreased production of cortisol and the secondary ACTH-driven increased production of precursor steroids that have precursor-specific activity at the mineralocorticoid or androgen receptors.

CONGENITAL LIPOID HYPERPLASIA

The StAR mobilizes cholesterol from the outer mitochondrial membrane to the inner mitochondrial membrane, where the rate-limiting steroid side-chain cleavage enzyme (P450scc) cleaves cholesterol to pregnenolone. Pathogenic variants in the genes encoding either StAR or P450scc result in congenital lipoid adrenal hyperplasia, the most severe form of CAH. This disorder is characterized by a deficiency in all adrenal and gonadal steroid hormones and an ACTH-driven buildup of cholesterol esters in the adrenal cortex. Congenital lipoid adrenal hyperplasia is an autosomal recessive disorder usually caused by pathogenic variants in the gene that encodes StAR. The steroidogenic defect progresses with age, suggesting that the cholesterol ester accumulation causes further dysfunction of the adrenocortical cells.

3β-HYDROXYSTEROID DEHYDROGENASE DEFICIENCY

Pregnenolone is converted to progesterone by 3β-HSD by a reaction involving dehydrogenation of the 3-hydroxyl group to a keto group and isomerization of the double bond at C5. The type I isoenzyme of 3β-HSD (3β-HSD1) is present in the placenta, liver, and brain, and the type II isoenzyme of 3β-HSD (3β-HSD2) is present in the adrenal cortex and gonads. Pathogenic variants in the 3β-HSD2 gene (*HSD3B2*) cause a rare form of CAH associated with deficiencies in cortisol, aldosterone, and gonadal steroids. Because of the block at 3β-HSD2, there is an accumulation of Δ^5-pregnenolone, 17α-hydroxypregnenolone, DHEA, and DHEA-S.

17α-HYDROXYLASE DEFICIENCY

Progesterone is hydroxylated to 17-hydroxyprogesterone through the activity of 17α-hydroxylase (P450c17). 17-Hydroxylation is a prerequisite for glucocorticoid synthesis (the zona glomerulosa does not express P450c17). P450c17 also possesses 17,20-lyase activity, which results in the production of the C19 adrenal androgens (DHEA and androstenedione). Deficiency of P450c17 is another rare form of CAH caused by pathogenic variants in *CYP17A1*. It is inherited in an autosomal recessive fashion and causes an ACTH-driven increased production of 11-deoxycorticosterone and corticosterone—both of which have some activity at the mineralocorticoid receptor—leading to hypokalemia and hypertension. The deficiency in 17,20-lyase activity results in decreased androgen and estrogen production because the androgen substrate is not present to be aromatized to estrogens.

21-HYDROXYLASE DEFICIENCY

21-Hydroxylation of either progesterone in the zona glomerulosa or 17-hydroxyprogesterone in the zona fasciculata is performed by 21-hydroxylase (P450c21) to yield 11-deoxycorticosterone or 11-deoxycortisol, respectively. Deficiency of P450c21 is the most common form of CAH, accounting for more than 90% of cases. Pathogenic variants in the *P450c21* gene result in 21-hydroxylase deficiency, which is inherited in an autosomal recessive fashion and leads to an ACTH-driven increased production of progesterone, 17-hydroxyprogesterone, and adrenal androgens.

11β-HYDROXYLASE DEFICIENCY

The final step in cortisol biosynthesis is the conversion of 11-deoxycortisol to cortisol by 11β-hydroxylase (P450c11β). Deficiency of P450c11β is the second most common form of CAH. 11β-Hydroxylase deficiency is inherited in an autosomal recessive fashion and leads to an ACTH-driven buildup of 11-deoxycortisol, 11-deoxycorticosterone, and adrenal androgens. This disorder is caused by pathogenic variants in the *CYP11B1* gene.

Additional Enzymatic Steps

In the zona glomerulosa, aldosterone synthase (P450c11AS) converts corticosterone to aldosterone via the intermediate 18-hydroxycorticosterone. Whereas aldosterone secretion is confined to the zona glomerulosa through the restricted expression of aldosterone synthase, the zona glomerulosa cannot synthesize cortisol because it does not express 17α-hydroxylase. In the zona reticularis, high levels of cytochrome b5 facilitate 17,20-lyase activity on P450c17 and the production of DHEA. DHEA is either converted to androstenedione by 3β-HSD or sulfated in the zona reticularis by the DHEA sulfotransferase to form DHEA-S. Androstenedione may be converted to testosterone by 17β-ketosteroid reductase (17β-HSD3) in the adrenal glands or gonads. The interconversion of cortisol and cortisone via 11β-HSD regulates local corticosteroid hormone action. There are two distinct 11β-HSD isozymes. 11β-HSD1 is expressed primarily in the liver and converts cortisone to cortisol; 11β-HSD2 is found in the MR in the kidney, colon, and salivary glands and inactivates cortisol to cortisone.

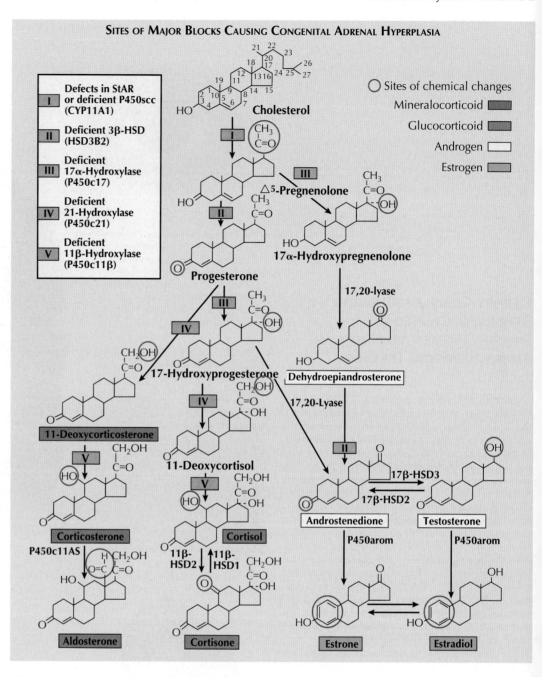

SITES OF MAJOR BLOCKS CAUSING CONGENITAL ADRENAL HYPERPLASIA

Plate 3.14

Adrenal

CLASSIC CONGENITAL ADRENAL HYPERPLASIA

CAH refers to the clinical disorders associated with the decreased production of cortisol because of blocks in the cortisol synthetic enzyme pathway (see Plate 3.13). With decreased cortisol production, there is a secondary ACTH-driven buildup of precursor steroids that have precursor-specific activity at the mineralocorticoid or androgen receptors. In addition, depending on the site of enzymatic deficiency, deficiency of mineralocorticoid or androgen production may occur. Depending on the mutation and resultant degree of protein dysfunction, the deficiency in adrenal enzyme activity may be severe or mild. The most severe forms of CAH are referred to as *classic,* and the milder forms of CAH are referred to as *late-onset* or *nonclassic* (see Plate 3.16).

CONGENITAL LIPOID HYPERPLASIA

Pathogenic variants in the genes encoding either the StAR or the steroid side-chain cleavage enzyme (P450scc) result in congenital lipoid adrenal hyperplasia, the most severe form of CAH. This disorder is characterized by a deficiency in all adrenal and gonadal steroid hormones and an ACTH-driven buildup of cholesterol esters in the adrenal cortex. Neonates with congenital lipoid hyperplasia usually present with signs and symptoms of marked adrenocortical insufficiency (e.g., hyperemesis, hypotension, hyperkalemia, hyponatremia) shortly after birth. Because of the lack of testicular androgen production, infants with a 46,XY karyotype have female external genitalia (see Plates 4.13 and 4.15). Laboratory testing shows low serum cortisol and PACs and increased serum ACTH concentration and PRA. If not recognized and treated, congenital lipoid hyperplasia is lethal. Treatment consists of glucocorticoid and mineralocorticoid replacement.

3β-HYDROXYSTEROID DEHYDROGENASE DEFICIENCY

Pregnenolone is converted to progesterone by 3β-HSD. Pathogenic variants in the 3β-HSD2 gene (*HSD3B2*) cause a rare form of CAH associated with deficiency in cortisol, aldosterone, and gonadal steroids. The clinical presentation of CAH caused by 3β-HSD deficiency is similar to that of StAR deficiency—infants present with signs and symptoms of both cortisol and aldosterone deficiencies. The excess DHEA may cause mild virilization in infants with a 46,XX karyotype. The phenotype in infants with a 46,XY karyotype varies from normal to hypospadias to female external genitalia. Late-onset forms of 3β-HSD also exist (see Plate 3.16). In addition to hyperkalemia, hyponatremia, cortisol deficiency, and aldosterone deficiency, laboratory studies show increased baseline blood concentrations of DHEA and DHEA-S. Because most of the adrenal androstenedione production is dependent on the conversion of DHEA to androstenedione by 3β-HSD, androstenedione levels are

not increased in this form of CAH. Exaggerated increases in the blood concentrations of Δ^5-pregnenolone and DHEA are observed with the cosyntropin-stimulation test. Patients who are affected are treated with glucocorticoid and mineralocorticoid replacement and, at puberty, with gonadal steroid replacement.

17α-HYDROXYLASE DEFICIENCY

Progesterone is hydroxylated to 17-hydroxyprogesterone through the activity of 17α-hydroxylase (P450c17). 17α-Hydroxylase deficiency is a rare form of CAH caused by pathogenic variants in *CYP17A1.* It is inherited in an autosomal recessive fashion and causes ACTH-driven increased production of 11-deoxycorticosterone and corticosterone—both of which have some activity at the mineralocorticoid receptor—leading to hypokalemia and hypertension. The deficiency in 17,20-lyase activity results in decreased androgen and estrogen production because the androgen substrate is not present to be aromatized to estrogens. The clinical presentation may not occur until puberty when individuals with a 46,XX karyotype are found to have primary amenorrhea, absent secondary sexual development, hypertension, and hypokalemia. Individuals with a 46,XY karyotype, who are phenotypically female, are usually not evaluated until the lack of pubertal development; they have female external genitalia, intraabdominal testes, short vagina, absent uterus and fallopian tubes, hypertension, and hypokalemia (see Plate 4.15). Laboratory studies show hypokalemia, low PRA, and low PAC. Blood concentrations of ACTH, progesterone, 11-deoxycorticosterone, LH, and follicle-stimulating hormone are increased. Decreased blood concentrations of 17-hydroxyprogesterone, 11-deoxycortisol, cortisol, DHEA, DHEA-S, androstenedione, testosterone, and estradiol are observed. Treatment includes replacement of glucocorticoid and gonadal steroids.

21-HYDROXYLASE DEFICIENCY

21-Hydroxylation of either progesterone in the zona glomerulosa or 17-hydroxyprogesterone in the zona fasciculata is performed by 21-hydroxylase (P450c21) to yield DOC or 11-deoxycortisol, respectively. Deficiency of P450c21 is the most common form of CAH, accounting for more than 90% of all cases. Classic 21-hydroxylase deficiency presents in infancy with typical signs and symptoms of adrenal insufficiency and androgen excess. Ambiguous genitalia are found in infants with a 46,XX karyotype (see Plate 4.12). Depending on the severity of the enzymatic defect and its effect on the mineralocorticoid synthetic pathway, classic 21-hydroxylase deficiency may be referred to as *salt wasting* or *simple virilizing.* In both forms of classic 21-hydroxylase deficiency, a markedly increased (greater than sixfold above the upper limit of the reference range) blood concentration of 17-hydroxyprogesterone is diagnostic. In borderline cases, a cosyntropin-stimulation test may be needed to demonstrate the enzymatic block. Additional blood tests

usually show low blood concentrations of 11-deoxycortisol, cortisol, 11-deoxycorticosterone, and aldosterone (the latter two in the salt-wasting form). Increased blood concentrations of the following are usually observed: progesterone, 17-hydroxyprogesterone, androstenedione, and ACTH. PRA is usually increased. Newborn screening for 21-hydroxylase deficiency by measuring 17-hydroxyprogesterone in a dried blood sample is routinely performed in the United States and in many other countries.

11β-HYDROXYLASE DEFICIENCY

Deficiency of 11β-hydroxylase (P450c11β) is the second most common form of CAH. With more severe defects in 11β-hydroxylase function, neonates with a 46,XX karyotype are born with ambiguous genitalia, and neonates with a 46,XY karyotype are born with penile enlargement. With *CYP11B1* pathogenic variants that result in decreased, but not absent, 11β-hydroxylase activity, individuals who are affected may present later in childhood with hypertension and precocious puberty or in young adulthood with hypertension, acne, hirsutism, and oligomenorrhea or amenorrhea. Although 11-deoxycortisol has no glucocorticoid activity, 11-deoxycorticosterone has mineralocorticoid activity, and when produced in excess, it can cause hypertension, hypokalemia, low PRA, and low PAC. Additional findings on laboratory testing in patients with 11β-hydroxylase deficiency include increased blood concentrations of 11-deoxycortisol, 11-deoxycorticosterone, DHEA, DHEA-S, androstenedione, and testosterone.

APPARENT MINERALOCORTICOID EXCESS

The interconversion of cortisol and cortisone via 11β-HSD regulates local corticosteroid hormone action. There are two distinct 11β-HSD isozymes. 11β-HSD1 converts cortisone to cortisol; 11β-HSD2 inactivates cortisol to cortisone. Apparent mineralocorticoid excess is the result of impaired 11β-HSD2 activity. Cortisol can be a potent mineralocorticoid, and as a result of the enzyme deficiency, high levels of cortisol accumulate in the kidneys. Thus 11β-HSD2 normally excludes physiologic glucocorticoids from the nonselective MR by converting them to the inactive 11-keto compound, cortisone. Decreased 11β-HSD2 activity may be hereditary or secondary to pharmacologic inhibition of enzyme activity by glycyrrhizic acid, the active component of licorice root (*Glycyrrhiza glabra*) or treatment with triazole antifungals (e.g., posaconazole and itraconazole). The clinical phenotype of patients with apparent mineralocorticoid excess includes hypertension, hypokalemia, metabolic alkalosis, low PRA, low PAC, and normal plasma cortisol levels. The diagnosis is confirmed by demonstrating an abnormal ratio of cortisol to cortisone (e.g., >10:1) in a 24-hour urine collection. The apparent mineralocorticoid excess state caused by ectopic ACTH secretion, seen in patients with Cushing syndrome, is related to the high rates of cortisol production that overwhelm 11β-HSD2 activity.

Plate 3.14

Endocrine System: VOLUME 2

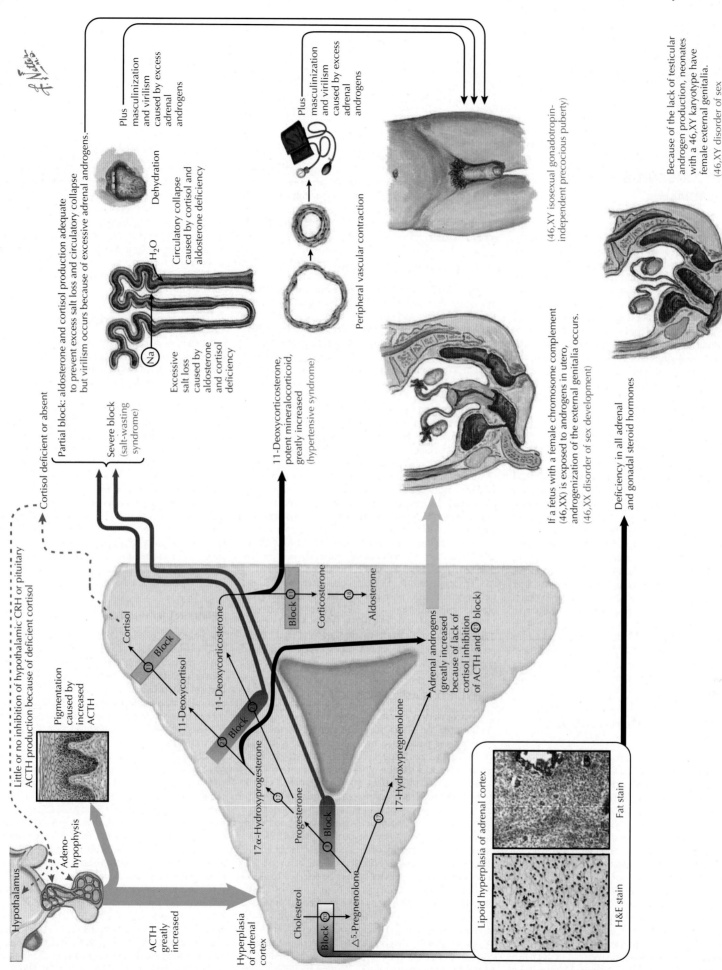

Little or no inhibition of hypothalamic CRH or pituitary ACTH production because of deficient cortisol

Cortisol deficient or absent

Partial block: aldosterone and cortisol production adequate to prevent excess salt loss and circulatory collapse but virilism occurs because of excessive adrenal androgens.

Plus masculinization and virilism caused by excess adrenal androgens

Dehydration

Circulatory collapse caused by cortisol and aldosterone deficiency

Severe block (salt-wasting syndrome)

H₂O

Na

Excessive salt loss caused by aldosterone and cortisol deficiency

11-Deoxycorticosterone, potent mineralocorticoid, greatly increased (hypertensive syndrome)

Plus masculinization and virilism caused by excess adrenal androgens

Peripheral vascular contraction

If a fetus with a female chromosome complement (46,XX) is exposed to androgens in utero, androgenization of the external genitalia occurs. (46,XX disorder of sex development)

(46,XY isosexual gonadotropin-independent precocious puberty)

Because of the lack of testicular androgen production, neonates with a 46,XY karyotype have female external genitalia. (46,XY disorder of sex development)

Pigmentation caused by increased ACTH

Cortisol

Block

11-Deoxycortisol

11-Deoxycorticosterone

Block

17α-Hydroxyprogesterone

Progesterone

Block

Cholesterol

Block

Δ⁵-Pregnenolone

17-Hydroxypregnenolone

Adrenal androgens (greatly increased because of lack of cortisol inhibition of ACTH and block)

Corticosterone

Aldosterone

Block

Deficiency in all adrenal and gonadal steroid hormones

Hypothalamus

Adeno-hypophysis

ACTH greatly increased

Hyperplasia of adrenal cortex

Lipoid hyperplasia of adrenal cortex

Fat stain

H&E stain

Plate 3.15   Adrenal

BIOLOGIC ACTIONS OF ADRENAL ANDROGENS

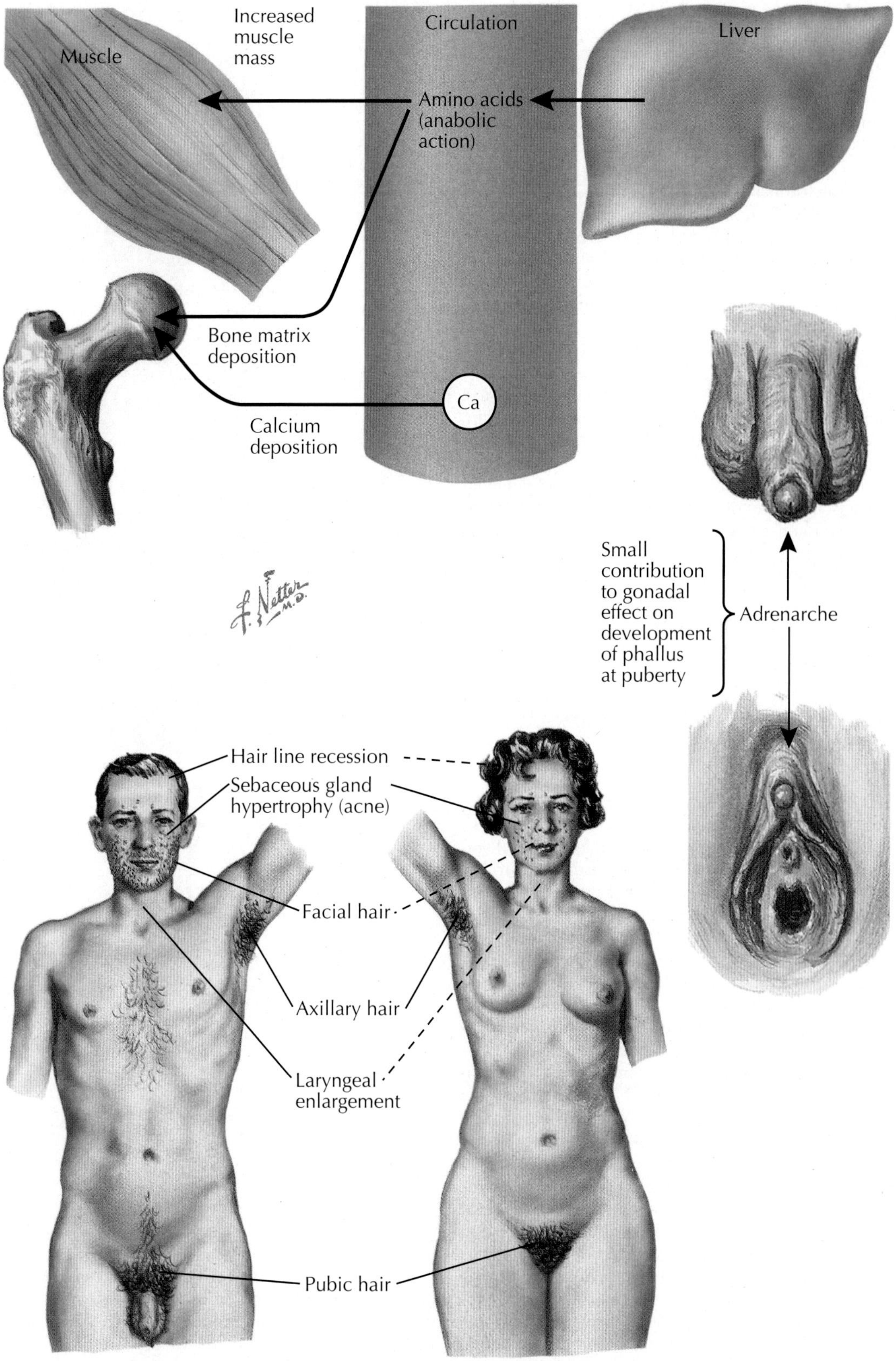

Androgens produced by the adrenal cortex in both sexes include DHEA, DHEA-S, androstenedione, and testosterone. In varying degrees, adrenal androgens have an anabolic effect leading to increased muscle mass. They stimulate male sex characteristics, including an increase in facial hair, recession of the scalp hairline, hypertrophy of sebaceous glands and acne, enlargement of larynx resulting in the deep male voice, secondary sex hair growth in axillary and pubic regions, hair growth over the chest and around the nipples, and development of the phallus in puberty. Although the main source of androgens in males is gonadal, in most females, the adrenal glands are the primary source of androgens. Indeed, a key sign of primary adrenal failure in females is loss of axillary and pubic hair.

Adrenarche is a biochemical event, defined as the increase in adrenal androgens that occurs between 6 and 8 years of age. Pubarche is a phenotypic event, defined as the growth of sexual hair in the suprapubic area and the axillae. Adrenal androgens are the primary factors that facilitate pubic and axillary hair growth in girls; labial hair usually precedes axillary hair growth. In boys, the role of adrenal androgens is not as clear because of the dominant role of testicular testosterone production. Adrenal androgens appear to be an important factor in the onset of puberty and the maturation of the hypothalamic-pituitary-gonadal complex. Adrenarche and pubarche are considered premature when pubic hair growth appears before age 8 years in girls and before age 9 years in boys. Premature adrenarche, which is more common in girls, is associated with taller height, increased body odor and acne, and a bone age that is advanced by 1 to 2 years.

Adrenal androgens may have additional physiologic roles yet to be delineated. DHEA-S may serve as a large sex steroid depot. DHEA-S is converted to testosterone and estradiol in peripheral tissues; a sulfatase converts DHEA-S to DHEA, which is then converted to androstenedione by 3β-hydroxysteroid dehydrogenase. Androstenedione is metabolized to either testosterone or estradiol by 17β-hydroxysteroid dehydrogenase and P450 aromatase, respectively. DHEA may also act as a neurosteroid in the central nervous system (CNS); however, a DHEA-specific receptor has not yet been identified.

Androgenic (anabolic) steroids have been used surreptitiously by athletes to increase muscle mass and to enhance physical performance. The prevalence of their use is difficult to determine, but approximately 6% of high school boys and 2% of high school girls have reported using androgenic steroids at least once. Anabolic steroids are prohibited by the International Olympic Committee and the National Collegiate Athletic Association for use in competition. Athletes often take several performance-enhancing drugs in various patterns (e.g., simultaneously, consecutively, escalating doses, or intermittently) in an attempt to increase the overall effect on performance. Adverse effects include suppression of endogenous testicular function

(resulting in transient infertility and decreased testicular size), gynecomastia (because testosterone is aromatized to estradiol), erythrocytosis, increased liver enzymes and peliosis hepatitis (only with oral 17-α-alkylated androgens), mood disorders and aggressive behavior, decreased serum high-density lipoprotein cholesterol concentrations, increased low-density lipoprotein cholesterol concentrations, virilization in females (e.g., hirsutism, temporal hair recession, acne,

deepening of the voice, and clitoral enlargement), premature epiphyseal fusion, and stunting of growth in adolescents. Athletes may take additional agents to mask the visible side effects of high-dose anabolic steroids; for example, athletes may take hCG to counteract the decrease in testicular size, an aromatase inhibitor or estrogen receptor antagonist to counteract the gynecomastia, and a 5α-reductase inhibitor to prevent balding and acne.

Plate 3.16

Endocrine System: VOLUME 2

ADULT ANDROGENITAL SYNDROMES

Adult adrenogenital syndromes are disorders associated with excess adrenal androgen effects in adults. The causes of adrenal androgen excess in adults include late-onset (nonclassic) CAH, familial glucocorticoid resistance, Cushing syndrome, and androgen-secreting adrenal neoplasms. Because of the presence of more potent testicular androgens, adrenal androgen excess in males may go undetected because of lack of symptomatology. However, females with adrenal androgen excess usually present with varying degrees of masculinization and menstrual dysfunction (see Plates 4.14 and 4.15).

Hirsutism is defined as excessive male-pattern coarse hair growth in females (e.g., cheeks, upper lip, chin, midline chest, male escutcheon, inner thighs, and midline lower back). Virilization, reflecting a more severe form of androgen excess, is defined as the development of signs and symptoms of masculinization in females. The signs and symptoms of masculinization include increased muscle bulk, loss of female body contours, deepening of the voice, breast atrophy, clitoromegaly, temporal balding, and androgenic flush (plethora of the face, neck, and upper chest). The normal size of the clitoris is smaller than 10 mm in length and smaller than 7 mm in width.

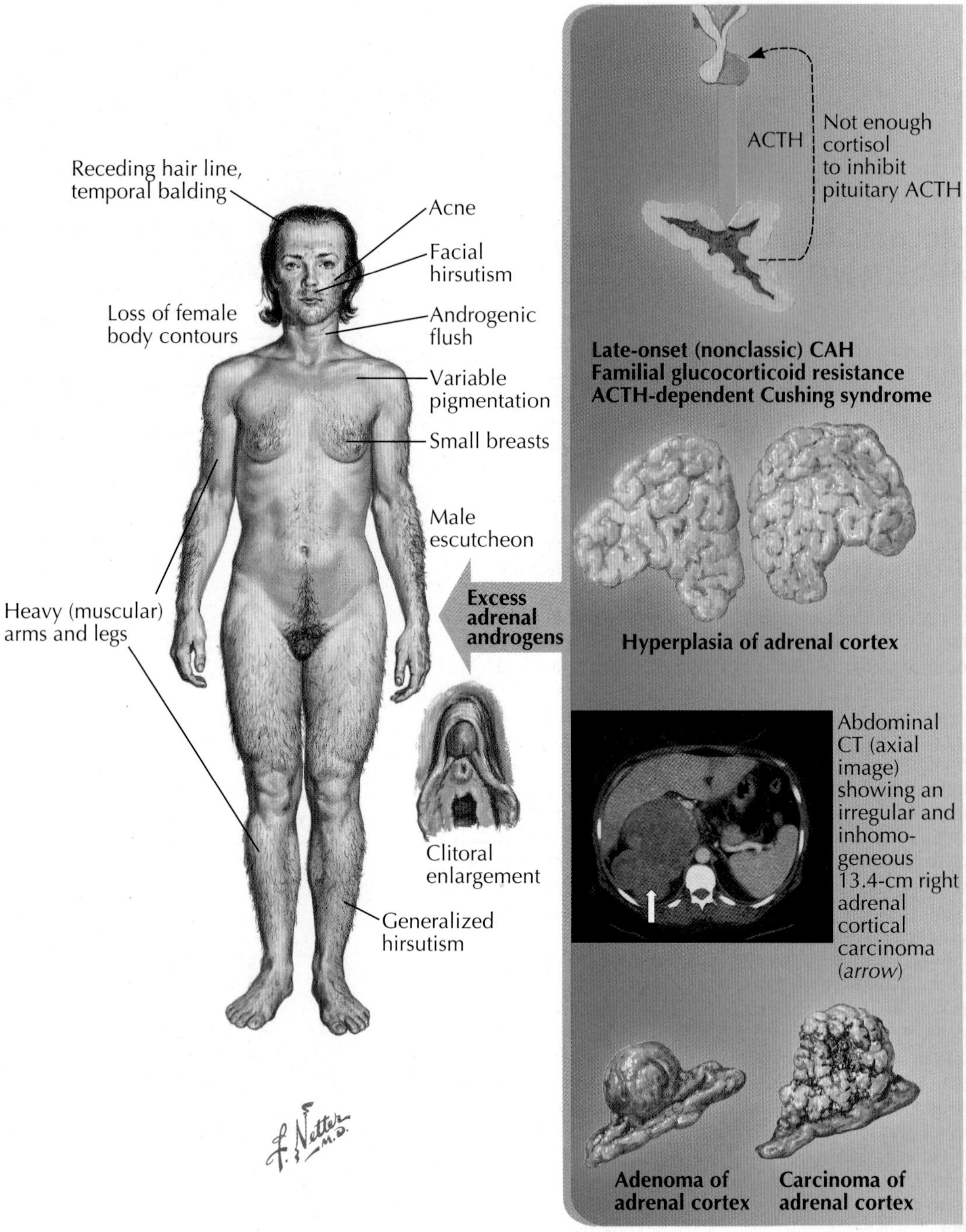

LATE-ONSET (NONCLASSIC) CONGENITAL ADRENAL HYPERPLASIA

Partial enzymatic blocks in 3β-HSD, 21-hydroxylase, and 11β-hydroxylase may all present in late-onset or nonclassic forms (also referred to as *adult-onset, attenuated, incomplete, and cryptic adrenal hyperplasia*) and be responsible for hirsutism, menstrual irregularities, and varying degrees of virilization. Late-onset 3β-HSD deficiency should be suspected in symptomatic females who have markedly increased blood concentrations of DHEA-S and low levels of androstenedione. The diagnosis can be confirmed with cosyntropin-stimulation testing and demonstration of a marked increase in 17-hydroxypregnenolone and DHEA but no increase in 17-hydroxyprogesterone and androstenedione. Late-onset 21-hydroxylase deficiency may have an identical presentation to that of 3β-HSD deficiency, but the laboratory profile is different. With 21-hydroxylase deficiency, the baseline levels of progesterone, 17-hydroxyprogesterone, and androstenedione are increased above the reference range, and all three increase dramatically after cosyntropin stimulation. A partial block at 11β-hydroxylase is associated with increased blood concentrations of 11-deoxycortisol, 11-deoxycorticosterone, DHEA, and androstenedione. In addition to symptoms related to androgen excess, individuals with partial 11β-hydroxylase deficiency may have hypertension and hypokalemia. Cosyntropin-stimulation testing may be needed to confirm the block at 11β-hydroxylase. Treatment for late-onset CAH includes glucocorticoid replacement to suppress the excess ACTH secretion, with the goal of avoiding overtreatment and resultant Cushing syndrome.

FAMILIAL GLUCOCORTICOID RESISTANCE

Familial glucocorticoid resistance is caused by pathogenic variants in the glucocorticoid receptor gene. These pathogenic variants inhibit the action of cortisol, leading to increased ACTH secretion and

adrenocortical hyperplasia. With the increased mass action of cortisol production, there is increased production of adrenal androgens (e.g., DHEA) and mineralocorticoids (e.g., 11-deoxycorticosterone). Thus individuals with familial glucocorticoid resistance present clinically in a very similar way to those with late-onset 11β-hydroxylase deficiency with signs and symptoms of androgen excess, hypertension, and hypokalemia.

ACTH-DEPENDENT CUSHING SYNDROME

The hypersecretion of ACTH in patients with ACTH-dependent Cushing syndrome leads to the production of excess adrenal androgens and weak mineralocorticoids (see Plate 3.9).

ANDROGEN-SECRETING ADRENAL NEOPLASMS

Androgen-secreting adrenal neoplasms are rare. Androgen hypersecretion occurs more often with ACC than with adrenal adenomas. The most common hypersecreted androgen is DHEA, followed by androstenedione and testosterone. The distinction between adenoma and carcinoma can usually be made before surgery on the basis of the imaging phenotype on CT. Whereas testosterone-secreting adenomas are usually small (e.g., 1 cm in diameter), homogeneous, and low unenhanced CT attenuation (e.g., <10 Hounsfield units [HU]), androgen-secreting ACCs are almost always more than 4 cm in diameter (average diameter, 10 cm), are inhomogeneous, and have a high unenhanced CT attenuation (e.g., >20 HU).

Receding hair line, temporal balding

Acne

Facial hirsutism

Androgenic flush

Loss of female body contours

Variable pigmentation

Small breasts

Male escutcheon

Heavy (muscular) arms and legs

Clitoral enlargement

Generalized hirsutism

ACTH — Not enough cortisol to inhibit pituitary ACTH

Late-onset (nonclassic) CAH
Familial glucocorticoid resistance
ACTH-dependent Cushing syndrome

Excess adrenal androgens

Hyperplasia of adrenal cortex

Abdominal CT (axial image) showing an irregular and inhomogeneous 13.4-cm right adrenal cortical carcinoma (*arrow*)

Adenoma of adrenal cortex

Carcinoma of adrenal cortex

Plate 3.17   Adrenal

BIOLOGIC ACTIONS OF ALDOSTERONE

Aldosterone secretion is stimulated by angiotensin II, hyperkalemia, and (to a lesser extent) corticotropin; aldosterone secretion is inhibited by atrial natriuretic factor and hypokalemia. Approximately 50% to 70% of aldosterone circulates bound to either albumin or weakly to corticosteroid-binding globulin; 30% to 50% of total plasma aldosterone is free. Thus aldosterone has a relatively short half-life of 15 to 20 minutes. In the liver, aldosterone is rapidly inactivated to tetrahydroaldosterone. The normal peripheral blood concentration of aldosterone ranges between 0 and 21 ng/dL.

The classic functions of aldosterone are regulation of extracellular volume and control of potassium homeostasis. These effects are mediated by binding of free aldosterone to the MR in the cytosol of epithelial cells, principally the distal tubules in the kidney, where it facilitates the exchange of sodium for potassium and hydrogen ions. The action of angiotensin II on aldosterone involves a negative feedback loop that also includes extracellular fluid volume. The main function of this feedback loop is to modify sodium homeostasis and, secondarily, to regulate blood pressure. Thus sodium restriction activates the renin-angiotensin-aldosterone axis. The effects of angiotensin II on both the adrenal cortex and the renal vasculature promote renal sodium conservation. Conversely, with suppression of renin release and suppression of the level of circulating angiotensin, aldosterone secretion is reduced and renal blood flow is increased, thereby promoting sodium loss. The renin-angiotensin-aldosterone loop is very sensitive to dietary sodium intake. Sodium excess enhances the renal and peripheral vasculature responsiveness and reduces the adrenal responsiveness to angiotensin II. Sodium restriction has the opposite effect. Thus sodium intake modifies target tissue responsiveness to angiotensin II, a fine-tuning that appears to be critical to maintaining normal sodium homeostasis without a chronic effect on blood pressure.

Mineralocorticoid receptors have tissue-specific expression. For example, the tissues with the highest concentrations of these receptors are the distal nephron, colon, and hippocampus. Lower levels of mineralocorticoid receptors are found in the rest of the gastrointestinal tract, sweat glands, salivary glands, and heart. Transport to the nucleus and binding to specific binding domains on targeted genes lead to their increased expression. Aldosterone-regulated kinase appears to be a key intermediary, and its increased expression leads to modification of the apical sodium channel, resulting in increased sodium ion transport across the cell membrane. The increased luminal negativity augments tubular secretion of potassium by the tubular cells and hydrogen ion by the interstitial cells. Glucocorticoids and mineralocorticoids bind equally to the mineralocorticoid receptor. Specificity of action is provided in many tissues by the presence of a glucocorticoid-degrading enzyme, 11β-HSD, which prevents glucocorticoids from interacting with the receptor. Mineralocorticoid "escape" refers to the counterregulatory mechanisms that are manifested after 3 to 5 days of excessive mineralocorticoid administration. Several mechanisms contribute to this escape, including renal hemodynamic factors and an increased level of atrial natriuretic peptide.

In addition to the classic genomic actions mediated by aldosterone binding to cytosolic receptors, mineralocorticoids have acute, nongenomic actions caused by

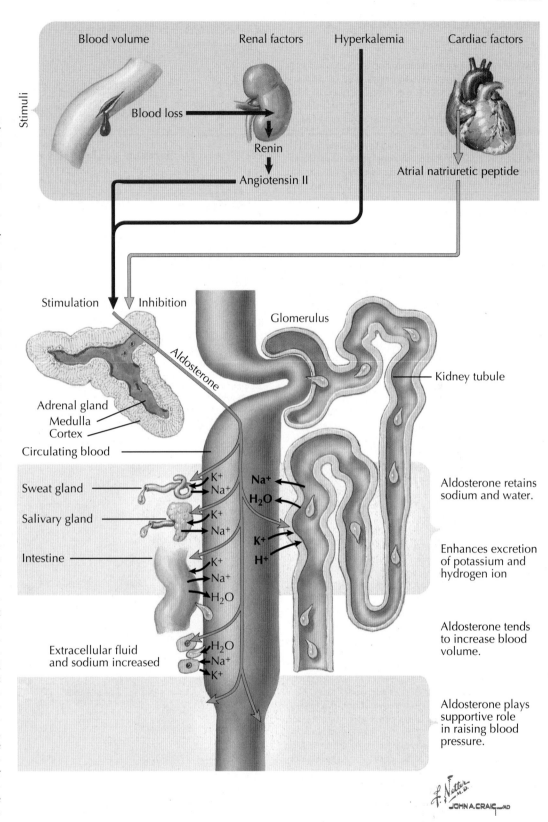

activation of an unidentified cell surface receptor. This action involves a G protein signaling pathway and probably modification of the sodium-hydrogen exchange activity. This effect has been demonstrated in both epithelial and nonepithelial cells.

Aldosterone has additional, nonclassic effects primarily on nonepithelial cells. These actions, although probably genomic and therefore mediated by activation of the cytosolic mineralocorticoid receptor, do not include modification of sodium-potassium balance.

Aldosterone-mediated actions include the expression of several collagen genes; genes controlling tissue growth factors, such as transforming growth factor β and plasminogen activator inhibitor type 1; or genes mediating inflammation. The resultant actions lead to microangiopathy; acute necrosis; and fibrosis in various tissues such as the heart, vasculature, and kidney. Increased levels of aldosterone are not necessary to cause this damage; an imbalance between the volume or sodium balance state and the level of aldosterone appears to be the critical factor.

Plate 3.18

Endocrine System: VOLUME 2

PRIMARY ALDOSTERONISM

Hypertension, suppressed renin, and increased aldosterone secretion characterize the syndrome of primary aldosteronism (PA), which was first described in 1955 by Jerome Conn. Bilateral idiopathic hyperaldosteronism (IHA) and aldosterone-producing adenoma (APA) are the most common subtypes of PA. A much less common form, unilateral adrenal hyperplasia (UAH), is caused by zona glomerulosa hyperplasia of predominantly one adrenal gland. Familial hyperaldosteronism (FH) is an uncommon subset of PA. There are five forms of FH: FH type I or glucocorticoid-remediable aldosteronism due to a *CYP11B1/CYP11B2* chimeric gene; FH type II caused by germline *CLCN2* pathogenic variants; FH type III caused by germline *KCNJ5* pathogenic variants; FH type IV caused by germline *CACNA1H* pathogenic variants; and primary aldosteronism with seizures and neurologic abnormalities caused by germline *CACNA1D* pathogenic variants. Very rarely, excessive aldosterone may be secreted by a neoplasm outside of the adrenal gland (e.g., ovary).

PA is the most common form of identifiable secondary hypertension, affecting 5% to 10% all patients with hypertension. Most patients with PA do not have hypokalemia and present with asymptomatic hypertension, which may be mild or severe. Aldosterone excess results in the renal loss of potassium and hydrogen ions. When hypokalemia does occur, it is usually associated with alkalosis, and patients may present with nocturia and polyuria (caused by hypokalemia-induced failure in renal concentrating ability), palpitations, muscle cramps, or positive Chvostek and Trousseau signs. Identifying PA is important because of its prevalence and association with a higher rate of cardiovascular morbidity and mortality compared with age- and sex-matched patients with primary hypertension and the same degree of blood pressure elevation. In patients diagnosed with PA, surgical cure or treatment with MR antagonists results in reversal or improvement of the hypertension and resolution of the increased cardiovascular risk. Thus all people with hypertension should be tested for PA at least once.

Case detection testing can be completed with a morning (8–10 AM) blood test for measurement of PAC and PRA (or plasma renin concentration [PRC]) in a seated, ambulatory patient. The patient may take any antihypertensive drugs except MR antagonists or high-dose amiloride. A positive case detection test consists of documenting that the PRA or PRC is suppressed (e.g., PRA < 1 ng/mL/h; PRC less than the lower limit of reference range) and that the PAC is inappropriately high for the PRA or PRC (typically >10 ng/dL). Patients with a positive case detection test should undergo confirmatory testing, a step completed with aldosterone-suppression testing (e.g., oral sodium loading, saline-suppression testing, captopril-stimulation testing, or fludrocortisone-suppression testing).

Unilateral adrenalectomy in patients with APA or UAH results in normalization of hypokalemia in all; hypertension is improved in all and is cured in approximately 30% to 60% of these patients. In IHA, unilateral or bilateral adrenalectomy seldom corrects the hypertension. IHA and most patients with familial PA should be treated medically. Therefore for patients who want to pursue a surgical cure, the accurate distinction between the subtypes of PA is a critical step. The subtype evaluation may require one or more tests, the first of which is imaging the adrenal glands with CT. When a small, solitary, hypodense macroadenoma (>1 cm and <2 cm) and normal contralateral adrenal

Mechanisms in primary aldosteronism

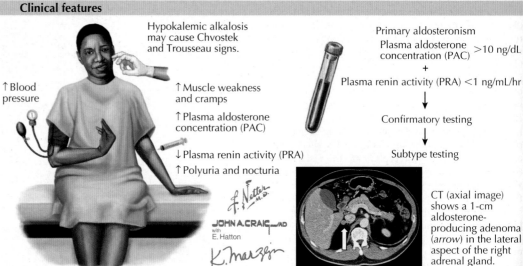

Angiotensinogen

↓ Renin secretion

Angiotensin I

Angiotensin II

Autonomous excessive secretion of aldosterone

↑ Plasma volume
↓ Urinary Na⁺

Stimulation of mineralocorticoid receptors

Atrial natriuretic peptide

Major natriuretic effect in medullary collecting duct

Aldosterone

Autonomous secretion of aldosterone by adrenal adenoma or hyperplasia results in stimulation of renal mineralocorticoid receptors, causing increased sodium and water reabsorption and leading to increased cardiac output. Increased potassium excretion also results.

Increased cardiac output and increased peripheral vascular resistance result in hypertension. Increased vascular resistance results from autoregulation of blood flow as cardiac output increases. Aldosterone also has direct effects on the vasculature.

↑ K⁺, H⁺ excretion
↑ Na⁺ H₂O reabsorption

↑ Plasma volume

Na⁺ excretion (aldosterone escape)

Other natriuretic hormones, pressure natriuresis, and increase in NaCl transporters are activated and favor sodium excretion, preventing peripheral edema.

Increased urinary excretion of potassium

↑ Peripheral vascular resistance   ↑ Cardiac output

Hypokalemia

↑ Blood pressure

Clinical features

Hypokalemic alkalosis may cause Chvostek and Trousseau signs.

↑ Blood pressure

↑ Muscle weakness and cramps

↑ Plasma aldosterone concentration (PAC)

↓ Plasma renin activity (PRA)

↑ Polyuria and nocturia

Primary aldosteronism
Plasma aldosterone concentration (PAC) >10 ng/dL
+
Plasma renin activity (PRA) <1 ng/mL/hr

Confirmatory testing

Subtype testing

CT (axial image) shows a 1-cm aldosterone-producing adenoma (*arrow*) in the lateral aspect of the right adrenal gland.

morphology are found on CT in a patient younger than 35 years with severe PA (e.g., spontaneous hypokalemia and PAC > 30 ng/dL), unilateral adrenalectomy is a reasonable therapeutic option. However, in most cases, the patient is older and the CT may show normal-appearing adrenal glands, minimal unilateral adrenal limb thickening, unilateral microadenomas (≤1 cm), or bilateral macroadenomas. Thus adrenal venous sampling (AVS) is usually essential to direct appropriate therapy in patients with PA who want to pursue a surgical treatment option (see Plate 3.19).

The treatment goal is to prevent the morbidity and mortality associated with hypertension, hypokalemia, and cardiovascular damage. The cause of the PA helps to determine the appropriate treatment. Normalization of blood pressure should not be the only goal in managing patients with PA. In addition to the kidney and colon, MRs are present in the heart, brain, and blood vessels. Excessive secretion of aldosterone is associated with increased cardiovascular morbidity. Therefore normalization of circulating aldosterone concentrations or MR blockade should be part of the management plan for all patients with PA. Unilateral laparoscopic adrenalectomy is an excellent treatment option for patients with APA or UAH. Patients with IHA and most familial forms of PA should be treated medically with an MR antagonist.

Plate 3.19

Adrenal

ADRENAL VENOUS SAMPLING FOR PRIMARY ALDOSTERONISM

Multiple studies have shown that the accuracy of adrenal CT in localizing the source of aldosterone excess is poor (~50%) and that in patients with PA who wish to pursue the surgical option for hypertension management, AVS is a key step.

The keys to successful AVS include appropriate patient selection, careful patient preparation, focused technical expertise, a defined protocol, and accurate data interpretation. A center-specific, written protocol is mandatory. Many centers use a continuous cosyntropin infusion (50 μg/h started 30 minutes before sampling and continued throughout the procedure) during AVS for the following reasons: (1) to minimize stress-induced fluctuations in aldosterone secretion (due to endogenous corticotropin) during nonsimultaneous AVS, (2) to maximize the gradient in cortisol from adrenal vein to IVC and thus confirm successful sampling of the adrenal veins, and (3) to maximize the secretion of aldosterone from an APA.

The adrenal veins are sequentially catheterized through the percutaneous femoral vein approach under fluoroscopic guidance. Correct catheter tip location is confirmed with injection of a small amount of contrast medium. Blood is obtained by gentle aspiration from both adrenal veins.

The right adrenal vein enters the IVC posteriorly several centimeters above the right renal vein. It is more difficult to cathetcrize than the left one for a variety of reasons—it is short, small in caliber, and often has an angulated path causing the catheter tip to impact the intima, making blood aspiration problematic. Because of its short length, sometimes it does not support a stable catheter position during respiratory motion. Rarely, it arises in conjunction with a hepatic vein branch and needs to be separately engaged using a specific catheter shape to match the anatomy. Additionally, some interventional radiologists confuse the right adrenal vein with adjacent small hepatic vein branches, which are frequently encountered entering the IVC near the adrenal vein region.

The left adrenal vein is a tributary of the inferior phrenic vein, which enters the roof of the left renal vein near the lateral margin of the vertebral column in almost all patients. The venous sample from the left side is typically obtained from the common inferior phrenic trunk vein close to the junction of the adrenal vein. Usually, it is rapidly catheterized, and the blood aspiration is easy to achieve.

The final sample needs to be from a pure background source isolated from any possible contamination from the adrenal venous drainage. Traditionally, it is stated to be the "IVC" sample, although it should be from the external iliac vein.

To minimize the time lag between the sampling of the adrenal veins, the right adrenal vein is sampled first because it is usually more time-consuming and will be quickly followed by the left sample in almost all cases. The final sample is from the external iliac vein. This approach allows all three samples to be close in physiologic time frame. Aldosterone and cortisol concentrations are measured in the blood from all three sites (i.e., right adrenal vein, left adrenal vein, and IVC). All of the blood samples should be assayed at 1:1, 1:10, and 1:50

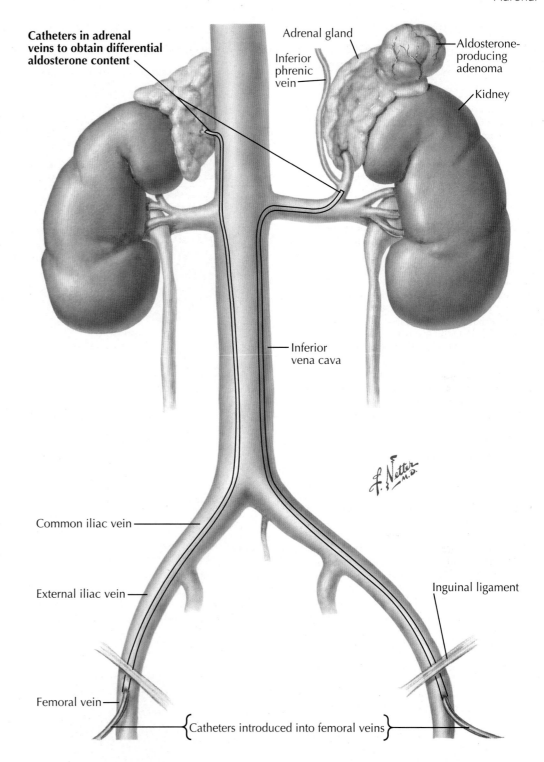

Catheters in adrenal veins to obtain differential aldosterone content

Adrenal gland

Inferior phrenic vein

Aldosterone-producing adenoma

Kidney

Inferior vena cava

Common iliac vein

External iliac vein

Inguinal ligament

Femoral vein

Catheters introduced into femoral veins

dilutions; absolute values for aldosterone and cortisol are mandatory.

The cortisol concentrations from the adrenal veins and IVC are used to confirm successful cannulation of both adrenal veins. With the cosyntropin infusion protocol, an adrenal vein-to-IVC cortisol ratio ≥ 5:1 is required to be confident that the adrenal veins were successfully catheterized. Dividing the right and left adrenal vein aldosterone concentrations by their respective cortisol concentrations corrects for the dilutional effect of the inferior phrenic vein flow into the left adrenal vein. An aldosterone lateralization ratio (dominant adrenal aldosterone/cortisol ratio divided by the nondominant adrenal aldosterone/cortisol ratio) ≥ 4:1 is consistent with unilateral adrenal aldosterone excess, whereas an aldosterone lateralization ratio ≤ 3:1 is consistent with bilateral adrenal aldosterone hypersecretion. In addition, in most patients with unilateral adrenal disease, the contralateral adrenal aldosterone-to-cortisol ratio is less than the aldosterone-to-cortisol ratio in the IVC and is termed *contralateral suppression*.

At centers with experience with AVS, the complication rate is 2.5% or less. Complications can include symptomatic groin hematoma, adrenal hemorrhage, and dissection of an adrenal vein.

Plate 3.20

Endocrine System: VOLUME 2

RENIN-ANGIOTENSIN-ALDOSTERONE SYSTEM AND RENOVASCULAR HYPERTENSION

Aldosterone is secreted from the zona glomerulosa under the control of angiotensin II, potassium, and corticotropin. Renin is an enzyme produced primarily in the juxtaglomerular apparatus of the kidney, and its release into the circulation is the rate-limiting step in the renin-angiotensin-aldosterone system. Renal renin release is controlled by four factors: (1) the macula densa, a specialized group of distal convoluted tubular cells that function as chemoreceptors for monitoring the sodium and chloride loads present in the distal tubule; (2) juxtaglomerular cells acting as pressure transducers that sense stretch of the afferent arteriolar wall and thus renal perfusion pressure; (3) the sympathetic nervous system, which modifies the release of renin, particularly in response to upright posture; and (4) humoral factors, including potassium, angiotensin II, and atrial natriuretic peptides. Thus renin release is maximized in conditions of low renal perfusion pressure or low tubular sodium content (e.g., renal artery stenosis, hemorrhage, dehydration). Renin release is suppressed by elevated perfusion pressure at the kidney (e.g., hypertension) and high-sodium diets. Renin release is increased directly by hypokalemia and decreased by hyperkalemia.

Angiotensinogen, an α_2-globulin synthesized in the liver, is the substrate for renin and is broken down into the angiotensin peptides. The action of renin on angiotensinogen produces angiotensin I. Angiotensin I is composed of the first 10 amino acids of the sequence after the presegment and does not appear to have biologic activity. Angiotensin II, the main form of biologically active angiotensin, is formed by cleavage of the two carboxyl-terminal peptides of angiotensin I by angiotensin-converting enzyme (ACE). ACE is localized to cell membranes in the lung and intracellular granules in certain tissues that produce angiotensin II. Angiotensin II functions through the angiotensin receptor to maintain normal extracellular volume and blood pressure by (1) increasing aldosterone secretion from the zona glomerulosa by increasing transcription of aldosterone synthase (CYP11B2); (2) constricting vascular smooth muscle, thereby increasing blood pressure and reducing renal blood flow; (3) releasing norepinephrine and epinephrine from the adrenal medulla; (4) enhancing the activity of the sympathetic nervous system by increasing central sympathetic outflow, thereby increasing norepinephrine discharge from sympathetic nerve terminals; and (5) promoting the release of vasopressin.

The classic functions of aldosterone are regulation of extracellular volume and control of potassium homeostasis. These effects are mediated by binding of free aldosterone to the MR in the cytosol of epithelial cells, principally in the kidney. Mineralocorticoid receptors have a tissue-specific expression. For example, the tissues with the highest concentrations of these receptors are the distal nephron, colon, and hippocampus. Lower levels of mineralocorticoid receptors are found in the rest of the gastrointestinal tract and heart.

Excess aldosterone secretion causes hypertension through two main mechanisms: (1) mineralocorticoid-induced expansion of plasma and extracellular fluid volume and (2) increase in total peripheral vascular resistance. Renovascular disease, which is caused by atherosclerosis or fibromuscular dysplasia, is a correctable cause of secondary hypertension. It should be

PATHOPHYSIOLOGY OF RENOVASCULAR HYPERTENSION IN UNILATERAL RENAL ARTERY STENOSIS

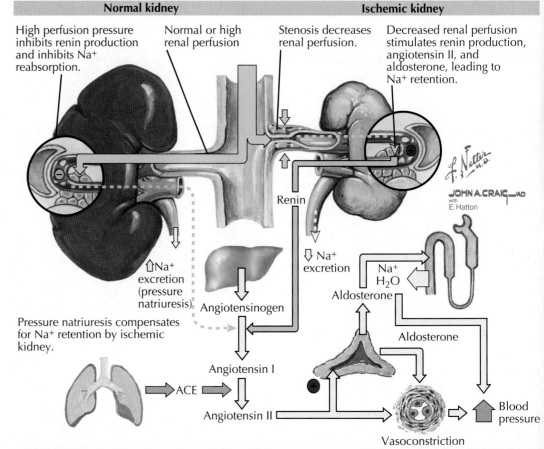

Normal kidney

High perfusion pressure inhibits renin production and inhibits Na$^+$ reabsorption.

Normal or high renal perfusion

Ischemic kidney

Stenosis decreases renal perfusion.

Decreased renal perfusion stimulates renin production, angiotensin II, and aldosterone, leading to Na$^+$ retention.

$\uparrow$Na$^+$ excretion (pressure natriuresis)

Pressure natriuresis compensates for Na$^+$ retention by ischemic kidney.

Renin

$\downarrow$ Na$^+$ excretion

Na$^+$ H$_2$O

Aldosterone

Angiotensinogen

Aldosterone

Angiotensin I

ACE

Angiotensin II

Vasoconstriction

Blood pressure

Causes of renovascular hypertension

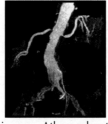

Atherosclerotic renal artery stenosis

Severe concentric atherosclerosis of renal artery with lipid deposition, calcification, and thrombosis

Fibromuscular dysplasia

Longitudinal section of fibromuscular dysplasia demonstrating variations in mural thickness

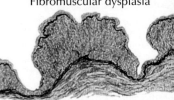

Atherosclerosis is most common cause of renal artery stenosis.

CT angiogram. Atherosclerotic bilateral renal artery ostial stenoses.

Renal arteriogram is criterion standard in diagnosis and assessment of severity of renal artery stenosis.

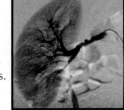

Renal arteriogram. Characteristic beaded appearance caused by alternating stenoses and aneurysmal dilations.

suspected in patients with onset of hypertension before the age of 30 years (especially if there is no family history and no other risk factors for hypertension such as obesity); onset of severe hypertension ($\geq$160/100 mm Hg) after the age of 55 years; an acute elevation in blood pressure over a previously stable baseline; moderate to severe hypertension and an unexplained atrophic kidney; or an acute elevation in serum creatinine that occurs shortly after the institution of therapy with an ACE inhibitor or angiotensin-receptor blocker. The criterion standard for diagnosing renal artery stenosis is renal arteriography. However, several less invasive tests may be used for case-detection purposes (e.g., magnetic resonance angiography, computed tomographic angiography, duplex Doppler ultrasonography).

Plate 3.21

Adrenal

ACUTE ADRENAL FAILURE: ADRENAL CRISIS

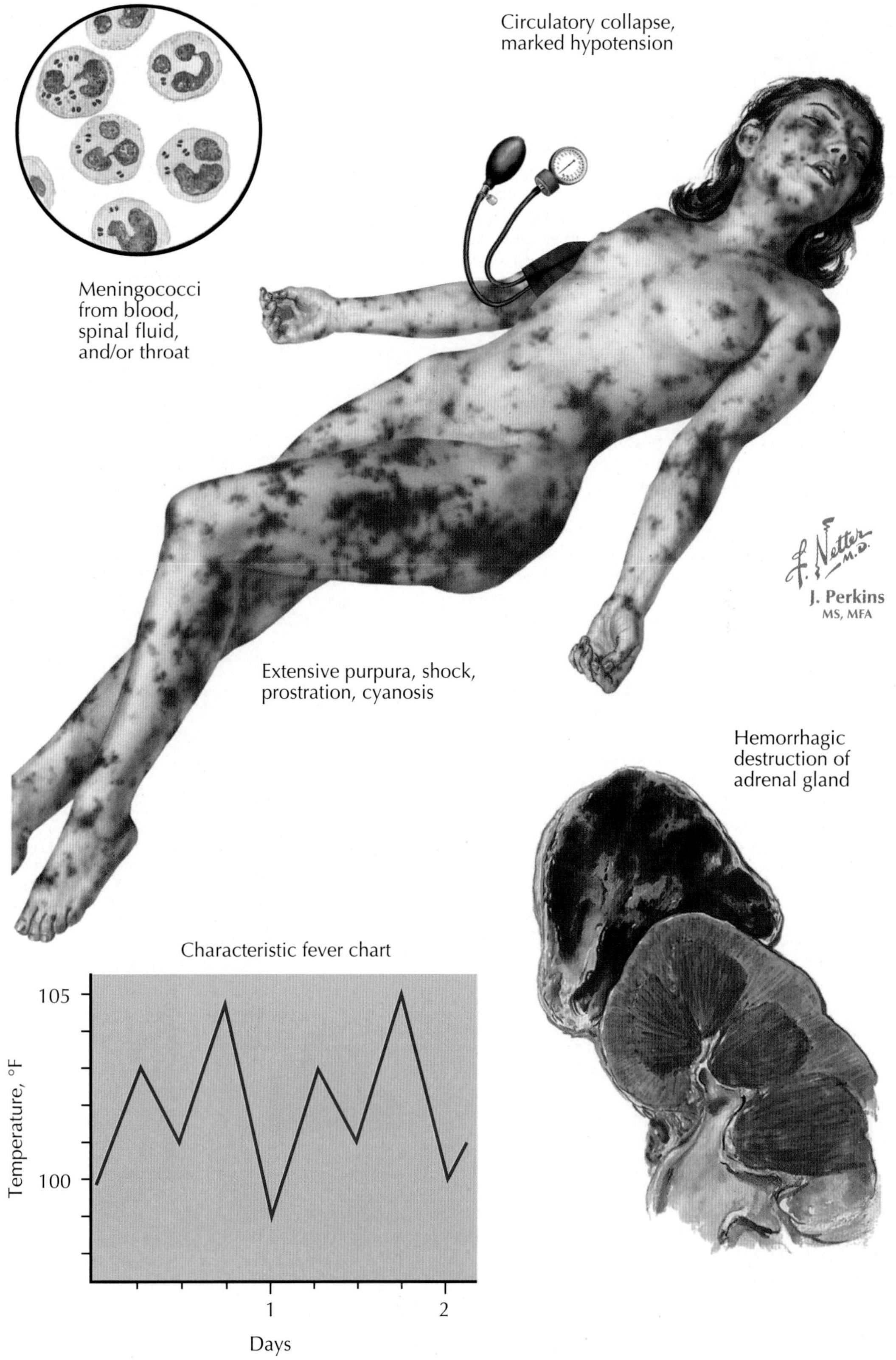

Acute adrenal failure or adrenal crisis is an endocrine emergency and is fatal if untreated. The presentation of adrenal crisis is dominated by dehydration and cardiovascular collapse. Adrenal crisis may occur in the following clinical settings: patients with known primary adrenal failure who have omitted glucocorticoid replacement therapy or who have not increased their replacement dosage for physical illness; patients with undiagnosed primary adrenal insufficiency undergoing a major physical stress (e.g., infection, surgery); and patients with necrosis of the adrenals caused by intraadrenal hemorrhage or infarction. Although much less common because of intact mineralocorticoid secretion, adrenal crisis can also be seen in these settings in patients with secondary adrenal insufficiency (e.g., hypopituitarism).

Adrenal hemorrhage should be considered in the setting of circulatory collapse and known underlying infection, trauma, anticoagulant therapy (e.g., heparin or warfarin), or coagulopathy (e.g., antiphospholipid syndrome). Adrenal hemorrhage may be associated with upper back, flank, or abdominal pain. Intraadrenal bleeding may occur in severe septicemia, especially in children with *Pseudomonas aeruginosa* septicemia. Fulminating meningococcal septicemia may result in hemorrhagic destruction of both adrenal glands and is known as *Waterhouse-Friderichsen syndrome*, most often occurring in children and young adults. These patients present with extensive purpura, meningitis, prostration, and shock. The initial presentation of meningitis caused by *Neisseria meningitidis* consists of sudden onset of fever (typically biphasic), nausea, vomiting, headache, cognitive dysfunction, and myalgias. There may be rapid progression to disseminated intravascular coagulation (DIC) and purpura fulminans, which occurs in 20% of patients with meningococcemia. Purpura fulminans is characterized by cutaneous hemorrhage and necrosis caused by vascular thrombosis and DIC.

In addition to shock, patients with adrenal crisis usually have additional symptoms that include anorexia, nausea, emesis, generalized abdominal pain, lethargy, fever, or confusion. The symptoms and signs of previously undiagnosed primary adrenal insufficiency may also be present (e.g., hyperpigmentation, weight loss, hyponatremia, hyperkalemia). When these signs are not recognized and when the presentation is dominated by fever and abdominal pain, it may lead to the misdiagnosis of acute surgical abdomen and result in disastrous surgical misadventure.

Empiric treatment for possible adrenal failure should be considered in all patients who are severely ill with shock that is refractory to volume expansion and pressor agents. If adrenal failure has not been diagnosed, the following guidelines for treatment should not be postponed pending the results of tests for diagnosing adrenal insufficiency. The therapeutic approach to acute adrenal insufficiency should include (1) hydrocortisone sodium succinate at a dose of 100 mg administered intravenously as a bolus; (2) rapid intravascular volume repletion with dextrose in isotonic saline (~2–4 L over the first 4 hours) depending on the degree of dehydration, presence of other cardiovascular

or renal disorders, and the clinical response; (3) diagnostic assessment for the precipitating cause (e.g., infection); and (4) frequent monitoring of serum electrolytes, acid-base balance, blood glucose level, and renal function. The dosage of hydrocortisone sodium succinate is continued at 100 mg intravenously every 8 hours until remission of the underlying illness; the dose may then be decreased by 50% per day until maintenance doses are achieved.

For each patient, all of the causes of adrenal insufficiency should be considered; the possibility of autoimmune adrenal disease should be considered, and patients should be assessed for other glandular dysfunction (primary thyroid failure, diabetes mellitus, hypoparathyroidism, and gonadal failure). Adrenal crisis may be precipitated by other acute illnesses such as infectious diseases. Each patient should be evaluated for an underlying triggering disease.

Meningococci from blood, spinal fluid, and/or throat

Circulatory collapse, marked hypotension

J. Perkins
MS, MFA

Extensive purpura, shock, prostration, cyanosis

Hemorrhagic destruction of adrenal gland

Characteristic fever chart

Plate 3.22

Endocrine System: VOLUME 2

CHRONIC PRIMARY ADRENAL FAILURE: ADDISON DISEASE

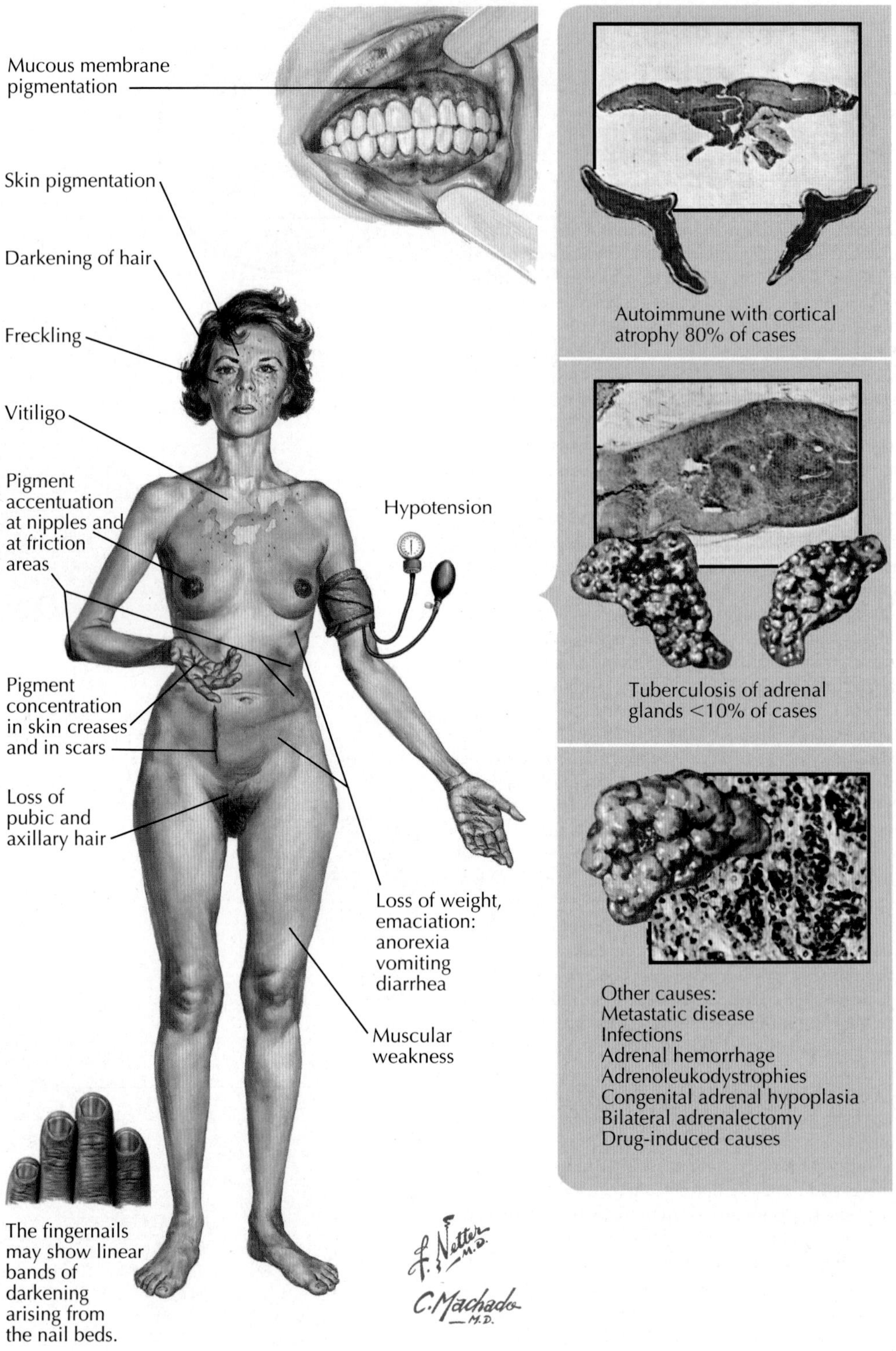

The normal adrenal cortex has a remarkable functional reserve; adrenal failure does not become clinically evident until more than 90% of the cortex has been destroyed. Thus the clinical presentation of adrenal insufficiency depends on both the rate and extent of adrenocortical destruction. If it is slowly progressive, the patient may not come to clinical detection until an illness (e.g., infection) or other stress (e.g., trauma, surgery) precipitates an adrenal crisis. The typical chronic signs and symptoms relate to both glucocorticoid and mineralocorticoid insufficiency, and these include fatigue, generalized weakness, diffuse myalgias and arthralgias, anorexia, weight loss, nausea, emesis, abdominal pain, psychiatric symptoms, auricular cartilage calcification (in males), postural lightheadedness, hypotension, hyperpigmentation (skin and hair), hyponatremia, hyperkalemia, and anemia. The hyponatremia is dilutional in nature and caused by inappropriate secretion of antidiuretic hormone and decreased renal free-water clearance. Low blood pressure and postural lightheadedness are associated with both mineralocorticoid and glucocorticoid deficiencies; some patients may present with spontaneous resolution of long-standing hypertension. Hypoglycemia, which is more common in children with adrenal insufficiency, may occur in the setting of a prolonged fast. The recognition of early adrenal insufficiency may be difficult because of the nonspecific nature of its symptoms.

Generalized hyperpigmentation is caused by ACTH-driven increased melanin production in the epidermal melanocytes. The extensor surfaces (e.g., knees, knuckles, elbows) and other friction areas (e.g., belt line, brassiere strap) tend to be even more hyperpigmented. Other sites of prominent hyperpigmentation include the inner surfaces of the lips, buccal mucosa, gums, hard palate, recent surgical scars, areolae, freckles, and palmar creases (the latter may be a normal finding in individuals with darker skin). The fingernails may show linear bands of darkening arising from the nail beds. With adequate glucocorticoid replacement, the hyperpigmentation resolves over several months; however, the hyperpigmentation in scars may be permanent. Vitiligo (depigmented skin), which is caused by autoimmune destruction of melanocytes, is seen in approximately 20% of patients with autoimmune primary adrenal failure.

In females with primary adrenal failure, secondary sex hair (axillary and pubic hair) may be lost and libido decreased because of loss of adrenal androgen secretion. These findings are not present in males because the testicles are the main source of androgens.

The most common cause of primary adrenal failure has evolved over time, from tuberculosis in 1855 when Thomas Addison first described the clinical features and autopsy findings in 11 patients with primary adrenal failure, to autoimmune disease in the 21st century (in ~80% of cases). Other less common causes of primary adrenal failure include metastatic disease (e.g., lymphoma, lung cancer, breast cancer, melanoma), infections (e.g., fungal, HIV, tuberculosis), adrenal hemorrhage, adrenoleukodystrophies, congenital adrenal hypoplasia (e.g., *NR0B1* [DAX1] or *NR5A1* [SF-1] pathogenic variants), bilateral adrenalectomy, and drug-induced causes (e.g., mitotane, ketoconazole, mifepristone, metyrapone, osilodrostat). Antibodies directed against 21-hydroxylase can be found in nearly all patients with autoimmune primary adrenal failure,

and they are absent in patients with other causes of adrenal insufficiency.

Approximately half of patients with autoimmune adrenal failure have one or more other autoimmune endocrine disorders. In such patients, the cause of their findings may be autoimmune polyglandular syndrome type II (APS2). Patients who are affected typically present between the ages of 20 to 40 years with primary adrenal insufficiency as the main manifestation. Autoimmune thyroid disease (e.g., Hashimoto thyroiditis, Graves disease) and type 1 diabetes mellitus are common in patients with APS2. APS2 was previously referred to as Schmidt syndrome and is three times

more common in females than in males. The inheritance can be autosomal recessive, autosomal dominant, or polygenic.

APS1 is a rare autosomal recessive disorder that most commonly affects females and is most prevalent in individuals of Finnish and Sardinian descent (see Plate 8.6). It is less common than APS2 and is caused by pathogenic variants in the autoimmune regulator (*AIRE*) gene. Hypoparathyroidism or chronic mucocutaneous candidiasis is usually the first manifestation that typically appears during childhood or early adolescence and is followed shortly thereafter (average age, 15 years) by primary adrenal insufficiency.

Mucous membrane pigmentation

Skin pigmentation

Darkening of hair

Freckling

Vitiligo

Pigment accentuation at nipples and at friction areas

Pigment concentration in skin creases and in scars

Loss of pubic and axillary hair

The fingernails may show linear bands of darkening arising from the nail beds.

Hypotension

Loss of weight, emaciation: anorexia vomiting diarrhea

Muscular weakness

Autoimmune with cortical atrophy 80% of cases

Tuberculosis of adrenal glands <10% of cases

Other causes:
Metastatic disease
Infections
Adrenal hemorrhage
Adrenoleukodystrophies
Congenital adrenal hypoplasia
Bilateral adrenalectomy
Drug-induced causes

Plate 3.23

Adrenal

LABORATORY FINDINGS AND TREATMENT OF PRIMARY ADRENAL INSUFFICIENCY

In addition to the cortisol deficiency associated with primary adrenal insufficiency, there is a loss of aldosterone and adrenal androgens. Therefore primary adrenal insufficiency is also associated with hyponatremia and hyperkalemia. The hyponatremia is associated with an inappropriate increase in vasopressin secretion and a cortisol-related decreased free-water clearance at the kidney. The hyperkalemia is a direct result of lack of aldosterone effect at the mineralocorticoid receptor. Aldosterone concentrations in the blood and urine are inappropriately low for the degree of hyperkalemia and the increased levels of PRA. The hypotension and dehydration may lead to secondary renal insufficiency and an increase in serum creatinine. Normochromic-normocytic anemia and neutropenia with relative lymphocytosis are usually present.

Blood levels of the adrenal androgens—DHEA-S and androstenedione—are low, and the 24-hour urinary excretion of 17-ketosteroids is low. The decreased adrenal androgen secretion leads to loss of axillary and pubic hair in females.

The serum cortisol concentrations are low in the presence of the high blood concentration of ACTH. In addition, the 24-hour urinary cortisol excretion is low. In patients who are symptomatic, all that is needed to confirm the diagnosis is an 8 AM serum ACTH concentration greater than 500 pg/mL (normal, 10–60 pg/mL) and a simultaneous serum cortisol concentration less than 5 μg/dL (normal, 7–25 mcg/dL). In this setting, stimulation testing with cosyntropin is not needed. When the 1-hour cosyntropin-stimulation test is performed in patients with primary adrenal failure, the serum cortisol concentration does not change from baseline (the baseline value is typically <5 μg/dL, and the increment after cosyntropin administration is <7 μg/dL), and the peak value remains below 18 μg/dL.

For guidance on maintenance glucocorticoid replacement, see Plate 3.24. Patients should be told to (1) increase the replacement dosage of glucocorticoids two- to threefold during major physical stress (e.g., fever > 101° F, acute illness, tooth extraction); (2) seek medical care if more than 3 days of stress glucocorticoid coverage is required; (3) avoid long-term supraphysiologic dosages because of the potential for iatrogenic Cushing syndrome; (4) be aware that increased glucocorticoid dosage is not required for mental stress, headaches, or minor illness; (5) administer the increased glucocorticoid dose intramuscularly if it cannot be taken orally because of nausea or emesis; and (6) carry and wear medical identification (a wallet card and bracelet or necklace) that includes the diagnosis ("adrenal insufficiency") and the words "give cortisone," so that appropriate glucocorticoid treatment can be given if the patient is found unconscious. Complete patient understanding of these instructions is key to successful treatment.

Three syringes, each to be filled with 4 mg (4 mg/mL) of dexamethasone, should be prescribed for patients to keep at home, at work, and with them if possible (they should avoid exposure to extreme heat). A single dose may be repeated in 8 hours if symptoms of the underlying illness persist and a physician is not available. Instructions on self-injection technique should be given and periodically reviewed. Expired medication should be replaced promptly.

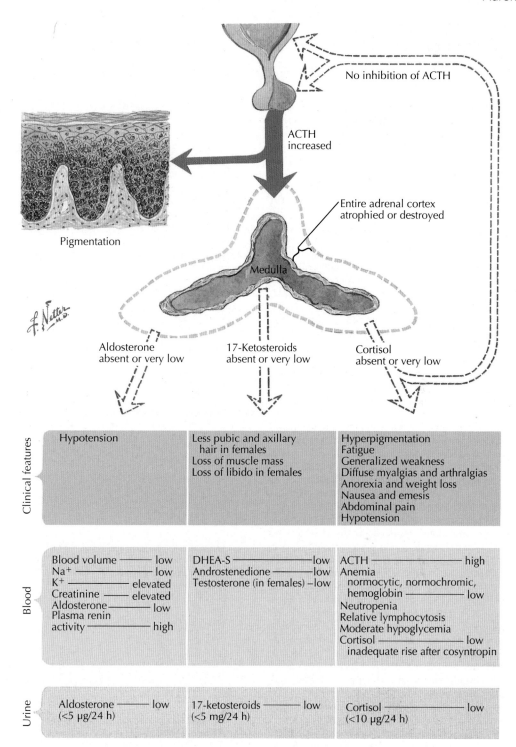

No inhibition of ACTH

ACTH increased

Pigmentation

Entire adrenal cortex atrophied or destroyed

Medulla

Aldosterone absent or very low

17-Ketosteroids absent or very low

Cortisol absent or very low

	Clinical features		
	Hypotension	Less pubic and axillary hair in females Loss of muscle mass Loss of libido in females	Hyperpigmentation Fatigue Generalized weakness Diffuse myalgias and arthralgias Anorexia and weight loss Nausea and emesis Abdominal pain Hypotension

Blood	Blood volume —— low
	Na+ —— low
	K+ —— elevated
	Creatinine —— elevated
	Aldosterone —— low
	Plasma renin activity —— high
		DHEA-S —— low
		Androstenedione —— low
		Testosterone (in females) –low
			ACTH —— high
			Anemia
			  normocytic, normochromic,
			  hemoglobin —— low
			Neutropenia
			Relative lymphocytosis
			Moderate hypoglycemia
			Cortisol —— low
			  inadequate rise after cosyntropin

Urine	Aldosterone —— low (<5 μg/24 h)	17-ketosteroids —— low (<5 mg/24 h)	Cortisol —— low (<10 μg/24 h)

Surgical procedures with general anesthesia require coverage with stress doses of glucocorticoid. A standard glucocorticoid preparation preoperatively is 20 to 40 mg of methylprednisolone sodium succinate administered intramuscularly the morning of the operation and again the evening of the operation; the dosage is tapered to 20 mg and 10 mg intramuscularly every 12 hours on the first and second postoperative days, respectively. The patient's clinical condition is the guide to how much further to taper the dosage to parallel clinical improvement and when to reinstate maintenance glucocorticoid therapy. Patients who take fludrocortisone daily do not usually require supplemental mineralocorticoid until oral intake is resumed postoperatively.

In secondary adrenal failure, the renin-angiotensin-aldosterone axis is intact, and mineralocorticoid replacement is not needed. However, in primary adrenal insufficiency, mineralocorticoid replacement is important. Aldosterone is not available for therapeutic use. Fludrocortisone, a very potent steroid, is the only medication commonly used for this purpose. Typically, 50 to 200 μg (100 μg/day is the usual dosage) is administered orally in a single dose daily. The dosage is titrated to achieve a normal serum level of potassium. Inadequate dosage causes dehydration, hyponatremia, and hyperkalemia. Excessive dosage results in hypertension, weight gain, and hypokalemia. Most patients are advised to maintain a sodium intake of approximately 150 mEq/day.

Plate 3.24

Endocrine System: VOLUME 2

LABORATORY FINDINGS AND TREATMENT OF SECONDARY ADRENAL INSUFFICIENCY

The clinical features of secondary (pituitary ACTH deficiency) or tertiary (hypothalamic CRH deficiency) adrenal insufficiency are similar to those of primary adrenal insufficiency, with a few notable exceptions. ACTH has a melanocyte-stimulating effect, and patients with primary adrenal insufficiency (high ACTH levels) have a "muddy" type of hyperpigmentation (especially in the palmar creases and over extensor surfaces) and tan easily in the sun. In contrast, secondary adrenal insufficiency (low ACTH levels) is associated with relative pallor and sun sensitivity. In addition, aldosterone secretion and normokalemia are maintained in secondary adrenal insufficiency because the renin-angiotensin-aldosterone axis is intact. Thus dehydration is less common in secondary adrenal insufficiency.

Hyponatremia may be present and is caused by an inappropriate increase in vasopressin secretion and by decreased free-water clearance at the kidney. Hypoglycemia in children is more common in secondary adrenal insufficiency, in part because of concomitant growth hormone deficiency. Normochromic-normocytic anemia and neutropenia with relative lymphocytosis are usually present.

Recognizing that the presentation and laboratory findings in secondary adrenal insufficiency may be dominated by the sellar or hypothalamic process and the associated hormonal deficiencies or tumoral hypersecretion is important. Thus the presentation may be complicated by hypothyroidism, diabetes insipidus, growth hormone deficiency, and secondary hypogonadism. Because of the decreased free-water clearance associated with adrenal insufficiency, diabetes insipidus may only become evident after glucocorticoid replacement. Mass-effect symptoms (e.g., visual field loss, headaches) related to the sellar or hypothalamic mass may also be observed. In panhypopituitarism, the patient may have the characteristic facies with fawn-colored skin, fine facial wrinkling and crow's feet around the eyes, and thinning of the lateral third of the eyebrows that is associated with hypothyroidism and hypogonadism. In addition, ACTH may be the only pituitary hormone that is deficient (isolated secondary adrenal insufficiency) and usually associated with lymphocytic hypophysitis.

Aldosterone concentrations in the blood and urine are usually normal for the prevailing renin secretion. Blood levels of the adrenal androgens—DHEA-S, androstenedione, and testosterone—are low, and the 24-hour urinary excretion of 17-ketosteroids is low. The decreased adrenal androgen secretion leads to loss of axillary and pubic hair in females.

The serum cortisol concentration is low because of the low blood concentration of ACTH. In addition, the 24-hour urinary cortisol excretion is low. In patients who are symptomatic, all that is needed to confirm the diagnosis of secondary adrenal insufficiency is an 8 AM serum ACTH concentration that is undetectable and a simultaneous serum cortisol concentration less than 5 μg/dL. In this setting, stimulation testing with insulin-induced hypoglycemia or cosyntropin is not needed. When the cosyntropin-stimulation test is performed in patients with secondary adrenal failure, the serum cortisol concentration may start to change from baseline at the 60-minute time point, but the peak value typically remains less than 18 μg/dL.

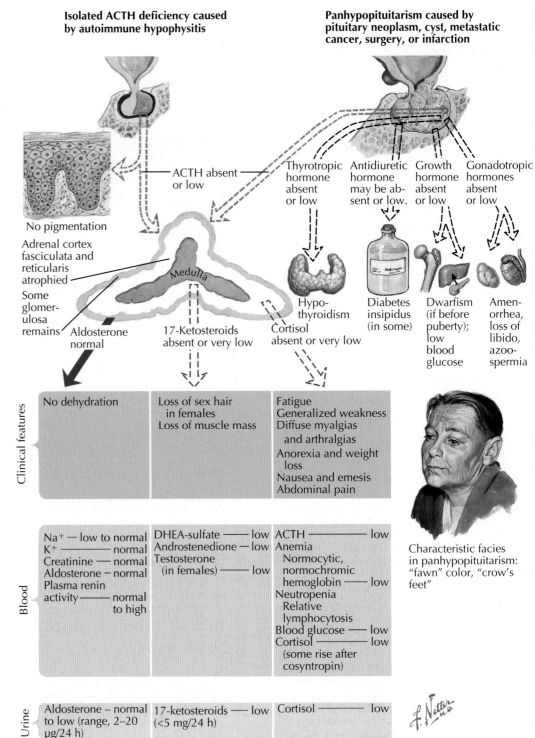

Isolated ACTH deficiency caused by autoimmune hypophysitis

Panhypopituitarism caused by pituitary neoplasm, cyst, metastatic cancer, surgery, or infarction

Characteristic facies in panhypopituitarism: "fawn" color, "crow's feet"

ACTH is not used for replacement therapy because of the need for parenteral administration, the potential for allergic reactions, and the increased cost. Hydrocortisone, cortisone acetate, and prednisone are the most frequently used preparations in standard replacement therapy. The catabolism of synthetic steroids is affected by interindividual variability and the effects of concomitantly administered drugs. For these reasons, most clinicians prefer the major glucocorticoid secreted by the adrenal cortex, hydrocortisone. In an attempt to replicate the normal glucocorticoid circadian rhythm, two-thirds of the glucocorticoid dose (hydrocortisone, 10 or 15 mg) is administered in the morning, and one-third (hydrocortisone, 5 or 10 mg) is administered before the evening meal. Giving the afternoon dose later in the evening may cause insomnia. Lower doses or a single morning dose of hydrocortisone may be given to patients who have partial ACTH deficiency. Clinical judgment and lack of symptoms of glucocorticoid deficiency or excess are the primary means for determining dosage adequacy. Hepatic enzyme inducers such as rifampin and phenobarbital may accelerate hepatic glucocorticoid catabolism and necessitate an increased maintenance dosage. Because of the short half-life of hydrocortisone, serum cortisol concentration is not a useful index for dosage adequacy. For guidance on stress dosage management, see Plate 3.23.

Plate 3.25

Adrenal

ADRENAL MEDULLA AND CATECHOLAMINES

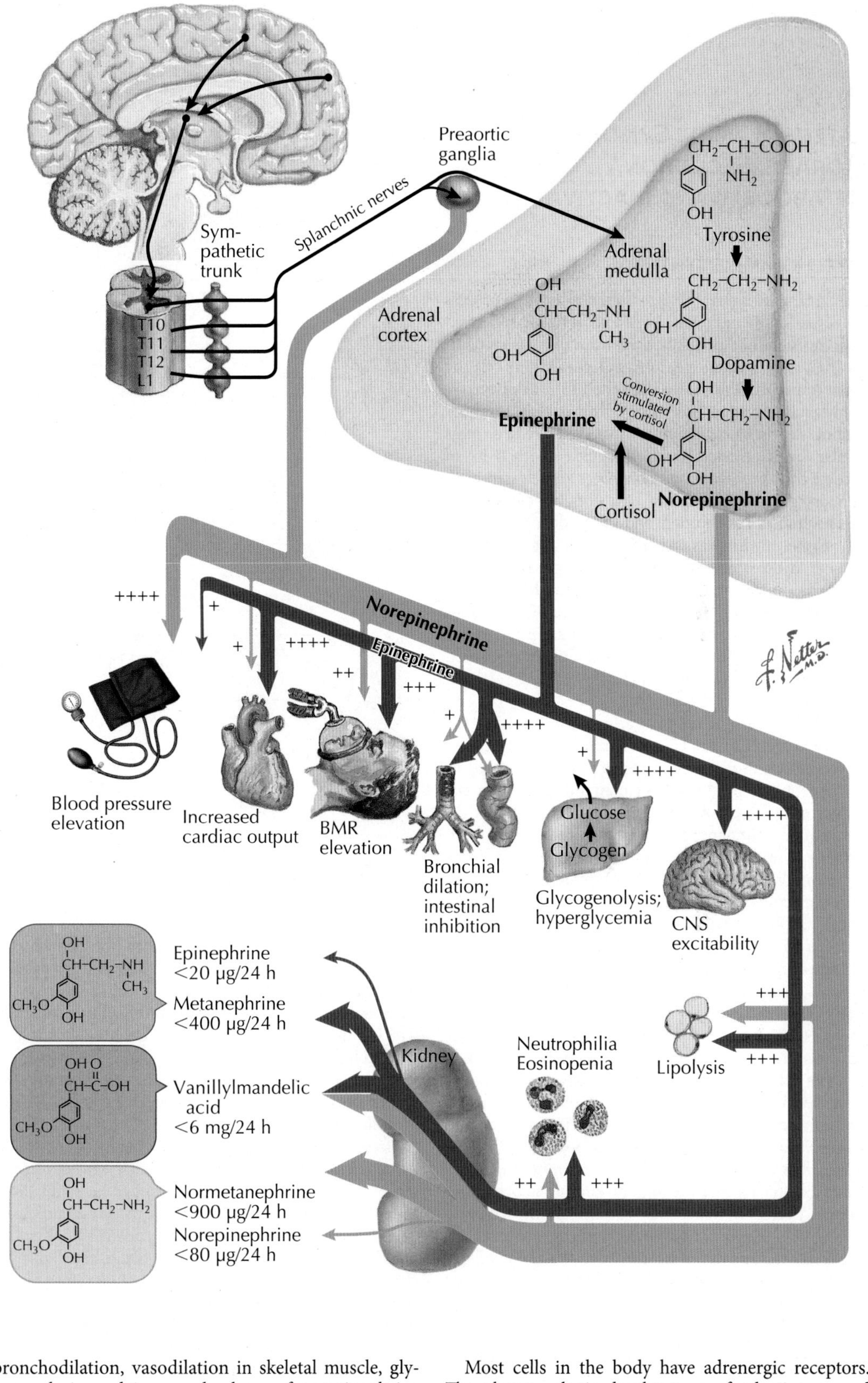

The adrenal medulla occupies the central portion of the adrenal gland and accounts for 10% of the total adrenal gland volume. Adrenomedullary cells are called *chromaffin cells* (which stain brown with chromium salts) or *pheochromocytes*. Cytoplasmic granules turn dark when stained with chromic acid because of the oxidation of epinephrine and norepinephrine to melanin. Chromaffin cells differentiate in the center of the adrenal gland in response to cortisol; some chromaffin cells also migrate to form paraganglia, collections of chromaffin cells on both sides of the aorta. The preganglionic sympathetic neurons receive synaptic input from neurons within the pons, medulla, and hypothalamus, providing regulation of sympathetic activity by the brain. Axons from the lower thoracic and lumbar preganglionic neurons (from T10 to L1), via splanchnic nerves, directly innervate the cells of the adrenal medulla. Stressful stimuli (e.g., myocardial infarction, anesthesia, hypoglycemia) trigger adrenal medullary catecholamine secretion. Acetylcholine from preganglionic sympathetic fibers stimulates nicotinic cholinergic receptors and causes depolarization of adrenomedullary chromaffin cells. Depolarization leads to activation of voltage-gated calcium channels, which results in exocytosis of secretory vesicle contents.

The term *catecholamine* refers to substances that contain catechol (ortho-dihydroxybenzene) and a side chain with an amino group—the catechol nucleus. Epinephrine is synthesized and stored in the adrenal medulla and released into the systemic circulation. Norepinephrine is synthesized and stored not only in the adrenal medulla but also in the peripheral sympathetic nerves. DA, the precursor of norepinephrine found in the adrenal medulla and peripheral sympathetic nerves, acts primarily as a neurotransmitter in the CNS.

Catecholamines affect many cardiovascular and metabolic processes, including increasing the heart rate, blood pressure, myocardial contractility, and cardiac conduction velocity. Specific receptors mediate the biologic actions. The three types of adrenergic receptors (α, β, DA) and their receptor subtypes (α_1, α_2, β_1, β_2, β_3, DA_1, DA_2) have led to an understanding of the physiologic responses to exogenous and endogenous administration of catecholamines. The α_1 subtype is a postsynaptic receptor that mediates vascular and smooth muscle contraction; stimulation causes vasoconstriction and increased blood pressure. The α_2 receptors are located on presynaptic sympathetic nerve endings and, when activated, inhibit release of norepinephrine; stimulation causes suppression in central sympathetic outflow and decreased blood pressure. For example, the central α_2-agonists clonidine, α-methyldopa, and guanfacine are used as antihypertensive agents. There are three main β-receptor subtypes. The β_1 receptor mediates cardiac effects and is more responsive to isoproterenol than to epinephrine or norepinephrine; stimulation causes positive inotropic and chronotropic effects on the heart, increased renin secretion in the kidney, and lipolysis in adipocytes. The β_2 receptor mediates bronchial, vascular, and uterine smooth muscle relaxation; stimulation causes

bronchodilation, vasodilation in skeletal muscle, glycogenolysis, and increased release of norepinephrine from sympathetic nerve terminals. The β_3 receptor regulates energy expenditure and lipolysis. DA_1 receptors are localized to the cerebral, renal, mesenteric, and coronary vasculatures; stimulation causes vasodilation in these vascular beds. DA_2 receptors are presynaptic and localized to sympathetic nerve endings, sympathetic ganglia, and brain; stimulation inhibits the release of norepinephrine, ganglionic transmission, and prolactin release, respectively.

Most cells in the body have adrenergic receptors. The pharmacologic development of selective α- and β-adrenergic agonists and antagonists has advanced the pharmacotherapy for various clinical disorders. For example, β_1-antagonists, such as atenolol and metoprolol, are considered standard therapies for angina pectoris, hypertension, and cardiac arrhythmias. Administration of β_2-agonists (terbutaline, formoterol fumarate, and albuterol) causes bronchial smooth muscle relaxation; these agents are commonly prescribed in inhaled formulations for the treatment of asthma.

Plate 3.26

Endocrine System: VOLUME 2

CATECHOLAMINE SYNTHESIS, STORAGE, SECRETION, METABOLISM, AND INACTIVATION

CATECHOLAMINE SYNTHESIS

Catecholamines are synthesized from tyrosine by a process of hydroxylation and decarboxylation. Tyrosine is derived from ingested food or synthesized from phenylalanine in the liver, and it enters neurons and chromaffin cells by active transport. Tyrosine is converted to 3,4-dihydroxyphenylalanine (dopa) by tyrosine hydroxylase, the rate-limiting step in catecholamine synthesis. Increased intracellular levels of catechols downregulate the activity of tyrosine hydroxylase; as catecholamines are released from secretory granules in response to a stimulus, cytoplasmic catecholamines are depleted, and the feedback inhibition of tyrosine hydroxylase is released. Transcription of tyrosine hydroxylase is stimulated by glucocorticoids, cAMP-dependent protein kinases, calcium/phospholipid-dependent protein kinase, and calcium/calmodulin-dependent protein kinase. α-Methyl-paratyrosine (metyrosine) is a tyrosine hydroxylase inhibitor that may be used therapeutically in patients with catecholamine-secreting tumors.

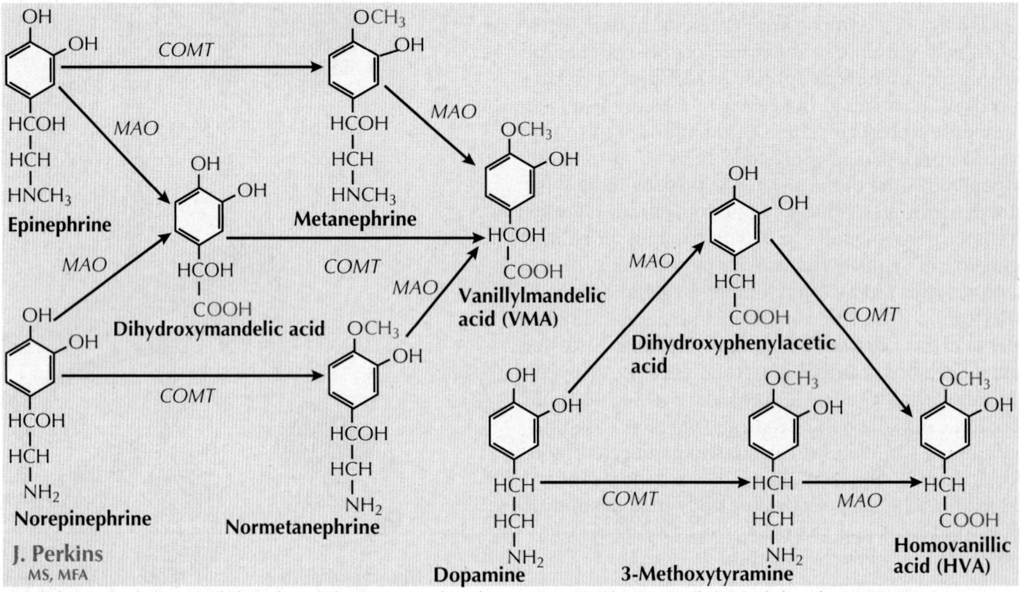

Aromatic L-amino acid decarboxylase catalyzes the decarboxylation of dopa to DA. DA is actively transported into granulated vesicles to be hydroxylated to norepinephrine by the copper-containing enzyme DA β-hydroxylase. Ascorbic acid is a cofactor and hydrogen donor. The enzyme is structurally similar to tyrosine hydroxylase, and they may share similar transcriptional regulatory elements. Both are stimulated by glucocorticoids and cAMP-dependent kinases. These reactions occur in the synaptic vesicle of adrenergic neurons in the CNS, the peripheral nervous system, and the chromaffin cells of the adrenal medulla. In the adrenal medulla, norepinephrine is released from the granule into the cytoplasm, where the cytosolic enzyme phenylethanolamine N-methyltransferase (PNMT) converts it to epinephrine. Epinephrine is then transported back into another storage vesicle. The N-methylation reaction by PNMT involves S-adenosylmethionine as the methyl donor, as well as oxygen and magnesium. PNMT expression is regulated by the presence of glucocorticoids, which are in high concentration in the adrenal medulla through the corticomedullary portal system. Thus catecholamine-secreting tumors that secrete primarily epinephrine are localized to the adrenal medulla. In normal adrenal medullary tissue, approximately 80% of the catecholamine released is epinephrine.

CATECHOLAMINE STORAGE AND SECRETION

Catecholamines are found in the adrenal medulla and sympathetically innervated organs. Catecholamines are stored in electron-dense granules that also contain adenosine triphosphate (ATP), neuropeptides (e.g., adrenomedullin, ACTH, vasoactive intestinal polypeptide), calcium, magnesium, and chromogranins. Uptake into the storage vesicles is facilitated by active transport using vesicular monoamine transporters (VMATs). The VMAT ATP-driven pump maintains a steep electrical gradient. For every monoamine transported, ATP is

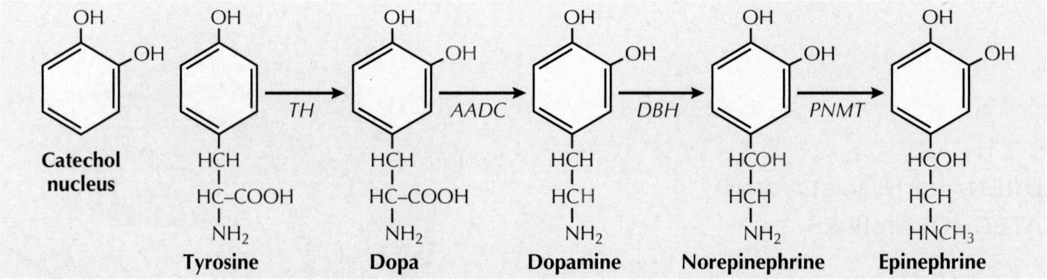

Biosynthetic pathway for catecholamines. The term catecholamine comes from the catechol (orthodihydroxybenzene) structure and a side chain with an amino group — the "catechol nucleus" (shown on *left*). Tyrosine is converted to 3,4-dihydroxyphenylalanine (dopa) in the rate-limiting step by tyrosine hydroxylase (TH); this step provides the clinician with the option to treat patients with pheochromocytoma with a TH inhibitor, α-methyl-para-tyrosine (metyrosine). Aromatic L-amino acid decarboxylase (AADC) converts dopa to dopamine. Dopamine is hydroxylated to norepinephrine by dopamine β-hydroxylase (DBH). Norepinephrine is converted to epinephrine by phenylethanolamine N-methyltransferase (PNMT); cortisol serves as a cofactor for PNMT, and this is why epinephrine-secreting pheochromocytomas are almost exclusively localized to the adrenal medulla.

Catecholamine metabolism. Metabolism of catecholamines occurs through two enzymatic pathways. Catechol-O-methyltransferase (COMT) converts epinephrine to metanephrine and converts norepinephrine to normetanephrine by meta-O-methylation. Metanephrine and normetanephrine are oxidized by monoamine oxidase (MAO) to vanillylmandelic acid (VMA) by oxidative deamination. MAO also may oxidize epinephrine and norepinephrine to dihydroxymandelic acid, which is then converted by COMT to VMA. Dopamine is also metabolized by MAO and COMT with the final metabolite, homovanillic acid (HVA).

hydrolyzed, and two hydrogen ions are transported from the vesicle into the cytosol. Iodine-123 and ^{131}I-labeled metaiodobenzylguanidine (MIBG) are imported by VMATs into the storage vesicles in the adrenal medulla, which makes ^{123}I-MIBG useful for imaging localization of catecholamine-secreting tumors and ^{131}I-MIBG potentially useful in treating malignant catecholamine-secreting tumors. Catecholamine uptake, as well as MIBG, is inhibited by reserpine.

Stressful stimuli (e.g., myocardial infarction, anesthesia, hypoglycemia) trigger adrenal medullary catecholamine secretion. Acetylcholine from preganglionic sympathetic fibers stimulates nicotinic cholinergic receptors and causes depolarization of adrenomedullary chromaffin cells. Depolarization leads to activation of voltage-gated calcium channels, which results in exocytosis of secretory vesicle contents. A calcium-sensing receptor appears to be involved in the process of exocytosis. During exocytosis, all the granular contents are released into the extracellular space. Norepinephrine modulates its own release by activating the α_2-receptors on the presynaptic membrane. Stimulation of the presynaptic α_2-receptors inhibits norepinephrine release (the mechanism of action of some antihypertensive medications such as clonidine and guanfacine). Catecholamines are among the shortest-lived signaling molecules in plasma; the initial biologic half-life of circulating catecholamines is between 10 and 100 seconds. Approximately half of the catecholamines circulate in plasma in loose association with albumin. Thus plasma concentrations of catecholamines fluctuate widely.

CATECHOLAMINE METABOLISM AND INACTIVATION

Catecholamines are removed from the circulation either by reuptake by sympathetic nerve terminals or by metabolism through two enzyme pathways, followed by sulfate conjugation and renal excretion. Most of the metabolism of catecholamines occurs in the same cell in which they are synthesized. Almost 90% of catecholamines released at sympathetic synapses are taken up locally by the nerve endings, termed *uptake-1*. Uptake-1 can be blocked by cocaine, tricyclic antidepressants, and phenothiazines. Extraneuronal tissues also take up catecholamines, and this is termed *uptake-2*. Most of these catecholamines are metabolized by catechol O-methyltransferase (COMT).

Although COMT is found primarily outside neural tissue, O-methylation in the adrenal medulla is the predominant source of metanephrine (COMT converts epinephrine to metanephrine) and a main source of normetanephrine (COMT converts norepinephrine to normetanephrine) by methylating the 3-hydroxy group. S-Adenosylmethionine is used as the methyl donor, and calcium is required. Metanephrine and normetanephrine are oxidized by monoamine oxidase (MAO) to vanillylmandelic acid (VMA) by oxidative deamination. MAO may also oxidize epinephrine and norepinephrine to 3,4-dihydroxymandelic acid, which is then converted by COMT to VMA. In the storage vesicle, norepinephrine is protected from metabolism by MAO. MAO and COMT metabolize DA to homovanillic acid.

Plate 3.27

Adrenal

Pheochromocytoma and Paraganglioma

Catecholamine-secreting tumors that arise from chromaffin cells of the adrenal medulla and the sympathetic ganglia are referred to as *pheochromocytomas* and *catecholamine-secreting paragangliomas,* respectively. Because the tumors have similar clinical presentations and are treated with similar approaches, many clinicians use the term *pheochromocytoma* to refer to both adrenal pheochromocytomas and catecholamine-secreting paragangliomas. However, the distinction between pheochromocytoma and paraganglioma is an important one because of implications for associated neoplasms, risk for malignancy, and genetic testing. Catecholamine-secreting tumors are rare, with an annual incidence of 2 to 8 cases per million people. Nevertheless, it is important to suspect, confirm, localize, and resect these tumors because (1) the associated hypertension is curable with surgical removal of the tumor; (2) a risk of lethal paroxysm exists; (3) at least 10% of the tumors are malignant; and (4) 40% of the tumors are familial, and detection of this tumor in the proband may result in early diagnosis in other family members.

The association between adrenal medullary tumors and symptoms was first recognized by Fränkel in 1886. He described Fräulein Minna Roll, age 18 years, who had intermittent attacks of palpitation, anxiety, vertigo, headache, chest pain, cold sweats, and vomiting. She had a hard, noncompressible pulse and retinitis. Despite champagne therapy and injections of ether, she died. At autopsy, bilateral adrenal tumors were initially thought to be angiosarcomas, but a positive chromaffin reaction later confirmed the pheochromocytoma lesion.

The term *paraganglioma,* introduced in 1908, was defined as an extraadrenal chromaffin tumor arising in a paraganglion. The term *pheochromocytoma,* proposed by Pick in 1912, comes from the Greek words *phaios* (dusky), *chroma* (color), and *cytoma* (tumor) because of the dark staining reaction that is caused by the oxidation of intracellular catecholamines when exposed to dichromate salts. In 1926 Roux in Lausanne, Switzerland, and Mayo in Rochester, Minnesota, successfully surgically removed adrenal pheochromocytomas. In 1929 it was discovered that pheochromocytomas contain an excess amount of a pressor agent. Subsequently, epinephrine (in 1936) and norepinephrine (in 1949) were isolated from pheochromocytoma tissue. In 1950 it was observed that patients with pheochromocytoma excreted increased amounts of epinephrine, norepinephrine, and DA in the urine.

Catecholamine-secreting tumors occur with equal frequency in both sexes, primarily in the third, fourth, and fifth decades of life. These tumors are rare in children, and when discovered, they may be multifocal and associated with a hereditary syndrome. When symptoms are present, they are attributable to the pharmacologic effects of excess concentrations of circulating catecholamines. The resulting hypertension may be sustained (in about one-half of patients) or paroxysmal (in about one-third of patients). The remaining patients have normal blood pressure. The lability in blood pressure is attributed to episodic release of catecholamines, chronic volume depletion, and impaired sympathetic reflexes. Symptoms of orthostatic hypotension (e.g., lightheadedness, presyncope, syncope) may dominate the presentation, especially in patients with epinephrine-predominant or DA-predominant tumors.

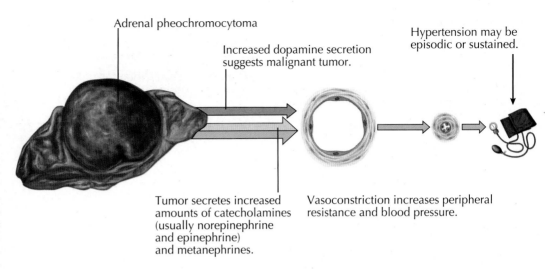

Adrenal pheochromocytoma

Increased dopamine secretion suggests malignant tumor.

Hypertension may be episodic or sustained.

Tumor secretes increased amounts of catecholamines (usually norepinephrine and epinephrine) and metanephrines.

Vasoconstriction increases peripheral resistance and blood pressure.

Pheochromocytoma is a chromaffin cell tumor secreting excessive catecholamines resulting in increased peripheral vascular resistance and hypertension.

Clinical features of pheochromocytoma

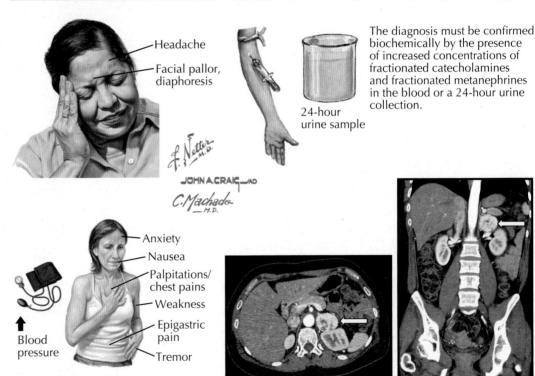

Headache

Facial pallor, diaphoresis

24-hour urine sample

The diagnosis must be confirmed biochemically by the presence of increased concentrations of fractionated catecholamines and fractionated metanephrines in the blood or a 24-hour urine collection.

Anxiety

Nausea

Palpitations/chest pains

Weakness

Epigastric pain

Tremor

Blood pressure

Symptoms are secondary to excessive catecholamine secretion and are usually paroxysmal. However, because of the increased use of CT imaging and familial testing, pheochromocytoma is diagnosed in more than 60% of patients before any symptoms develop.

Computer-assisted imaging of the abdomen and pelvis with CT or MRI should be the first localization test in a patient with a biochemically confirmed catecholamine-secreting tumor. A left adrenal pheochromocytoma (*arrow*) can be seen on the axial (*above left*) and coronal (*above right*) images of a contrast-enhanced CT scan of the abdomen.

Episodic symptoms may occur in spells, or paroxysms, that can be extremely variable in presentation but typically include forceful heartbeat, pallor, tremor, headache, and diaphoresis. The spell may start with a sensation of a rush in the chest and a sense of shortness of breath followed by a pounding heartbeat in the chest that typically progresses to a throbbing headache. Peripheral vasoconstriction with a spell results in cool or cold hands and feet and facial pallor. Increased sense of body heat and sweating are common symptoms that occur toward the end of the spell. Spells may be either spontaneous or precipitated by postural change, anxiety, medications (e.g., metoclopramide, corticosteroids, β-adrenergic blockers, anesthetic agents), exercise, or maneuvers that increase intraabdominal pressure (e.g., change in position, lifting, defecation, exercise, colonoscopy, pregnancy, trauma). Although the types of spells experienced across the patient population are highly variable, spells tend to be stereotypical for each patient. Spells may occur multiple times daily or as infrequently as once monthly.

Plate 3.28

Endocrine System: VOLUME 2

PHEOCHROMOCYTOMA AND PARAGANGLIOMA (Continued)

The typical duration of a pheochromocytoma-related spell is 15 to 20 minutes, but it may be much shorter or last several hours. However, the clinician must recognize that most patients with spells do not have a pheochromocytoma.

Additional clinical signs of catecholamine-secreting tumors include hypertensive retinopathy, orthostatic hypotension, angina, nausea, constipation (megacolon may be the presenting symptom), hyperglycemia, diabetes mellitus, hypercalcemia, Raynaud phenomenon, livedo reticularis, erythrocytosis, and mass effects from the tumor. Although the hypercalcemia may be a sign of multiple endocrine neoplasia type 2 (MEN 2), it is usually isolated and resolves with resection of the catecholamine-secreting tumor. Calcitonin secretion is a catecholamine-dependent process, and serum calcitonin concentrations are frequently elevated in patients with catecholamine-secreting tumors and are usually unrelated to MEN 2. Fasting hyperglycemia and diabetes mellitus are caused in part by the α-adrenergic inhibition of insulin release. Painless hematuria and paroxysmal attacks induced by micturition and defecation are associated with urinary bladder paragangliomas. Some of the cosecreted hormones that may dominate the clinical presentation include ACTH (Cushing syndrome), parathyroid hormone-related peptide (hypercalcemia), vasopressin (syndrome of inappropriate antidiuretic hormone secretion), vasoactive intestinal peptide (watery diarrhea), and growth hormone-releasing hormone (acromegaly). Cardiomyopathy and congestive heart failure are the symptomatic presentations caused by pheochromocytoma that perhaps are most frequently unrecognized by clinicians. The cardiomyopathy, whether dilated or hypertrophic, may be totally reversible with tumor resection. Myocarditis and myocardial infarction with normal coronary arteries seen on angiography are cardiac-based presentations that may not be recognized as being caused by pheochromocytoma. The myocarditis is characterized by infiltration of inflammatory cells and focal contraction-band necrosis. Many physical examination findings are associated with genetic syndromes that predispose to pheochromocytoma; these findings include retinal angiomas, marfanoid body habitus, café au lait spots, axillary freckling, subcutaneous neurofibromas, and mucosal neuromas on the eyelids and tongue. Some patients with pheochromocytoma may be asymptomatic despite high circulating levels of catecholamines, likely reflecting adrenergic receptor desensitization related to chronic stimulation.

Because of the increased use of computerized imaging (e.g., CT and MRI) and familial testing, pheochromocytoma is diagnosed in more than 60% of patients before any symptoms develop. Although these incidentally discovered tumors in patients are typically small (e.g., <3 cm), they may be as large as 10 cm.

The diagnosis must be confirmed biochemically by the presence of increased concentrations of fractionated catecholamines and fractionated metanephrines in the blood or a 24-hour urine collection. Localization studies should not be initiated until biochemical studies have confirmed the diagnosis of a catecholamine-secreting tumor.

Pheochromocytomas are localized to the adrenal glands and, when symptomatic, have an average diameter of 4.5 cm. Paragangliomas occur where there

POTENTIAL SITES OF PHEOCHROMOCYTOMA AND PARAGANGLIOMA

Secreting norepinephrine

Secreting epinephrine and norepinephrine

Sympathetic trunk

Arch of aorta

Diaphragm

Spleen

Adrenal medulla

Abdominal aorta

Kidney

Organ of Zuckerkandl

Ovary

Bladder wall

Testis

is chromaffin tissue, including along the para-aortic sympathetic chain, within the organs of Zuckerkandl (at the origin of the inferior mesenteric artery), in the wall of the urinary bladder, and along the sympathetic chain in the neck or mediastinum. During early postnatal life, the extraadrenal sympathetic paraganglionic tissues are prominent; they then degenerate, leaving residual foci associated with the vagus nerves, carotid vessels, aortic arch, pulmonary vessels, and mesenteric arteries. Unusual locations for paragangliomas include the intraatrial cardiac septum, spermatic cord, vagina, scrotum, and sacrococcygeal region. Whereas paragangliomas in the skull base and neck region (e.g., carotid body tumors, glomus tumors, chemodectomas) usually arise from parasympathetic tissue and typically do not hypersecrete catecholamines and metanephrines, paragangliomas in the mediastinum, abdomen, and pelvis usually arise from sympathetic chromaffin tissue and typically do hypersecrete catecholamines and metanephrines.

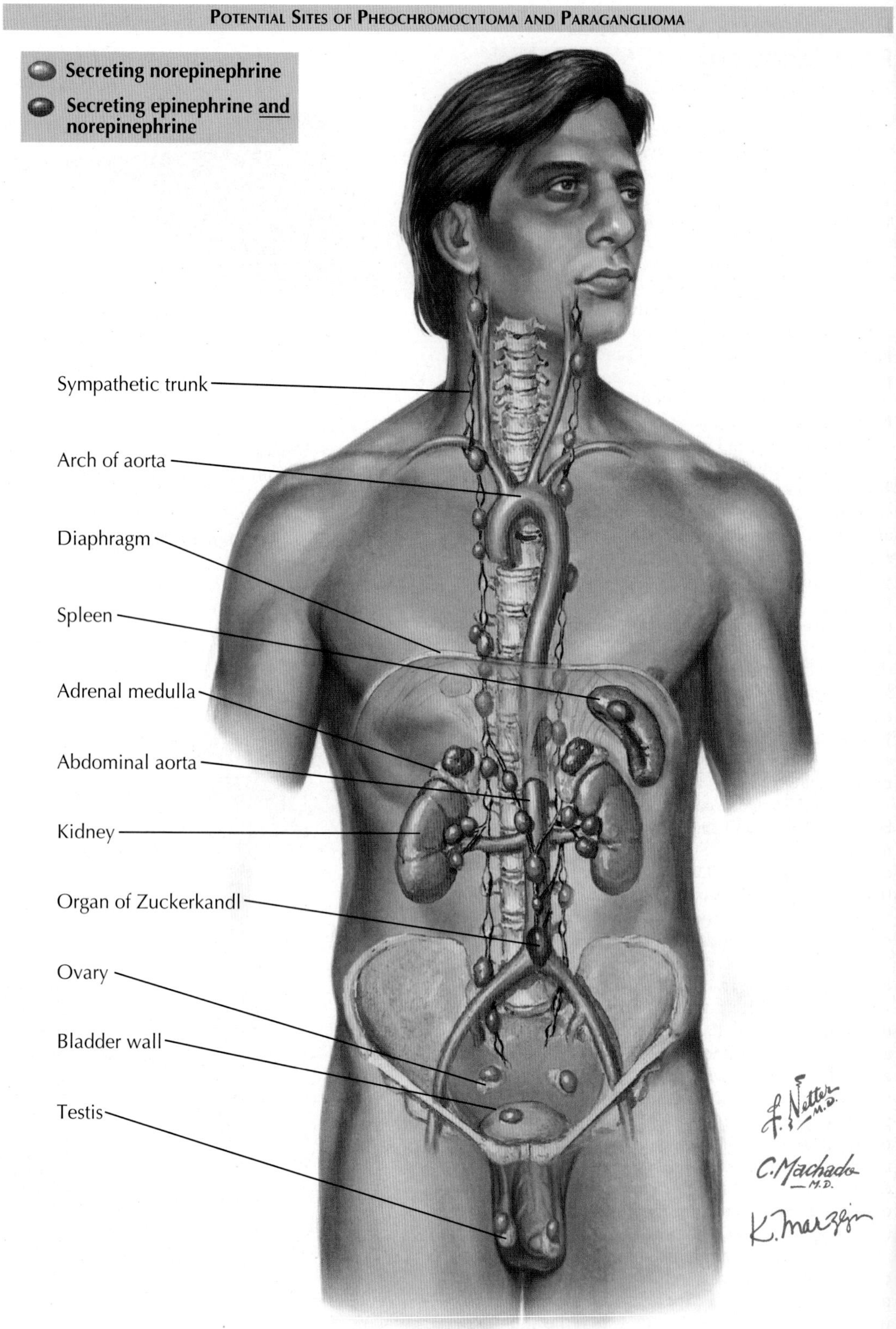

Plate 3.29

Adrenal

METASTATIC PHEOCHROMOCYTOMA AND PARAGANGLIOMA

The World Health Organization classification of tumors of endocrine organs advises that all pheochromocytomas and paragangliomas (PPGLs) have malignant potential—a potential that is only confirmed when metastatic disease is documented. Most patients with metastatic PPGL have sporadic tumors, whereas succinate dehydrogenase subunit B (*SDHB*) pathogenic variants are the most frequent form heritable PPGL in those patients who develop metastatic disease. In the Mayo Clinic series of 272 patients with metastatic PPGL, the median age at initial tumor diagnosis was 39 years (range, 7–83 years), and in 65% of patients the metastases developed at a median of 5.5 years (range, 0.3–53.4 years) from the initial diagnosis.

Metastatic sites of PPGL can be identified with gallium-68 (^{68}Ga) 1,4,7,10-tetraazacyclododecane-1,4,7,10-tetraacetic acid (DOTA)-octreotate (DOTATATE) positron emission tomography (PET) CT or ^{18}F-fluorodeoxyglucose (FDG) PET CT. MRI may be helpful in better defining size and anatomic associations of the metastatic sites identified on PET imaging studies.

The overall prognosis for patients with metastatic PPGL can be better than that reported for other metastatic malignancies. In the Mayo Clinic series, the median overall and disease-specific survivals were 24.6 and 33.7 years, respectively. Success in extending life is associated with a multimodality, multidisciplinary, and individualized approach to control catecholamine-dependent symptoms, local mass effect symptoms from the tumor, and overall tumor burden. The aggressiveness of the metastatic PPGL should be matched by the escalation in the use of treatment options—a process of "matching the penalty (treatment) to the crime (tumor)." Because there is no cure and because all treatment options carry risk, in patients with indolent disease the best treatment may be observation with periodic biochemical testing and imaging. In patients with a limited number of metastases (e.g., <6), targeted treatments are preferred over systemic treatment options. Treatment options include observation, surgery, thermal ablation, external radiotherapy, somatostatin analogs, cytotoxic chemotherapy, tyrosine kinase inhibitors, therapeutic doses of high-specific activity ^{131}I-metaiodobenzylquanidine, immunotherapy, and peptide receptor radiotherapy.

Metastatic sites include local tissue invasion, bone, liver, lung, omentum, and lymph nodes. Metastatic lesions should be resected, if possible, to decrease tumor burden. Skeletal metastatic lesions that are painful or threaten structural function can be treated with external radiotherapy, thermal ablation, or approached surgically. Thermal ablation may also be used to treat small (e.g., ≤3 cm in diameter) liver metastases. Because of the risk of massive catecholamine release, ablative therapy should be performed with great caution and only at centers with experience with these techniques; in addition to α- and β-adrenergic blockade, these patients are usually pretreated with α-methyl-paratyrosine (metyrosine) to decrease catecholamine stores in the tumor sites. External radiotherapy can also be used to treat unresectable soft tissue lesions. In selected cases, long-acting octreotide has been beneficial.

If the metastatic PPGL is considered aggressive and tumor burden has exceeded that which can be managed with targeted treatment options, cytotoxic chemotherapy with cyclophosphamide, vincristine, and dacarbazine can provide disease stabilization. Chemotherapy is typically administered for 6 months unless new lesions develop or there is a significant (e.g., >25%) increase in size of known tumor sites.

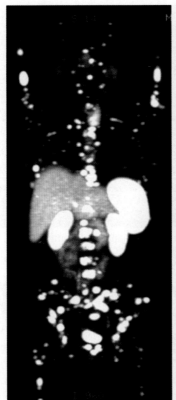
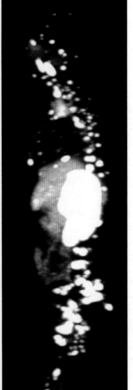

Coronal (*left*) and sagittal (*right*) images from Ga-68 DOTATATE PET CT scan. Markedly DOTATATE avid bone metastases are seen throughout the axial and appendicular skeleton in this patient with metastatic pheochromocytoma. Normal DOTATATE avidity is seen in the spleen, kidneys, liver, urinary bladder, and pituitary gland.

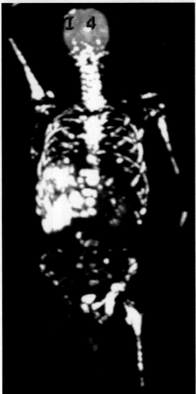

Coronal image from ^{18}F-FDG PET CT scan. Marked and diffuse FDG avid bone metastases are seen throughout the axial and appendicular skeleton and liver in this patient with metastatic pheochromocytoma. The cervical vertebral bodies and ribs are nearly totally replaced with metastatic disease.

Plate 3.30

Endocrine System: VOLUME 2

ADRENOCORTICAL CARCINOMA

ACC is an aggressive malignancy with an annual incidence of 1 to 2 cases per million individuals. ACC has a bimodal distribution, with peaks in the first and fifth decades of life (median age ≈ 55 yrs). Approximately 50% to 75% of patients present with signs and symptoms of adrenal steroid hormone excess—primarily glucocorticoids and androgens and less commonly mineralocorticoids and estrogens. A minority of ACCs (25%–50%) are hormonally silent.

The four stages of ACC at initial diagnosis include:

Stage I: <5 cm, no local extension or metastatic disease

Stage II: >5 cm, no local extension or metastatic disease

Stage III: any size with local extension (e.g., lymph nodes or periadrenal adipose tissue)

Stage IV: any size with distant metastatic disease (e.g., liver, lung, bone)

Approximately 40% of patients present with Stage I or II disease, 30% Stage III, and 30% with Stage IV. The median overall survivals are 14 years for Stage I, 6 years for Stage II, 4 years for Stage III, and 1 year for Stage IV disease. Complete surgical resection is the only possible curative treatment for ACC.

The "imaging phenotype" of an adrenal mass refers to its appearance on CT or MRI. The unenhanced CT attenuation measured in Hounsfield units (HU) is an excellent method to assess lipid content. Most adrenal cortical adenomas are lipid-rich with an unenhanced CT attenuation of <10 HU, whereas ACCs are lipid poor with unenhanced CT attenuations of >20 HU. In addition, most adrenal adenomas are small (e.g., <3 cm in diameter) and most ACCs are large (e.g., >4 cm in diameter). In addition to large size, the ACC imaging phenotype includes inhomogeneous appearance, irregular borders, speckled calcifications, tumor thrombus extension into the renal vein and IVC, and invasion of surrounding structures and/or lymph node enlargement. ^{18}F-fluorodeoxyglucose (FDG) PET may be helpful in assessing the extent of disease and the presence of metastases.

Before surgery, patients should have a hormonal assessment to determine the secretory activity of the tumor. Biochemical tests include measurements of cortisol in the blood and urine, measurements of adrenal androgens (e.g., DHEA-S and androstenedione), estrogens (e.g., estradiol and estrone), and mineralocorticoids (e.g., aldosterone and DOC). Additional testing may be needed to confirm Cushing syndrome or PA (see Plates 3.10 and 3.18).

Surgery should be performed by an expert adrenal surgeon to minimize the risk of incomplete resection. An oncologic en bloc resection of involved organs may be needed. Intracaval tumor thrombus is not a contraindication to surgery, and resection may require cardiopulmonary bypass.

The Weiss scoring system is based upon nine histopathologic features (nuclear grade, mitotic rate, atypical mitoses, clear cell component, diffuse architecture, tumor necrosis, invasion of venous or sinus structures, or tumor capsule). Each Weiss criterion is scored 0 when absent and 1 when present. Adrenal neoplasms with three or fewer features are considered as benign, and a Weiss score of 4 or higher is consistent with ACC. In addition, high-grade ACC is characterized by a high mitotic rate and/or Ki67 score >20%.

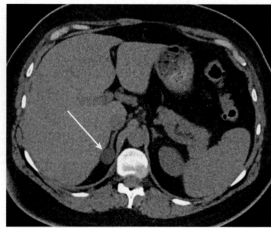

Axial image from an unenhanced abdominal CT scan shows a 1.9-cm lipid-rich (2.9 Hounsfield units) adrenal adenoma.

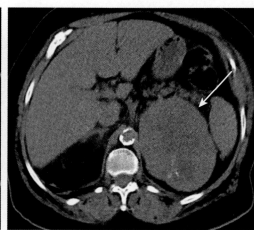

Axial image from an unenhanced abdominal CT scan shows an 11.4-cm lipid-poor (31 Hounsfield units) adrenal carcinoma.

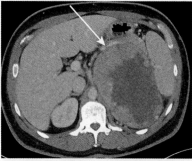

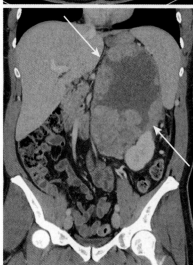

Abdominal CT scan (axial image *above*, coronal image *below*) shows a partially necrotic 16.1 cm × 11.2 cm × 22.3 cm adrenocortical carcinoma (*arrows*).

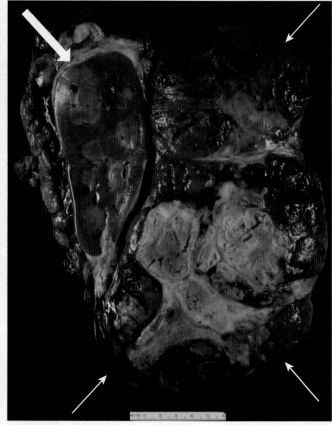

Gross pathology cut section of the adrenocortical carcinoma (*arrows*) and kidney (*thick arrow*) en bloc resection. Margins were free of tumor.

Mitotane (o,p′-DDD) is the initial treatment option for those patients with incomplete tumor resection. In addition, adjuvant mitotane treatment should be considered for patients at the highest risk of recurrence based on histologic findings (e.g., Ki67 staining of >10% of tumor cells and/or >20 mitotic figures per 50 HPF) or for those who had intraoperative tumor spillage or fracture. Due to its adrenolytic effects on the remaining normal adrenal gland, glucocorticoid replacement is indicated in all patients treated with mitotane. Postoperative radiation therapy should be considered for patients with incompletely resected ACC and those who have tumor spillage at the time of resection. There is no curative therapy for metastatic or recurrent ACC. For patients with unresectable metastatic disease, treatment with mitotane in combination with etoposide, doxorubicin, and cisplatin should be considered. Immunotherapy-based treatments, tyrosine kinase inhibitors, and other anticancer agents are under investigation.

Plate 3.31

Adrenal

TUMORS METASTATIC TO THE ADRENAL GLANDS

Metastatic disease to the adrenal glands is common. Although the reason for its frequency is not clear, it likely relates to the high concentrations of glucocorticoids and the rich sinusoidal blood supply. At autopsy, adrenal metastases are found in 50% of patients with disseminated lung or breast cancer, in 30% of patients with melanoma, and in 15% of patients with stomach or colon cancer. The adrenal metastases are bilateral in approximately half of the cases. However, clinically evident adrenal metastases or adrenal insufficiency is seen in only 4% of patients with tumors metastatic to the adrenal glands because most of the adrenal cortex of both adrenal glands must be destroyed before hypofunction becomes symptomatic.

In the past, when metastatic disease to the adrenal glands was detected during life, the most common clinical presentation was an insidious onset of signs and symptoms related to primary adrenal insufficiency (e.g., fatigue, myalgias, nausea, anorexia, orthostatic hypotension, hyperpigmentation) or flank pain. However, asymptomatic metastases to the adrenal glands are becoming more commonly detected during life because of the widespread use of CT imaging and PET in staging malignancies. Adenocarcinoma is the most common cell type. The most common organ locations for the primary malignancy (in order of frequency) are the lung, stomach, kidney, breast, colon, skin (melanoma), and pancreas. Adrenal metastases from primary tumors of the esophagus, liver, and bile ducts are more common in individuals of Asian ancestry. In approximately 70% of cases, the adrenal metastasis is discovered concurrently with the primary malignancy; in the remaining patients, the adrenal metastases are typically found over a median duration of 7 to 30 months after the detection of the primary tumor. The longest interval between the diagnosis of primary cancer and the discovery of the adrenal metastasis is found in patients with lymphoma, breast cancer, renal cell carcinoma, and colorectal carcinoma.

Accurate identification of the type of metastatic lesion usually relies on image-guided fine-needle aspiration biopsy and use of adjunctive immunocytochemical techniques on the biopsy specimen. The possibility of an incidentally discovered adrenal pheochromocytoma should be excluded with biochemical tests before proceeding with any biopsy procedure.

Nearly 100% of these patients have metastatic disease to sites in addition to the adrenal glands.

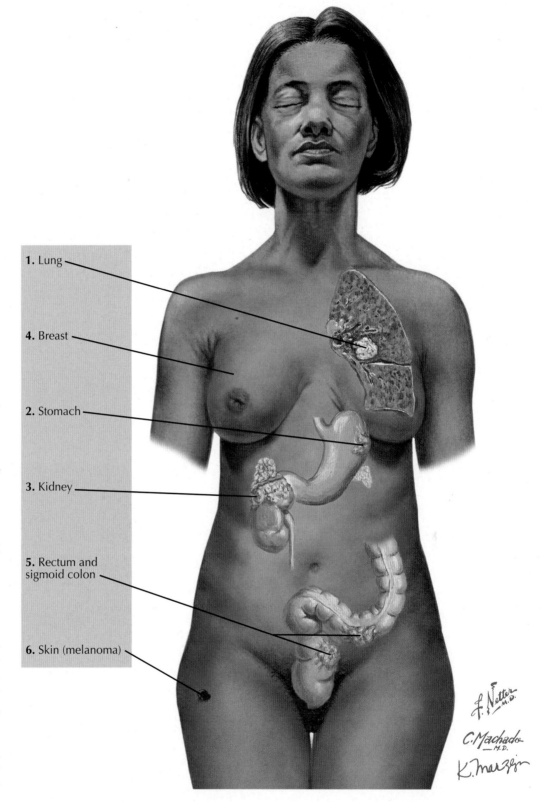

1. Lung
4. Breast
2. Stomach
3. Kidney
5. Rectum and sigmoid colon
6. Skin (melanoma)

Metastatic disease to the adrenal glands is a poor prognostic sign; the 1-year mortality rate is 80%. However, patients with adrenal metastases that are removed surgically have better survival rates than patients who do not have surgery. Long-term survivors after surgical treatment for adrenal metastasis have been reported. More recently, adrenal ablative therapy has been used for the management of small (<5 cm in largest lesional diameter) adrenal masses. Percutaneous thermal ablation offers an effective minimally morbid intervention for patients who are poor surgical candidates. Ablative techniques include radiofrequency ablation, microwave ablation, cryoablation, and chemical ablation. Most of these procedures can be performed under percutaneous radiographic guidance in the outpatient setting. Potential complications at the time of ablative therapy include hypertensive crisis and damage to adjacent tissues.

REPRODUCTION

Plate 4.1

Endocrine System: VOLUME 2

DIFFERENTIATION OF GONADS

FACTORS INFLUENCING NORMAL AND ABNORMAL GONADAL DIFFERENTIATION

Whether the primordial gonad differentiates as a testis or as an ovary is determined by genetic information coded on the X and Y chromosomes. The differentiation of all the other anatomic and functional features that distinguish male from female stem secondarily from the effect of testicular or ovarian secretions on their respective primordial structures. The Y chromosome possesses male-determining genes that direct the primitive gonad to develop as a testis, even in the presence of more than one X chromosome. Two X chromosomes are essential for the formation of normal ovaries; individuals with a single X chromosome (karyotype, 45,XO; Turner syndrome) develop gonads that usually display only the most rudimentary form of differentiation.

Although many patients with congenitally defective gonads have an abnormal karyotype caused by meiotic nondisjunction, similar patients may have normal-appearing sex chromosomes or chromosomal abnormalities not explainable on this basis. In individuals with chromosomal mosaicism, the various tissues may have multiple cell lines of differing chromosomal makeup. Mosaicism arises from mitotic nondisjunction or chromosomal loss occurring after fertilization. Other patients may have deletions or translocations of small chromosomal fragments. If these rearrangements disrupt the sex-determining genes, the effect on gonadal structure may be as devastating as in instances where a total chromosome is lost. In other individuals, pathogenic variants in sex-determining genes may cause a specific enzymatic error, leading to defective gonadal structure or hormonal secretion.

STAGES IN GONADAL DIFFERENTIATION

Undifferentiated Stage

At the sixth week of gestation, the primitive gonad is represented by a well-demarcated genital ridge running along the dorsal root of the mesentery. The cortical portion of the ridge consists of a cloak of coelomic epithelial cells. The mature ovary is derived principally from these cortical cells. Large primordial germ cells are also found in these superficial layers that are capable of differentiating as either oogonia or spermatogonia.

The medullary, or interior, portion of the primitive gonad is composed of a mesenchyme, in which sheets of epithelial cells are condensed to form the primary sex cords. This medullary portion has the potential to further differentiate as a testis.

Testicular Differentiation

Testicular differentiation is determined by the Y chromosome *SRY* gene and a related homeobox gene, *SOX9* (an autosomal gene). *SRY* regulates *SOX9* expression. *SOX9* in turn directly regulates transcription of antimüllerian hormone (AMH) by Sertoli cell precursors. AMH causes müllerian duct regression. As the primitive gonad becomes a testis, the inner portion of the primary sex cords becomes a collecting system connecting the seminiferous tubules with the mesonephric, or wolffian, duct. The peripheral portions of the sex cords join with ingrowths of coelomic epithelium (containing primordial germ cells) to form seminiferous tubules. Most of the cortex, however, becomes isolated by the tunica albuginea and the tunica vaginalis, which

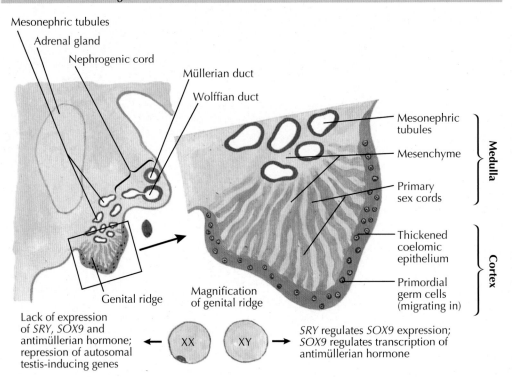

Undifferentiated stage

Mesonephric tubules
Adrenal gland
Nephrogenic cord
Müllerian duct
Wolffian duct
Genital ridge
Magnification of genital ridge

Mesonephric tubules
Mesenchyme
Primary sex cords
— Medulla

Thickened coelomic epithelium
Primordial germ cells (migrating in)
— Cortex

Lack of expression of *SRY*, *SOX9* and antimüllerian hormone; repression of autosomal testis-inducing genes ← XX | XY → *SRY* regulates *SOX9* expression; *SOX9* regulates transcription of antimüllerian hormone

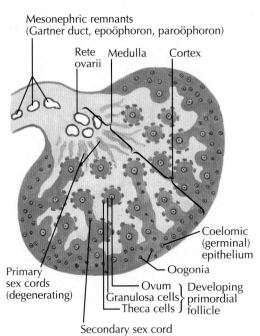

Female (primitive ovary)

Mesonephric remnants (Gartner duct, epoöphoron, paroöphoron)
Rete ovarii
Medulla
Cortex
Primary sex cords (degenerating)
Coelomic (germinal) epithelium
Oogonia
Ovum
Granulosa cells
Theca cells
Developing primordial follicle
Secondary sex cord

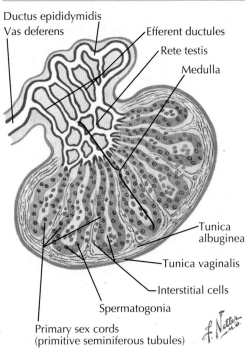

Male (primitive testis)

Ductus epididymidis
Vas deferens
Efferent ductules
Rete testis
Medulla
Tunica albuginea
Tunica vaginalis
Interstitial cells
Spermatogonia
Primary sex cords (primitive seminiferous tubules)

are the only cortical vestiges in the mature testis. Interstitial cells of Leydig become abundant at about 8 weeks and secrete androgenic hormone necessary for the development of male external genitalia. Leydig cells disappear shortly after birth and are not seen again until the onset of adolescence.

Ovarian Differentiation

Ovarian development occurs several weeks later than testicular differentiation. Ovarian differentiation is determined by the lack of expression of *SRY*, *SOX9*, and AMH. There is likely a mechanism to repress autosomal

testis-inducing genes (e.g., *SOX9*) and to activate ovary-inducing genes (e.g., *WNT4* and *NR0B1* [*DAX1*]). At this time, the cortex undergoes intense proliferation, and strands of epithelial cells (called *secondary sex cords*) push into the interior of the gonad. Primordial germ cells are carried along in this inward migration. Clumps from the secondary sex cords fragment off to form primordial follicles. While the ovary is thus forming, the primary sex cords recede to the hilum, leaving stromal and connective tissue cells behind. Leydig cells and the rete ovarii persist as medullary remnants in the ovary. Proliferation of the cortex ceases at about 6 months.

Plate 4.2   Reproduction

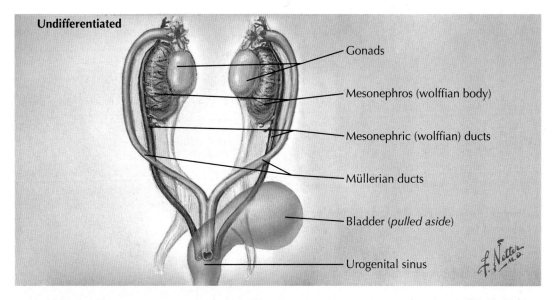

Undifferentiated
- Gonads
- Mesonephros (wolffian body)
- Mesonephric (wolffian) ducts
- Müllerian ducts
- Bladder (*pulled aside*)
- Urogenital sinus

Female
- Ovary
- Wolffian duct degenerates and müllerian duct persists in absence of *SRY*.
- Fallopian tube
- Gartner duct
- Epoöphoron
- Appendix vesiculosa
- Paroöphoron
- Ovary
- Uterus
- Round lig.
- Upper vagina
- Wolffian duct remnant
- Urethra
- Lower vagina
- Skene duct
- Bartholin gland

Male
- Testis
- Degenerating müllerian duct
- Persistent wolffian duct (vas deferens)
- Vas deferens
- Seminal vesicle
- Prostatic utricle
- Prostate gland
- Bulbourethral gland
- Vas deferens
- Appendix epididymis
- Appendix testis
- Epididymis
- Vasa efferentia
- Testis
- Gubernaculum

DIFFERENTIATION OF GENITAL DUCTS

The early embryo of either sex is equipped with identical primitive gonads that have the capacity to develop into either testes or ovaries. In the case of the internal genital ducts, however, the early embryo has both a male and a female set of primordial structures. The müllerian ducts have the potential to develop into fallopian tubes, a uterus, and the upper portion of the vagina. The mesonephric, or wolffian, ducts have the capacity to develop into the vas deferens and the seminal vesicles. The large wolffian body, containing the proximal mesonephric ducts, becomes the epididymis.

During the third fetal month, either the müllerian or the wolffian structures normally complete their development, and involution occurs simultaneously in the other set. Vestigial remnants of the other duct system, however, persist into adult life. In females, the mesonephric structures are represented by the epoöphoron, paroöphoron, and the ducts of Gartner. In males, the only müllerian remnant normally present is the appendix testis.

The direction in which these genital ducts develop is a direct consequence of the gonadal differentiation that occurred somewhat earlier. Testicular differentiation is determined by the Y chromosome *SRY* gene and a related homeobox gene, *SOX9* (an autosomal gene). *SRY* regulates *SOX9* expression. *SOX9* in turn directly regulates transcription of AMH by Sertoli cell precursors. AMH causes müllerian duct regression through apoptosis and mesenchymal-epithelial cell remodeling. Müllerian ducts are nearly completely absent by 10 weeks; then the derivatives of the mesonephric system complete their normal male development.

Ovarian differentiation is determined by the lack of expression of *SRY*, *SOX9*, and AMH. There is likely a mechanism to repress autosomal testis-inducing genes (e.g., *SOX9*) and to activate ovary-inducing genes (e.g., *WNT4* and *NR0B1* [*DAX1*]). In this setting, the müllerian structures proceed to become the uterus and fallopian tubes, and the mesonephric structures become vestigial. It should be emphasized that female development is not dependent on any ovarian secretion because in the absence of any gonads at all, the uterus and fallopian tubes develop normally.

In the female, ovarian differentiation is determined by the lack of expression of *SRY*, *SOX9*, and antimüllerian hormone. Müllerian structures proceed to become the uterus and fallopian tubes, and the wolffian ducts become vestigial.

In the male, the Y chromosome–encoded *SRY* regulates *SOX9* expression. *SOX9* regulates transcription of antimüllerian hormone, causing the müllerian ducts to degenerate and wolffian ducts to persist and differentiate.

It is clear that *SRY* is the key factor in testis determination. However, multiple other factors must be repressed or activated for normal testicular development. This concept is evidenced by the findings of 46,XX males with testes who do not have a Y chromosome and by 46,XY females with gonadal dysgenesis who have an intact *SRY* gene. Thus non–Y chromosomal factors must contribute in a clinically important way to testis determination.

Plate 4.3

Endocrine System: VOLUME 2

DIFFERENTIATION OF EXTERNAL GENITALIA

Before the ninth week of gestation, both sexes have a urogenital sinus and an identical external appearance. At this undifferentiated stage, the external genitalia consist of a genital tubercle beneath which is a urethral groove, bounded laterally by urethral folds and labioscrotal swellings. The male and female derivatives of these structures are shown in Plate 4.3.

The urogenital slit is formed at an even earlier stage when the perineal membrane partitions it from a single cloacal opening. Thereafter, the bladder and both genital ducts find a common outlet in this sinus.

The vagina develops as a diverticulum of the urogenital sinus in the region of the müllerian tubercle and becomes contiguous with the distal end of the müllerian ducts. About two-thirds of the vagina originates in the urogenital sinus, and about one-third is of müllerian origin.

In normal male development, the vaginal remnant is tiny because the müllerian structures atrophy before this diverticulum develops very far. In male pseudohermaphroditism, however, a sizable remnant of this vaginal diverticulum may persist as a blind vaginal pouch.

In normal female development, the vagina is pushed posteriorly by a downgrowth of connective tissue, so that by the 12th fetal week, it has acquired a separate external opening. In female pseudohermaphroditism, the growth of this septum is inhibited, leading to persistence of the urogenital sinus.

The principal distinctions between male and female external genitalia at this stage of development are the location and size of the vaginal diverticulum, the size of the phallus, and the degree of fusion of the urethral folds and labioscrotal swellings.

As in the case of the genital ducts, there is an inherent tendency for the external genitalia to develop along feminine lines. Masculinization of the external genitalia is brought about by exposure to androgenic hormones during the process of differentiation. Normally, the androgenic hormone is testosterone, derived from the Leydig cells of the fetal testis. The critical factor in determining whether masculinization will occur, however, is not the source of the androgen but rather its timing and its amount. In female pseudohermaphroditism caused by congenital adrenal hyperplasia (CAH), the fetal adrenal glands secrete sufficient androgen to bring about some masculinization of the external genitalia. In other instances, androgenic hormone may be derived from the maternal circulation.

By the 12th fetal week, the vagina has migrated posteriorly, and androgens will no longer cause fusion of the urethral and labioscrotal folds. Clitoral hypertrophy, however, may occur at any time in fetal life or even after birth.

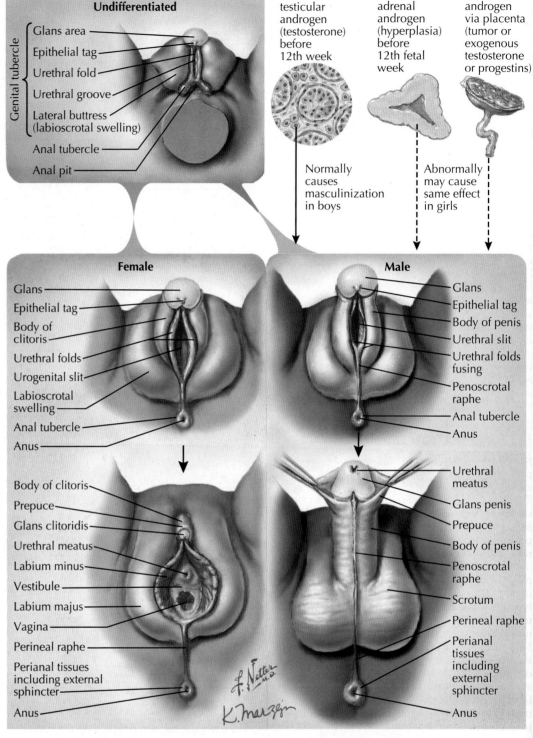

Female and male derivatives of urogenital sinus and external genitalia

Female derivative	Primordial structure	Male derivative
Vagina (lower two-thirds) Paraurethral glands (of Skene) Bartholin glands	Urogenital sinus	Prostatic utricle (vagina masculina) Prostate Bulbourethral glands (of Cowper)
Clitoris Corpora cavernosa Glands clitoridis	External genitalia *Genital tubercle*	Penis Corpora cavernosa Glans penis
Labia minora	Urethral folds	Corpus spongiosum (enclosing penile urethra)
Labia majora	Labioscrotal swellings	Scrotum

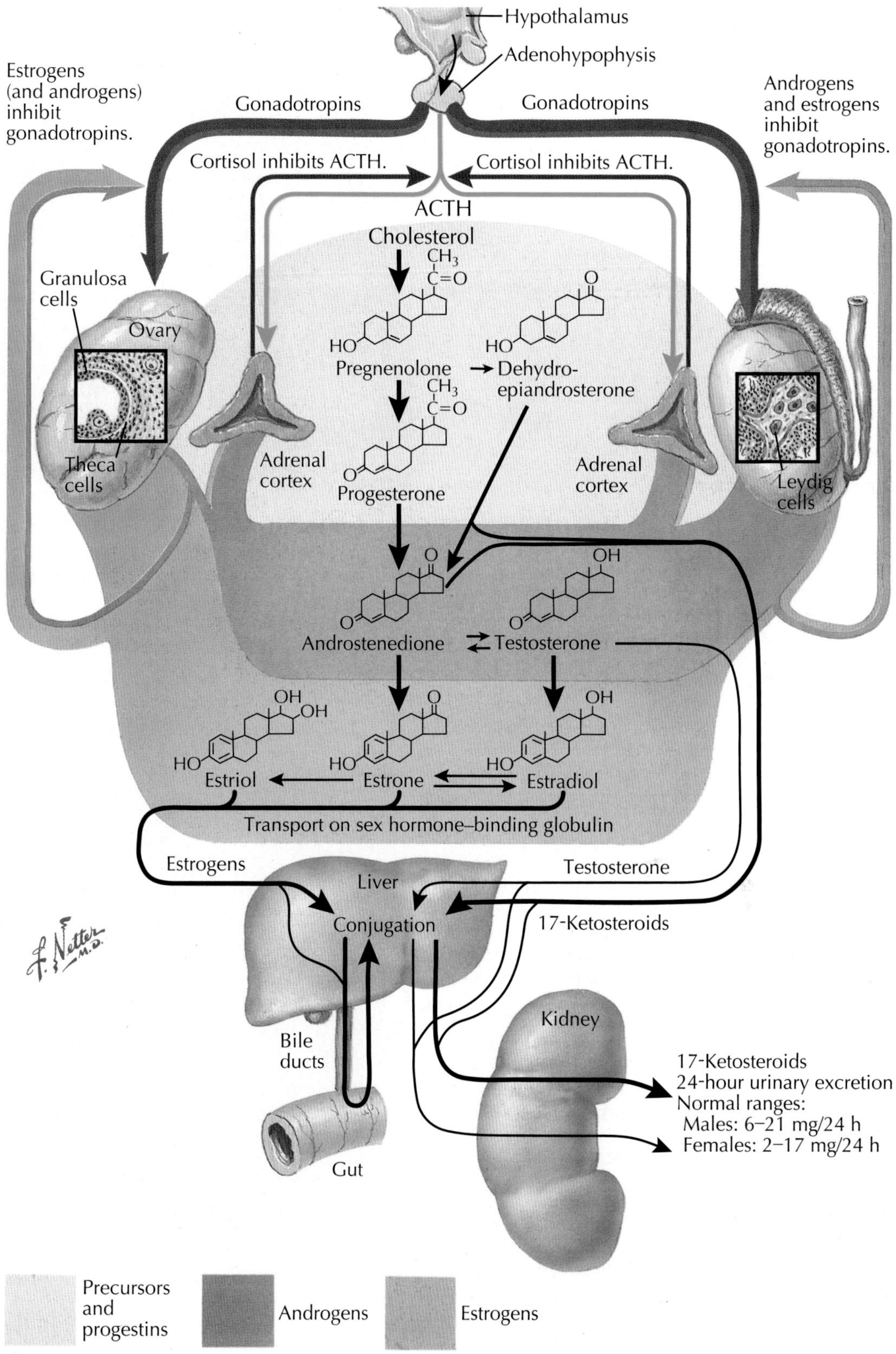

Plate 4.4

Reproduction

TESTOSTERONE AND ESTROGEN SYNTHESIS

Three glands that originate in the coelomic cavity—the adrenal cortex, the ovary, and the testis—produce steroids under the influence of tropic hormones of the anterior pituitary, corticotropin (adrenocorticotropic hormone [ACTH]) and gonadotropins. Cleaving cholesterol into pregnenolone (the C_{21} precursor of all active steroid hormones) and isocaproaldehyde is the critical first step, and it occurs in a limited number of sites in the body (adrenal cortex, testicular Leydig cells, ovarian theca cells, trophoblast cells of the placenta, and certain glial and neuronal cells of the brain). The roles of different steroidogenic tissues are determined by how this process is regulated and how pregnenolone is subsequently metabolized. Androgens have 19 carbon atoms (C19 steroids), and estrogens have 18 carbon atoms (C18 steroids).

Pregnenolone is converted to 17α-hydroxypregnenolone by 17α-hydroxylase (P450c17). P450c17 also possesses 17,20-lyase activity, which results in the production of the C19 adrenal androgens (dehydroepiandrosterone [DHEA] and androstenedione). Most of the adrenal androstenedione production is dependent on the conversion of DHEA to androstenedione by 3β-hydroxysteroid dehydrogenase. Androstenedione may be converted to testosterone by 17β-ketosteroid reductase (17β-HSD3) in the adrenal glands or gonads. Androstenedione and testosterone are secretory products of the Leydig cells, which are found in abundance in the testis but are present in only small numbers in the hilar region of the ovary. In males, 95% of testosterone (7 mg/day) is produced by the testicles under the control of luteinizing hormone (LH). The local effect of testosterone can be amplified by conversion via type 2 5α-reductase to the more potent dihydrotestosterone. This local amplification system occurs at the hair follicle and the prostate gland. Testosterone is bound to sex hormone-binding globulin (SHBG) in the blood. Conjugation with glucuronic acid takes place in the liver. Much of the conjugated testosterone is excreted in its water-soluble form by the kidney with a little free, unconjugated testosterone.

DHEA, a precursor of androstenedione and testosterone, is found mostly in the 17-ketosteroid fraction in the urine and is derived largely from the adrenal cortex. It is a weak androgen that makes up more than 60% of the 17-ketosteroids. The normal excretion value for 17-ketosteroids is higher in males than in females, presumably because of the contribution by the testis of some DHEA and a variety of other C17-ketosteroids.

The ovary contains at least three differential secretory zones: the granulosa cells of the follicle, engaged in estrogen formation; the theca cells, having a tendency to produce somewhat more androgens; and the hilar cells, predominantly involved in androgen formation. The balance of these cellular elements ensures a normal

degree of femininity; conversely, an imbalance leads to androgenicity. Within the ovary there are also the cells of the corpus luteum, which produce the bulk of progesterone.

Testosterone and androstenedione, respectively, are precursors of estradiol and estrone. Hydroxylation of the 19-carbon initiates a series of reactions that aromatize the A ring of the steroid nucleus, and this aromatization is, in fact, characteristic of estrogens. Estradiol is

more potent than estrone; estriol is purely an excretory product, which is extremely weak biologically.

The estrogens are bound in blood by SHBG and albumin. Inactivation of estrogen occurs in the liver through conversion to less active estrogens (i.e., estradiol to estrone to estriol), oxidation to totally inert compounds, or conjugation to glucuronic acid. There is considerable enterohepatic circulation because estrogens are excreted in the bile.

Plate 4.5

Endocrine System: VOLUME 2

TANNER STAGES OF BREAST DEVELOPMENT

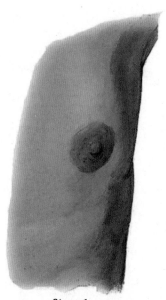

Stage 1
Elevation of papilla only

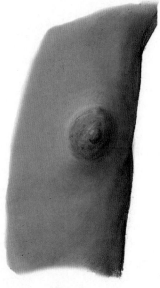

Stage 2
Breast bud: elevation of
breast and papilla as a small
mound and enlargement
of areolar diameter

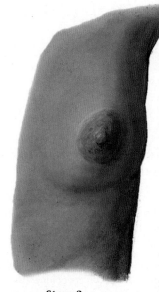

Stage 3
Additional enlargement
of breast and areola with
no separation of their
contours

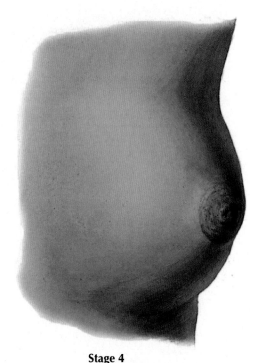

Stage 4
Areola and papilla project from surface
of breast to form secondary mound.

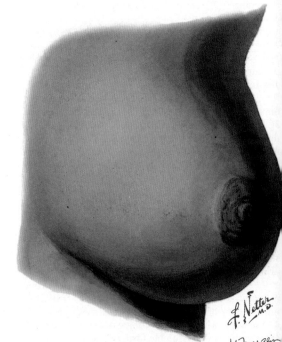

Stage 5
Mature stage with projection of papilla only with recession
of the areola to the general contour of the breast

NORMAL PUBERTY

TIMING OF PUBERTY

Although it is often thought of as a distinct event, puberty is part of a lifelong process of hypothalamic-pituitary-gonadal development. Puberty is a biologic transition during which secondary sex characteristics develop, a linear growth spurt occurs, fertility is realized, and psychosocial changes occur. *Adrenarche* refers to the adrenal component of pubertal maturation and usually occurs earlier than gonadarche (the maturation of the hypothalamic-pituitary-gonadal system). *Thelarche* refers to pubertal breast development.

Before the onset of puberty, conspicuous physical differences between boys and girls are largely confined to the anatomy of their genital organs. The mean age of puberty onset is 10.6 years (range, 7–13 years) in White girls and 8.9 years (range, 6–13 years) in African American girls. The mean age of puberty onset in boys is 11 years (range, 9–14 years); some African American boys start puberty between 8 and 9 years.

The factors that lead to the maturation of the GnRH pulse generator and thus trigger the onset of puberty are multiple and not yet fully understood. For example, body weight is one factor that triggers puberty, and the mechanism may involve leptin, a hormone produced in adipocytes. Puberty does not occur in animal models that are deficient in leptin but can be induced by leptin administration.

Most of the physical changes that begin at puberty are attributable to an increase in androgens and estrogens from the gonads and reticular zone of the adrenal cortex. The gonads are activated by pituitary LH and follicle-stimulating hormone (FSH), which, until this time, are not secreted in clinically important amounts in normally developing children. Corticotropin (ACTH) and a yet to be identified adrenal androgen-stimulating factor (perhaps of pituitary origin) appear to be responsible for adrenarche.

The capacity to secrete both androgens and estrogens is inherent in the adrenal glands as well as in the gonads of both sexes. Enlargement of the reticular zone of the adrenal cortex and increased secretion of adrenal androgens occur at about the same time that the ovaries exhibit heightened activity. Androgenic hormones from both the adrenals and ovaries increase the growth rate and the development of pubic hair, later axillary hair, and seborrhea

and acne. Both androgens and estrogens have a stimulatory effect on epiphysial maturation, and as fusion occurs, the rate of linear growth rapidly decelerates.

Approximately 18% of total adult height accrues during the pubertal growth spurt. Although the pubertal growth velocity is slightly lower in girls, they reach their peak height velocity about 2 years earlier than

boys. In boys, the peak height velocity is approximately 9.5 cm per year at an average age of 13.5 years, whereas in girls, the peak height velocity is approximately 8.3 cm per year at an average age of 11.5 years. Because of a longer duration of pubertal growth, boys on average gain 10 more centimeters of increased height than girls through the pubertal growth spurt, thus accounting for the general difference in sex-dependent adult

Plate 4.6

Reproduction

TANNER STAGES OF FEMALE PUBIC HAIR DEVELOPMENT

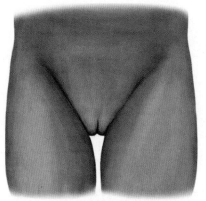

Stage 1
The vellus over the pubes is the same as that over the anterior abdominal wall.

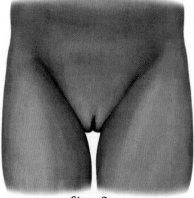

Stage 2
Sparse slightly pigmented, downy hair along the labia that is straight or only slightly curled

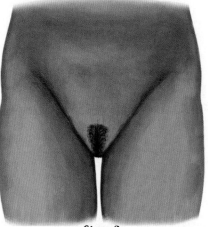

Stage 3
Hair spreads sparsely over the pubic region and is darker, coarser, and curlier.

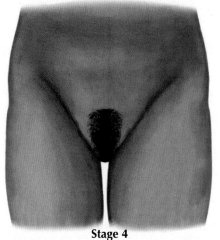

Stage 4
Hair is adult type, but the area covered is smaller than in most adults, and there is no spread to the medial surface of the thighs.

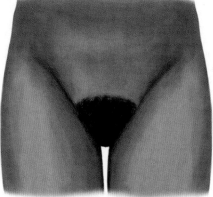

Stage 5
Hair is adult in quantity and type, distributed as an inverse triangle, and spreads to the medial surface of the thighs but not up the midline anterior abdominal wall.

NORMAL PUBERTY (Continued)

height. Normal growth spurt in girls is dependent on growth hormone (GH), insulin-like growth factor 1 (IGF-1), and estrogen. In boys, growth is dependent on GH, IGF-1, estrogen, and testosterone. Increased pubertal blood estradiol concentrations appear to trigger hypothalamic-pituitary activity that results in increased GH pulse amplitude and frequency. Serum IGF-1 concentrations peak during puberty and remain increased for approximately 2 years after the pubertal growth spurt before falling into the adult reference ranges.

The upper body to lower body segment ratio (U:L ratio) is defined as the distance from the top of the head to the top of the pubic ramus, divided by the length from the bottom of the feet to the top of the pubic ramus. The U:L ratio is approximately 1.7 at birth, 1.4 at 1 year of age, 1.0 at 10 years of age, 0.92 in White adults, and 0.85 in African American adults. The U:L ratios are the same in females and males. Eunuchoid proportions (decreased U:L ratio) develop in patients with hypogonadism, in whom epiphyseal fusion is delayed and the extremities grow for a prolonged period of time. Eunuchoid proportions are also seen patients with estrogen receptor deficiency or defects in estrogen synthesis. Patients who produce excess estrogen (aromatase excess), however, have advanced skeletal maturation, an increased U:L ratio, and short adult height.

Almost 50% of total body calcium in girls and slightly more than 50% in boys is laid down in bone mineral during puberty. After puberty, boys have 50% more total body calcium than girls. During puberty, the hips enlarge more in girls, and the shoulders become wider in boys. The pelvic inlet widens in girls because of the growth of the os acetabuli. Males have 50% more lean body mass and skeletal mass than females, and females generally have twice the amount of body adipose tissue (distributed in the upper arms, thighs, and upper back) than males. Cardiovascular changes that occur during puberty include a greater aerobic reserve.

Marshall and Tanner developed a staging system to document the sequence of changes of secondary sexual characteristics. The Tanner stages are based on visual criteria to document five stages of pubertal development with regard to breast and pubic hair development in girls and genital and pubic hair development in boys. Stage 1 is the prepubertal state, and stage 5 is the adult state.

FEMALE PUBERTY

The three main phenotypic pubertal events in girls are increased height velocity, breast development (thelarche, under the control of ovarian estrogen secretion), and growth of axillary and pubic hair (under the control of androgens secreted by the ovaries and adrenal glands). An increase in height velocity is usually the first sign of puberty in girls. Most girls grow only approximately 2.5 cm in height after menarche. The stages of breast and pubic hair development usually progress in concert, but discordance may occur, and they are best classified separately. The mean age of puberty onset is 10.6 years (range, 7–13 years) in White girls and 8.9 years (range, 6–13 years) in African American girls.

Pubertal breast enlargement (thelarche) is associated with increased amounts of glandular and connective tissue. The size and shape of breasts are determined by

Plate 4.7

Endocrine System: VOLUME 2

TANNER STAGES OF MALE PUBIC HAIR AND GENITAL DEVELOPMENT

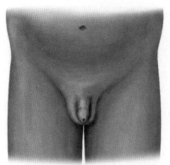

Stage 1

Penis, testes, and scrotum are the same size and proportion as in early childhood.

The vellus hair over the pubic region is the same as that on the abdominal wall.

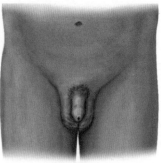

Stage 2

Testes and scrotum enlarge, and scrotal skin shows a change in texture and reddening.

Sparse growth of straight or slightly curled pigmented hair appearing at the base of the penis

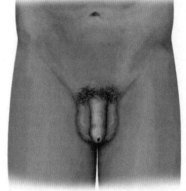

Stage 3

Penile growth in length more than width; further growth of the testes and scrotum

Hair is coarser, curlier, and darker, spread sparsely over the junction of the pubes.

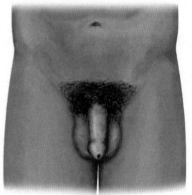

Stage 4

Further penile growth and development of the glans; further enlargement of testes and scrotum

Adult-type hair, but area covered less than in most adults; no spread to the medial surface of the thighs

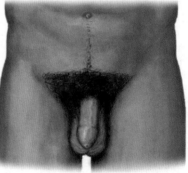

Stage 5

Genitalia are adult in size and shape.

Adult in quantity and type of hair, distributed as an inverse triangle; spread is to the medial surface of the thighs.

NORMAL PUBERTY (Continued)

genetic factors, nutritional factors, and exposure to estrogen. Initially, breast development may be unilateral and then asynchronous. In the prepubertal girl (Tanner stage 1), there is elevation of papilla (see Plate 4.5). Tanner stage 2 is the breast bud stage, with enlargement of the areolar diameter and elevation of breast and papilla as a small mound. The mean age of onset of Tanner stage 2 breast development is 10.3 years in White girls and 9.5 years in African American girls. In Tanner stage 3, there is further enlargement of breast and areola, but with no separation of their contours. In Tanner stage 4, the areola and papilla project above the level of the breast to form a secondary mound. In Tanner stage 5, the mature breast has formed, there is recession of the areola, and only the papilla projects from the surface of the breast. The diameter of the papilla increases from 3 to 4 mm (in Tanner breast stages 1 through 3) to an average diameter of 9 mm in Tanner stage 5.

In the prepubertal girl (Tanner pubic hair stage 1), there is vellus-type hair over the pubic region, but it is not different from that over the anterior abdominal wall (see Plate 4.6). In Tanner stage 2, early pubic hair becomes evident; it is slightly pigmented and straight or slightly curled, appearing along the labia. The mean age of onset of Tanner stage 2 pubic hair development is 10.4 years in White girls and 9.4 years in African American girls. During Tanner stage 3, the hair spreads sparsely over the pubic region, and it becomes coarser, darker, and curlier. In Tanner stage 4, the hair is adult in type, but it covers a smaller area than in most adults and it does not appear on the medial surface of the thighs. In Tanner stage 5, the appearance is that of an adult in distribution (including the medial surface of the thighs), quantity, and type.

During the progression through the pubic hair stages, the vaginal mucosa undergoes changes because of estrogen effects. The vaginal mucosa loses its prepubertal reddish glistening form and becomes thickened and dull because of cornification of the vaginal epithelium. Several months before menarche, there is vaginal secretion of clear or whitish discharge. The length of the vagina increases, and the labia minor and majora become thickened and rugated. There is a rounding of body contours, a fat pad develops in the mons pubis, and the clitoris increases in size. The uterus enlarges from a prepubertal length of 3 cm to a postpubertal

length of 8 cm. The endometrium begins to proliferate during the first stages of puberty.

In White girls in the United States, the average age of menstruation (menarche) onset is 12.8 years; it is 6 months earlier in African American girls. Menarche occurs 1 to 3 years after the onset of puberty, typically during Tanner stage 4. Ovulation does not occur until some additional months have elapsed. Until then, the menses are often erratic, and even then, anovulatory cycles are common for the first 2 years after menarche.

Progesterone is secreted only as corpora lutea are formed after ovulation. When this occurs, the proliferative endometrium is transformed into a secretory type. The peak in ovarian primordial follicles is reached at 20 weeks of fetal life, and no additional germ cells develop after this time point. Under gonadotropin stimulation during puberty, the ovaries become microcystic with the development of follicles more than 4 mm in diameter. The ovarian volume increases from a prepubertal size of 0.2 to 1.6 mL to 2.8 to 15 mL during puberty.

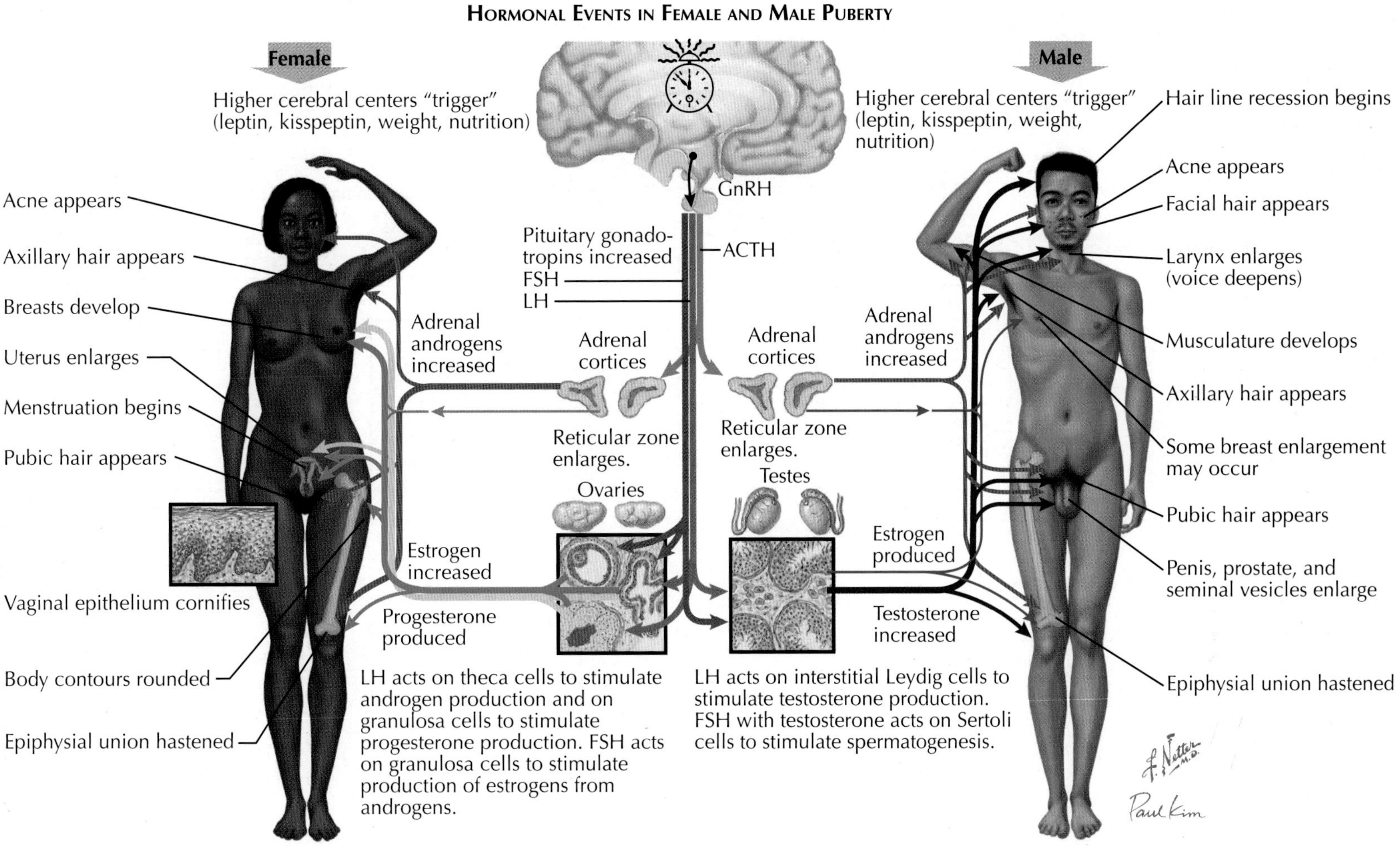

Plate 4.8

Reproduction

HORMONAL EVENTS IN FEMALE AND MALE PUBERTY

Female

Higher cerebral centers "trigger" (leptin, kisspeptin, weight, nutrition)

Acne appears

Axillary hair appears

Breasts develop

Uterus enlarges

Menstruation begins

Pubic hair appears

Vaginal epithelium cornifies

Body contours rounded

Epiphysial union hastened

GnRH

Pituitary gonado-tropins increased
FSH
LH

ACTH

Adrenal androgens increased

Adrenal cortices

Reticular zone enlarges.

Ovaries

Estrogen increased

Progesterone produced

Adrenal cortices

Adrenal androgens increased

Reticular zone enlarges.

Testes

Estrogen produced

Testosterone increased

LH acts on theca cells to stimulate androgen production and on granulosa cells to stimulate progesterone production. FSH acts on granulosa cells to stimulate production of estrogens from androgens.

LH acts on interstitial Leydig cells to stimulate testosterone production. FSH with testosterone acts on Sertoli cells to stimulate spermatogenesis.

Male

Higher cerebral centers "trigger" (leptin, kisspeptin, weight, nutrition)

Hair line recession begins

Acne appears

Facial hair appears

Larynx enlarges (voice deepens)

Musculature develops

Axillary hair appears

Some breast enlargement may occur

Pubic hair appears

Penis, prostate, and seminal vesicles enlarge

Epiphysial union hastened

NORMAL PUBERTY (Continued)

Axillary hair development is evident by age 12 years in more than 90% of African American girls and 70% of White girls. The development of acne—sometimes the most obvious initial sign of puberty in a girl—is caused by adrenal and ovarian androgen secretion. Acne represents a dysfunction of the pilosebaceous unit, where there is follicular occlusion and inflammation as a result of androgenic stimulation. Facial changes occur during puberty in both boys and girls with enlargement of the nose, mandible, maxilla, and frontal sinuses. In girls, the pituitary gland increases in height from an average of 6 mm before puberty to an average of 10 mm by Tanner stage 5.

MALE PUBERTY

The three main phenotypic pubertal events in boys are increased height velocity, genitalia development (under the control of pituitary gonadotropins and testicular testosterone secretion), and growth of axillary and pubic hair (under the control of androgens secreted by the testicles and adrenal glands). The first sign of puberty in boys is usually testicular growth; in the United States, this occurs approximately 6 months after the onset of breast development in girls.

Testicular volume, which correlates with the stages of puberty, can be measured by comparing the testes with model ellipsoids (orchidometer) that have volumes ranging from 1 to 35 mL. The increase in size is primarily caused by seminiferous tubule growth. The main cell type in the seminiferous cords before

puberty is the Sertoli cell, whereas in mature males, germ cells are the predominant cell type. With the increased LH levels with puberty, adult-type Leydig cells appear. Spermatogenesis starts between ages 11 and 15 years. Onset of puberty is predicted when a testis is more than 4 mL in volume. In adults, the average testicle has a volume of 29 mL; the right testis is usually slightly larger than the left, and the left testis is usually located lower in the scrotum than the right testis. When the phallus is measured, it should be flaccid and stretched. The phallus length is approximately 6 cm prepubertally and 12 cm in White males. The male areolar diameter also increases during puberty. The normal age range for onset of puberty in boys is 9 to 14 years.

In Tanner genital development stage 1 (prepubertal), the penis, testes, and scrotum are the same as in early childhood (see Plate 4.7). In Tanner stage 2, the testes and scrotum start to enlarge, and the scrotal skin starts to redden and change in texture. The average age at Tanner genital stage 2 is 11.2 years. In Tanner stage 3, penile growth has started, more evident in length than width, and there is also further enlargement of the testes and scrotum. In Tanner stage 4, the penis increases in size (both length and width), and the glans of the penis starts to develop; the testicles and scrotum continue to enlarge, and the scrotal skin becomes darker. In Tanner stage 5, the genitalia are adult in size and shape, and no further enlargement occurs.

In Tanner pubic hair development stage 1 in boys, the hair over the pubic region is vellus in type and is

the same as that on the abdominal wall (see Plate 4.7). In Tanner stage 2, there is sparse, straight or slightly cured, lightly pigmented hair that appears at the base of the penis. In Tanner stage 3, the hair is spread sparsely over the pubic area, and it is curlier, darker, and coarser. In Tanner stage 4, the hair, although adult in type, covers a smaller area than in most adults, and it has not yet spread to the medial surface of the thighs. In Tanner stage 5, the hair is adult in type and quantity and is distributed to the medial surface of the thighs.

The vocal cords lengthen during puberty, and the larynx, cricothyroid cartilage, and laryngeal muscles enlarge. The pitch of the voice changes dramatically between Tanner genital stages 3 and 4. The average age when the adult voice is reached is 15 years. During Tanner pubic hair stage 3, facial hair starts to appear, initially at the corners of the upper lip and cheeks, then spreading to below the lower lip and eventually (after achieving Tanner pubic and genital stages 5) extending to the sides of the cheeks and chin. Axillary hair development is evident at age 14 years in boys. Acne, caused by testicular and adrenal androgen secretion, appears at an average age of 12 years (range, 9–15 years) and progresses through puberty. Pubertal gynecomastia occurs in about 50% of normally developing boys at an average age of 13 years, and it usually resolves spontaneously over 1 to 2 years (see Plate 4.26).

Facial changes occur during puberty in both boys and girls with enlargement of the nose, mandible, maxilla, and frontal sinuses.

Plate 4.9

Endocrine System: VOLUME 2

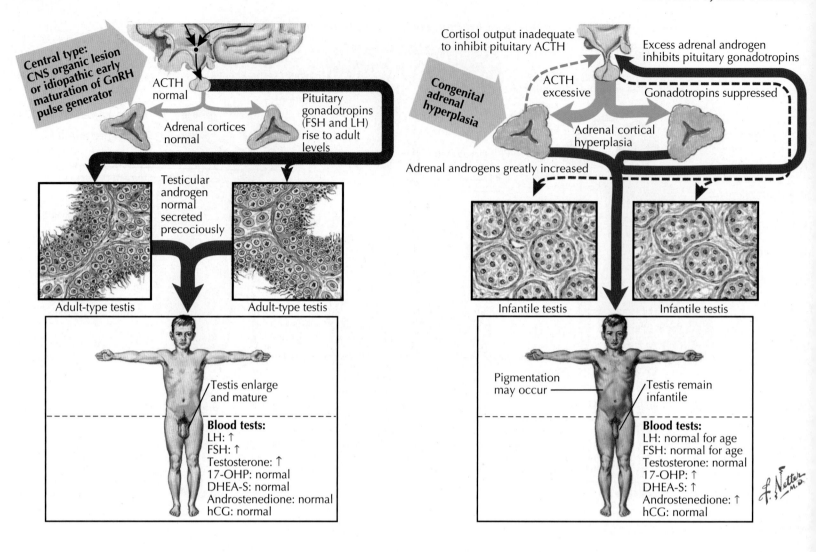

Central type: CNS organic lesion or idiopathic early maturation of GnRH pulse generator

ACTH normal

Adrenal cortices normal

Pituitary gonadotropins (FSH and LH) rise to adult levels

Testicular androgen normal secreted precociously

Adult-type testis

Adult-type testis

Testis enlarge and mature

Blood tests:
LH: ↑
FSH: ↑
Testosterone: ↑
17-OHP: normal
DHEA-S: normal
Androstenedione: normal
hCG: normal

Cortisol output inadequate to inhibit pituitary ACTH

Excess adrenal androgen inhibits pituitary gonadotropins

Congenital adrenal hyperplasia

ACTH excessive

Gonadotropins suppressed

Adrenal cortical hyperplasia

Adrenal androgens greatly increased

Infantile testis

Infantile testis

Pigmentation may occur

Testis remain infantile

Blood tests:
LH: normal for age
FSH: normal for age
Testosterone: normal
17-OHP: ↑
DHEA-S: ↑
Androstenedione: ↑
hCG: normal

PRECOCIOUS PUBERTY

Precocious puberty is the initiation of puberty before the age of 8 years in girls and 9 years in boys. The cause may be benign (normal variant early adrenarche) or more serious (malignant germinoma). When the sexual characteristics are appropriate for the child's sex, it is termed *isosexual precocious puberty*. Inappropriate virilization in girls or feminization in boys is termed *contrasexual precocious puberty*. Precocious puberty is 10-fold more common in girls, in whom the cause is usually central in nature.

GONADOTROPIN-DEPENDENT PRECOCIOUS PUBERTY

Central or true precocious puberty is gonadotropin-dependent and attributable to early maturation of the gonadotropin-releasing hormone (GnRH) pulse generator, a finding that is 20-fold more common in girls than in boys. Although this form of precocious puberty may be triggered by a central nervous system (CNS) process, the cause cannot be identified in 90% of affected girls. This development leads to premature breast (thelarche) and pubic hair (pubarche) changes in girls and premature pubarche and testicular enlargement (gonadarche) in boys.

When pubertal changes start, they progress at a pace and in an order found in puberty that starts at a normal age. The blood concentrations of LH, FSH, testosterone, and estradiol are characteristic of those seen in normal puberty. These patients have an advanced bone age and accelerated growth for their age.

Although the etiology is usually idiopathic in girls, head magnetic resonance imaging (MRI) is indicated to exclude a CNS disorder. In boys with central precocious puberty, the etiology is idiopathic in half and a CNS abnormality in the other half. Some considerations in this setting include hamartomas of the tuber cinereum that contain GnRH neurosecretory neurons and function as an ectopic GnRH pulse generator; astrocytoma; ependymoma; hypothalamic or optic gliomas in patients with neurofibromatosis type 1; any neoplasm in the hypothalamic region (e.g., craniopharyngioma) that impinges on the posterior hypothalamus; an adverse effect of CNS radiotherapy (e.g., for tumors or leukemia); hydrocephalus; CNS inflammatory disorder (e.g., sarcoidosis); congenital midline defects; and pineal neoplasms. Hamartomas of the tuber cinereum are not actually tumors but rather congenital malformations that appear on MRI as an isodense fullness of the prepontine, interpeduncular, and posterior suprasellar cisterns. When the diameter of the hamartoma exceeds 1 cm, there is a high risk

for seizures, which may be gelastic (laughing), petit mal, or generalized tonic-clonic. A rare cause is a gonadotropin-secreting pituitary tumor. Exposure to androgens (exogenous or endogenous) can trigger maturation of the GnRH pulse generator and central precocious puberty.

GONADOTROPIN-INDEPENDENT PRECOCIOUS PUBERTY

Peripheral or gonadotropin-independent precocious puberty (also referred to as *pseudoprecocious puberty*) is caused by excess secretion of estrogen or testosterone from gonadal or adrenal sources. These patients usually do not follow the normal sequence and pace of puberty (e.g., menstrual bleeding may be the first sign). Depending on the type of sex hormone excess, gonadotropin-independent precocious puberty may be isosexual or contrasexual. Blood concentrations of LH and FSH are suppressed in these patients.

The possible causes of isosexual gonadotropin-independent precocious puberty in girls include exogenous estrogen (e.g., estrogen-containing creams and ointments), follicular ovarian cysts, ovarian neoplasms (e.g., granulosa-cell tumors, gonadoblastoma, and Leydig cell tumors), estrogen-secreting adrenal neoplasms,

Plate 4.10

Reproduction

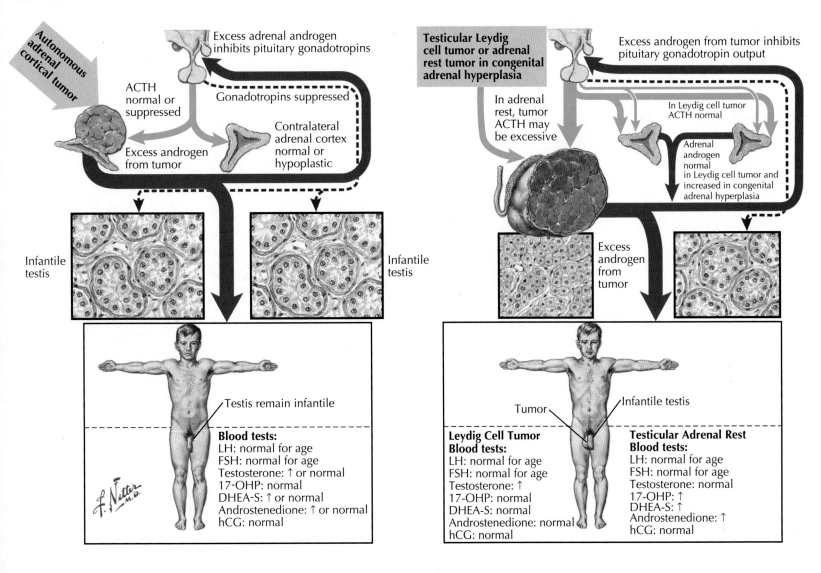

PRECOCIOUS PUBERTY
(Continued)

and McCune-Albright syndrome (see Plate 8.8). McCune-Albright syndrome is associated with pathogenic variants in the *GNAS* gene that encodes the α-subunit of the guanosine triphosphate (GTP)-binding protein (Gs) that is involved in adenylate cyclase activation. The disorder is caused by a postzygotic somatic mutation, thus the extent of tissue involvement depends on how early in development the mutation occurs. The clinical presentation of McCune-Albright syndrome is the triad of gonadotropin-independent precocious puberty, irregularly edged café au lait spots that usually do not cross the midline, and bony fibrous dysplasia (e.g., hyperostosis of the skull base and facial asymmetry) (see Plate 4.11). Based on the tissue distribution of the somatic mutation, other endocrine hyperfunction disorders may be seen in patients with McCune-Albright syndrome (see Plate 8.8), including Cushing syndrome (bilateral adrenal hyperplasia), thyrotoxicosis, hyperparathyroidism (adenoma or hyperplasia), hypophosphatemic vitamin D-resistant rickets, and gigantism (mammosomatotroph hyperplasia). McCune-Albright syndrome-related sexual precocity usually begins in the first 2 years of life with menstrual

bleeding caused by autonomously functioning ovarian luteinized follicular cysts.

In boys with isosexual peripheral precocious puberty, the diagnostic considerations include testicular Leydig cell tumors (usually benign) and human chorionic gonadotropin (hCG)-secreting germ cell tumors (hCG is an LH receptor agonist) that arise from sites of embryonic germ cells (pineal region of the brain, posterior mediastinum, liver [malignant hepatoma and hepatoblastoma], retroperitoneum, and testicles). Germ cell tumors are malignant but may be indolent (e.g., dysgerminoma) or more aggressive (e.g., choriocarcinoma, embryonal cell carcinoma). Androgen-secreting adrenal tumors and CAH (e.g., 21-hydroxylase deficiency or, less commonly, 11β-hydroxylase deficiency) are additional considerations of isosexual gonadotropin-independent precocious puberty. Boys can also have a germline autosomal dominant activating pathogenic variant in the LH receptor gene that predisposes to early Leydig cell development and testosterone secretion (testotoxicosis). McCune-Albright syndrome does occur in boys, although its occurrence is 50% less common than in girls.

Causes of contrasexual gonadotropin-independent precocious puberty in girls include exogenous androgens (e.g., testosterone gel), androgen-secreting adrenal neoplasms, and CAH. Causes of contrasexual

gonadotropin-independent precocious puberty in boys include exogenous estrogen (e.g., estrogen-containing creams and ointments) and adrenal estrogen-secreting neoplasms.

INCOMPLETE PRECOCIOUS PUBERTY

Incomplete precocious puberty is the descriptor used for premature thelarche or premature adrenarche, both of which may be variants of normal puberty. Usually bone age is not advanced in these settings. Thus premature thelarche may occur in isolation in normally developing girls, with no other signs of puberty. However, a subset of girls with premature thelarche or premature adrenarche may progress to gonadotropin-dependent precocious puberty. In addition, incomplete precocious puberty may be caused by long-standing, untreated primary hypothyroidism.

DIAGNOSTIC EVALUATION AND TREATMENT

A focused history and physical examination usually provide clues as to the cause of precocious puberty. For example, headaches, visual changes, or symptoms of diabetes insipidus should increase the suspicion for a mass in the hypothalamic region. All previous height

Plate 4.11

Endocrine System: VOLUME 2

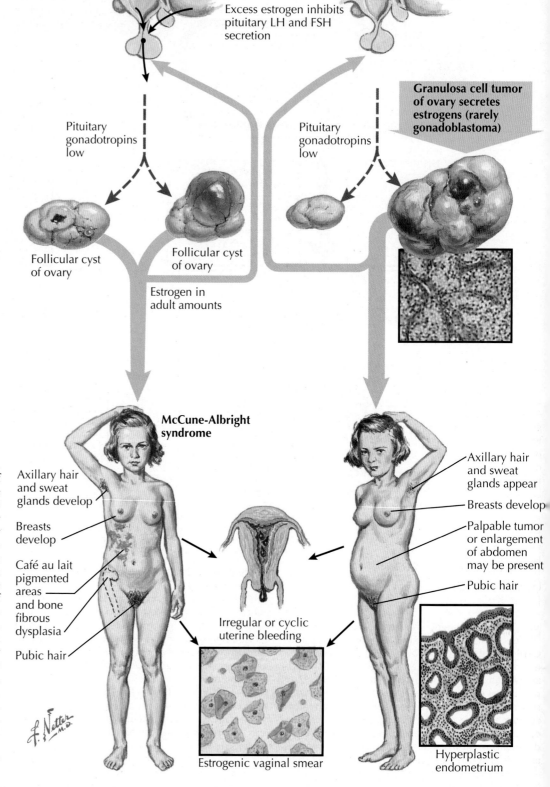

Excess estrogen inhibits
pituitary LH and FSH
secretion

**Granulosa cell tumor
of ovary secretes
estrogens (rarely
gonadoblastoma)**

Pituitary
gonadotropins
low

Pituitary
gonadotropins
low

Follicular cyst
of ovary

Follicular cyst
of ovary

Estrogen in
adult amounts

**McCune-Albright
syndrome**

Axillary hair
and sweat
glands develop

Breasts
develop

Café au lait
pigmented
areas
and bone
fibrous
dysplasia

Pubic hair

Axillary hair
and sweat
glands appear

Breasts develop

Palpable tumor
or enlargement
of abdomen
may be present

Pubic hair

Irregular or cyclic
uterine bleeding

Estrogenic vaginal smear

Hyperplastic
endometrium

PRECOCIOUS PUBERTY (Continued)

measurements should be plotted on a growth chart. On physical examination, a detailed description of secondary sexual characteristics on the basis of the Tanner staging should be documented (see Plates 4.5 to 4.7). Measurements should be made of testicular volume and penile length in boys and of diameter of breast tissue in girls. The patient should be examined for the presence of multiple café au lait spots; in neurofibromatosis type 1, they are smoother in outline ("coast of California" appearance) than those associated with McCune-Albright syndrome ("coast of Maine" appearance). Complete neurologic examination may provide clues to an underlying CNS process. The abdominal and pelvic examination may detect a hepatic or ovarian mass. Testicular examination may show symmetric testicular enlargement in patients with central precocious puberty or a unilateral nodular enlargement in boys with Leydig cell tumors. Bone age should be evaluated to see if it is advanced compared with chronologic age. Basal blood concentrations of LH, FSH, estradiol, testosterone, 17-hydroxyprogesterone (17-OHP), dehydroepiandrosterone sulfate (DHEA-S), and androstenedione distinguish between central and peripheral precocious puberty. Serum thyrotropin should be measured in all patients with precocious puberty. Blood concentrations of β-hCG and α-fetoprotein may be measured in select cases. Performing a GnRH stimulation test for LH may be necessary to confirm central precocious puberty, in which LH is expected to increase after GnRH administration.

Head MRI is indicated in patients with gonadotropin-dependent precocious puberty. Abdominal and gonadal imaging are indicated in patients with gonadotropin-independent precocious puberty.

Treatment is determined by the cause and pace of precocious puberty. If a CNS lesion is discovered in patients with gonadotropin-dependent precocious puberty, treatment options are usually clear. For example, a dysgerminoma is usually confirmed by biopsy and then treated with radiation therapy, chemotherapy, or both. In patients with idiopathic gonadotropin-dependent precocious puberty (a diagnosis of exclusion), treatment with a GnRH agonist is an effective option to arrest pubertal development, and it improves final adult height compared with final height of patients who are not treated.

The treatment of patients with gonadotropin-independent precocious puberty is directed at the source of sex hormone excess. For example, androgen excess associated with CAH caused by 21-hydroxylase deficiency is very effectively treated with glucocorticoid replacement.

DISORDERS OF SEX DEVELOPMENT

CLASSIFICATION

The distinction between the male and female phenotypes at birth is usually clear. However, ambiguous genitalia—found in every one of 4000 births—may delay sex assignment. Disorders of sex development (DSD) occur when there is a congenital discrepancy between external genitalia and the gonadal and chromosomal sex. For clinical purposes, the three main categories of DSD are:

1. **Sex chromosome DSD**
   - Turner syndrome: 45,X
   - Klinefelter syndrome: 47,XXY
   - Mixed gonadal dysgenesis: 45,X/46,XY
   - Chimerism: 46,XX/46,XY
2. **46,XX DSD (virilized XX female)**
   - Disorders of gonadal development (gonadal dysgenesis, ovotesticular DSD, testicular DSD)
   - Androgen excess (fetal, maternal)
3. **46,XY DSD (undervirilized XY male)**
   - Disorders of testis development (complete or partial gonadal dysgenesis, ovotesticular DSD, testis regression)
   - Disorders of androgen synthesis or action (CAH, LH receptor pathogenic variants, 5α-reductase 2 deficiency)

Sex determination can be considered to have three main components: chromosomal sex (e.g., 46,XX or 46,XY), phenotypic sex (e.g., male or female external genitalia), and gonadal sex (e.g., presence of ovaries or testicles). Psychosocial development is superimposed on these three components. DSD are congenital disorders in which the development of chromosomal, phenotypic, or gonadal sex is atypical. For example, ambiguous genitalia in a newborn may be caused by CAH, in which case it should be classified as 46,XX DSD. If the cause is PAIS, it should be classified as 46,XY DSD. For conceptual and practical purposes, DSD can be divided into sex chromosome DSD, disorders of testicular development and androgenization (46,XY DSD [male pseudohermaphroditism]), and disorders of ovarian development and androgen excess (46,XX DSD [female pseudohermaphroditism]).

CHROMOSOMAL SEX

Chromosomal sex is determined at fertilization and usually results in 46,XY (male) or 46,XX (female) zygotes. However, meiotic nondisjunction may lead to gain or loss of sex chromosomal material in the ova or sperm—sex chromosome aneuploidy—resulting in zygotes with chromosome complements such as 47,XXY (Klinefelter syndrome) and 45,X (Turner syndrome). Mitotic nondisjunction can occur in a zygote and lead to chromosomal mosaicism (e.g., 45,X/46,XX).

GONADAL SEX

Gonadal sex is determined by the presence of ovaries or testicles. *SRY* is the testis-determining gene on the Y chromosome (see Plates 4.1 and 4.2). *SRY* and *SOX9* expression in the embryo leads to cellular proliferation and migration of mesonephric cells into the developing testis. However, many factors have a role in normal testicular development. Normal ovarian development is dependent on both expression of factors that prevent testis development and lack of expression of AMH.

46,XX DSD: ANDROGEN EXCESS

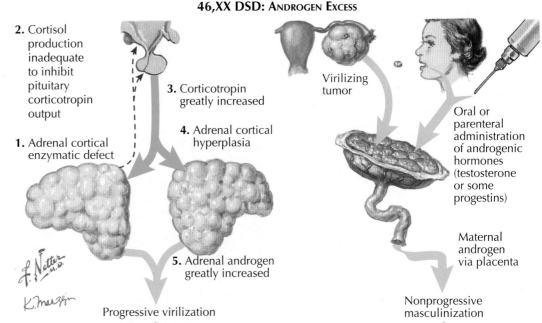

2. Cortisol production inadequate to inhibit pituitary corticotropin output

3. Corticotropin greatly increased

4. Adrenal cortical hyperplasia

1. Adrenal cortical enzymatic defect

5. Adrenal androgen greatly increased

Virilizing tumor

Oral or parenteral administration of androgenic hormones (testosterone or some progestins)

Maternal androgen via placenta

Progressive virilization

Nonprogressive masculinization

Degree of genital masculinization dependent on fetal stage when androgen exposure occurs

Early (before 12th week: severe)

Late (mild)

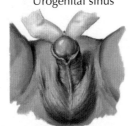

Fallopian tubes
Ovaries
Uterus

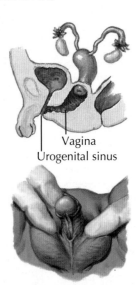

Vagina
Urogenital sinus

Vagina
Urogenital sinus

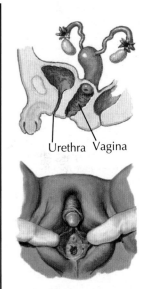

Urethra Vagina

Penile urethra (hypospadiac or normal); vagina opening into urethra (urogenital sinus); labial fusion (scrotum)

Enlarged clitoris: vagina opening into urogenital sinus with orifice at base of clitoris; partly fused labia (bifid scrotum)

Simple enlargement of clitoris; genitalia otherwise normal

PHENOTYPIC SEX

Male Sexual Differentiation

Sexual differentiation is mediated by the secretion of several steroid and peptide hormones. For example, Sertoli cells produce AMH and inhibin B. The secretion of AMH (under the regulation of *SOX9* and other transcription factors) starts in the seventh week of gestation and causes regression of müllerian structures (uterus, fallopian tubes, and the upper two-thirds of the vagina). If a fetus with a male chromosome complement (46,XY) has pathogenic variants in either AMH or its receptor or if there is Sertoli cell dysfunction, persistent müllerian duct syndrome (PMDS) and undescended testes (46,XY

DSD) can result (see Plate 4.14). If a defect is limited to Leydig cell steroidogenesis, PMDS does not occur because Sertoli cell production of AMH is not affected.

Fetal Leydig cells start to secrete androgens by the ninth week of gestation and are stimulated by placental hCG during the first two trimesters and by fetal pituitary LH in the last trimester of pregnancy. Cholesterol is taken up into Leydig cells, and LH stimulates the steroidogenic acute regulatory protein to generate its movement from the outer to the inner mitochondrial membrane. The cholesterol side chain is then cleaved by $P450_{scc}$ (CYP11A1) to produce pregnenolone. Pregnenolone is converted to either progesterone by 3β-hydroxysteroid dehydrogenase type 2 (HSD3B2) or to

DISORDERS OF SEX DEVELOPMENT (Continued)

17-hydroxypregnenolone by 17α-hydroxylation by P450c17 (CYP17). Then 17-hydroxypregnenolone is converted to DHEA by P450c17. DHEA is then converted to androstenedione by 3β-hydroxysteroid dehydrogenase type 2, and androstenedione is converted to testosterone by 17β-hydroxysteroid dehydrogenase type 3 (HSD17B3). Testosterone is converted to dihydrotestosterone (DHT) by 5α-reductase type 2. DHT has high affinity for the androgen receptor and is the mediator of androgenization of the external genitalia and urogenital sinus. Testosterone production stabilizes the wolffian structures (vas deferens, epididymis, and seminal vesicles) (see Plate 4.2). The urogenital sinus becomes the prostate and prostatic urethra. The genital tubercle becomes the glans penis. The urogenital folds fuse to become the shaft of the penis. The urogenital swellings become the scrotum. Testicular descent has two stages: transabdominal and transinguinal. The transabdominal descent is initiated by the testicles and starts at 12 weeks' gestation and is dependent on the contraction and thickening of the gubernacular ligament. The transinguinal descent is triggered by LH and androgens.

Female Sexual Differentiation

In females, the müllerian structures form the uterus, the upper portion of the vagina, and the fallopian tubes. Without local testosterone production from the testes, the wolffian structures degenerate. Normal uterine development can occur without the presence of ovaries. The urogenital sinus becomes the lower portion of the vagina and the urethra (see Plate 4.2). The genital tubercle becomes the clitoris. The urogenital folds become the labia minora, and the urogenital swellings become the labia majora. The ovaries express receptors for LH and FSH at approximately 16 weeks' gestation. Circulating fetal FSH levels peak at week 20, and primary follicles form in the ovaries. Very little estrogen is secreted by fetal ovaries.

If a fetus with a female chromosome complement (46,XX) is exposed to androgens in utero (e.g., from the adrenal glands in the setting of CAH), androgenization of the external genitalia occurs (see Plate 4.12). In this setting, a uterus is present, and the testosterone concentrations are usually not high enough to stabilize wolffian structures.

PSYCHOSOCIAL DEVELOPMENT

Gender identity is an individual's self-identification as female or male, and *gender role* refers to sex-specific behaviors (e.g., physical aggression, toy preferences, peer group interactions). *Sexual orientation* refers to the inclination of an individual with respect to heterosexual, homosexual, bisexual, pansexual, and asexual behavior. Psychosocial development is complex and depends in part on prenatal endocrine and innate chromosomal factors. It appears that the Y chromosome is not a major factor; for example, phenotypic females with complete androgen insensitivity syndrome (CAIS) have female psychosocial development despite an 46,XY karyotype. Psychosocial development may evolve; for example, children with 5α-reductase deficiency may change their gender roles in adolescence.

46,XY DSD: ANDROGEN INSENSITIVITY SYNDROME

Normal female external genitalia (or slightly masculinized); vagina ends blindly.

Relatively normal female habitus (inguinal herniae)

Testes operatively exposed in groins; laparotomy reveals complete absence of uterus, fallopian tubes, and ovaries.

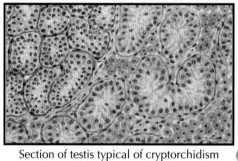

Section of testis typical of cryptorchidism (in situ neoplasia in upper left corner)

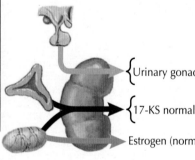

Urinary gonadotropins normal

17-KS normal or slightly elevated

Estrogen (normal levels for female)

The presenting phenotype in DSD is extremely variable and depends on the underlying condition. Defining the basis for DSD is important with respect to gender assignment, treatment, and associated medical implications.

SEX CHROMOSOME DISORDERS OF SEX DEVELOPMENT

Sex chromosome aneuploidy is sex chromosome DSD. The most common examples are Klinefelter syndrome (47,XXY) and Turner syndrome (45,X) (see Plates 4.17 to 4.20).

Mixed Gonadal Dysgenesis

The 45,X/46,XY mosaic karyotype is a form of mixed gonadal dysgenesis that is associated with a wide range of external genitalia phenotypes (normal female external genitalia, clitoromegaly, ambiguous genitalia, hypospadias, or normal male external genitalia).

The gonadal phenotypes range from ovary-like stroma with primordial follicles to intraabdominal

DISORDERS OF SEX DEVELOPMENT (Continued)

streak gonads to normal testes in the scrotum. When AMH production by Sertoli cells is impaired, müllerian structures may be evident. Physical features can range from those seen with Turner syndrome (e.g., short stature) to those characterizing a normal male phenotype.

In this setting, the infant is usually raised as a girl if there is only minimally androgenized genitalia. In this circumstance, the dysgenic intraabdominal gonads should be removed, and estrogen replacement should be initiated at the time of puberty. If a uterus is present, a progestational agent should be added.

When the ambiguous genitalia are limited to hypospadias, the infant is usually raised as a boy. The hypospadias is repaired, and if the testicles have not descended, orchiopexy should be performed. Exogenous testosterone therapy may be needed at the time of puberty.

When the genitalia are highly ambiguous, a multidisciplinary approach and parental involvement are needed because management is complex. When raised as girls, these patients require urogenital surgery and gonadectomy, and they are infertile because they lack a uterus. When raised as boys, they require gonadectomy and surgery for hypospadias, and they have poor erectile function.

Chimerism

46,XX/46,XY chimerism results from double fertilization or from ovum fusion and can result in ovarian and testicular tissue in the same or opposite gonads (true hermaphroditism) (see discussion under 46,XX DSD).

46,XX DISORDERS OF SEX DEVELOPMENT

The causes of 46,XX DSD include disorders of ovarian development (gonadal dysgenesis, ovotesticular DSD, testicular DSD) and androgen excess (CAH, gestational hyperandrogenism). However, it should be recognized that most causes of XX virilization remain undefined.

Congenital Adrenal Hyperplasia

CAH is the most common cause of virilized infants with a female chromosome complement (46,XX) (see Plate 4.12). The most frequent steroid synthetic enzymatic defect is in 21α-hydroxylase (CYP21A2), followed by 11β-hydroxylase and 3β-hydroxysteroid dehydrogenase deficiencies (see Plates 3.13 and 3.14).

Gestational Hyperandrogenism

Exposure of an XX fetus to excess maternal androgens during development can lead to virilization with normal female internal anatomy (see Plate 4.12). In addition to CAH, causes include theca-lutein cysts and placental aromatase enzyme deficiency.

Testicular Disorders of Sex Development

46,XX DSD with evidence of functioning testicular tissue may be caused by translocation of *SRY* or by *SOX9* duplication. These abnormalities may be detected by using fluorescence in situ hybridization (FISH) probes for the *SRY* and *SOX9* genes.

Ovotesticular Disorders of Sex Development (True Hermaphroditism)

Ovotesticular DSD is defined as the presence of both testicular and ovarian tissue in the opposite or the same

46,XY DSD

Left fallopian tube — Left testis — Left vas deferens

Infantile uterus

Right fallopian tube

Right testis

Persistent müllerian duct syndrome with testes, uterus, and fallopian tubes in hernial sac

Normal male habitus with inguinal hernia

Testes usually atrophic, characteristic of cryptorchidism; spermatogenesis occasionally present

Some variations in male sexual differentiation

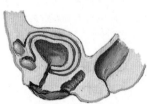

Androgen insensitivity syndrome with normal antimüllerian hormone secretion and function

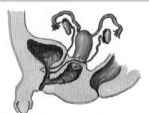

Testicular dysgenesis with varying deficiencies of androgens and antimüllerian hormone resulting in a wide range of findings

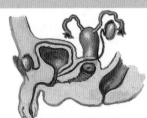

Persistent müllerian duct syndrome caused by Sertoli cell dysfunction or mutations in either the antimüllerian hormone gene or its receptor

gonads (see Plate 4.15). Most of these patients have a 46,XX karyotype, and there are probably multiple underlying causes. Less commonly, they have 46,XX/46,XY chimerism that results from double fertilization or ovum fusion. Most patients with ovotesticular DSD have a unilateral ovotestis on one side and an ovary or testis on the other side. Approximately 30% of affected patients have ovarian and testicular tissue bilaterally (e.g., ovotestes). The least common form of ovotesticular DSD is characterized by a testis on one side and an ovary on the other side. When an ovary is present, it is

typically in the usual anatomic location. However, a testis or ovotestis is usually undescended. The genital ducts typically develop as does the gonad. For example, a hemiuterus is usually present on the side of the ovary or ovotestis. Menses and pubertal breast development may occur.

When there is a clinically important amount of testicular tissue, the male changes at puberty may dominate. Gender assignment in infants with ovotesticular DSD follows similar steps as those highlighted in the discussion on mixed gonadal dysgenesis.

DISORDERS OF SEX DEVELOPMENT (Continued)

46,XY DISORDERS OF SEX DEVELOPMENT

The causes of undervirilization of male infants (46,XY DSD) include abnormalities in testicular development, androgen synthesis, or androgen action. Complete testicular dysgenesis (Swyer syndrome) may be caused by insufficient AMH production or action and results in persistent müllerian structures and lack of androgenization of the external genitalia (see Plate 4.14). Partial testicular dysgenesis may result in ambiguous genitalia with or without a uterus and vagina. Milder variants may present with hypospadias, micropenis, or infertility. Although the cause of testicular dysgenesis is infrequently found, many molecular genetic abnormalities have been identified (pathogenic variants in the following genes: *SRY,* nuclear receptor subfamily 5 group A member 1 [*NR5A1;* encoding steroidogenic factor 1], mitogen-activated protein kinase 1 [*MAP3K1*], DEAH-box helicase 37 [*DHX37*], androgen receptor gene [*AR*], LH receptor gene [*LHCGR*], Wilms tumor-related gene [*WT1*], sex-determining region Y-box 9 gene [*SOX9*], DM domain transcription factor [*DMRT1*], desert hedgehog homolog gene [*DHH*], aristaless-related homeobox gene [*ARX*], TSPY-like 1 gene [*TSPYL1*]).

Decreased androgen synthesis may also result from CAH caused by 17α-hydroxylase deficiency, 3β-hydroxysteroid dehydrogenase deficiency, P450 side-chain cleavage deficiency, and steroidogenic acute regulatory protein deficiency (lipoid hyperplasia). LH receptor defects (resulting in Leydig cell hypoplasia), 5α-reductase deficiency, and 17β-hydroxysteroid dehydrogenase type 3 deficiency (the most common defect in testosterone synthesis) can also cause abnormal androgen production. Steroid 5α-reductase deficiency is an autosomal recessive disorder in which individuals with a male chromosome complement (46,XY) who have bilateral testes and normal testosterone formation have impaired external virilization during embryogenesis because of defective conversion of testosterone to dihydrotestosterone.

Causes of decreased androgen action include androgen insensitivity syndrome (AIS), which may be partial (PAIS) or complete (CAIS) (see Plate 4.13). In the past, CAIS was termed *complete testicular feminization.* AIS is associated with pathogenic variants in the androgen receptor gene (*AR*) so that despite the presence of testes and normal testosterone production, there is absent (CAIS) or partial (PAIS) virilization. PAIS, referred to in the past as *incomplete testicular feminization,* may be diagnosed in infants with ambiguous genitalia, adolescent girls who become virilized, adolescent boys with pubertal delay or gynecomastia, and males with infertility. CAIS typically does not present until inguinal hernias or labial masses are noted in young girls or primary amenorrhea becomes evident. These phenotypic females lack secondary sex hair and a uterus; the karyotype is 46,XY, and the serum testosterone level is in the reference range for a male. Gonadectomy should be performed to prevent tumor formation in cryptorchid testes.

EVALUATION AND TREATMENT

The evaluation of infants with ambiguous genitalia should include a history to ascertain whether there are

other affected family members and to document maternal treatments and exposures during pregnancy; physical examination to document external genitalia findings and to check for gonads in the labia or inguinal canal; laboratory tests to assess for CAH (e.g., serum electrolytes, corticotropin, 17-OHP, 11-deoxycortisol, cortisol, and DHEA); karyotype analysis, including FISH with *SRY* probe; and ultrasonography of pelvic and abdominal structures to determine whether a uterus, gonads, and a vagina are present. The initial goal

is to determine whether the infant has sex chromosome DSD, 46,XX DSD, or 46,XY DSD; additional tests (e.g., targeted gene panel sequencing, massively parallel sequencing, and whole genome sequencing) are recommended on the basis of this distinction.

The cause of DSD has important implications for gender assignment, treatment, risk of tumor formation in cryptorchid testes, determination of future fertility options, and counseling of patients and their families.

OVOTESTICULAR DSD

True hermaphrodite with male habitus

True hermaphrodite with female habitus

Ovary

Ovotestis (ovumlike body in seminiferous tubule)

Unicornuate uterus

Ovary

Testis

Plate 4.16

Reproduction

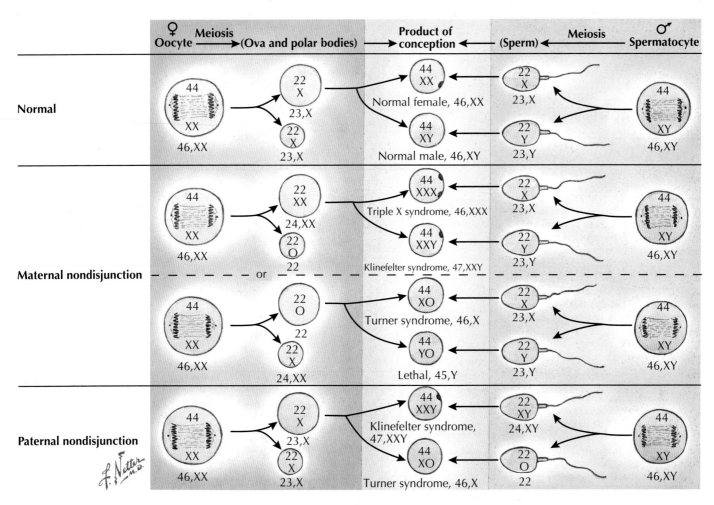

Errors in Chromosomal Sex

Many abnormalities in sex differentiation can be attributed to errors in chromosomal number or to morphologic abnormalities in the sex chromosomes. Humans have 46 chromosomes—22 pairs of autosomes (numbered 1–22 based on size) and one pair of sex chromosomes (XX or XY). During mitosis, each of the 46 chromosomes replicates itself exactly, so that each daughter cell again has the diploid number. A different process occurs in the production of germ cells, in which each primary spermatocyte or primary oocyte undergoes two meiotic divisions, to form, respectively, either four sperm cells or two ova and two polar bodies. Each of these cells contains the haploid number of 23 chromosomes. Chromosomal sex is determined at fertilization, in which two haploid gametes—sperm and ova—fuse to produce a diploid zygote with 46 chromosomes. A normal ova has one X chromosome, and a normal sperm has either a single X chromosome or a single Y chromosome. This process, in a single meiotic division, is illustrated in the upper section of the plate.

Errors in chromosomal number may be caused by faulty cell division of the parental gametocytes in meiosis or by faulty cell division in the zygote after fertilization (mitosis). Although exact halving of the chromosome number during meiosis and exact replication of the

46 chromosomes during mitosis ideally takes place, occasionally a chromosome becomes misplaced on the spindle and migrates to the wrong pole. In such instances, one daughter cell contains an extra chromosome, and the other daughter cell is deficient. This phenomenon, known as *nondisjunction,* may occur during either meiosis or mitosis. Fertilization of these abnormal gametes results in a zygote with an abnormal sex chromosome number. Examples of sex chromosome aneuploidy include 45,X; 47,XXY; 47,XXX; and 45,Y. Zygotes that lack X chromosomal material (e.g., 45,Y) are not viable.

The 45,X karyotype (Turner syndrome), which occurs in approximately 1 in 2500 live-born phenotypic female births, is caused by nondisjunction or chromosome loss during gametogenesis in either parent. The paternal X chromosome (X^p) is retained in one-third of patients, and the maternal X chromosome (X^m) is retained in the remaining two-thirds. Approximately 25% of patients with Turner syndrome have chromosome mosaicism (e.g., 45,X/46,XX) caused by mitotic errors that occurred in a zygote with an initially normal chromosome complement.

Klinefelter syndrome, which occurs in approximately 1 in 1000 live-born phenotypic male births, is the result of extra X chromosome material—most commonly 47,XXY and less commonly 48,XXXY; 46,XY/47,XXX mosaicism; and 46,XX (phenotypic males). The 47,XXY karyotype is caused by nondisjunction

of sex chromosomes during the meiotic division of gametogenesis in either parent. Mosaicism such as 46,XY/47,XXY results when mitotic errors occur in a zygote with an initially normal chromosome complement.

Triple X syndrome (47,XXX), also called *trisomy X,* occurs in 1 in 1000 newborn girls. Although triple X syndrome does not have an abnormal phenotype, individuals with this chromosome complement may be taller than average; have an increased risk of learning disabilities; and have delayed development of speech, language, and motor skills. These individuals have normal sexual development and are fertile.

The karyotype—an analysis of chromosome number and morphology—is determined from DNA in peripheral blood leukocytes. Cytogenetic techniques used to detect sex chromosome abnormalities include examination of chromosome number, banding patterns, Y-chromatin fluorescence, and FISH. In some cases, the documentation of mosaic status requires karyotyping other tissues (e.g., skin or gonads). However, even with these additional analyses, sometimes additional molecular genetic techniques are required. For example, the sex-determining region Y gene (*SRY*) on the Y chromosome may be translocated to the X chromosome, resulting in a 46,XX male. In addition, pathogenic variants in *SRY* may result in 46,XY females with gonadal dysgenesis. Molecular genetic testing can identify the presence of an abnormal *SRY* sequence.

Plate 4.17

Endocrine System: VOLUME 2

KLINEFELTER SYNDROME

Klinefelter syndrome is the most common genetic cause of primary hypogonadism, occurring in approximately 1 in 1000 live-born phenotypic male births. Klinefelter syndrome is the result of extra X-chromosome material—most commonly 47,XXY and less commonly 48,XXXY; 46,XY/47,XXY mosaicism; and 46,XX (phenotypic male). The 47,XXY karyotype is caused by nondisjunction of sex chromosomes during the meiotic division of gametogenesis in either parent (see Plate 4.16). Mosaicism such as 46,XY/47,XXY results when mitotic errors occur in a zygote with an initially normal chromosome complement. The extra X chromosome produces little or no abnormality until adolescence, when patients who are affected develop small, firm testes with hyalinized seminiferous tubules and clumped Leydig cells; azoospermia; small phallus; gynecomastia; mild to moderate degrees of eunuchoidism; decreased virilization; and elevations in blood concentrations of LH and FSH.

The eunuchoid body proportions are attributable to testosterone deficiency and delayed epiphyseal fusion. Although nearly always infertile, these males may show a spectrum of inadequate masculinization ranging from moderately severe eunuchoidism to an almost normal male phenotype. Blood concentrations of LH and FSH are usually elevated because of Leydig cell and seminiferous tubule dysfunction, respectively. The degree of gynecomastia is highly variable and is associated with the degree of testosterone deficiency.

Characteristically, the gonads exhibit an irregular distribution of tubules and tubular scars, separated by loose connective tissue and clumps of Leydig cells. The number of Leydig cells is often increased, and nests of them may assume the configuration of adenomas. There is considerable variation in the size of nonhyalinized tubules; some contain only Sertoli cells, and others reveal germ cells in early stages of maturation. The basement membrane of the seminiferous tubules is thickened and sclerosed, and many tubules contain large depositions of hyalin. The elastic membrane is frequently absent or poorly developed. Before adolescence, the testes are relatively normal, although subtle changes may be apparent to a pathologist skilled in testicular histopathology.

Males with Klinefelter syndrome usually do not have multiple congenital abnormalities (as in Turner syndrome), but they may have mild mental impairment, anxiety, or depression. In addition, psychosocial issues are common. For example, they may lack insight, have difficult social interactions, demonstrate poor judgment, and have cognitive deficits in verbal processing.

These individuals are also at increased risk for the development of pulmonary disorders (e.g., emphysema, bronchiectasis), cancer (e.g., mediastinal germ cell tumors, breast cancer), diabetes mellitus, and varicose veins.

Phenotypic males with a 46,XX karyotype have a similar phenotype to Klinefelter syndrome, with the exception of hypospadias and short stature. This disorder results from the translocation of the SRY gene from the Y chromosome to the short arm of the X chromosome.

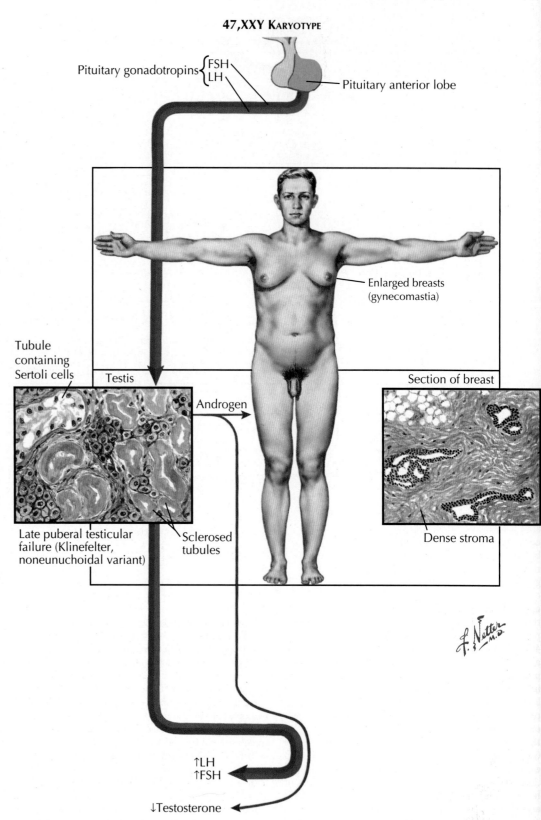

47,XXY KARYOTYPE

Pituitary gonadotropins { FSH / LH

Pituitary anterior lobe

Enlarged breasts (gynecomastia)

Tubule containing Sertoli cells

Testis

Section of breast

Androgen

Late puberal testicular failure (Klinefelter, noneunuchoidal variant)

Sclerosed tubules

Dense stroma

↑LH
↑FSH

↓Testosterone

The 47,XYY karyotype results in phenotypically normal males. Testicular function is usually normal, and they are fertile. Males with this karyotype do seem to have an increased risk of learning disabilities and delayed speech and language development.

The diagnosis of Klinefelter syndrome should be suspected in tall adolescent or adult males with gynecomastia and small testicles. The clinical suspicion can be confirmed with peripheral leukocyte karyotype. Blood levels of testosterone and inhibin-B are low. Serum estradiol levels are in the reference range for males. Blood concentrations of LH and FSH are increased. Semen analysis typically shows azoospermia, although spontaneous fertility may occur in patients with 46,XY/47,XXY mosaicism.

Testosterone replacement usually effectively treats the signs and symptoms associated with hypogonadism. The testosterone dosage should be adjusted for a midnormal serum testosterone concentration.

Plate 4.18

Reproduction

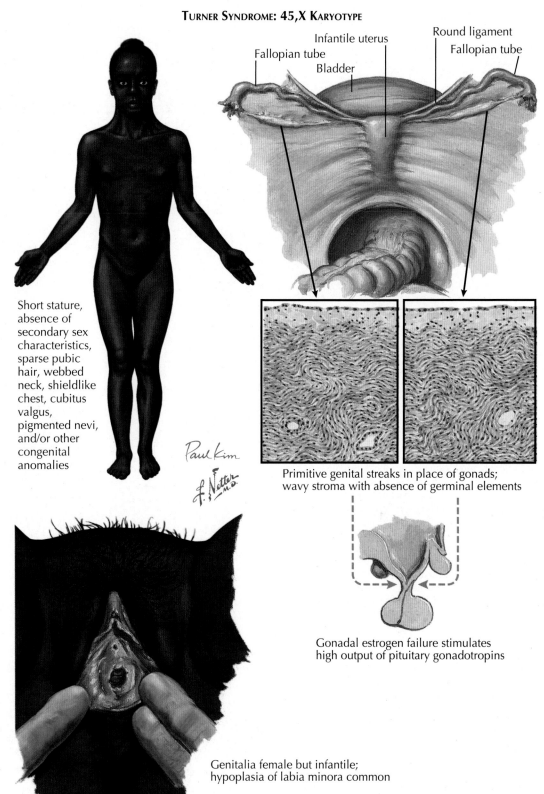

TURNER SYNDROME: 45,X KARYOTYPE

Fallopian tube

Infantile uterus

Round ligament
Fallopian tube

Bladder

Short stature, absence of secondary sex characteristics, sparse pubic hair, webbed neck, shieldlike chest, cubitus valgus, pigmented nevi, and/or other congenital anomalies

Paul Kim

F. Netter M.D.

Primitive genital streaks in place of gonads; wavy stroma with absence of germinal elements

Gonadal estrogen failure stimulates high output of pituitary gonadotropins

Genitalia female but infantile; hypoplasia of labia minora common

TURNER SYNDROME (GONADAL DYSGENESIS)

Turner syndrome (gonadal dysgenesis), or X-chromosome monosomy, is an important clinical consideration in young females with short stature and primary amenorrhea. As classically described by Turner in 1938, patients with this syndrome are short and may display a variety of visible congenital abnormalities such as a short, webbed neck (pterygium colli); cubitus valgus; and a broad, shieldlike chest. This disorder occurs in approximately 1 in 2500 live-born phenotypic female births. The 45,X karyotype appears to be caused by nondisjunction or chromosome loss during gametogenesis in either parent (see Plate 4.16). The paternal X chromosome (X^p) is retained in one-third of patients, and the maternal X chromosome (X^m) is retained in the remaining two-thirds. Approximately 25% of patients with Turner syndrome have mosaicism (e.g., 45,X/46,XX) caused by mitotic errors that occurred in a zygote that initially had a normal chromosome complement. The short stature in Turner syndrome, present in nearly all patients who are affected, is associated with loss of the short stature homeobox gene (*SHOX*) on the pseudoautosomal region of the short arms of the X chromosome (Xp22), where it encodes an osteogenic factor. Haploinsufficiency of *SHOX* is also the cause of other skeletal anomalies in Turner syndrome, such as cubitus valgus and short fourth metacarpals.

At puberty, most patients with Turner syndrome have primary amenorrhea and do not develop secondary sex characteristics. However, some patients with 45,X/46,XX mosaic karyotypes experience pubertal development and have secondary amenorrhea, and others may have normal menstrual cycles. Pelvic exploration usually reveals a normal but infantile uterus and fallopian tubes, with only rudimentary gonadal development. The gonads are usually represented by fibrous streaks in the broad ligament. However, as inferred by the diverse clinical presentations and the potential for mosaicism, the extent of ovarian defects is variable.

Patients with classic Turner syndrome rarely reach 5 feet in stature and are usually abnormally short at birth and throughout childhood. The upper-to-lower body segment ratio is increased in most patients. Congenital lymphedema of the hands and feet in a phenotypic female neonate is an early sign of this genetic disorder. In addition to short stature, the characteristic physical appearance includes two or more of the following: a short, webbed neck; high, arched palate; broad, shieldlike chest; widely spaced, hypoplastic nipples; shortened fourth metacarpal bones; and cubitus valgus. Additional findings include micrognathia, "fishmouth" appearance, low-set or deformed ears, hypoplastic nails, and a hairline in back that extends downward to the shoulders. Pigmented nevi, telangiectasias, and abnormalities of the eyes (e.g., strabismus, amblyopia, ptosis) and ears (e.g., eustachian tube anomalies resulting in frequent otitis media) are common. Coarctation of the aorta and other congenital cardiac malformations (e.g., bicuspid aortic valve, elongation of the transverse aortic arch), hypertension,

Plate 4.19

Endocrine System: VOLUME 2

TURNER SYNDROME: 45,X/46,XX KARYOTYPE

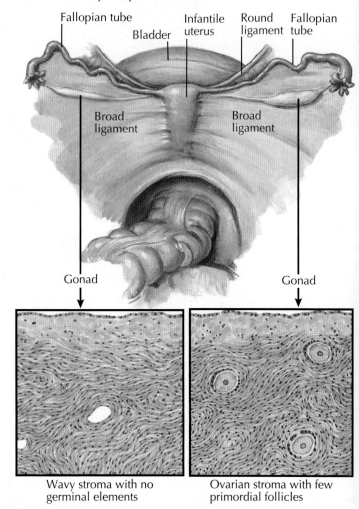

Fallopian tube — Bladder — Infantile uterus — Round ligament — Fallopian tube

Broad ligament — Broad ligament

Gonad — Gonad

Wavy stroma with no germinal elements

Ovarian stroma with few primordial follicles

TURNER SYNDROME (GONADAL DYSGENESIS) (Continued)

aortic dissection, renal abnormalities (e.g., horseshoe kidney, ureteropelvic junction anomalies), and a variety of other defects have been reported.

Although intelligence is usually normal, forms of neurocognitive dysfunction (e.g., attention-deficit disorder, visual-spatial organization) may be evident. Neurocognitive dysfunction is more common in individuals whose sole X chromosome is an X^m rather than an X^p. An example of abnormal social cognition in such patients is the difficulty in inferring affective intention from facial appearance. Head MRI and positron emission tomography show decreased tissue volumes and glucose metabolism in the right parietal and occipital lobes, findings consistent with the visual-perceptual spatiotemporal processing abnormalities. Intellectual disability is associated with the rare small ring X chromosome (karyotype 46,X,r[X]). Hypothyroidism (Hashimoto thyroiditis), sensorineural hearing loss, celiac disease, and liver function test abnormalities are common. The frequent bone fractures and osteoporosis in females with Turner syndrome appear to be multifactorial, with contributions from estrogen deficiency and haploinsufficiency for bone-related genes on the X chromosome. Finally, patients with Turner syndrome frequently develop keloids at sites of surgical incisions.

In patients with 45,X/46,XX mosaicism, the gonad may differentiate beyond its primitive state, and the cortex may differentiate to the extent of forming primordial follicles that are normal in appearance but are diminished in number. Girls with primordial follicles eventually may experience some breast enlargement and scanty menstrual periods. However, these estrogenic manifestations usually develop late, and at the usual age of adolescence, the classic picture is that of sexual infantilism. Such girls may or may not exhibit characteristic stigmata of Turner syndrome, and often they are tall and eunuchoid rather than short. In individuals who are affected least severely, only infertility and subnormal development of the estrogen-dependent sex characteristics may be present. Pregnancy is possible in a few of these patients.

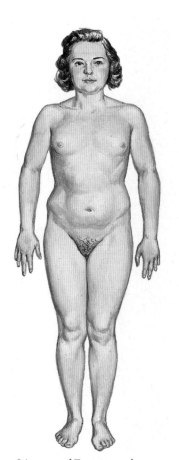

Stigmata of Turner syndrome may or may not be present

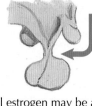

Gonadal estrogen may be adequate to prevent high pituitary gonadotropin output.

Genitalia are relatively normal but infantile; aplasia or hypoplasia of labia minora is common.

If virilization occurs, it is likely caused by mixed gonadal dysgenesis because of Y-chromosome mosaicism (45,X/46,XY) (see Plate 4.14). Other karyotypes (e.g., 45,X/47,XYY; 45,X/46XY/47,XYY) in this setting are observed much less frequently. These individuals may have typical gonadal dysgenesis, clitoral enlargement, ambiguous genitalia, hypospadiac phallus, or a normal-appearing penis (see Plate 4.20). The testicular differentiation in these patients ranges from streak gonads to functioning testes. Gender assignment may be difficult

and is usually dictated by the appearance of the external genitalia. If Y-chromosome mosaicism is confirmed, prophylactic gonadectomy is indicated. Malignant germ cell tumors (e.g., dysgerminomas) may arise from the gonadoblastoma or dysgenic gonads.

If the medullary component of the primitive gonad develops beyond its rudimentary stage in patients with 45,X/46/XY mosaicism, the secretion of duct-organizing substances and androgen is expected to parallel the morphologic development of the testis. If the testis

Plate 4.20

Reproduction

TURNER SYNDROME AND MIXED GONADAL DYSGENESIS: 45,X/46,XY KARYOTYPE

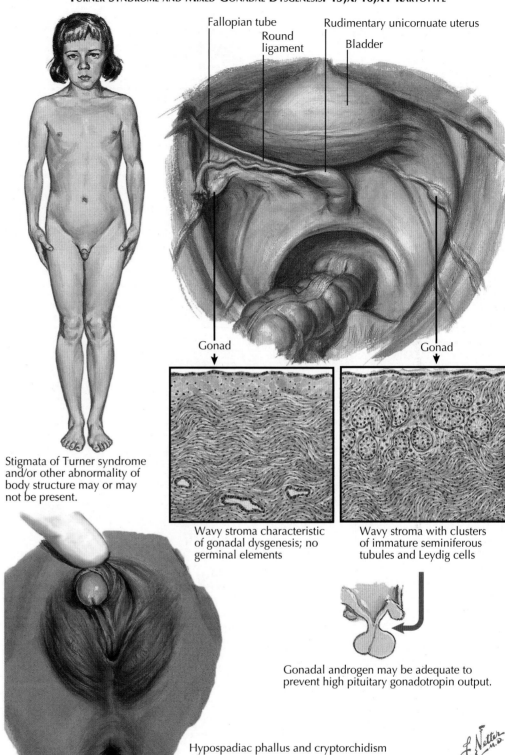

Stigmata of Turner syndrome and/or other abnormality of body structure may or may not be present.

Wavy stroma characteristic of gonadal dysgenesis; no germinal elements

Wavy stroma with clusters of immature seminiferous tubules and Leydig cells

Gonadal androgen may be adequate to prevent high pituitary gonadotropin output.

Hypospadiac phallus and cryptorchidism

TURNER SYNDROME (GONADAL DYSGENESIS) (Continued)

remains rudimentary, the genital ducts and external genitalia likewise are ambiguous or hermaphroditic in appearance. Because the duct-organizing substance secreted from a testis exerts its action unilaterally, asymmetric duct development is expected to occur if the two testes do not mature equally.

In the most primitive of such rudimentary testes, only rete tubules and nests of Leydig cells can be identified. In other instances, solid cords of cells resembling the primary sex cords are enmeshed within an abundant mesenchymal matrix. The spectra of testicular development in these cases find their counterparts in all the stages through which a normal testis passes in its embryonic differentiation. The hormonal pattern that emerges at adolescence is frequently a recapitulation of the performance of the Leydig cells in utero. Thus if these cells were sufficiently abundant to produce virilization of the external genitalia in utero, at adolescence they may be expected to produce androgenic hormones and bring about male secondary sex characteristics. Likewise, gonads in which the cortical elements have differentiated beyond the primitive stage may be expected to bring about some degree of feminization at adolescence.

The time in life when Turner syndrome becomes clinically evident is variable. For example, Turner syndrome may be evident at birth with the typical physical anomalies and lymphedema of the extremities and cutis laxa. It may be diagnosed in childhood because of growth failure, in adolescence with pubertal failure and primary amenorrhea, or later in life with secondary amenorrhea. Turner syndrome should be suspected in all prepubertal girls who are of short stature (<2 standard deviations below the mean height for age) and have at least two of the physical stigmata. In the past, a buccal smear for assessment of Barr bodies (nuclear heterochromatin) was performed in this setting. However, because this technique lacks sensitivity and specificity, it is no longer performed. If Turner syndrome is suspected, a peripheral blood karyotype analysis is indicated. A 46,X karyotype is documented in approximately 75% of patients with Turner syndrome, and the remainder proves

to have mosaic forms (e.g., 45,X/46,XX). Blood concentrations of LH and FSH are increased above normal in most of these patients throughout all age groups.

Treatment depends in part on the age at diagnosis and the presence of congenital anomalies. Although the short stature is not caused by GH deficiency, the administration of recombinant human GH in childhood—typically initiated when height falls below the 5th percentile for age—enhances growth and final adult height (the typical height gain is between 2 and 6 inches). The reasons for estrogen replacement therapy

include inducing sexual development, optimizing adolescent bone development, and optimizing cognitive function. Typically, low-dose estrogen replacement is started around age 13 to 14 years. A progestin is given with the estrogenic agent to prevent endometrial hyperplasia. Treatment of the adult patient with Turner syndrome includes surveillance for potential cardiovascular anomalies with periodic echocardiography. Because of the high risk for hypothyroidism, annual measurement of serum thyrotropin concentration is indicated.

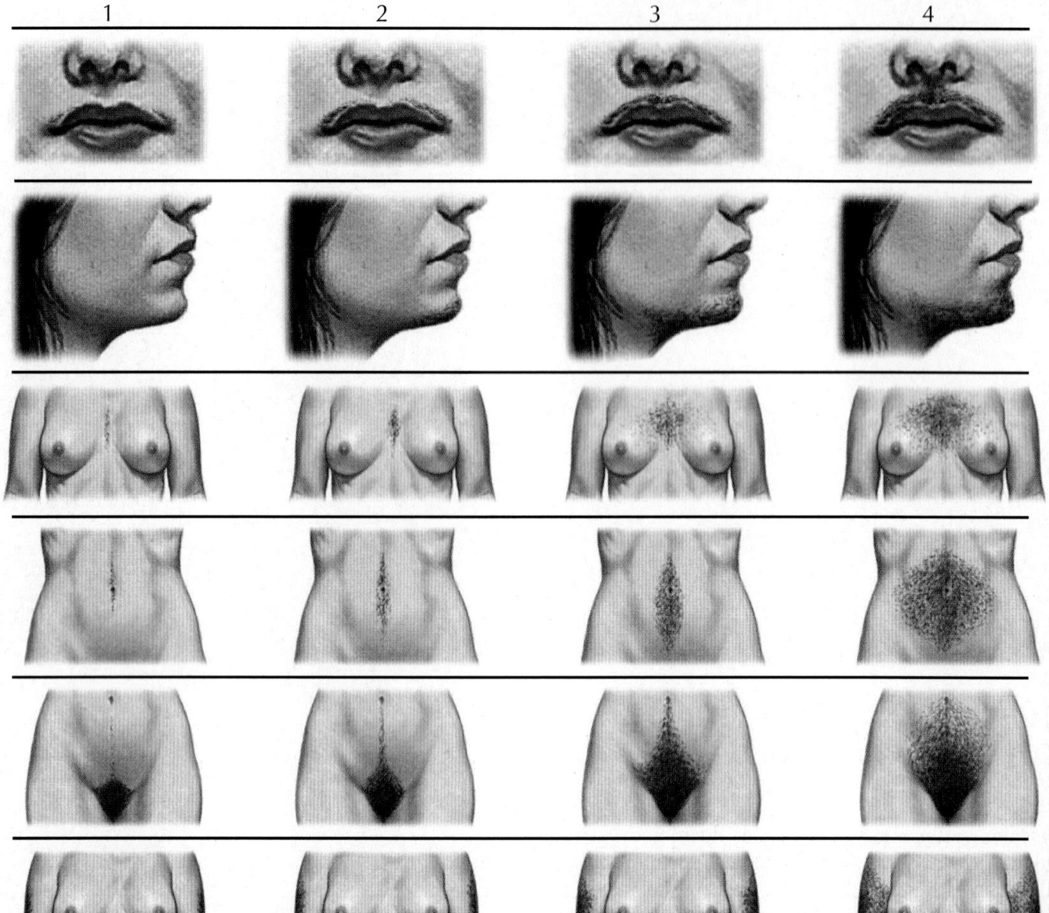

Plate 4.21

Endocrine System: VOLUME 2

HIRSUTISM AND VIRILIZATION

Hirsutism is defined as excessive male-pattern hair growth in females. The causes of hirsutism are many and diverse—from an ethnic or hereditary disposition toward superfluous hair growth to hyperplasia or neoplasia of the adrenal gland or ovaries. Virilization, reflecting a more severe form of androgen excess, is defined as the development of signs and symptoms of masculinization in females (increased muscle bulk, loss of female body contours, deepening of the voice, breast atrophy, clitoromegaly, temporal balding) (see Plate 3.16). Hypertrichosis is not true hirsutism but rather a diffuse increase in total body hair in females or males that may be drug induced (e.g., minoxidil) or associated with other conditions (e.g., anorexia nervosa, malnutrition).

Hair growth has three phases: growth phase (anagen), involution phase (catagen), and rest phase (telogen). Although hair follicle number does not change over time, the size and shape of the hair follicles can change. Hair is either vellus (not pigmented, fine, soft) or terminal (pigmented, thick, coarse). Vellus hair is present on most of the skin. Androgens, in addition to increasing hair follicle size and hair diameter, increase the proportion of time that terminal hairs remain in growth phase at androgen-sensitive body sites. Thus hirsutism is the development of terminal hair in areas where it does not usually occur in females (e.g., face, midline chest, abdomen, and back). At the scalp, androgens reduce the time that hair is in the growth phase and can result in hair thinning.

The degree of male-pattern terminal hair growth in a female can be assessed with a modified scale originally developed by Ferriman and Gallwey. The degree of terminal hair growth is graded at nine body areas: upper lip, chin, chest, upper back, lower back, upper abdomen, lower abdomen, upper arms, and thighs. Each area is scored 0 to 4 (0 = no growth of terminal hair and 4 = complete and heavy cover). The sum of these numbers is the modified Ferriman Gallwey hirsutism score. Most females have a modified Ferriman Gallwey hirsutism score of less than 8 (maximum score, 36), but 5% to 10% of females have scores above 8, a level consistent with the diagnosis of hirsutism. Ethnicity has a major influence on body hair in females. For example, despite equivalent circulating androgen levels, most American Indian and Asian females have little body hair, and females of Mediterranean descent have much more.

Hirsutism is usually caused by increased androgen effect, associated with either increased circulating androgen levels or increased local conversion of testosterone to the more potent DHT at the hair follicle. The conversion of testosterone to DHT is catalyzed by 5α-reductase and amplifies the androgenic effect. DHT is produced primarily by target tissues. Thus androgen action is determined in part by the target tissue androgen receptors and 5α-reductase activity. The adrenal glands produce DHEA and androstenedione. DHEA has no direct androgenic effects but rather serves as a substrate for conversion to androstenedione (which is also androgenically inactive) and then to testosterone. In the ovary, much of the testosterone is aromatized to estradiol. Blood testosterone concentrations in premenopausal females are determined by direct ovarian secretion (one-third of total) and by the peripheral conversion of androstenedione to testosterone in adipose tissue and skin (two-thirds of total). Increased blood testosterone concentrations usually originate from the ovaries, and increased DHEA sulfate (DHEA-S) concentrations usually originate from the adrenal glands. Excess androstenedione secretion can come from either the adrenal glands or the ovaries.

Polycystic ovary syndrome (PCOS) is the most common cause of clinically evident androgen excess. Hirsutism is often concomitant with obesity, amenorrhea, and infertility. These females typically have anovulatory, irregular menstrual cycles; signs of excess androgen effect (e.g., hirsutism, acne); or increased blood concentrations of androgens. PCOS usually becomes evident shortly after the onset of puberty, and the signs and symptoms gradually progress with age.

Hyperthecosis, a severe variant of PCOS, is caused by increased ovarian stromal tissue with luteinized theca cells distributed among sheets of fibroblast-like cells. There is a positive correlation between the degree of

Plate 4.22

Reproduction

HIRSUTISM AND VIRILIZATION (Continued)

hyperthecosis and insulin resistance. The hyperinsulinism appears to stimulate proliferation of thecal interstitial cells. Virilization occurs in some patients with hyperthecosis because of the markedly increased serum testosterone levels.

Idiopathic hirsutism is the second most common diagnosis in females with hirsutism. It is associated with normal menstrual cycles and normal blood androgen concentrations, and no other cause of hirsutism can be identified on evaluation. It may be that these patients have increased cutaneous 5α-reductase activity.

Congenital causes of virilization of female neonates include CAH, which is characterized by an enzymatic defect in cortisol metabolism (see Plates 3.13 and 3.14). In this setting, corticotropin from the pituitary gland is not inhibited by the normal feedback mechanism, and in an effort to produce cortisol, the adrenal glands continue to produce DHEA and other androgenic precursors. As a result, clitoral hypertrophy and hirsutism may be apparent in the newborn. Similar to exogenous androgenic hormones in pill or injected forms taken in early pregnancy, an excess of androgenic steroids from a secretory ovarian or adrenal tumor in the pregnant mother may cause the same fetal changes because these steroids can cross the placental barrier into the fetal circulation. Patients with late-onset or nonclassic CAH (usually caused by partial 21-hyroxylase deficiency) may not present until after puberty with hirsutism and oligomenorrhea (see Plate 3.16). Thus the clinical presentation of late-onset CAH is very similar to that of PCOS. CAH is more common in persons of Ashkenazi Jewish, central European, and Hispanic descent.

Androgen-secreting Sertoli-Leydig cell tumors (arrhenoblastoma), granulosa-theca cell tumors, and hilum-cell tumors are associated with rapidly progressive signs and symptoms of androgen excess and markedly increased serum testosterone concentrations. In patients who present with signs and symptoms of androgen excess, Sertoli-Leydig cell tumors are usually large, but hilum-cell ovarian tumors are small and may escape detection with imaging studies. Adrenal androgen-secreting tumors—much less common than androgen-secreting neoplasms that arise from the ovary—are usually adrenocortical carcinomas producing excess DHEA. Rarely, benign adrenal cortical adenomas or adrenocortical carcinomas hypersecrete testosterone.

In old age, facial hair is considered to be the result of adrenal androgens that are not balanced by any of the estrogenic hormones after ovarian failure at menopause.

Hirsutism and virilization can result from androgenic medications (e.g., anabolic steroids). Rare causes of hirsutism include Cushing syndrome and glucocorticoid resistance syndrome.

EVALUATION OF FEMALES WITH HIRSUTISM

In the circulation, testosterone exists in three forms: tightly bound to SHBG, loosely bound to albumin, or unbound (free). The biologically active testosterone fraction includes the loosely bound and free fractions and is termed the *bioavailable fraction*. Some disorders (e.g., obesity, hypothyroidism, liver disease) decrease SHBG binding and increase bioavailable testosterone

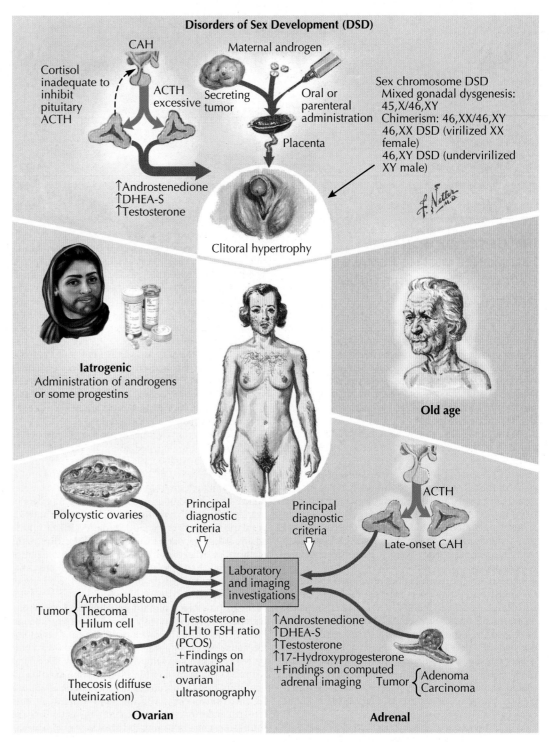

levels. Thus the measurement of bioavailable testosterone concentrations in the blood provides a more accurate assessment of the testosterone effect than the measurement of total testosterone.

When serum testosterone levels are increased in a female with hirsutism, the five most likely causes are PCOS, nonclassic CAH, hyperthecosis, hypothyroidism, or an androgen-secreting ovarian or adrenal tumor. An androgen-secreting neoplasm should be suspected when serum testosterone concentrations are more than threefold above the upper limit of the reference range. Tests that may be needed to differentiate among these diagnostic possibilities include

serum DHEA-S and androstenedione concentrations (increased in most patients with androgen-secreting adrenal tumors and in some patients with CAH), serum thyrotropin concentration (to exclude hypothyroidism), serum 8 AM 17-OHP concentration at baseline and after cosyntropin administration (abnormal in most patients with CAH), serum concentrations of LH and FSH (an increased ratio of LH to FSH is consistent with PCOS), 24-hour urinary-free cortisol excretion (to exclude Cushing syndrome), and imaging with transvaginal ultrasonography (ovary) or computed tomography (adrenal) to assess for neoplasia.

Plate 4.23

Endocrine System: VOLUME 2

INFLUENCE OF GONADAL HORMONES ON THE FEMALE REPRODUCTIVE CYCLE FROM BIRTH TO OLD AGE

From birth to old age, all female mammals exhibit a succession of biologic events characterized by the phases of infancy, childhood, puberty (sexual maturation), adult reproductive years, and, finally, postmenopause and senility. The physiologic indices that differentiate one phase from another are induced primarily by the secretion of ovarian estrogens.

Although ovulation may be considered the chief function of the ovaries, their production of estrogens and progestogens is no less essential to maintain and nourish all parts of the procreative apparatus and to also contribute to the function and maintenance of skin, hair growth, and the skeletal, vascular, and electrolyte systems. Finally, the effects of these hormones in achieving emotional stability during adolescence have their counterpart in psychologic changes associated with estrogen deficiency after menopause and after oophorectomy.

In neonates, the placenta does not block exposure to the high concentration of maternal estrogens before parturition. A female infant's breasts may show some enlargement, and "witch's milk" can occasionally be expressed from the nipples. The external genitalia are precociously developed, and the endometrium has been stimulated to proliferate. The vaginal mucosa is a many-celled layer of stratified epithelium. Vaginal smears show the large, flat, polygonal cells characterized as estrogen stimulated by their small pyknotic nuclei and extensive cornification.

Within 1 week or so after birth, all the above stigmata of estrogen stimulation recede. The newborn ovaries are small structures made up entirely of primordial follicles, disclosing no elements capable of producing estrogens.

In the decade of childhood, from the postnatal recessional changes to the time of puberty, the ovaries gradually show a buildup of interstitial tissue from an accumulation of fibrous stroma, as a constant succession of primordial follicles degenerate in atresia. The vaginal smear shows predominantly basal and parabasal cells mixed with bacteria and amorphous debris. The breasts remain infantile.

In the initiation of puberty, the uterus is first to respond to estrogenic hormones. The endometrium proliferates with the development of straight, tubular glands. Next, the vagina thickens and becomes stratified, with cornified superficial estrogenic cells appearing in the vaginal smear. In the ovary, primordial

follicles progress beyond the stage of a one- or two-layer granulosa with a tiny antrum and exhibit identifiable several cell thickness granulosa and theca interna layers. In the breast, the areolae show pigmentation along with a domelike change, becoming elevated as a conical protuberance (see Plate 4.5). Fat is deposited about the shoulder girdle, hips, and buttocks, and the patterns of adult pelvic and, later, axillary hair typical of the female begin to develop.

An intricate balance of stimulation and response between pituitary gonadotropins and ovarian steroids is essential for the proper sequence of events that result in normal ovulatory cycles. In adolescence as well as at menopause, minor disturbances are responsible for irregular, anovulatory uterine bleeding.

In the mature cycle, the upper two-thirds of the endometrium are sloughed away in the first 48 to 72 hours of menstruation; the bleeding surface is rapidly repaired in the next 2 or 3 days from a spreading proliferation of epithelium from broken glands and arterioles under the stimulus of estrogen secreted by numbers of ovarian follicles in response to FSH from the anterior pituitary. By day 12 in a typical 28-day cycle, one follicle attains ascendancy and exhibits a rapid growth toward maturity, associated with thickening of the proliferative endometrium and increased desquamation of precornified and cornified cells from the vagina. The release of LH at midcycle on day 14 is responsible for ovulation of the mature follicle and for initiation of progesterone secretion from the rapidly forming corpus luteum. Endometrial glands become saw-toothed and secretory; the vaginal smear shows a regression toward intermediate cell types that are clumped together, with folded and wrinkled cytoplasm. If fertilization and implantation do not occur, the corpus luteum degenerates on about day 26, and, consequently, with the rapid withdrawal of its estrogen and progesterone secretion, the endometrium shrinks, becomes ischemic, and breaks away with bleeding on day 28.

Through the changes described above, the juvenile breast has become mature, with branching and extension of both ducts (estrogens) and alveoli (progesterone). Toward the latter half of the cycle, there is often congestion of the lobules, with an increased sensitivity of the areolae and nipples.

Both estrogen and, to a lesser extent, progesterone are associated not only with the transient accumulation of edema fluid in the endometrium (most marked in the secretory phase) but, at times, also with a diffuse premenstrual edema in peripheral tissues, clinically recognized by subjective descriptions of bloating, increased girth, and weight gain.

In the decade of adolescence, the skeletal system reacts to estrogen, first, by an accelerated growth rate of the long bones, and, second, by a hastening of epiphyseal closure, the balance affecting final height.

When conception occurs, the early secretion of chorionic gonadotropin from the chorionic elements of a securely implanted embryo maintains the corpus luteum, preventing it from degenerating in 2 weeks. In pregnancy, the peak production of chorionic hormone is seen by about day 90 after the last menstrual period, declining thereafter to a plateau. The corpus luteum is responsible for increasing progesterone and estrogens throughout the first 3 months, after which the placenta takes over until the end of the pregnancy. The augmentation of both estrogen and progesterone is approximately linear throughout the 9 months of gestation, accounting for the cessation of any demonstrable ovarian activity through the suppression of pituitary FSH and LH secretion. The breasts react to the increasing steroid stimulation and pituitary prolactin secretion with an extension of both ductile and alveolar growth, and there is congestion without actual lactation. The vaginal smear shows the marked effect of the increased progesterone level, with massive clumping of the cells and the appearance of a particular form from the intermediate layer, called the *navicular cell of pregnancy*.

The puerperium is an inconstant phase of endocrine readjustment. The massive withdrawal of estrogen after placental delivery and the psychoneural mechanisms initiated by the suckling reflex bring about the release of oxytocin and prolactin. Breast tissues, already conditioned by growth, respond with milk production and letdown. Ovarian activity is held in abeyance during lactation and nursing, for several months in many cases and even for 1 year or more. However, reestablishment of the pituitary-ovarian cycle can, and often does, take place before weaning, so that another conception can occur before the advent of a menstrual flow. The raw and bleeding endometrial bed of the placental attachment takes from days to weeks to reepithelialize. The vaginal mucosa is thin, and the smear is relatively atrophic until ovarian estrogen is again produced.

Menopause—defined as the cessation of menstrual periods—normally occurs at a mean age of 51.4 years. Premature ovarian failure is defined as primary hypogonadism in a female younger than 40 years. The ovaries no longer contain any follicles capable of responding to pituitary gonadotropins. Increasing amounts of FSH are secreted because of the lack of negative feedback from inhibin and ovarian estrogen secretion. This estrogen deficiency is reflected by senile changes in the breasts, uterus, vagina, skin, bony skeleton, and vascular system.

Childhood and senility represent phases of tranquility in gonadal activity. Proper hormonal interactions through the menstrual cycle, pregnancy, and puerperium are determined fundamentally by appropriate modulations of estrogenic secretions.

Plate 4.23

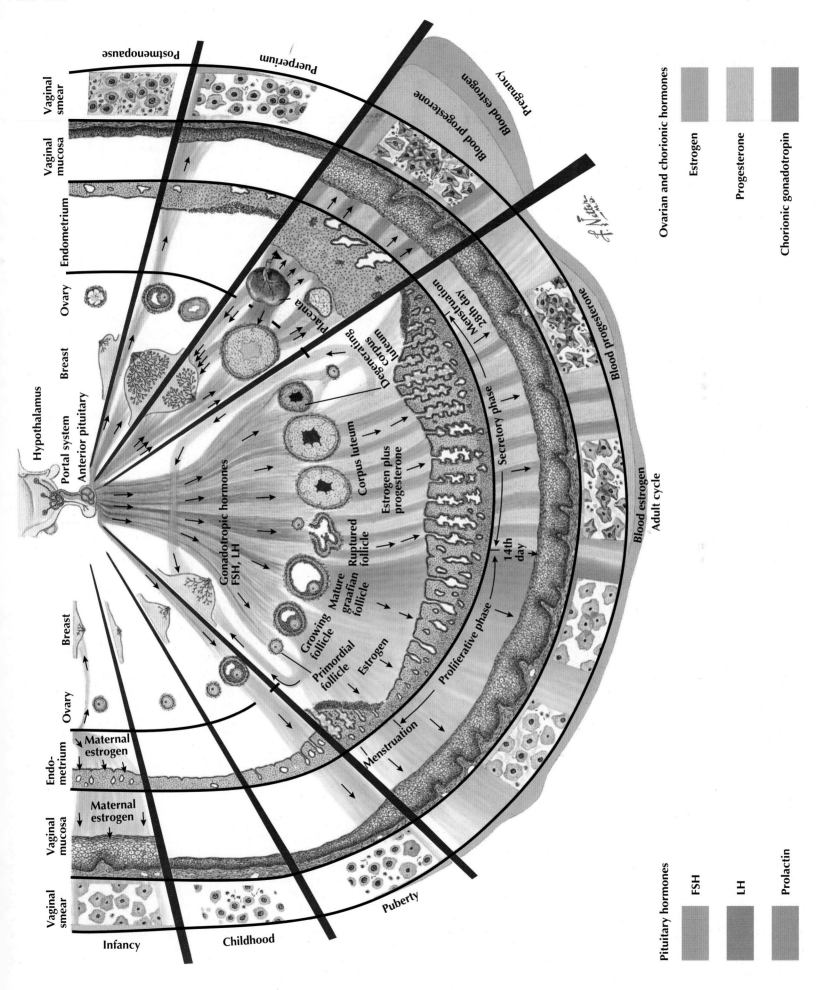

Ovarian and chorionic hormones

Estrogen

Progesterone

Chorionic gonadotropin

Postmenopause

Vaginal smear

Vaginal mucosa

Endometrium

Ovary

Breast

Hypothalamus

Portal system
Anterior pituitary

Puerperium

Blood progesterone

Blood estrogen

Pregnancy

Placenta

Degenerating corpus luteum

Corpus luteum

Estrogen plus progesterone

Ruptured follicle

Mature graafian follicle

Growing follicle

Primordial follicle

Estrogen

Gonadotropic hormones FSH, LH

Menstruation 28th day

Secretory phase

14th day

Proliferative phase

Menstruation

Blood progesterone

Blood estrogen

Adult cycle

Breast

Ovary

Endo-metrium

Maternal estrogen

Vaginal mucosa

Maternal estrogen

Vaginal smear

Infancy

Childhood

Puberty

Pituitary hormones

FSH

LH

Prolactin

Plate 4.24

Endocrine System: VOLUME 2

FUNCTIONAL AND PATHOLOGIC CAUSES OF UTERINE BLEEDING

The uterine mucosa is the only tissue in the body in which the regular, periodic occurrence of necrosis and desquamation with bleeding is usually a sign of health rather than of disease. This periodic blood loss is controlled through a delicate balance of pituitary and ovarian hormones and results from the specific response of the target tissue, the endometrium. The normal ebb and flow of estrogen and progesterone, through a monthly cycle, first builds up and then takes away, in regular sequence, the support of the endometrium; therefore a menstrual flow characterized by repeated regularity in timing, amount, and duration of bleeding bears witness to a normal and ordered chain of endocrine events for that individual. Irregularity in any of these characteristics suggests a functional disturbance or an organic pathology. The main categories of pathologic states that can cause or be accompanied by either menorrhagia (heavy or prolonged flow) or metrorrhagia (spotting or bleeding between menstrual flows) are discussed below.

The concept of bleeding caused by a decrease or withdrawal of ovarian steroids explains the unpredictable flow associated with persistent estrogen phases and anovulatory cycles. Anovulatory uterine bleeding is noncyclical and variable in duration and flow. Common causes of anovulation include adolescent age, perimenopausal state, PCOS, weight loss, strenuous exercise, thyroid dysfunction, and advanced liver or renal disease. In the normal cycle, a progressive increase in estrogen production, with a sharp rise from the maturing follicle toward the 14th day, causes parallel development of all elements in the endometrium—the stroma, glands, and coiled superficial arteries. At or soon after ovulation, the advent of progesterone from the corpus luteum slows growth and proliferation and modifies the tissue into a secretory pattern. If conception and pregnancy do not occur, the corpus luteum regresses in 14 days. Its production of both estrogen and progesterone wanes, and the following are observed: shrinkage of the endometrium, congestion of the nutrient arteries, anoxemia, necrosis, and desquamation. Duration of flow is typically 2 to 7 days with a volume less than 80 mL. Occasionally, irregular shedding from an imbalance of the estrogen-to-progesterone ratio, producing a mixed endometrium with both proliferative and secretory glands in an abnormal luteal phase pattern, may cause menorrhagia. Persistent estrogen production from a series of follicles that fail to ovulate tends to build up a hyperplastic endometrium in which nests of anaplastic glands may develop. The circulating level of estrogen fluctuates in accordance with haphazard spurts of follicle growth. Sporadic reduction in circulating estrogen, spontaneously or because of medication, undermines the vascular support of the uterine mucosa and initiates the changes inevitably followed by necrosis and bleeding. In old age, the hypoplastic, estrogen-deficient endometrium sometimes breaks down and bleeds from a vulnerability to mild trauma or infection.

In addition to the uterus, abnormal bleeding in the genital area may arise from the ovaries, fallopian tubes, cervix, vagina, vulva, urethra, urinary bladder, or bowel. Local ovarian or adnexal disorders may involve primary malignancies, including cystic or solid ovarian tumors that secrete steroids. Cervical lesions are usually not responsible for heavy bleeding but rather are sporadic and caused by postcoital spotting.

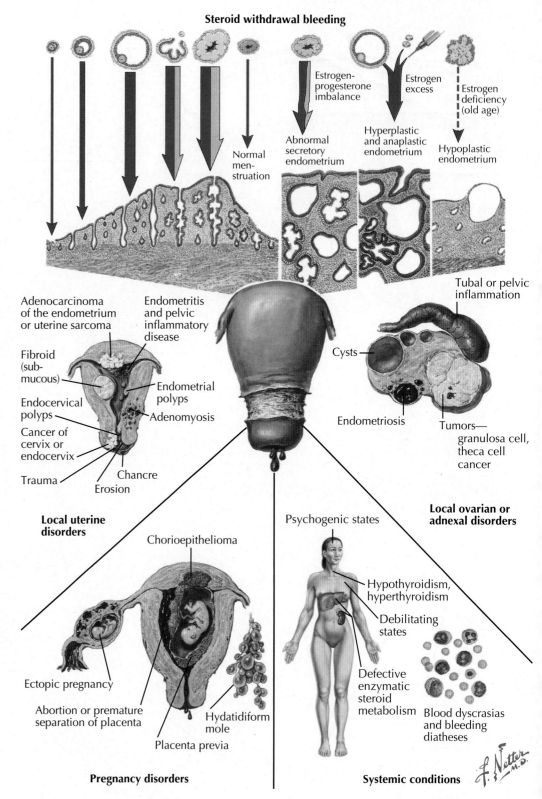

Local uterine disorders causing abnormal bleeding include uterine polyps, uterine leiomyomas (fibroids), adenomyosis (ectopic endometrial tissue in the uterine musculature), hysterotomy scar, adenocarcinoma of the endometrium, uterine sarcoma, metastatic disease to the endometrium, uterine arteriovenous malformation, cancer of the cervix or endocervix, trauma, or endometritis and pelvic inflammatory disease.

Pregnancy-related disorders caused not only by placenta previa, premature placental separation, abortion, or deficiencies as illustrated under systemic conditions but also by ectopic gestation or gestational trophoblastic disease constitute frequent causes of uterine hemorrhage.

A variety of systemic conditions may be responsible for abnormal bleeding. Conditions such as bleeding diatheses (e.g., von Willebrand disease, clotting factor deficiencies, and platelet abnormalities), acute leukemia, advanced liver disease, or anticoagulant therapy usually show signs of bleeding elsewhere. Chronic disease states such as hypothyroidism, hyperthyroidism, hyperprolactinemia, and Cushing syndrome can produce abnormal flow as well as undermine placental function.

Plate 4.25

Reproduction

GYNECOMASTIA

Enlargement of the male breast, caused by an increase in its glandular component, is known as *gynecomastia*. The degree of enlargement is variable, ranging from a barely visible, small, central, subareolar disk of mammary tissue to the proportions of a normal female adolescent breast. It may be unilateral or bilateral and is often painful and tender. Its presence is sometimes difficult to ascertain in males with obesity because their breast enlargement may be caused entirely, or in large part, by fat deposition (pseudogynecomastia). The first step in the evaluation of apparent gynecomastia is to differentiate true gynecomastia (glandular tissue) from pseudogynecomastia (adipose tissue) and breast cancer.

The histopathology is characterized by stimulation of ducts and proliferation of stroma. The ducts undergo lengthening and branching, with budding and formation of new ducts but no alveoli. Epithelial hyperplasia occurs. Simultaneously, there is an increase in the bulk of the stromal tissue, which is often hyalinized. These changes are caused by a decreased ratio of androgen to estrogen activity. The cause is physiologic (e.g., pubertal gynecomastia) or pathologic (e.g., hypogonadism, medication related, cirrhosis, malnutrition).

PHYSIOLOGIC STATES

Neonatally, slight transitory breast enlargement is common in both sexes—this is presumably caused by high levels of maternal estrogen. Pubertal gynecomastia, often slight, bilateral, and painful, occurs in about 50% of boys during puberty and is the single most common cause of gynecomastia. The cause appears to be enhanced aromatization of androgens to estrogens; blood estrogen concentrations reach the range expected for healthy males before testosterone reaches adult levels. Pubertal gynecomastia subsides spontaneously within 1 to 2 years in more than 90% of affected adolescent boys. When it persists into adulthood, it is termed *persistent pubertal gynecomastia*. Involutional breast enlargement occurs in some males later in life, presumably caused by the gradual decline in testosterone production with age.

PATHOLOGIC CONDITIONS

Medications are a common cause of gynecomastia. Less common causes include hypogonadism (primary or secondary), cirrhosis, malnutrition, testicular tumors, and hyperthyroidism. Often a cause for gynecomastia is not found, and it is termed *idiopathic gynecomastia*.

Medications that may cause gynecomastia include antiandrogens (e.g., flutamide, spironolactone), antibiotics (e.g., isoniazid, ketoconazole), oncologic agents (e.g., alkylating agents, imatinib), antiulcer drugs (e.g., cimetidine), cardiovascular agents (e.g., digoxin, methyldopa), illicit drugs (e.g., marijuana, heroin), hormonal drugs (e.g., estrogens, androgens, anabolic steroids, hCG), and psychoactive agents (e.g., haloperidol, phenothiazines). Some of these agents have multiple mechanisms of action. For example, spironolactone blocks the effect of testosterone at the testosterone receptor, enhances the aromatization of testosterone to estradiol, decreases testicular testosterone secretion, and increases the clearance of testosterone.

Hypogonadism, whether primary (testicular failure) or secondary (pituitary failure), is a common cause of gynecomastia. Primary hypogonadism may be caused by a genetic abnormality (e.g., Klinefelter syndrome; see Plate 4.17) or by some other process that affects testicular function (e.g., infection, trauma). Secondary hypogonadism is most commonly caused by illness or a

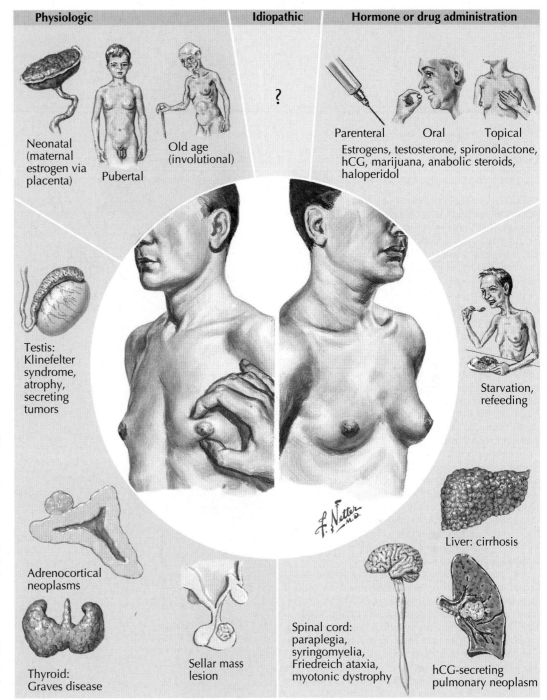

nonfunctioning pituitary macroadenoma that destroys or inhibits the function of the pituitary gonadotrophs. Prolactin-secreting pituitary tumors cause gynecomastia by prolactin-induced decreases in LH and FSH. Prolactin does not directly cause gynecomastia.

Persons with cirrhosis have increased adrenal androgen production and enhanced aromatization to estrogens. In addition, many patients with cirrhosis are treated with spironolactone.

With severe illness and starvation, secondary hypogonadism develops, but adrenal estrogen production is unaffected. Thus the ratio between androgens and estrogens declines in these settings and predisposes to gynecomastia. With improved nutrition, the secondary hypogonadism recovers and recreates the pubertal-like state with enhanced gynecomastia.

Germ cell tumors of the testis hypersecrete hCG, which increases testicular testosterone production but also enhances Leydig cell aromatase activity. hCG may also be hypersecreted by neoplasms in the lung, stomach, kidney, and liver.

More than 25% of men with hyperthyroidism have gynecomastia. These patients have increased LH secretion that leads to both increased Leydig cell testosterone production and aromatization. The peripheral aromatization of androgens to estrogens is also enhanced in these patients. In addition, SHBG is increased, which decreases free testosterone concentrations.

Rarely, patients with gynecomastia have an estrogen-secreting tumor of the adrenal gland; most of these are adrenocortical carcinomas.

Plate 4.26

Endocrine System: VOLUME 2

GALACTORRHEA

Galactorrhea (abnormal lactation) refers to the inappropriate mammary secretion of milky fluid that occurs more than 6 months' postpartum in a female who is not breastfeeding. It is usually bilateral but may be unilateral and spontaneous or expressible. The onset may date back to normal postpartum lactation that failed to stop. Galactorrhea is extremely rare in males.

For normal lactation and galactopoiesis (maintenance of lactation), the basic requirements include optimal amounts of prolactin from the anterior pituitary gland and estrogen and progesterone from the ovaries for duct formation and lobule-alveolar development, respectively. Blood prolactin concentrations increase progressively through pregnancy and peak at the time of delivery to levels approximately 10 times the upper limit of the reference range for individuals who are not lactating. The increasing blood estrogen levels in pregnancy promote prolactin secretion by binding to a prolactin response element in the pituitary lactotroph cell. Suckling has a dual action in the promotion and maintenance of lactation; it stimulates the release of prolactin and oxytocin. The latter leads to the contraction of the myoepithelial cells of the mammary acini, thereby allowing the free flow of milk into the larger ducts. Prolactin secretion is inhibited by dopamine, the prolactin-inhibiting factor that is continuously released by the hypothalamus and reaches the pituitary lactotrophs via the pituitary stalk.

The causes of galactorrhea are quite diverse, but a common pathway is hyperprolactinemia. Any process (e.g., hypothalamic mass, pituitary stalk lesions, or pituitary macroadenomas) that interferes with the transmission of dopamine from the hypothalamus to the anterior pituitary lactotrophs may result in hyperprolactinemia. Frequently, the initial presentation of a prolactin-secreting pituitary tumor (prolactinoma) is galactorrhea (see Plate 1.21). Drugs that block the effect of dopamine at the dopamine receptors on the lactotrophs (e.g., risperidone, phenothiazines, metoclopramide) can cause hyperprolactinemia. Hyperprolactinemia also occurs in patients with primary hypothyroidism when increased hypothalamic thyrotropin-releasing hormone stimulates lactotroph prolactin release. Chronic renal failure causes hyperprolactinemia because of increased prolactin secretion and decreased metabolic clearance.

Anything that simulates the effect of a suckling infant (e.g., chronic nipple stimulation) can result in galactorrhea. This mechanism is also responsible for galactorrhea associated with thoracotomy and healing chest wall wounds, chest wall injuries, cervical spine lesions, and herpes zoster affecting the chest wall.

Approximately 50% of females with acromegaly have galactorrhea, frequently in the absence of hyperprolactinemia. GH is a potent lactogen itself.

The most common cause of galactorrhea, accounting for approximately 50% of cases, is end organ breast hypersensitivity in which the serum prolactin

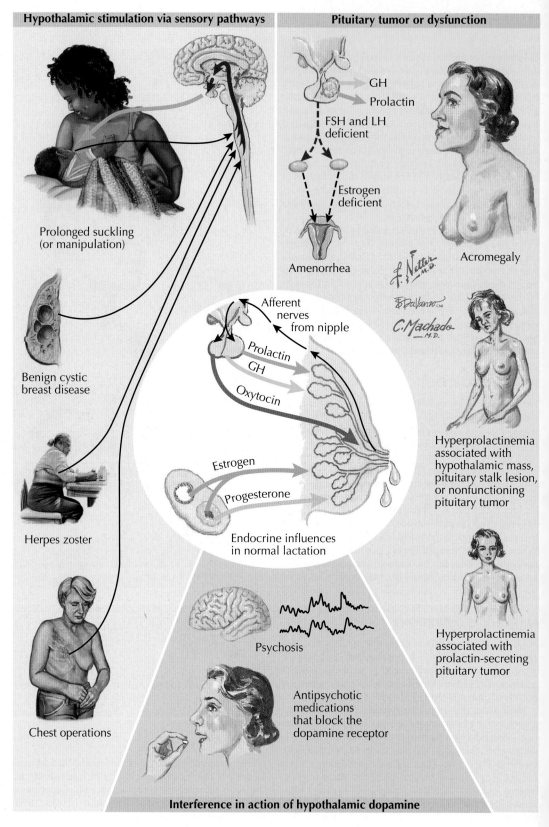

Hypothalamic stimulation via sensory pathways

Prolonged suckling (or manipulation)

Benign cystic breast disease

Herpes zoster

Chest operations

Pituitary tumor or dysfunction

GH
Prolactin
FSH and LH deficient
Estrogen deficient
Amenorrhea
Acromegaly

Afferent nerves from nipple
Prolactin
GH
Oxytocin
Estrogen
Progesterone
Endocrine influences in normal lactation

Hyperprolactinemia associated with hypothalamic mass, pituitary stalk lesion, or nonfunctioning pituitary tumor

Hyperprolactinemia associated with prolactin-secreting pituitary tumor

Psychosis

Antipsychotic medications that block the dopamine receptor

Interference in action of hypothalamic dopamine

concentration is normal. In this setting, the menstrual cycles are typically regular. This form of idiopathic galactorrhea usually occurs postpartum and persists when the menses restart.

In general, galactorrhea is most effectively treated by correcting the hyperprolactinemia. Dopamine agonists (e.g., bromocriptine, cabergoline) are the treatment of choice for patients with prolactin-secreting pituitary tumors (see Plate 1.21). These agents normalize serum prolactin and resolve galactorrhea. Although hyperprolactinemia associated with stalk effect of nonfunctioning pituitary tumors can be corrected with a dopamine agonist, these agents do not address the tumor itself. When a medication is identified as the cause of hyperprolactinemia, an alternative medication should be prescribed.

PANCREAS

Plate 5.1

Endocrine System: VOLUME 2

PANCREAS ANATOMY AND HISTOLOGY

The pancreas is a retroperitoneal organ that lies in an oblique position, where it slopes upward from the duodenum to the hilum of the spleen. The pancreas is 15 to 20 cm long and weighs 75 to 100 g. The four general regions of the pancreas are the head, neck, body, and tail. The head of the pancreas is located in the C-loop of the duodenum, posterior to the transverse mesocolon and anterior to the vena cava, right renal artery, and both renal veins. The uncinate process is the posterior and medial aspects of the head of the pancreas, and it lies behind the portal vein and superior mesenteric vessels. The neck of the pancreas is anterior to the portal vein and first and second lumbar vertebral bodies. The body of the pancreas lies anterior to the aorta at the origin of the superior mesenteric artery. The body and tail of the pancreas lie anterior to the splenic artery and vein. The tail of the pancreas is anterior to the left kidney. The anterior surface of the pancreas is covered by peritoneum. The base of the transverse mesocolon attaches to the inferior margin of the body and tail of the pancreas.

The embryologic origin of the pancreas is the result of fusion of the ventral and dorsal buds. The duct from the smaller ventral bud connects directly to the common bile duct and becomes the duct of Wirsung. The ventral bud becomes the inferior portion of the pancreatic head and uncinate process. The duct from the larger dorsal bud drains directly into the duodenum and becomes the duct of Santorini. The dorsal bud becomes the body and tail of the pancreas. The ducts from each anlage fuse in the pancreatic head so that most of the exocrine pancreas drains through the duct of Wirsung or the main pancreatic duct and then into the common channel formed by the bile duct and pancreatic duct to empty at the ampulla of Vater on the medial aspect of the second portion of the duodenum. The flow of pancreatic and biliary secretions is controlled by the sphincter of Oddi, a group of muscle fibers at the ampulla of Vater.

The blood supply to the pancreas includes multiple branches from the superior mesenteric and celiac arteries. The gastroduodenal artery comes off the common hepatic artery and supplies the head and uncinate process. The body and tail of the pancreas are supplied by multiple branches of the splenic artery. The inferior pancreatic artery arises from the superior mesenteric artery. Three arteries that connect the splenic and inferior pancreatic arteries run perpendicular to the long axis of the pancreas and form an arterial arcade supplying the body and tail of the pancreas. The venous drainage includes an anterior and posterior venous arcade within the head of the pancreas that drains into the portal and mesenteric veins. The venous outflow from the body and tail of the pancreas drains into the splenic vein. The lymphatic drainage of the pancreas includes a profuse network of lymphatic vessels and lymph nodes.

Both the sympathetic and parasympathetic nervous systems innervate the acinar cells (exocrine secretion), islet cells (endocrine secretion), and islet vasculature.

Low-power section of pancreas
1. Acini, **2.** islet, **3.** interlobular septum, **4.** interlobular duct

High magnification: acini, intercalated duct, and zymogen granules

Pancreatic islet: **A** (α-cell), **B** (β-cell), and **C** (δ-cell). **1.** Reticulum, **2.** acini.

In general, the parasympathetic system stimulates endocrine and exocrine secretions, and the sympathetic system inhibits secretions. The neurons that innervate the pancreas also release unique transmitters that include peptides and amines (e.g., somatostatin, galanin, vasoactive intestinal polypeptide, and calcitonin gene-related peptide). A rich supply of afferent sensory nerve fibers is responsible for the intense abdominal pain associated with pancreatic inflammation.

The distribution of pancreatic mass is 85% exocrine, 2% endocrine, 10% extracellular matrix, and 3% blood vessels and ducts. The exocrine cells are clustered in acini (lobules) divided by connective tissue and connected to a duct that drains into the pancreatic duct and into the duodenum. The acinar cells have a high content of endoplasmic reticulum (ER) and apically located eosinophilic zymogen granules. Small clusters of endocrine cells—islets of Langerhans—are embedded within the acini. The three main types of endocrine cells are β-cells (75% of endocrine cell mass) that produce insulin, α-cells (20% of endocrine cell mass) that produce glucagon, and the δ-cells (5% of endocrine cell mass) that secrete somatostatin. Within the islet, the β-cells are in the center and surrounded by the α-cells and δ-cells.

Plate 5.2

Pancreas

Normal adult stool (average values):
N excretion = 10%–15% of intake; 1–2 g/d
Fat excretion = 2%–7% of intake; 3–7 g/d

Exocrine Functions of the Pancreas

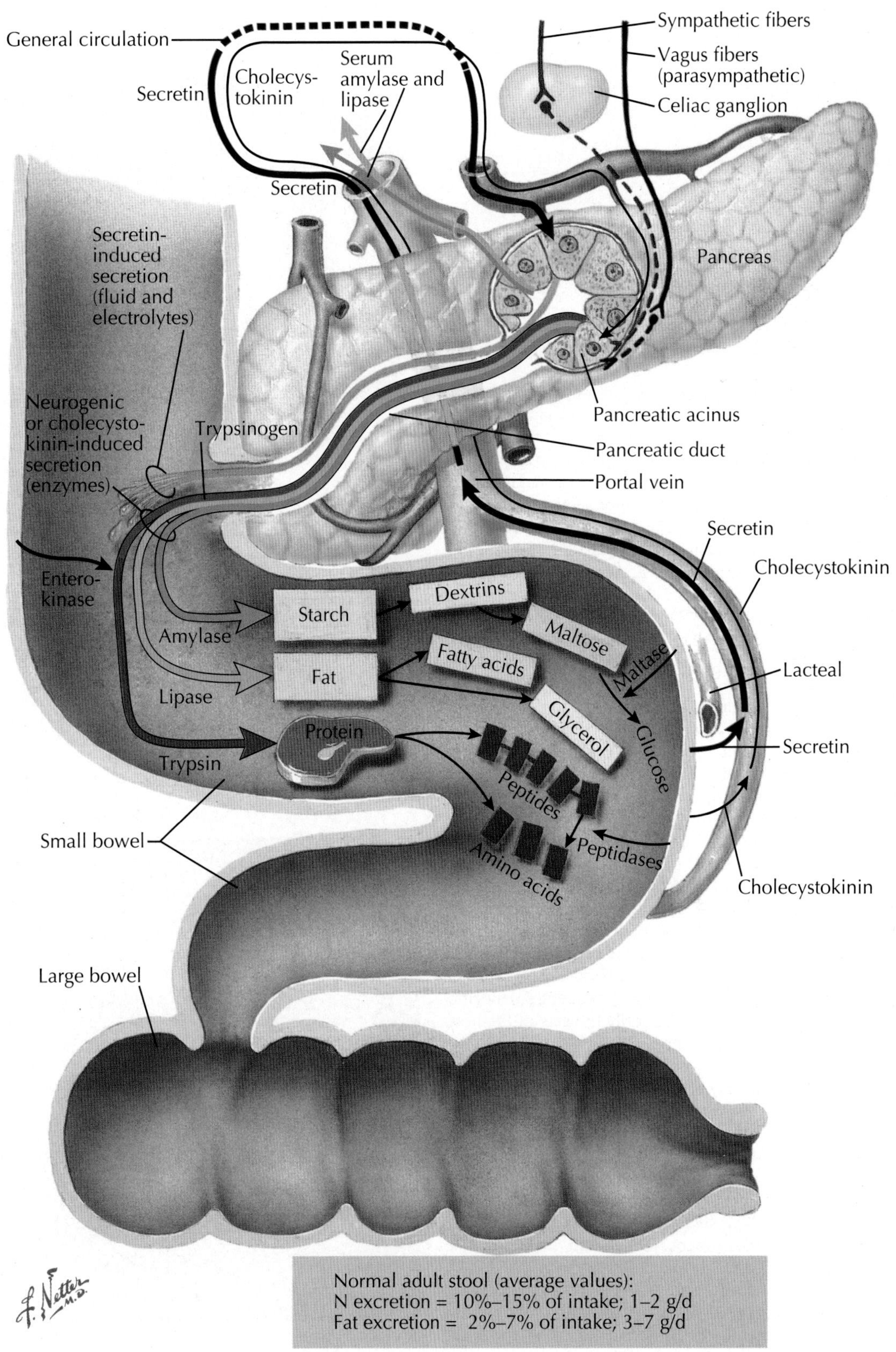

Each day the pancreas secretes approximately 1 L of alkaline isosmotic pancreatic juice that originates from the pancreatic acinar cells and pancreatic ducts. The colorless, bicarbonate-rich, and protein-rich pancreatic juice plays key roles in duodenal alkalinization and food digestion. The acinar cells secrete the enzymes required for the digestion of the three main food types: amylase for carbohydrate (starch) digestion, proteases (e.g., trypsin) for protein digestion, and lipases for fat digestion. The acinar cells are pyramidal in shape with the apices facing the lumen of the acinus, where the enzyme-containing zymogen granules fuse with the apical cell membrane for release. Acinar cells, unlike the endocrine cells of the pancreas, are not specialized and produce all three types of pancreatic enzymes from the same cell type.

Amylase is secreted in its active form and hydrolyzes starch and glycogen to the simple sugars of dextrins and maltose; maltose is then metabolized to glucose by intestinal maltase. The proteolytic enzymes are secreted as proenzymes and must be activated in the duodenum. For example, trypsinogen is converted in the duodenum to trypsin by enterokinase. Intrapancreatic conversion of trypsinogen is prevented by a pancreatic secretory trypsin inhibitor, a step that prevents pancreatic autodigestion. Another example of a proteolytic enzyme that is secreted as a proenzyme is chymotrypsinogen, which is activated in the duodenum to chymotrypsin. The actions of trypsin, chymotrypsin, and other proteolytic enzymes (e.g., elastase, carboxypeptidase A and B, intestinal peptidases) cleave bonds between amino acids in peptide chains, yielding smaller peptides that stimulate the intestinal endocrine cells to release cholecystokinin and secretin, which further stimulate the pancreas to release more digestive enzymes and bicarbonate. The amino acids and dipeptides are actively transported into enterocytes.

Pancreatic lipase is secreted in its active form, and it hydrolyzes triglycerides to fatty acids and glycerol. Phospholipase A cleaves the fatty acid off lecithin to form lysolecithin. Phospholipase B cleaves the fatty acid off lysolecithin to form glycerol phosphatidylcholine. Phospholipase A2 is activated by trypsin in the duodenum, where it serves to hydrolyze phospholipids. Hydrolyzed fat is organized in micelles and is transported into the enterocytes.

There are approximately 40 acinar cells per acinus. The acinar cells near the center of the acinus are termed *centroacinar cells*. Centroacinar cells and pancreatic duct cells secrete electrolytes, bicarbonate, and water into the pancreatic juice. At rest, secretion occurs at a

low basal rate (~2% of maximal). The pancreas' response to a meal occurs in three phases. The cephalic phase—in response to the smell, sight, and taste of food—accounts for 10% of meal-stimulated pancreatic secretion and is mediated by peripherally released acetylcholine. The gastric phase—in response to gastric distension from food—accounts for 10% of meal-stimulated pancreatic secretion. With gastric distension, gastrin is released, and vagal afferents are stimulated to directly mediate pancreatic enzyme secretion

and enhance gastric acid secretion and duodenal acidification. The intestinal phase accounts for 80% of meal-stimulated pancreatic secretion. The duodenal hormone secretin is released in response to acid chyme (pH <3.0) and bile passing into the duodenum. Secretin then stimulates increased production of centroacinar cell bicarbonate to buffer the acidic chyme. Cholecystokinin is also released in response to protein and fat in the proximal small intestine, and it enhances the centroacinar cell response to secretin.

Plate 5.3

Endocrine System: VOLUME 2

Normal Histology of Pancreatic Islets

The pancreas is the union of an endocrine gland (pancreatic islets) and an exocrine gland (acinar and ductal cells). Approximately 85% of pancreatic mass is exocrine, 2% endocrine, 10% extracellular matrix, and 3% blood vessels and ducts. The exocrine (acinar) cells are clustered in acini, divided by connective tissue, and connected to a duct that drains into the pancreatic duct and into the duodenum. Small clusters of endocrine cells—islets of Langerhans—are embedded within the acini of the pancreas. The three main types of endocrine cells are β-cells (75% of endocrine cell mass) that produce insulin, α-cells (20% of endocrine cell mass) that produce glucagon, and δ-cells (5% of endocrine cell mass) that secrete somatostatin. The δ_2-cells secrete vasoactive intestinal polypeptide. The pancreatic polypeptide-producing (PP) cells secrete pancreatic polypeptide. Within the islet, the β-cells are in the center and surrounded by the α-cells, δ-cells, and PP cells.

The adult pancreas contains about 1 million islets (varying in size from 40 to 300 μm) that are more densely distributed in the tail of the gland. The entire mass of islets in a single pancreas weighs only approximately 1 g. Each islet contains approximately 3000 cells. The β-cells are polyhedral in shape and are distributed equally in islets across the pancreas. The α-cells are columnar in shape and are located primarily in islets in the body and tail of the pancreas. The δ-cells are smaller than the α- and β-cells and are frequently dendritic. The PP cells are located primarily in islets in the head and uncinate process of the pancreas. The Gomori aldehyde fuchsin and Ponceau techniques stain the insulin-containing granules in β-cells a deep bluish-purple; the α-cells appear pink or red.

Insulin, discovered in 1920 by Banting and Best, is a 56–amino acid peptide with two chains (α and β chains) joined by two disulfide bridges. β-Cell synthesis of insulin is regulated by plasma glucose concentrations, neural signals, and paracrine effects. The enteric hormones glucose-dependent insulinotropic polypeptide (GIP), glucagon-like peptide-1 (GLP-1), and cholecystokinin also augment insulin secretion. Somatostatin, amylin, and pancreastatin inhibit insulin release. Cholinergic and β-adrenergic sympathetic innervation stimulate insulin release, and α-adrenergic sympathetic innervation inhibits insulin secretion. Insulin acts by inhibiting hepatic glucose production, glycogenolysis, fatty acid breakdown, and ketone formation. Insulin also facilitates glucose transport into cells and stimulates protein synthesis.

Glucagon is a 29–amino acid single-chain peptide hormone that counteracts the effects of insulin by promoting hepatic glycogenolysis and gluconeogenesis. Glucagon release is inhibited by increased levels of plasma glucose and by GLP-1, insulin, and somatostatin. Glucagon secretion is stimulated by the amino acids arginine and alanine. As with insulin, cholinergic and β-adrenergic sympathetic innervation stimulate glucagon release, and α-adrenergic sympathetic innervation inhibits glucagon secretion.

Somatostatin is a peptide that has two bioactive forms: 14–amino acid and 28–amino acid forms. In general, somatostatin inhibits pancreatic endocrine and exocrine secretions.

Pancreatic polypeptide is a 36–amino acid hormone that inhibits bile secretion, gallbladder contraction, and exocrine pancreatic secretion. Pancreatic polypeptide also regulates hepatic insulin receptor expression. Enteral protein and fat stimulate pancreatic polypeptide secretion.

Amylin (also referred to as *islet amyloid polypeptide*) is a 37–amino acid hormone secreted by β-cells in concert with insulin. Amylin is synergistic with insulin by slowing gastric emptying, inhibiting digestive secretions, and inhibiting glucagon release. The effects of amylin are centrally mediated.

Relative density of distribution of islets in various parts of pancreas

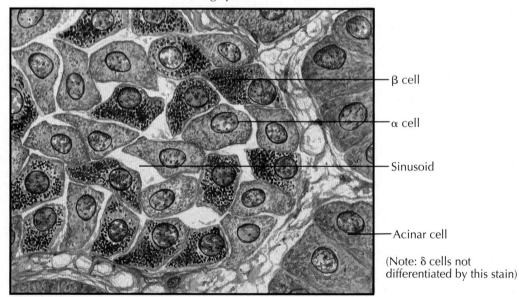

Section of an islet surrounded by acini (×220); Gomori aldehyde fuchsin and Ponceau stain: β granules stain deep purple; α cells, orange-pink

- β cell
- α cell
- Sinusoid
- Acinar cell

(Note: δ cells not differentiated by this stain)

Portion of islet greatly magnified (×1200); Gomori aldehyde fuchsin and Ponceau stain

Plate 5.4   Pancreas

INSULIN SECRETION

Pancreatic β-cell production of insulin is regulated by plasma glucose concentration, neural inputs, and the effects of other hormones by paracrine and endocrine actions. Proinsulin consists of an amino-terminal β-chain, a carboxy-terminal α-chain, and a connecting peptide (C-peptide) in the middle. C-peptide functions by allowing folding of the molecule and the formation of disulfide bonds between the α- and β-chains. C-peptide is cleaved from proinsulin by endopeptidases in the β-cell ER to form insulin. Insulin and C-peptide are packaged into secretory granules in the Golgi apparatus. The secretory granules are released into the portal circulation by exocytosis. Insulin is degraded in the liver, kidney, and target tissues; it has a circulating half-life of 3 to 8 minutes. C-peptide does not act at the insulin receptor and is not degraded by the liver; it has a circulating half-life of 35 minutes. Thus measurement of serum C-peptide concentration serves as a measure of β-cell secretory capacity. Defects in the synthesis and cleavage of insulin can lead to rare forms of diabetes mellitus (e.g., Wakayama syndrome, proinsulin syndromes).

Insulin is released in a pulsatile and rhythmic background pattern throughout the day and serves to suppress hepatic glucose production and mediates glucose disposal by adipose tissue. Superimposed on the background secretion of insulin is the meal-induced insulin release. There are two phases of caloric intake-induced insulin secretion. In the first phase, prestored insulin is released over 4 to 6 minutes. The second phase is a slower onset and longer sustained release because of the production of new insulin.

The regulators of insulin release include nutrients (e.g., glucose and amino acids), hormones (e.g., GLP-1, somatostatin, insulin, and epinephrine), and neurotransmitters (e.g., acetylcholine, norepinephrine). The β-cells are exquisitely sensitive to small changes in glucose concentration; maximal stimulation of insulin secretion occurs at plasma glucose concentrations more than 400 mg/dL. Glucose enters the β cells by a membrane-bound glucose transporter (GLUT 2). Glucose is then phosphorylated by glucokinase as the first step in glycolysis (leading to the generation of acetyl–coenzyme A (CoA) and adenosine triphosphate (ATP) through the Krebs cycle (see Plate 5.6). The rise in intracellular ATP closes (inhibits) the ATP-sensitive potassium (K^+) channels and reduces the efflux of K^+, which causes membrane depolarization and opening (activation) of the voltage-dependent calcium (Ca^{2+}) channels. The resultant Ca^{2+} influx increases the concentration of intracellular Ca^{2+}, which triggers the exocytosis of insulin secretory granules into the circulation. The β-cell Ca^{2+} concentrations can also be increased by the ATP generated from amino acid metabolism.

Insulin release from β-cells can be amplified by cholecystokinin, acetylcholine, GIP, glucagon, and GLP-1. Orally administered glucose stimulates a greater insulin response than an equivalent amount of glucose administered intravenously because of the release of enteric hormones (e.g., GLP-1, GIP) that potentiate insulin secretion. This phenomenon is referred to as the *incretin effect,* a finding that has led to new pharmacotherapeutic options in the treatment of patients with type 2 diabetes mellitus (see Plate 5.21). Acetylcholine and cholecystokinin bind to cell surface receptors and activate adenylate cyclase and phospholipase C, which leads to inositol triphosphate (IP_3) breakdown and mobilization of Ca^{2+} from intracellular stores; activation of protein kinase C also triggers

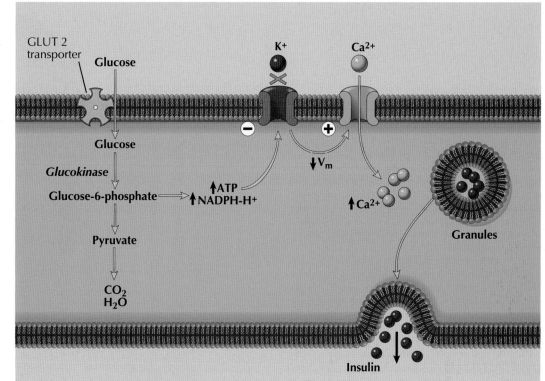

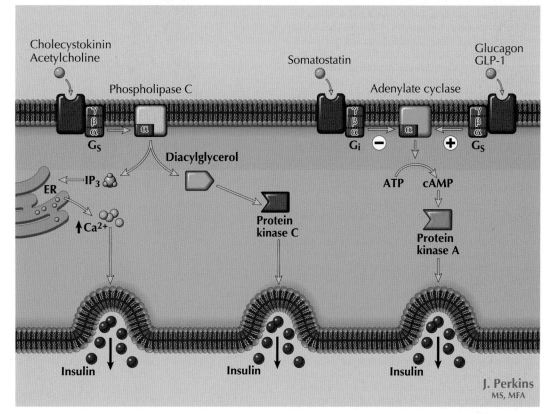

J. Perkins
MS, MFA

insulin secretion. GLP-1 receptor activation leads to increased cyclic adenosine monophosphate (cAMP) and activation of the cAMP-dependent protein kinase A; the Ca^{2+} signal is amplified by decreasing Ca^{2+} uptake by cellular stores and by activation of proteins that trigger exocytosis of insulin. Somatostatin and catecholamines inhibit insulin secretion through G-protein-coupled receptors and inhibition of adenylate cyclase.

Normal insulin secretion is dependent on the maintenance of an adequate number of functional β-cells (referred to as *β-cell mass*). The β-cells must be able to sense the key regulators of insulin secretion (e.g., blood glucose concentration). In addition, the rates of proinsulin synthesis and processing must be sufficient to maintain adequate insulin secretion. Defects in any of these steps in insulin secretion can lead to hyperglycemia and diabetes mellitus.

Plate 5.5

Endocrine System: VOLUME 2

ACTIONS OF INSULIN

Insulin is a 56–amino acid polypeptide that consists of two peptide chains (α and β) that are joined by two disulfide bridges. Insulin is secreted into the portal vein and delivered directly to the liver. Approximately 80% of insulin is cleared by the hepatic cell surface insulin receptors with the first pass through the liver. Insulin acts through the insulin receptor and has anabolic effects at target organs to promote synthesis of carbohydrate, fat, and protein.

The insulin receptor, a member of the growth factor receptor family, is a heterotetrameric glycoprotein membrane receptor that has two α- and two β-subunits that are linked by disulfide bonds. The α-subunits form the extracellular portion where insulin binds. The α-subunits form the transmembrane and intracellular portions of the receptor and contain an intrinsic tyrosine kinase activity. Insulin binding to the receptor triggers autophosphorylation on the intracellular tyrosine residues and leads to phosphorylation of insulin receptor substrates (IRS-1, IRS-2, IRS-3, and IRS-4). The phosphorylation of the IRS proteins activates the phophatidylinositol-3-kinase (PI₃ kinase) and mitogen-activated protein kinase (MAPK) pathways. The PI_3 kinase pathway mediates the metabolic (e.g., glucose transport, glycolysis, glycogen synthesis, and protein synthesis) and antiapoptotic effects of insulin. The MAPK pathway has primarily proliferative and differentiation effects. The number of insulin receptors expressed on the cell membrane can be modulated by diet, body type, exercise, insulin, and other hormones. Obesity and high serum insulin concentrations downregulate the number of insulin receptors. Exercise and starvation upregulate the number of insulin receptors.

Glucose oxidation is the major energy source for many tissue types. Cell membranes are impermeable to hydrophilic molecules such as glucose and require a carrier system to transport glucose across the lipid bilayer cell membrane. GLUT 1 is present in all tissues and has a high affinity for glucose to mediate a basal glucose uptake in the fasting state. GLUT 2 has a low affinity for glucose and functions primarily at high plasma glucose concentrations (e.g., after a meal). GLUT 3 is a high-affinity glucose transporter for neuronal tissues. GLUT 4 is localized primarily to muscle and adipose tissues.

In muscle, activation of the insulin receptor and the PI₃ kinase pathway leads to recruitment of the glucose transporter GLUT 4 from the cytosol to the plasma membrane. Increased expression of GLUT 4 leads to active transport of glucose across the myocyte cell membrane. Insulin promotes myocyte glycogen synthesis by increasing the activity of glycogen synthase and inhibiting the activity of glycogen phosphorylase. Insulin also enhances protein synthesis by increasing amino acid transport and by phosphorylation of a serine/threonine protein kinase.

In adipose tissue, insulin inhibits lipolysis by promoting dephosphorylation of hormone-sensitive (intracellular) lipase. The decreased breakdown of adipocyte triglycerides to fatty acids and glycerol leads to decreased substrate for ketogenesis. Insulin also induces the production of the endothelial cell-bound

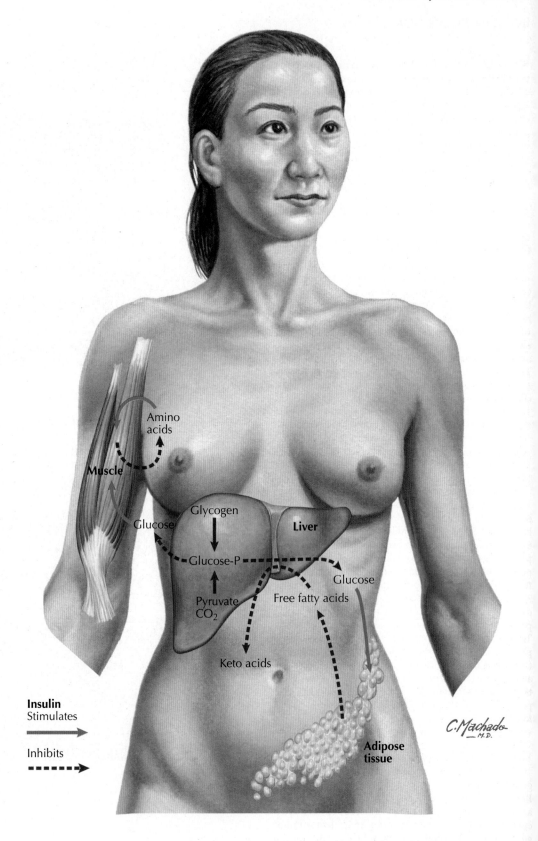

lipoprotein lipase, which hydrolyzes triglycerides from circulating lipoproteins to provide free fatty acids for adipocyte uptake. Insulin stimulates lipogenesis by activating acetyl-CoA carboxylase. Increased glucose transport into adipocytes increases the availability of α-glycerol phosphate that is used in the esterification of free fatty acids into triglycerides. The decreased fatty acid delivery to the liver is a key factor in the net impact of insulin to decrease hepatic gluconeogenesis and ketogenesis.

In the liver, insulin stimulates the synthesis of enzymes that are involved in glucose utilization (e.g., pyruvate kinase, glucokinase) and inhibits the synthesis of enzymes involved in glucose production (e.g., glucose 6-phospatase, phosphoenolpyruvate carboxykinase). Insulin enhances glycogen synthesis by increasing phosphatase activity, causing dephosphorylation of glycogen synthase and glycogen phosphorylase. Insulin also promotes hepatic synthesis of triglycerides, very low-density lipoprotein (VLDL), and proteins.

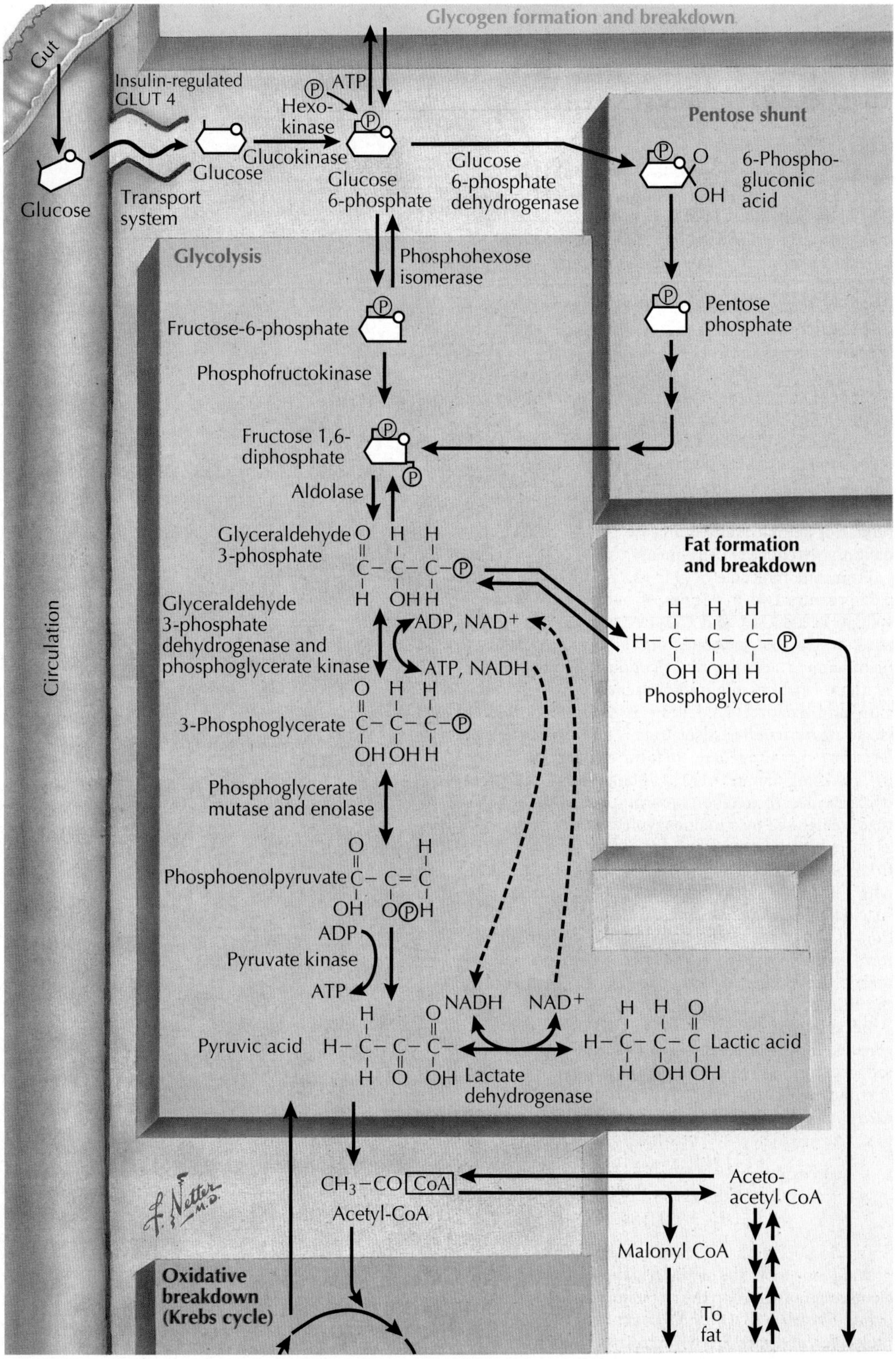

Plate 5.6

Pancreas

GLYCOLYSIS

Glycolysis is the major pathway for glucose metabolism, and it occurs in the cytosol of all cells. Glycolysis breaks down glucose (a 6-carbon molecule) into pyruvate (a 3-carbon molecule). Glycolysis can function either aerobically or anaerobically, depending on the availability of oxygen and the electron transport chain. The ability of glycolysis to provide energy in the form of ATP from adenosine diphosphate (ADP) in the absence of oxygen allows tissues to survive anoxia.

Glycolysis occurs when a molecule of glucose 6-phosphate is transformed to pyruvate:

$$\text{Glucose} + 2\,\text{ADP} + 2\,\text{NAD}^+$$
$$+ 2 \text{ Inorganic phosphate (P}_i\text{)}$$
$$\rightarrow 2 \text{ Pyruvate} + 2\,\text{ATP}$$
$$+ 2\,\text{NADH} + 2\,\text{H}^+ + 2\text{H}_2\text{O}$$

Glucose enters glycolysis by phosphorylation to glucose 6-phosophate, an irreversible reaction catalyzed by hexokinase, and ATP serves as the phosphate donor. Glucose 6-phosphate is converted to fructose-6-phosphate by phosphohexose isomerase. This intermediate is then phosphorylated to yield fructose-1,6-diphosphate. At this stage, the hexose molecule is cleaved by aldolase into two 3-carbon compounds: glyceraldehyde 3-phosphate and dihydroxyacetone phosphate. Dihydroxyacetone phosphate is quickly converted to glyceraldehyde 3-phosphate. The aldehyde group (CHO) of glyceraldehyde 3-phosphate is oxidized by a nicotinamide adenine dinucleotide (NAD)-dependent enzyme, and a phosphate group is attached, yielding 1,3-bisphosphoglycerate. The energy of this oxidative step now rests in the phosphate bond at position 1. This energy is transferred to a molecule of ADP, forming ATP.

$$\text{Glyceraldehyde 3-phosphate} + P_i + \text{NAD} + \text{ADP}$$
$$\rightarrow \text{3-Phosphoglycerate} + \text{NADH} + \text{ATP}$$

This reaction yields energy that is not immediately given off as heat but is stored in the form of ATP. Because two molecules of glyceraldehyde 3-phosphate are produced for every molecule of glucose, two molecules of ATP are formed at this step per molecule of glucose undergoing glycolysis. An ensuing transformation of phosphoenolpyruvate to pyruvate (catalyzed by pyruvate kinase) gives rise to another ATP (two molecules of ATP per molecule of glucose oxidized).

When a tissue possesses the systems for further oxidation of pyruvate, provided oxygen is present, pyruvate is cleaved to acetyl-CoA, and it enters the tricarboxylic acid (TCA) cycle (see Plate 5.7). However, when the oxidative systems are absent (e.g., in erythrocytes that lack mitochondria) or if oxygen is excluded or is present in insufficient amounts (e.g., under

anaerobic conditions), pyruvate is reduced to lactic acid by the enzyme lactate dehydrogenase. This system provides for the reoxidation of NADH and thus enables its participation again in oxidizing glyceraldehyde 3-phosphate; otherwise, the latter reaction would stop as soon as all the molecules of NAD were reduced.

(A) Glyceraldehyde 3-phosphate + NAD
 → 1,3-Diphosphoglycerate + NADH

(B) Pyruvate + NADH → Lactate + NAD

The coupling of these two reactions allows the provision of energy by carbohydrates in the absence of oxygen, albeit at the expense of considerable amounts of carbohydrate. Under aerobic conditions, approximately 30 molecules of ATP are generated per molecule of glucose that is oxidized to CO_2 and H_2O, but only two molecules of ATP when oxygen is absent. Glycolysis is regulated by the three enzymes that catalyze nonequilibrium reactions: hexokinase, phosphofructokinase, and pyruvate kinase.

Plate 5.7

Endocrine System: VOLUME 2

TRICARBOXYLIC ACID CYCLE

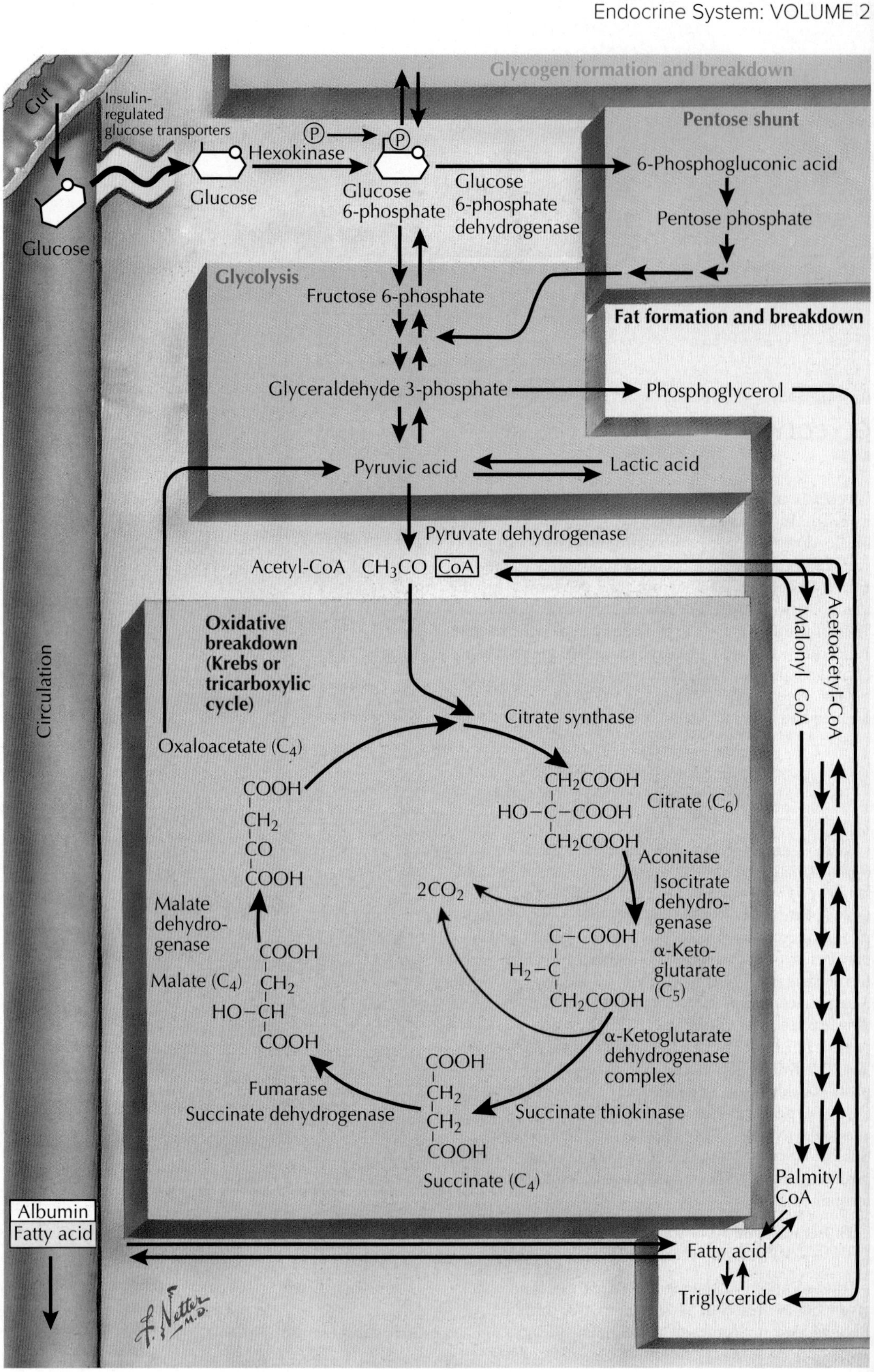

The TCA cycle, also referred to as the *citric acid cycle* or the *Krebs cycle*, is the final common pathway for oxidation of carbohydrate, lipid, and protein. Most of these nutrients are metabolized to acetyl-CoA or one of the intermediates in the TCA cycle. For example, in protein catabolism, proteins are broken down by proteases into their constituent amino acids. The carbon backbone of these amino acids can become a source of energy by being converted to acetyl-CoA and entering into the TCA cycle. The TCA cycle also provides carbon skeletons for gluconeogenesis and fatty acid synthesis.

The TCA cycle starts with a reaction between the acetyl moiety of acetyl-CoA and the 4-carbon dicarboxylic acid, oxaloacetate, to form a 6-carbon TCA, citrate. In the reactions that follow, two molecules of CO_2 are released and oxaloacetate is regenerated. This process is aerobic and requires oxygen as the final oxidant of the reduced coenzymes.

From one molecule of glucose, glycolysis (see Plate 5.6) provides two molecules of pyruvate. Pyruvate is split to acetyl-CoA and CO_2 by pyruvate dehydrogenase, a step that generates one molecule of reduced nicotinamide adenine dinucleotide (NADH). Citrate synthase catalyzes the initial reaction between acetyl-CoA and oxaloacetate. Citrate is then isomerized to isocitrate by aconitase. Isocitrate is dehydrogenated by isocitrate dehydrogenase to form oxalosuccinate and then α-ketoglutarate. α-Ketoglutarate then undergoes oxidative decarboxylation to form succinyl-CoA, a step that is catalyzed by a multienzyme complex referred to as the *α-ketoglutarate dehydrogenase complex*. Succinate thiokinase converts succinyl-CoA to succinate. Succinate is then dehydrogenated to fumarate by succinate dehydrogenase. Fumarase catalyzes the addition of water across the double bond of fumarate to form malate. Malate is converted to oxaloacetate by malate dehydrogenase. Oxaloacetate can then reenter the TCA cycle.

Because of the oxidations catalyzed by the dehydrogenases in the TCA cycle, three molecules of the reduced form of NADH and one molecule of flavin adenine dinucleotide H_2 (FADH$_2$) are produced for each molecule of acetyl-CoA catabolized in one turn of the cycle.

$$Acetyl\text{-}CoA + 3\,NAD^+ + FAD + ADP + P_i$$
$$+ 2\,H_2O \rightarrow CoA\text{-}SH + 3\,NADH + 3\,H^+$$
$$+ FADH_2 + ATP + 2\,CO_2$$

In addition, the pyruvate dehydrogenase step provides one molecule of NADH. These reducing equivalents are transferred to the respiratory chain, and reoxidation of each NADH results in approximately 2.5 ATP molecules, and each FADH$_2$ translates to approximately 1.5 ATP molecules. In addition, one ATP equivalent is generated from the phosphorylation step of succinyl-CoA catalyzed by succinate thiokinase. Thus including the pyruvate dehydrogenase step, approximately 12 ATP molecules are formed per turn of the TCA cycle.

Four of the B vitamins have key roles in the TCA cycle. Riboflavin (vitamin B$_2$) in the form of FAD is a cofactor for succinate dehydrogenase. Niacin (vitamin B$_3$) in the form of NAD is the electron acceptor for isocitrate dehydrogenase, α-ketoglutarate dehydrogenase, and malate dehydrogenase. Pantothenic acid (vitamin B$_5$) is part of CoA. Thiamine (vitamin B$_1$)

serves as the coenzyme for decarboxylation of the α-ketoglutarate dehydrogenase step.

Recent studies have shown a link between intermediates of the TCA cycle and the regulation of hypoxia-inducible factors (HIFs). HIFs have a key role in the regulation of oxygen homeostasis. HIFs are transcription factors that have broad targets, which include apoptosis, angiogenesis, vascular remodeling, glucose use, and iron transport. Dysregulation of HIFs appears

central to the development of paragangliomas and pheochromocytomas in individuals with von Hippel-Lindau syndrome, where the *VHL* tumor suppressor gene encodes a protein that regulates hypoxia-induced proteins (see Plate 8.4). In addition, the familial paraganglioma syndromes are associated with pathogenic variants in the genes that encode key subunits of succinate dehydrogenase (*SDHB, SDHD, SDHC, SDHA, SDHAF2*).

Plate 5.8

Pancreas

GLYCOGEN METABOLISM

Glycogen is a branched polymer of α-D-glucose and is the major depot of carbohydrates in the body, primarily in muscle and liver. Glycogen is the analog of starch, which is a less branched glucose polymer in plants.

GLYCOGENESIS

Glycogenesis occurs mainly in the liver and muscle. Catalyzed by glucokinase in the liver and hexokinase in the muscle, glucose is phosphorylated to glucose 6-phosphate. Glucose 6-phosphate is isomerized to glucose 1-phosphate by the action of phosphoglucomutase. Glucose 1-phosphate interacts with uridine triphosphate (UTP) to form uridine diphosphate glucose (UDPGlc) and pyrophosphate in a reaction catalyzed by UDPGlc pyrophosphorylase. Glycogen synthase catalyzes the bond between C_1 of the glucose of UDP-Glc with the C_4 terminal glucose residue ($1 \rightarrow 4$ linkage) of glycogen and uridine diphosphate (UDP) liberated in the process. This step keeps repeating until the glycogen chain is at least 11 glucose residues long; at that point, branching enzyme transfers six or more glucose residues to a neighboring chain to form a $1 \rightarrow 6$ linkage to establish a branch point.

GLYCOGENOLYSIS

The rate-limiting step of glycogenolysis is the cleavage of the $1 \rightarrow 4$ linkages of glycogen by glycogen phosphorylase to produce glucose 1-phosphate. This cleaving starts at the terminal glucosyl residues until four glucose residues remain on either side of a $1 \rightarrow 6$ linkage, at which point glucan transferase transfers a trisaccharide unit from one branch to the other to expose the $1 \rightarrow 6$ linkage. Debranching enzyme can then hydrolyze the $1 \rightarrow 6$ linkage, and further phosphorylase actions proceed to completely convert the glycogen chain to glucose 1-phosphate. The glucose 6-phosphate molecules have three possible fates: (1) transformation to glucose 1-phosphate by phosphoglucomutase and proceeding to glycogenesis; (2) hydrolyzation by glucose 6-phosphatase in the liver and kidney to produce glucose for release into the bloodstream; or (3) proceeding on to the glycolysis or the pentose phosphate (pentose shunt) pathways.

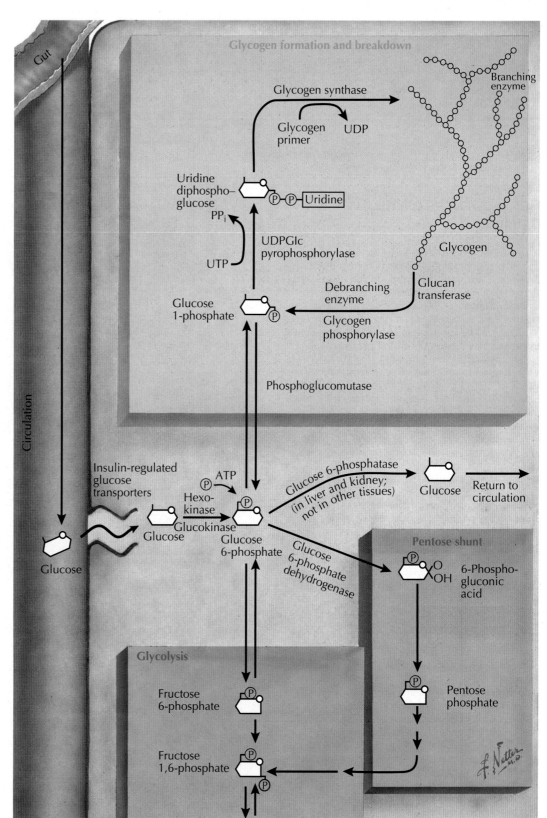

REGULATION OF GLYCOGENESIS AND GLYCOGENOLYSIS

The rate-limiting enzymes are glycogen synthase and glycogen phosphorylase. Glycogen serves as a rapid and short-term source of glucose. The liver releases glycogen-derived glucose during fasting. After ingesting a meal containing carbohydrates, blood glucose concentrations rise and stimulate the pancreas to release insulin. Insulin-regulated glucose transporters provide glucose to the hepatocyte. Insulin also stimulates glycogen synthase. Glucose continues to be added to the glycogen chains as long as glucose and insulin are supplied. After food digestion, blood glucose concentrations fall, and insulin release is decreased, leading to a cessation in glycogen synthesis. Approximately 4 hours after a meal, because of decreasing blood glucose levels, the pancreas begins to secrete glucagon. Glucagon and epinephrine are the main hormones that activate glycogenolysis.

Plate 5.9

Endocrine System: VOLUME 2

CONSEQUENCES OF INSULIN DEPRIVATION

The absence of insulin is incompatible with life. Insulin deprivation can result from surgical removal (pancreatectomy) or autoimmune destruction of β-cells (type 1 diabetes mellitus); both lead to absence or severe curtailment of insulin production and release. In these settings, insulin-sensitive tissues (e.g., muscle, adipose tissue, liver) are deprived of insulin and its actions. Cell membranes are impermeable to hydrophilic molecules such as glucose and require a carrier system (e.g., GLUT 1, 2, 3, 4) to transport glucose across the lipid bilayer cell membrane. Because of decreased insulin-induced activation of the cell membrane glucose transporters, the transit of glucose from the blood into cells is diminished. At the same time, in the absence of insulin, glycogenesis is slowed. The suppressive effect of insulin on glucagon is removed, and glucagon enhances hepatic gluconeogenesis, which is fueled by the increased availability of precursors (e.g., glycerol and alanine) from accelerated fat and muscle breakdown. Thus in the setting of insulin deprivation, there is impaired glucose utilization in peripheral tissues, increased glycogenolysis, and increased gluconeogenesis.

When the blood glucose concentration increases above 200 mg/dL, the renal tubules begin to exceed their capacity for glucose reabsorption (renal threshold). Excess glucose is lost in the urine (glucosuria) which, because of osmotic forces, takes water and sodium with it. Weight loss, thirst, polyuria, and hunger occur. Patients with indolent uncontrolled diabetes over months can present with wasting and cachexia similar to that seen in those with advanced malignancies.

In insulin-sensitive tissues, metabolic adjustments occur as a consequence of the curtailed glucose supply. Proteins are broken down faster than they can be synthesized; hence amino acids are liberated from muscle, brought to the liver, and transformed to urea. The nonprotein nitrogen excreted in the urine rises and a negative nitrogen balance results.

Lipolysis is enhanced in the setting of insulin deprivation. There is a net liberation of stored fat as free fatty acids, which are used by many tissues for energy production. Hepatic uptake and metabolism of fatty acids lead to excess production of the ketones acetoacetate and β-hydroxybutyrate, strong organic acids that lead to ketoacidosis (see Plate 5.10). Ketones provide an alternate energy source when the utilization of glucose is impaired. The circulating β-hydroxybutyrate and acetoacetate obtain their sodium from $NaHCO_3$, thus leading to a metabolic acidosis. In addition, acetoacetate and β-hydroxybutyrate are excreted readily by the kidney, accompanied by base, and fixed base is lost. The severity of the metabolic acidosis depends on the rate and duration of ketoacid production.

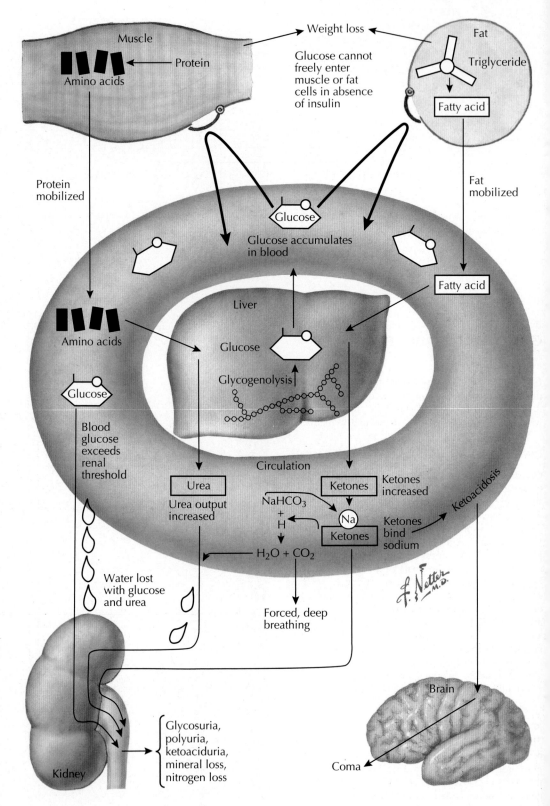

Insulin deprivation also leads to deficits in minerals. A potassium deficit results from urinary losses with the glucose osmotic diuresis and in an effort to maintain electroneutrality as ketoacid anions are excreted. A negative phosphate balance is a result of phosphaturia caused by hyperglycemic-induced osmotic diuresis.

The outcomes of severe insulin deprivation include negative nitrogen balance, weight loss, ketosis, and acidosis. These are the hallmarks of the most severe state of metabolic decompensation characteristic of insulin deprivation in individuals with no endogenous source of insulin (e.g., type 1 diabetes mellitus). Acidosis, when not compensated for, exerts its major effect on brain function. In addition, acidosis affects the contractile responses of the small blood vessels throughout the body that, when coupled with osmotic diuresis-induced volume loss, results in hypotension and vascular collapse. Thus diabetic coma and death—the fate of all those with type 1 diabetes mellitus before the advent of insulin replacement therapy—are the end result of uncompensated and untreated insulin deprivation.

Plate 5.10   Pancreas

DIABETIC KETOACIDOSIS

Diabetic ketoacidosis (DKA) is serious complication of diabetes mellitus characterized by the triad of hyperglycemia, anion gap metabolic acidosis, and ketonemia. DKA results from severe insulin deficiency with resultant hyperglycemia, excessive lipolysis, increased fatty acid oxidation, and excess ketone body production. The deficiency of insulin and the excess secretion of glucagon, catecholamines, glucocorticoids, and growth hormone stimulate glycogenolysis and gluconeogenesis while simultaneously impairing glucose disposal. DKA is primarily a complication of type 1 diabetes mellitus because it is usually only seen in the setting of severe insulin deficiency. DKA may be the initial presentation of new-onset type 1 diabetes mellitus.

Most patients with DKA have preceding symptoms of polyuria, polydipsia, and weight loss that result from a partially compensated state. However, with absolute insulin deficiency, metabolic decompensation can intervene rapidly over 24 hours. Typical DKA presenting symptoms include nausea, emesis, abdominal pain, lethargy, and hyperventilation with slow, deep breaths (Kussmaul respirations). On physical examination, most patients with DKA have a low-normal blood pressure (BP), increased heart rate, increased respiratory rate, signs of volume depletion (e.g., decreased skin turgor, low jugular venous pressure, and dry oral mucosa), and breath that smells of acetone (a fruity odor similar to nail polish remover). With profound dehydration, patients may be obtunded or comatose.

The laboratory profile in patients with DKA includes low serum bicarbonate (HCO_3^-) concentration (<10 mEq/L); increased serum concentrations of ketoacids (acetoacetate, β-hydroxybutyrate); increased anion gap (calculated by subtracting the sum of the serum concentrations of chloride and bicarbonate from that of sodium; reference range, <14 mEq/L; DKA usually >20 mEq/L); increased serum glucose concentration (500–900 mg/dL); and decreased arterial pH (<7.3).

The differential diagnosis of DKA includes other causes of metabolic acidosis (e.g., lactic acidosis, starvation ketosis, alcoholic ketoacidosis, uremic acidosis, and toxin ingestion [e.g., salicylate intoxication]).

TREATMENT

Keys to successful outcomes in DKA are prompt recognition and management. The three main thrusts of treatment are fluid repletion, insulin administration, and management of electrolyte abnormalities. All patients with DKA have some degree of volume contraction, which contributes to decreased renal clearance of ketone bodies and glucose. Most patients with DKA should be treated with 1 L of normal saline over the first hour followed by 200 to 500 mL per hour until volume repletion. The rate and type of volume repletion should be guided by clinical and laboratory responses. Insulin should be administered intravenously to avoid slow absorption from hypoperfused subcutaneous tissues. Insulin is usually started with a 10-U priming dose and followed by a low-dose continuous infusion (e.g., 0.1 U/kg body weight/h). Serum glucose usually decreases by 50 to 75 mg/dL per hour. As the serum glucose concentration decreases to approximately 200 mg/dL, the insulin infusion rate should be decreased so that hypoglycemia and cerebral edema are avoided (the latter can result from too rapid a correction from the hyperosmolar state). With volume repletion, resolving acidosis, and improving blood glucose concentrations, an

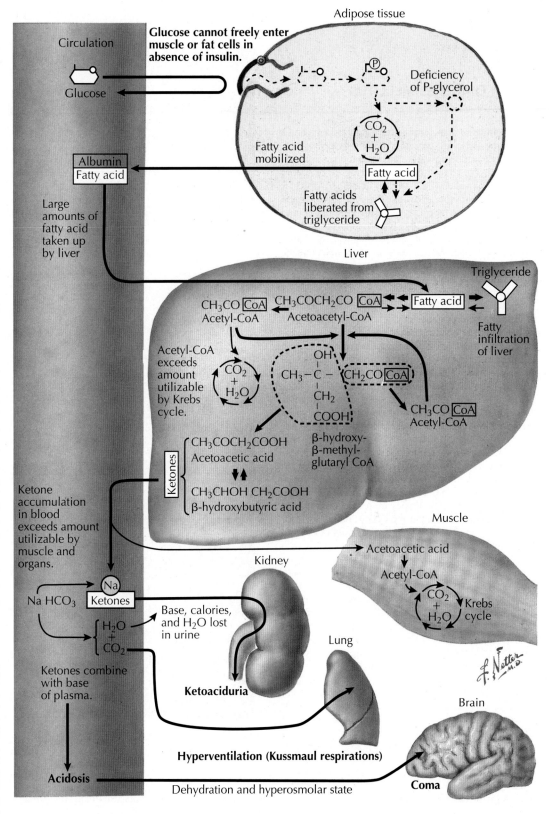

underlying potassium deficit usually becomes evident and should be replaced when the serum potassium concentration decreases below 5.3 mEq/L.

Most patients with DKA should be admitted to an intensive care unit setting in the hospital to facilitate close monitoring with continuous electrocardiography and hourly measurement of blood concentrations of glucose, potassium, chloride, and bicarbonate. Other blood parameters should be monitored every 2 hours

(e.g., calcium, magnesium, and phosphate). DKA can be corrected in most patients over 12 to 36 hours.

It is important to address the cause of DKA. The most common cause is noncompliance with insulin therapy in a patient with known type 1 diabetes mellitus. Underlying infection (e.g., pneumonia, meningitis, or urinary tract infection [UTI]) or severe illness (e.g., myocardial infarction [MI], cerebrovascular accident, or pancreatitis) may be a trigger for DKA in a patient with type 1 diabetes.

Plate 5.11

Endocrine System: VOLUME 2

ISLET CELL PATHOLOGY IN DIABETES

TYPE 1 DIABETES MELLITUS

The diagnosis of diabetes mellitus is established when a patient presents with typical symptoms of hyperglycemia (polyuria, polydipsia, weight loss) and has a fasting plasma glucose concentration of 126 mg/dL or higher or a random value of 200 mg/dL or higher, which is confirmed on another occasion. There are three general types of diabetes: type 1, type 2 (see Plate 5.12), and gestational (see Plate 5.20). Type 1 diabetes mellitus affects less than 10% of all patients diagnosed with diabetes. Type 1 diabetes mellitus is the result of pancreatic β-cell destruction; in more than 95% of the cases, it has an autoimmune basis caused by an apparent selected loss of immune tolerance. If untreated, type 1 diabetes is a fatal catabolic disorder (see Plate 5.10). Because of absolute insulin deficiency, all persons with type 1 diabetes require insulin replacement therapy.

Immune-mediated type 1 diabetes is most common in northern Europe, where the approximate annual incidence is 30 per 100,000 persons. The lowest incidence of type 1 diabetes is in China (1 per 100,000 persons per year). The peak life stage of onset is in children or young adults. The offspring of a mother with type 1 diabetes have a 3% risk of developing diabetes; the offspring of a father with type 1 diabetes have a 6% risk. Environmental factors (infectious or toxic environmental insult) have a major role in disease development; only 50% of identical twins of patients with type 1 diabetes develop diabetes. Individuals with certain human leukocyte antigen (HLA) types are predisposed to type 1 diabetes. HLA class II molecules DQ and DR code for antigens expressed on the surface of B lymphocytes and macrophages. Approximately 95% of individuals with type 1 diabetes have HLA-DR3, HLA-DR4, or both, findings present in 50% of nondiabetic control subjects. Some DQ alleles (e.g., HLA-DQA1*0102, HLA-DQB1*0602) are associated with a decreased risk of diabetes. Non-HLA genes also affect susceptibility to type 1 diabetes. For example, polymorphisms in a lymphocyte-specific tyrosine phosphatase (PTNN22) and in a promoter of the insulin gene are associated with an increased risk of type 1 diabetes.

The immune system mistakenly targets β-cell proteins that share homologies with viral or other foreign peptides, a concept termed *molecular mimicry*. Most patients with newly diagnosed type 1 diabetes have circulating antibodies (islet cell antibody, antibody to glutamic acid decarboxylase [GAD], antibody to tyrosine phosphatases [insulinoma-associated protein 2], cation efflux zinc transporter, or insulin autoantibody). GAD is an enzyme in pancreatic β-cells that has homology to coxsackievirus B.

The autoimmune destruction of β-cells progresses over months and years, during which time individuals who are affected are euglycemic and asymptomatic (termed the *latent period*). Impaired glucose tolerance usually precedes the onset of overt diabetes. By the time patients come to clinical attention, they have lost more than 90% of their β-cell mass. The progressive hyperglycemia has a toxic effect on the remaining islets, with increased rate of apoptosis and impaired insulin secretion. These toxic hyperglycemic effects can be reversed over the short term with exogenous insulin treatment; the pancreas seems to recover for a period of time,

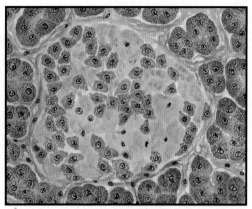

Partial hyalinization
(Mallory aniline blue stain)

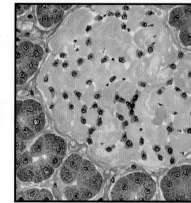

Complete hyalinization
(Mallory aniline blue stain)

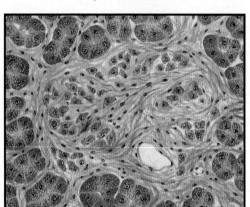

Fibrosis
(Mallory aniline blue stain)

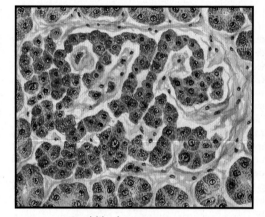

Cord-like formation
(Mallory aniline blue stain)

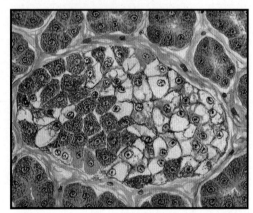

Hydropic change (vacuolization)
(Gomori aldehyde fuchsin and Ponceau stain)

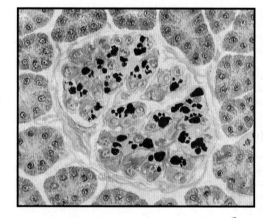
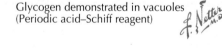

Glycogen demonstrated in vacuoles
(Periodic acid–Schiff reagent)

termed the *honeymoon period*. Eventually, the viability of the remaining β-cells is exhausted.

Histopathology studies from the 1960s showed that hydropic changes (vacuolization) were the initial step in islet destruction. This change was actually attributable to infiltration with glycogen as shown with periodic acid-Schiff reagent. There is a selective destruction of β-cells. At the time of clinical presentation, a chronic inflammatory infiltrate of the islets is present (insulitis). The inflammatory infiltrate consists primarily of T lymphocytes (CD8 cells outnumber CD4 cells). Eventually, the islets become hyalinized, a process that partially or completely replaces an islet.

CLINICAL PRESENTATION

Sustained hyperglycemia that exceeds the renal threshold for glucose reabsorption causes an osmotic diuresis, resulting in polyuria and polydipsia. The hyperosmolar state may also cause blurred vision caused by osmolar effects on lens and retina. Weight loss is caused by depletion of water, glycogen, fat, and muscle. Volume depletion may cause postural lightheadedness. Paresthesias are a result of neurotoxicity from sustained hyperglycemia. As insulin deficiency becomes nearly complete, the signs and symptoms of DKA predominate (see Plate 5.10).

Plate 5.12

Pancreas

Type 2 Diabetes Mellitus

The finding of fasting plasma glucose concentrations higher than 126 mg/dL on more than one occasion is diagnostic of diabetes. Individuals with fasting glucose levels from 100 to 125 mg/dL are considered to have impaired fasting glucose. Individuals with plasma glucose concentrations at or above 140 mg/dL, but not over 200 mg/dL, 2 hours after a 75-g oral glucose load are considered to have impaired glucose tolerance.

There are three general types of diabetes—type 1 (see Plate 5.11), type 2, and gestational (see Plate 5.20). Type 2 diabetes mellitus accounts for more than 90% of patients diagnosed with diabetes. Unlike type 1 diabetes, in which the individual has an absolute insulin deficiency, individuals with type 2 diabetes have a relative insulin deficiency in part because of a resistance to insulin action. Most patients with type 2 diabetes are obese and are diagnosed after the age of 30 years.

Insulin resistance in patients with type 2 diabetes is related to polygenic factors, abdominal visceral obesity, sedentary lifestyle, and aging. Approximately 40% of patients with type 2 diabetes have a least one parent with the disorder. The concordance of type 2 diabetes in monozygotic twins is 90%. Although many genetic factors are yet to be discovered, several common genetic polymorphisms increase the risk for type 2 diabetes. The basic pathogenesis of type 2 diabetes is inadequate pancreatic β-cell insulin secretory response for the prevailing blood glucose concentration. Sustained hyperglycemia magnifies the underlying insulin resistance and β-cell dysfunction, both of which improve with treatment and corrected glycemic control. The impaired insulin secretion in patients with type 2 diabetes is multifactorial but is partly attributable to decreased β-cell mass associated with increased β-cell apoptosis.

Obesity (body mass index [BMI] >30 kg/m²) is present in 80% of individuals with type 2 diabetes who are of European, North American, or African descent. Only 30% of individuals with type 2 diabetes of Japanese and Chinese descent are obese. The combination of abdominal obesity, hyperglycemia, hyperinsulinemia, dyslipidemia, and hypertension has been referred to as the *metabolic syndrome* (see Plate 7.15). Abdominal obesity aggravates insulin resistance that results in hyperglycemia leading to further hyperinsulinemia. Type 2 diabetes occurs when the hyperinsulinemia is insufficient to correct the hyperglycemia.

Diffuse damage to more than 70% of the pancreas can cause diabetes. Examples of such insults include pancreatitis, trauma, pancreatic carcinoma, hemochromatosis, and partial pancreatectomy. Excess production of the four insulin counterregulatory hormones can also cause diabetes. For example, diabetes may be the initial presentation of the following endocrine disorders: pheochromocytoma (catecholamines), acromegaly (growth hormone), glucagonoma (glucagon), and Cushing syndrome (glucocorticoids). Patients with thyrotoxicosis or somatostatinomas may also have diabetes. The hyperglycemia in patients with these endocrinopathies typically is cured by effective treatment of the underlying disorder.

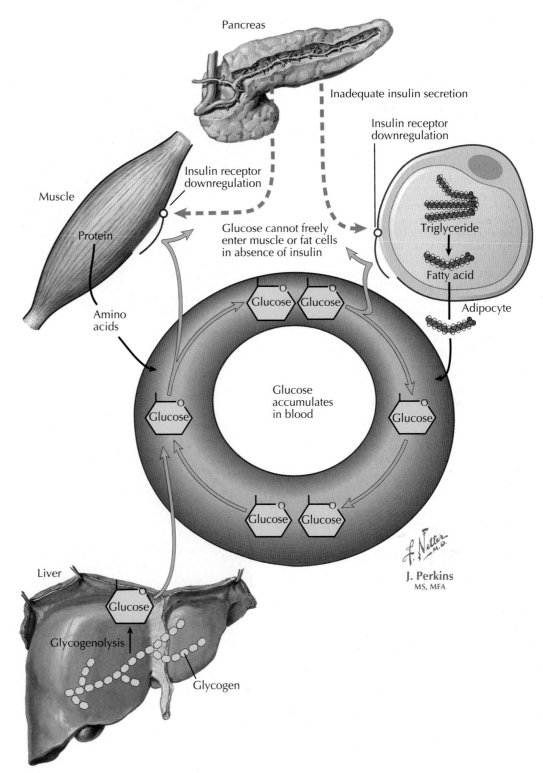

J. Perkins
MS, MFA

Approximately 5% of individuals with type 2 diabetes have monogenic diabetes (formerly called *maturity-onset diabetes of the young* [MODY]), resulting in a defect in glucose-induced insulin release. These individuals are usually not obese and are diagnosed with diabetes in late childhood or as young adults. Six types of autosomal dominant monogenic diabetes have been described. MODY 2 is caused by impaired conversion of glucose to glucose 6-phosphate in the β-cell because of a pathogenic variant in the gene (*GCK*) encoding the glucokinase enzyme. Glucokinase serves as a glucose sensor in the β-cell. The other forms of MODY are caused by pathogenic variants of genes that encode transcription factors that regulate β-cell gene expression. For example, MODY 3 (the most common form of MODY) and MODY 1 are caused by pathogenic variants in the genes that encode hepatocyte nuclear factor 1α (HNF-1α) and HNF-4α, respectively. MODY 4 is caused by pathogenic variants in insulin promoter factor-1 (IPF-1), which mediates insulin gene transcription and regulates other β-cell genes (e.g., glucokinase and glucose transporter 2). MODY 5 is caused by pathogenic variants in the gene encoding HNF-1β, and MODY 6 is caused by pathogenic variants in the gene encoding islet transcription factor neuroD1 (also referred to as BETA2).

Plate 5.13

Endocrine System: VOLUME 2

DIABETIC RETINOPATHY

Diabetic retinopathy (DR), a microvascular complication of chronic hyperglycemia, causes a 25-fold increased incidence of blindness in patients with diabetes compared with the general population. Vision loss is caused by retinal hemorrhage, macular edema, retinal detachment, or neovascular glaucoma. Patients with both type 1 and type 2 diabetes are at risk of developing DR. Nearly all patients with type 1 diabetes and more than 50% of patients with type 2 diabetes develop some degree of retinopathy within 20 years of their diagnosis.

The pathogenesis of DR is complex and related to abnormal retinal vessel permeability and vascular occlusion with ischemia. The retina is exquisitely sensitive to both ischemia and substrate imbalance. Chronic hyperglycemia causes impaired autoregulation of retinal blood flow, accumulation of advanced glycosylation end products, and accumulation of retinal cell sorbitol. Normally, retinal blood flow is tightly autoregulated. For example, retinal blood flow does not change in normal individuals unless the mean arterial BP is raised more than 40%. Hyperglycemia impairs this autoregulation, and retinal blood flow increases lead to greater shear stress, vascular leakage, and extracellular fluid accumulation. Retinal pericytes and microvascular cells become damaged and dysfunctional. Microaneurysms are saccular outpouchings that appear in retinal vessels at sites of retinal pericyte loss. Microthrombosis and occlusion of retinal capillaries lead to retinal ischemia and capillary leakage. Retinal ischemia triggers the release of vascular growth factors (e.g., vascular endothelial growth factor, platelet-derived growth factor, fibroblast growth factor, erythropoietin, and insulinlike growth factor 1). These growth factors promote the development of new blood vessels (neovascularization) in an attempt to revascularize ischemic retina. The two major forms of DR are nonproliferative and proliferative.

NONPROLIFERATIVE DIABETIC RETINOPATHY

Nonproliferative diabetic retinopathy (NPDR) is associated with the findings of microvascular abnormalities (e.g., dilated retinal veins, occluded vessels with resultant dot-and-blot hemorrhages, and microaneurysms), nerve fiber layer retinal infarcts (cotton-wool patches), intraretinal hemorrhages, macular edema, and hard exudates (leakage of lipid and proteinaceous material). The macular edema in patients with NPDR is responsible for vision loss. The severity of NPDR predicts the risk of progressing to proliferative retinopathy. For example, although the 1-year risk of progression to proliferative retinopathy for patients with mild NPDR is 5%, the risk is 75% for those with very severe NPDR.

PROLIFERATIVE DIABETIC RETINOPATHY

Proliferative diabetic retinopathy (PDR) is distinguished from NPDR by the presence of neovascularization that arises from retinal vessels or the optic disc. The neovascularization leads to acute vision loss caused by hemorrhage (preretinal and vitreous), fibrosis, and traction retinal detachment (see Plate 5.14). PDR usually arises from a background of NPDR. Arteriolar narrowing is usually evident on the fundus examination. The ischemia-induced release of vascular growth factors triggers the development of new vessels from adjacent retinal vessels. The intraluminal proliferation of cells results in vascular occlusion and rupture, resulting in the appearance of flame-shaped (occur in inner retina closer to the vitreous) and dot-and-blot hemorrhages (occur deeper in the

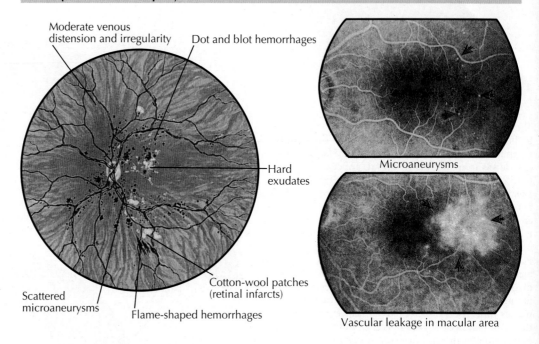

Nonproliferative retinopathy

Moderate venous distension and irregularity

Dot and blot hemorrhages

Hard exudates

Cotton-wool patches (retinal infarcts)

Scattered microaneurysms

Flame-shaped hemorrhages

Microaneurysms

Vascular leakage in macular area

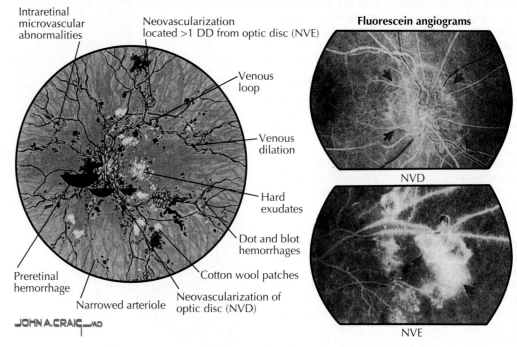

Proliferative retinopathy

Intraretinal microvascular abnormalities

Neovascularization located >1 DD from optic disc (NVE)

Venous loop

Venous dilation

Hard exudates

Dot and blot hemorrhages

Cotton wool patches

Neovascularization of optic disc (NVD)

Preretinal hemorrhage

Narrowed arteriole

JOHN A. CRAIG—AD

Fluorescein angiograms

NVD

NVE

retina) proximal to the occlusion and intraretinal infarcts (cotton-wool patches) distal to the occlusion. In the early stages of PDR, the new vessels can be seen as fine loops, and existing veins may become tortuous and beaded and develop loops. As PDR progresses, there is marked neovascularization covering more than 50% of the optic disc and an increased risk for preretinal and vitreous hemorrhage. If severe PDR is not treated, there is a 60% risk of progression to vision loss over 5 years. The findings of PDR are evident on the fundus examination. Intravenously administered fluorescein dye (fluorescein angiography) can assess areas of capillary underperfusion and leakage from sites of neovascularization. Neovascularization at the disc (NVD) refers to neovascularization occurring at or within 1500 μm (or ≤1 disc diameter [DD]) of

the optic disc. Neovascularization elsewhere (NVE) refers to neovascularization that is located more than 1500 μm (or >1 DD) away from the optic disc.

MACULAR EDEMA

Macular edema is retinal thickening and edema involving the macula, and it may complicate PDR or NPDR. Macular edema is the most common cause of vision loss from diabetes and can be diagnosed by stereoscopic fundus examination or fluorescein angiography. It is termed *clinically significant macular edema* when the thickening in the macular region is of sufficient extent and location to threaten central visual function.

Plate 5.14

Pancreas

COMPLICATIONS OF PROLIFERATIVE DIABETIC RETINOPATHY

PDR is associated with neovascularization that arises from retinal vessels or the optic disc. As PDR progresses, the marked neovascularization increases the risk for preretinal and vitreous hemorrhage. Severe PDR leads to acute vision loss caused by hemorrhage (preretinal and vitreous), fibrosis, and traction retinal detachment. If severe PDR is not treated, there is a 60% risk of progression to vision loss over 5 years. Puberty and pregnancy can accelerate retinopathy progression.

DR is usually asymptomatic until the late stages. Symptoms include decreased visual acuity related to macular edema, a "curtain falling" sensation with a vitreous hemorrhage, and floaters during the resolution phase of vitreous bleeds. Eye-directed therapy decreases the rate of disease progression. Thus annual screening for DR is important so that preventative therapy can be instituted. A comprehensive eye examination with slit-lamp biomicroscopy combined with indirect ophthalmoscopy on dilated fundi by an experienced ophthalmologist and seven-field digital stereoscopic retinal photography are standard screening methods. Eye examinations should be done more frequently during pregnancy.

The newly recruited vessels of neovascularization initially grow along the plane of the retina. However, as the vitreous gradually pulls away and detaches from the retina, the new vessels extend into the vitreous cavity. These aberrant vessels are fragile and at high risk for rupture with resultant vitreous hemorrhage. The neovascularization process can also lead to a fibrovascular proliferation that can distort the retina and predispose to retinal detachment.

Before the advent of tight glycemic control, studies showed that the prevalence of DR increased progressively in patients with increasing duration of diabetes; DR would start within 3 to 5 years of the diagnosis of type 1 diabetes. Subsequent studies documented that improved glycemic control dramatically decreased the development and progression of DR. Thus the first steps in treatment should be to prevent the development of DR or to prevent progression of existing DR by maximizing efforts at good glycemic control. In addition, if hypertension is present, treatment should be targeted for average BP less than 130/80 mm Hg.

In patients with established PDR, the treatment goals are to preserve vision, repair high-risk lesions, and reduce the rate of progression. Panretinal (scatter) laser photocoagulation is the primary treatment for patients with severe PDR. Administering approximately 1200 to 1800 laser burns (in a grid that targets peripheral retinal tissue and avoids large vessels and the optic disc) per eye over two to three sessions decreases the risk of severe vision loss by 50%. Panretinal laser treatment decreases viable hypoxic growth factor–generating cells, increases oxygen delivery to the inner retina, and increases relative perfusion to viable retina.

Focal laser photocoagulation is the optimal treatment for clinically significant macular edema. Laser treatment is directed at microaneurysms and the microvascular lesions around hard exudates, avoiding the fovea region.

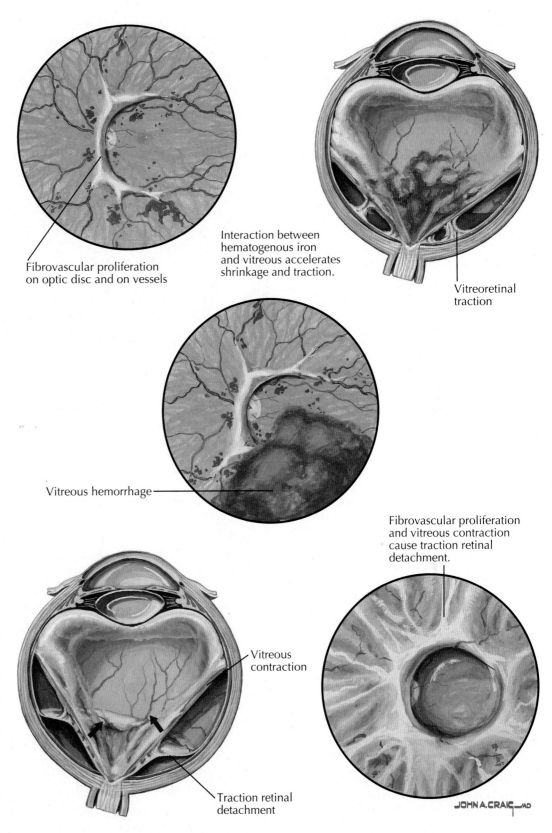

Fibrovascular proliferation on optic disc and on vessels

Interaction between hematogenous iron and vitreous accelerates shrinkage and traction.

Vitreoretinal traction

Vitreous hemorrhage

Fibrovascular proliferation and vitreous contraction cause traction retinal detachment.

Vitreous contraction

Traction retinal detachment

JOHN A. CRAIG_AD

Vitreous hemorrhage results from rupture of fragile new vessels or from contraction of the fibrovascular proliferation that causes avulsion of retinal vessels. Whereas blood that collects behind the detached posterior vitreous face is absorbed over many weeks, blood in the vitreous itself can turn white and is absorbed much more slowly. This opaque vitreous humor can be surgically removed.

Vitreal contraction also predisposes to traction retinal detachment, which leads to vision loss when the fovea or the macula is involved. Surgical vitrectomy can relieve vitreous traction.

Pharmacologic approaches for treating PDR are under investigation. Candidate agents include intravitreal administration of vascular endothelial growth factor inhibitors.

Plate 5.15

Endocrine System: VOLUME 2

DIABETIC NEPHROPATHY

Diabetic nephropathy is a major cause of morbidity and mortality in patients with type 1 or type 2 diabetes mellitus. Diabetic nephropathy is characterized as the triad of proteinuria, hypertension, and renal impairment. Approximately 40% of patients with type 1 diabetes and 20% of patients with type 2 diabetes develop some degree of diabetic nephropathy. Diabetes is the single most common cause of end-stage renal disease (ESRD).

Diabetic nephropathy can be considered in five stages or phases. The initial phase of diabetic nephropathy is hyperfiltration with increased capillary glomerular pressure and elevated glomerular filtration rate (GFR) (e.g., >150 mL/min). The glomerular hyperfiltration is associated with glomerular hypertrophy and increased renal size. The second stage is termed the *silent stage*. In this stage, although the GFR is normal and there is no proteinuria, glomerular basement membrane thickening and mesangial expansion are occurring. The third stage is termed *incipient nephropathy,* during which the urinary albumin excretion rate becomes abnormal (e.g., 30–300 mg/24 hr). Also at this stage, systemic hypertension may become evident. The fourth stage of diabetic nephropathy is the *overt nephropathy* or *macroalbuminuria* stage. In this stage, the 24-hour urinary albumin excretion is more than 300 mg, and creatinine levels in the blood rise. The majority of patients at this stage have systemic hypertension. Untreated hypertension can accelerate the decline in GFR, which in turn accelerates systemic hypertension. The fifth and final stage is *uremia*, the effective treatment of which requires renal replacement therapy.

As with DR, the pathogenesis of diabetic nephropathy is complex and related to a hyperglycemia-triggered cascade of mechanisms. Chronic hyperglycemia causes impaired autoregulation of renal blood flow with intraglomerular hypertension, accumulation of advanced glycosylation end products, generation of mitochondrial reactive oxygen species, activation of protein kinase C, and accumulation of sorbitol. Improved glycemic control in patients with diabetes can slow the development of nephropathy.

Glomerular basement membrane thickening and mesangial expansion are prominent glomerular abnormalities in diabetes that progress to nodular (Kimmelstiel-Wilson lesion) or diffuse glomerulosclerosis. Nodular glomerulosclerosis is associated with hyaline deposits in the glomerular arterioles. A diabetic tubulopathy can also develop and may result in a type IV renal tubular acidosis with hyperkalemia and hyperchloremic metabolic acidosis, an outcome associated with hyporeninemic hypoaldosteronism.

The cornerstones of treatment for diabetic nephropathy are optimizing glycemic control and hypertension management. Decreases in glycosylated hemoglobin are associated with a decreased risk of development of microalbuminuria and decreased rate of progression through the stages of diabetic nephropathy. Angiotensin-converting enzyme (ACE) inhibitors and angiotensin receptor blockers (ARBs) are the antihypertensive drug classes of choice because these agents appear to have renoprotective effects that exceed their antihypertensive effects. ACE inhibitors and ARBs decrease urinary albumin excretion by more than 30% and retard the progression from microalbuminuria to overt proteinuria. In addition, exposure to agents that have adverse effects on BP or renal function should be avoided. For example, nonsteroidal antiinflammatory drugs and cyclooxygenase-2 inhibitors should be avoided because of their adverse effects on hypertension. In addition, radiographic contrast dye should be

GLOMERULOSCLEROSIS

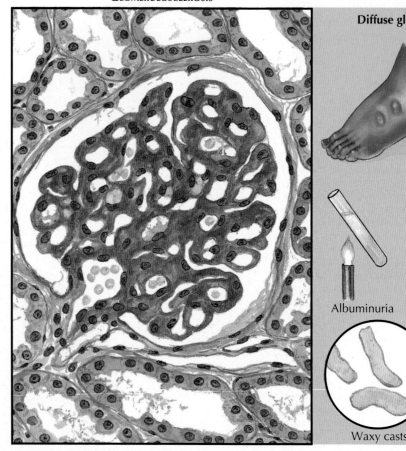

Diffuse glomerulosclerosis

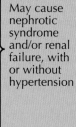

Edema

Albuminuria

Waxy casts

May cause nephrotic syndrome and/or renal failure, with or without hypertension

Nodular glomerulosclerosis

This nodular component (Kimmelstiel-Wilson lesions) associated with hyaline deposits in the glomerular arterioles is pathognomonic for diabetic nephropathy.

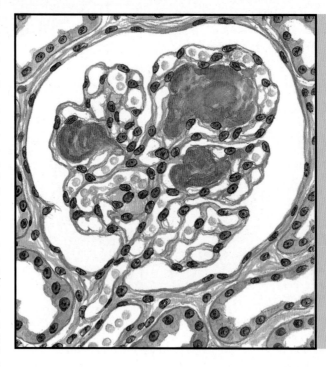

avoided because of its adverse effects on renal function and risk for acute renal failure.

Progressive diabetic nephropathy may result in severe proteinuria and associated symptoms that are referred to as *nephrotic syndrome*. Nephrotic syndrome is defined by urinary protein excretion of more than 3.5 g/1.73 m^2 per 24 hours, hypoalbuminemia (serum albumin concentration <3 g/dL), and

peripheral edema. Microscopic examination of the urine sediment may show waxy casts (degenerated cellular casts of collecting tubules), which are found in patients with severe chronic renal disease. For patients who progress to ESRD, renal replacement options include hemodialysis, peritoneal dialysis, renal transplantation, and combined pancreas-kidney transplantation.

Plate 5.16

Pancreas

DIABETIC NEUROPATHY

Approximately 50% of those with diabetes of more than 25 years' duration develop symptomatic diabetic neuropathy. Diabetic neuropathy is not a single disorder, but rather multiple disorders depending on the types of nerve fibers involved.

FOCAL NEUROPATHIES

In general, mononeuropathies occur in older patients with diabetes. Mononeuropathies are a result of vascular obstruction and are typically acute in onset, associated with pain and motor weakness, and self-limited (most resolve over 2 months). Nerves that are commonly involved include cranial nerves III, VI, and VII; the ulnar nerve; and the peroneal nerve. Patients may present with wrist drop or ankle drop. With third cranial nerve involvement, patients complain of diplopia, and examination shows ptosis and ophthalmoplegia. Diabetic polyradiculopathy is characterized by severe pain in the distribution of one or more nerve roots and may be accompanied by motor weakness. For example, intercostal or truncal radiculopathy presents with pain over the thorax or abdomen. Diabetic polyradiculopathy is usually self-limited and resolves over 1 year.

PROXIMAL MOTOR NEUROPATHIES

Proximal motor neuropathies (also known as *diabetic amyotrophy, proximal neuropathy, femoral neuropathy, diabetic neuropathic cachexia,* and *Ellenberg cachexia*) affect primarily older patients with type 2 diabetes. Symptoms usually start with thigh and pelvic girdle pains that progress to marked atrophy of the quadriceps muscles. Patients present with symptoms caused by lower extremity proximal muscle weakness (e.g., must use arms to assist them when rising from a chair). The signs and symptoms may start unilaterally but usually progress to bilateral involvement. Pain may be a predominant component of the clinical presentation, and profound weight loss and depression are common. Axonal loss is the primary pathophysiologic process, and electromyography shows lumbosacral plexopathy. Most of these patients prove to have chronic inflammatory demyelinating polyneuropathy, monoclonal gammopathy, ganglioside antibody syndrome, or an inflammatory vasculitis.

DISTAL SYMMETRIC POLYNEUROPATHY

Distal symmetric polyneuropathy (DSPN) is the most common form of diabetic neuropathy. The onset of DSPN is usually slow and involves small and/or large fibers of either sensory and/or motor nerves. Small-fiber neuropathy usually manifests as paresthesia, hyperalgesia (increased pain response to a normally painful stimulus), allodynia (pain response from a stimulus that is not normally painful), or hypesthesia involving the feet and lower extremities. The pain is usually described as burning. The paresthesias are described as pins and needles, numbness, tingling, cold, or burning. Physical examination usually reveals reduced pinprick and light touch sensations and loss of thermal sensitivity. An acute, painful small-fiber neuropathy may develop with the initiation of therapy to improve glycemic control.

Large-fiber neuropathies involve the myelinated and rapidly conducting sensory or motor nerves that are normally responsible for vibration perception,

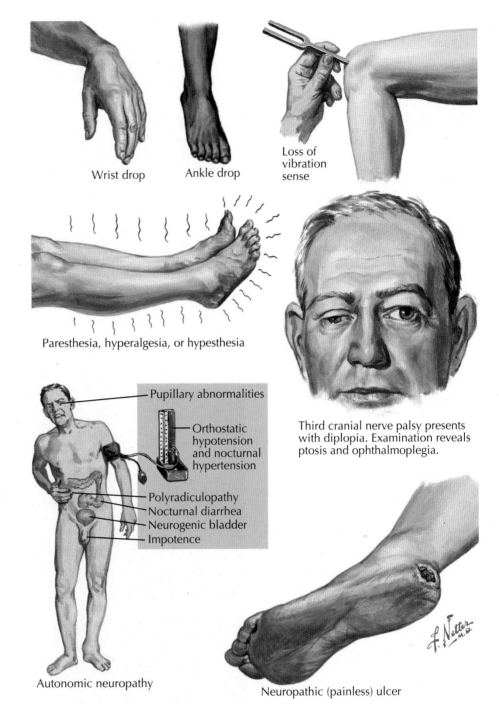

Wrist drop   Ankle drop   Loss of vibration sense

Paresthesia, hyperalgesia, or hypesthesia

Pupillary abnormalities

Orthostatic hypotension and nocturnal hypertension

Polyradiculopathy
Nocturnal diarrhea
Neurogenic bladder
Impotence

Autonomic neuropathy

Third cranial nerve palsy presents with diplopia. Examination reveals ptosis and ophthalmoplegia.

Neuropathic (painless) ulcer

cold thermal perception, position sense, and motor function. Typical initial symptoms include a sensation of walking on pebbles or cotton, inability to discriminate among coins, and trouble turning pages of a book. Large-fiber neuropathies are easily detected on physical examination (e.g., loss of vibration sense, loss of proprioception, loss of deep tendon reflexes). There may be wasting of the small muscles in the feet and hands.

Usually DSPN presents with signs and symptoms of both small- and large-fiber nerve damage. The longer nerves are especially vulnerable, and most patients have a stocking-and-glove type sensory loss that may spread proximally. Neuropathic foot ulcers and Charcot arthropathy (neurogenic arthropathy) can result from loss of proprioception, pain, and temperature perceptions (see Plate 5.19).

AUTONOMIC NEUROPATHY

Dysfunction of the sympathetic and parasympathetic nervous systems has the potential to cause malfunction of almost all body systems. Examples of organ systems that may be affected by autonomic neuropathy include pupillary abnormalities with Argyll-Robertson–type pupil and decreased diameter of dark-adapted pupil; cardiovascular system with orthostatic hypotension, nocturnal hypertension, resting tachycardia, silent MI, and heat and exercise intolerance; genitourinary system with erectile dysfunction, retrograde ejaculation, and neurogenic bladder with urinary retention; gastrointestinal system with gastroparesis, constipation, nocturnal diarrhea, and fecal incontinence; sweating disturbances with gustatory sweating, hyperhidrosis, and anhidrosis; and blunted adrenomedullary response to hypoglycemia, leading to hypoglycemic unawareness.

Plate 5.17

Endocrine System: VOLUME 2

ATHEROSCLEROSIS IN DIABETES

The type of macrovascular disease in patients with diabetes mellitus is similar to that in individuals without diabetes. However, the vascular disease is more extensive and rapidly progressive in the setting of diabetes, even when adjustments are made for other risk factors that are more prevalent in people with diabetes (e.g., hypertension and dyslipidemia). Glycosylated hemoglobin has been shown to be an independent risk factor for macrovascular disease. Thus diabetes should be considered a coronary heart disease (CHD) risk equivalent when assessing cardiovascular risk and designing treatment programs for hyperlipidemia (see Plate 7.5).

After adjusting for all known cardiovascular risk factors, insulin resistance is an independent risk factor for macrovascular disease. Insulin resistance at the adipocyte leads to increased free fatty acid release that stimulates hepatic VLDL secretion, which in turn leads to proatherogenic dyslipidemia, defined as low serum concentration of high-density lipoprotein cholesterol, high serum concentration of VLDL, and high serum concentration of small, dense low-density lipoprotein (LDL) cholesterol. Small, dense LDL cholesterol is more efficient at penetrating the blood vessel wall to prompt the atherogenic process (see Plates 7.12 and 7.13).

Insulin itself has proatherogenic properties. Insulin and hyperglycemia potentiate the effects of platelet-derived growth factor on vascular smooth muscle cell proliferation. Insulin also stimulates vascular smooth muscle cells to produce plasminogen activator inhibitor 1. Hyperglycemia inhibits endothelial cell nitric oxide production and potentiates collagen-induced platelet activation.

Mönckeberg arteriosclerosis (medial calcific sclerosis) is a form of arteriosclerosis that is more common in patients with diabetes. In advanced cases, the arteries become rigid and lose their distensibility and are referred to as *pipestem arteries*. The calcification may be evident on plain radiographs.

CARDIOVASCULAR RISK REDUCTION

Traditional CHD risk factors (dyslipidemia, obesity, hypertension, insulin resistance) are commonly present in individuals with type 2 diabetes. Thus the atherosclerosis risk in individuals with diabetes is multifactorial and likely synergistic. Intensive long-term treatment of these associated risk factors lowers the risk of macrovascular events by at least 50%. Lowering serum LDL cholesterol concentrations (even when pretreatment levels are in the reference range) with hydroxymethylglutaryl CoA reductase inhibitors (statins) reduces cardiovascular events in patients with diabetes. Thus lipid-directed pharmacologic therapy is a key intervention along with lifestyle modification (weight reduction, regular isotonic exercise, and smoking cessation), optimizing glycemic control, treatment of hypertension, and aspirin therapy.

The fatality rate with MI is twice as high in patients with diabetes than in those without diabetes. This increased risk is likely related to multiple factors (e.g., more severe underlying CHD, early reinfarction caused by impaired fibrinolysis, autonomic neuropathy predisposing to a sympathovagal imbalance, or maladaptive remodeling of the left ventricle). Blood glucose concentrations at the time of hospital admission are independently correlated with both early and late mortality after

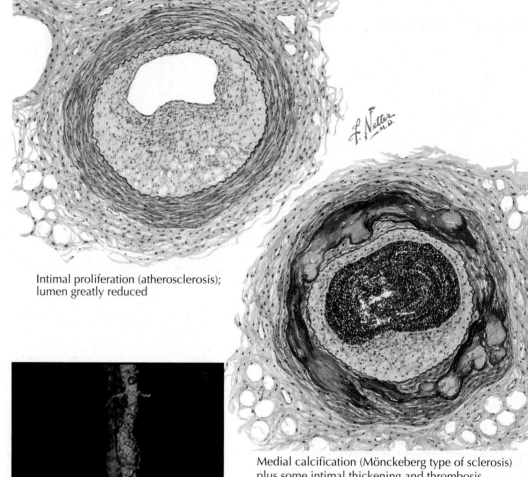

Intimal proliferation (atherosclerosis); lumen greatly reduced

Medial calcification (Mönckeberg type of sclerosis) plus some intimal thickening and thrombosis

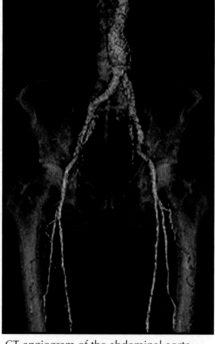

CT angiogram of the abdominal aorta shows the infrarenal abdominal aorta is mildly ectatic. There is a stenosis at the origin of the left internal iliac artery.

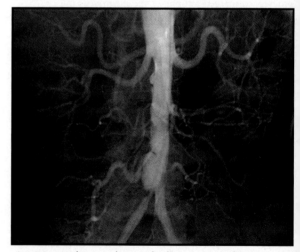

Aortogram shows advanced atheromatous disease involving the infrarenal abdominal aorta with multiple areas of ulceration. Tight atheromatous stenosis involves the origin of the right common iliac artery.

an MI. Optimizing glycemic control can improve myocardial cell metabolism by shifting from free fatty acid oxidation to glucose oxidation for generation of ATP. Treatment with an ACE inhibitor also decreases mortality in patients with diabetes after an MI. The mechanisms of this benefit are likely related to limitation of infarct size and improving endothelial cell function and fibrinolysis. Cardioselective β-adrenergic inhibitors are routinely given to patients with diabetes in the setting of

acute coronary syndromes to decrease mortality rates. The β-adrenergic inhibitors likely decrease the unrestrained sympathetic nervous system overactivity related to autonomic neuropathy. Aspirin has been shown to lower the risk of MI in individuals with diabetes. Thus aspirin (75–162 mg/day) is indicated for secondary macrovascular event protection in patients with diabetes and for primary prevention in any patient with diabetes at increased cardiovascular risk (10-year risk >10%).

Plate 5.18

Pancreas

DIABETES-RELATED DERMATOLOGIC MANIFESTATIONS

Cutaneous manifestations of diabetes mellitus are common and occur in 30% to 80% of patients with diabetes. The severity of the dermatologic manifestation varies from cometic to severe.

NECROBIOSIS LIPOIDICA DIABETICORUM

Necrobiosis lipoidica diabeticorum (NLD) is a rare, chronic granulomatous disease of the skin and occurs in 0.3% to 1.6% of individuals with type 2 diabetes and less commonly in patients with type 1 diabetes. When NLD occurs in the absence of diabetes, it is simply termed *necrobiosis lipoidica*. Onset is typically in the third to fourth decades of life and is more common in females (80% of cases). Typically pretibial in location, the lesions usually begin as red-brown or violaceous erythematous papules and rapidly progress to yellow-brown, atrophic, telangiectatic ovoid plaques with reddish-brown granulomatous borders. The lower legs, especially the shins, are the most common site of involvement, although it can also occur on the trunk, arms, and face. The NLD lesions may be asymptomatic, pruritic, or painful. NLD is a complication of microangiopathy and the lesions are asymptomatic. Biopsy shows palisading granulomas. Ulceration occurs in 10% to 20% of patients. Treatment options include high-potency topical corticosteroids, intralesional administration of corticosteroids, psoralen ultraviolet A radiation, pentoxifylline, antimalarial agents, and compression therapy. NLD usually has a chronic course characterized by slow progression and then stabilization over several years.

ACANTHOSIS NIGRICANS

Acanthosis nigricans is associated with hyperinsulinemic states (e.g., type 2 diabetes mellitus with insulin resistance) and is characterized by thickened, velvety to verrucous, gray-brown hyperpigmented, scaly symmetric patches and plaques, most commonly affecting the posterior neck, groin, and axilla. Acanthosis nigricans is asymptomatic and typically symmetric in distribution. The pathogenesis involves activation of insulinlike growth receptors leading to keratinocyte and dermal fibroblast hyperproliferation. Acanthosis nigricans improves with better glycemic control. Treatment with retinoids and keratolytics (e.g., urea cream) may improve the appearance.

SCLEREDEMA DIABETICORUM

A less well-known cutaneous marker of diabetes mellitus is scleredema. Affecting 3% to 14% of patients with diabetes, scleredema diabeticorum is characterized by a remarkable symmetric skin thickening and induration of the dermis of the neck and upper back. The prevalence is 10-fold higher in males and is associated with poor glycemic control. The dramatic increase in dermal thickness is obvious by simply palpating the involved skin, and it may have a peau d'orange appearance or erythematous tinge. Scleredema diabeticorum is typically asymptomatic but may be accompanied by pruritus, erythema, and hypoesthesia. When the skin over the deltoid muscles in involved, there may be decreased range of motion. Biopsy shows mucin containing thickened reticular dermis with thick collagen bundles. Treatment options are limited and include psoralen with ultraviolet A radiation and physical therapy.

GRANULOMA ANNULARE

Granuloma annulare affects 0.3% to 4% of patients with diabetes and is more common in females. The lesions

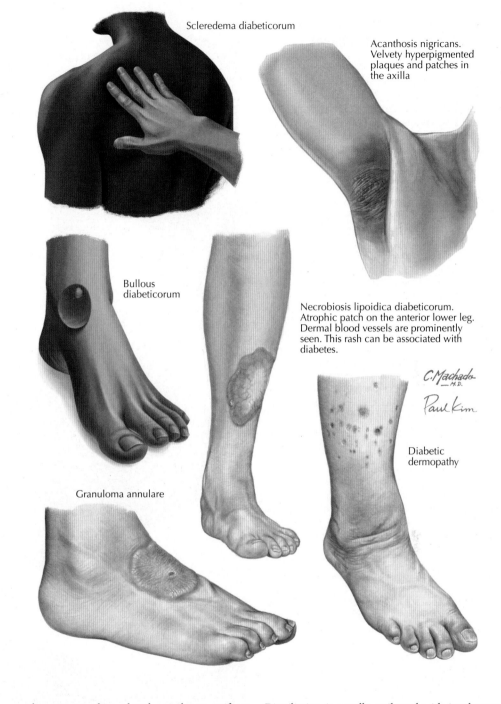

Scleredema diabeticorum

Acanthosis nigricans. Velvety hyperpigmented plaques and patches in the axilla

Bullous diabeticorum

Necrobiosis lipoidica diabeticorum. Atrophic patch on the anterior lower leg. Dermal blood vessels are prominently seen. This rash can be associated with diabetes.

C. Machado M.D.
Paul Kim

Diabetic dermopathy

Granuloma annulare

are erythematous or skin-colored, annular or arciform plaques with a moderately firm, rope-like border and central clearing. Most lesions are less than 5 cm in diameter and typically grow slowly in a centrifugal pattern. The granuloma annulare lesions are either asymptomatic or pruritic. Biopsy shows lymphohistiocytic granulomatous changes with increased mucin. Treatment options include local therapy with intralesional corticosteroid injections, high-potency topical corticosteroids, or a topical calcineurin inhibitor. For generalized disease, systemic treatment options include isotretinoin, dapsone, narrowband ultraviolet B phototherapy, adalimumab, infliximab, cyclosporine, or psoralen plus ultraviolet A photochemotherapy.

BULLOUS DIABETICORUM

Bullous diabeticorum affects 0.4% to 2% of patients with type 1 diabetes mellitus and presents as asymptomatic, tense bullae on otherwise normal-appearing skin.

Distribution is usually unilateral with involvement of the acral and distal surfaces of the lower extremities. Bullae characteristically arise rapidly overnight with no inflammation and resolve without scarring over 2 to 6 weeks. The risk of secondary infection necessitates close observation, and if present requires appropriate treatment with antibiotics and wound care.

DIABETIC DERMOPATHY

Diabetic dermopathy, also referred to as *shin spots*, is the most common diabetes-related skin disorder—affecting 40% to 50% of patients with type 1 and type 2 diabetes mellitus. The prevalence of diabetic dermopathy is more common in patients more than 50 years of age and in males. Occurring on the bilateral pretibial legs, the lesions are asymptomatic and start as red to pink ovoid papules or plaques that progress to atrophic brown macules. Diabetic dermopathy is asymptomatic and no specific therapy is indicated.

Plate 5.19

Endocrine System: VOLUME 2

Vascular Insufficiency in Diabetes: The Diabetic Foot

Diabetic foot ulcers occur in approximately 10% of patients with type 1 or type 2 diabetes mellitus. Approximately 1% of patients with diabetes require an amputation, a last-resort surgical step that is usually preceded by foot ulcers. Diabetes is the most common nontrauma cause of lower limb amputation. Diabetic foot ulcers are more common in patients who also have other evidence of other micro- or macrovascular disease (retinopathy, nephropathy, or CHD).

Diabetic neuropathy (see Plate 5.16) plays a key role in diabetic foot ulcers. For example, sympathetic autonomic neuropathy may result in dry skin (from decreased sweat production), leading to scaling, cracks, and fissures, which provide a portal for infection. Motor neuropathy affects the small intrinsic muscles of the feet so that the larger muscles in the anterior tibial compartment are unopposed, causing subluxation of the proximal interphalangeal-metatarsal joints (claw toe deformity). The prominent metatarsal heads become the point of effects of body weight and friction and a common site of diabetic foot ulcer development. Diabetic neuropathy–induced proprioceptive loss decreases the patient's recognition of these sites of irritation and inflammation. Plantar callus, which predisposes to ulceration, may build up at these high-pressure sites. The presence of neuropathy increases the risk of diabetic ulcer formation sevenfold.

Patients with diabetes should have annual comprehensive foot examinations to assess for evidence of neuropathic or vascular deficits, deformity, callus formation, or dry skin. Vibration sensation should be tested with a 128-Hz tuning fork at the great toe. Pressure sensation should be tested with a Semmes-Weinstein 5.07 (10-g) monofilament applied to buckling pressure on the plantar surface of the foot. In addition, the Achilles tendon reflex and temperature sensation should be checked. Vascular insufficiency can be evaluated with assessment of pulses (dorsal pedis, posterior tibial), skin temperature, presence of hair on skin, color of skin, and assessment for dependent rubor. Dependent rubor is present when the skin and nail beds are dark red because of the inadequate arterial flow and the presence of venous blood containing reduced hemoglobin in dilated venous capillaries; when the foot is raised above the level of the heart, the venous blood drains away and unmasks the pallid tissues supplied by insufficient arterial flow. Patients who are determined to have risk factors for foot ulcer formation should be advised by a foot care team that includes diabetes physician specialists, diabetes nurse educators, podiatrists, orthotic specialists, orthopedic surgeons, and vascular surgeons. Prophylactic measures to prevent diabetic foot ulcers include smoking cessation; avoiding walking barefoot; checking water temperature before stepping into a bath; keeping the toenails trimmed; inspecting the feet daily for blisters, swelling, or redness; and wearing properly fitting shoes.

The Wagner diabetic foot ulcer classification scheme is as follows:

Grade 0: No ulcer but high-risk (e.g., deformity, callus, insensitivity)

Grade 1: Superficial full-thickness ulcer

Grade 2: Deeper ulcer that penetrates tendons but does not involve bone

Grade 3: Deeper ulcer with bone involvement (osteitis)

Grade 4: Partial gangrene (e.g., toes and forefoot)

Grade 5: Gangrene of the whole foot

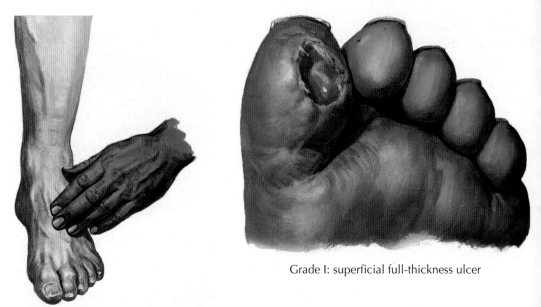

Dependent rubor, absence of dorsalis pedis pulsation

Grade I: superficial full-thickness ulcer

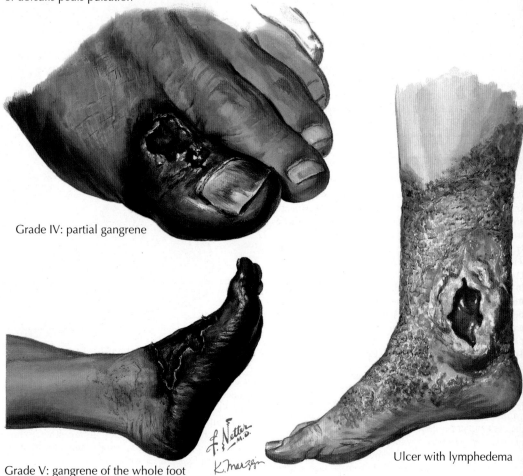

Grade IV: partial gangrene

Grade V: gangrene of the whole foot

Ulcer with lymphedema

Key steps to ensure effective healing of diabetic foot ulcers include confirming adequate arterial blood flow, treating underlying infection, removing pressure from the wound and surrounding area, and debriding all dead and macerated tissue. Pressure relief can usually be achieved with a removable cast boot. A nonhealing foot ulcer should be investigated for ischemia with noninvasive techniques and arteriography in some cases. If osteomyelitis is suspected, additional imaging is indicated with a combination of plain radiographs, magnetic resonance imaging, and bone scintigraphy. The treatment of osteomyelitis requires systemic antibiotic therapy and, in many cases, surgical removal of infected bone. Localized gangrene of a toe that is not associated with infection may be allowed to self-amputate. However, more extensive gangrene is a medical urgency that requires hospitalization, treatment of the underlying infection, optimization of glycemic control, vascular assessment, and consultation with vascular and orthopedic surgeons.

Plate 5.20

Pancreas

DIABETES MELLITUS IN PREGNANCY

Diabetes mellitus is the most common medical complication of pregnancy. Gestational diabetes mellitus (GDM) complicates 4% of pregnancies, and preexisting type 1 or type 2 diabetes mellitus (pregestational diabetes) complicates 0.5% of all pregnancies. Diabetes in pregnancy is associated with unique risks for the fetus and the mother. Poorly controlled diabetes is associated with high risks for spontaneous abortion, major congenital malformations, premature birth, preeclampsia, and stillbirths. Although maternal glucose crosses the placenta, insulin does not, resulting in increased fetal pancreas production of insulin, which leads to increased fetal somatic growth.

Fetal macrosomia (fetal birth weight >4500 g) can complicate delivery and predispose to birth trauma. To prevent these risks, pregestational diabetes should be under optimal glycemic control for months before conception and throughout pregnancy. In addition, all pregnant females should be tested for GDM and treated when identified.

In the first trimester of pregnancy, the increasing blood concentrations of estrogen and progesterone are associated with a decrease in fasting plasma glucose concentrations by an average of 15 mg/dL. Plasma glucose concentrations rise in the second and third trimesters of pregnancy, primarily because of increasing circulating levels of human chorionic somatomammotropin (hCS), also called *human placental lactogen*. The structure of hCS is very similar to that of human growth hormone and has most of the actions of growth hormone; hCS enhances lipolysis and decreases glucose utilization.

The diagnostic criteria for pregestational type 1 or type 2 diabetes are as outlined in Plates 5.11 and 5.12. GDM is defined as hyperglycemia or glucose intolerance with an onset or first recognition during pregnancy. All females without known diabetes should be tested for GDM between weeks 24 and 28 of gestation. Testing for GDM should be done earlier in pregnancy if risk factors are present (prepregnancy BMI >30 kg/m^2, history of GDM, prior infant with a major congenital malformation, or family history of diabetes in a first-degree relative). The initial screening test is a 50-g oral glucose challenge test (GCT) with measurement of plasma glucose 1 hour later. Glucose levels above 135 mg/dL should trigger confirmatory testing with a 3-hour 100-g oral glucose tolerance test (OGTT). If the 1-hour GCT glucose is more than 180 mg/dL and fasting plasma glucose is more than 95 mg/dL, then GDM is confirmed, and a 3-hour OGTT is not needed. In addition, GDM is confirmed on the 3-hour OGTT if two or more of the following plasma glucose concentrations are exceeded: fasting above 95 gm/dL, 1 hour above 180 mg/dL, 2 hours above 155 mg/dL, or 3 hours above 140 mg/dL.

Patients with GDM should be treated with daily exercise, diet (with relative carbohydrate restriction [33%–40% of calories] and guidance on caloric allotment and calorie distribution), and pharmacologic therapy if needed. Patients should self-monitor blood glucose (SMBG) at least four times daily (fasting and 1–2 hours postprandial) or wear a continuous glucose monitor. Target glucose levels during pregnancy are 70 to 95 mg/dL fasting and less than 120 mg/dL at 1 to 2 hours after a meal. Insulin treatment is needed in about 15% of females with GDM because they cannot achieve these glycemic targets with diet and exercise.

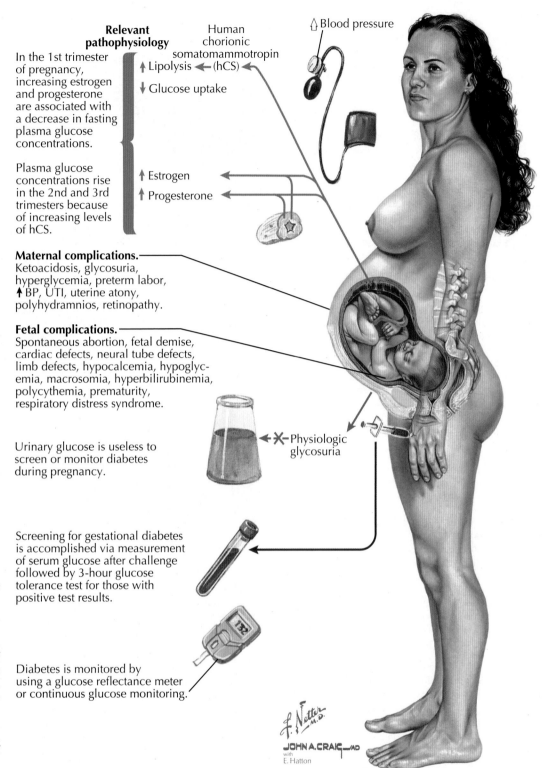

Relevant pathophysiology

In the 1st trimester of pregnancy, increasing estrogen and progesterone are associated with a decrease in fasting plasma glucose concentrations.

Plasma glucose concentrations rise in the 2nd and 3rd trimesters because of increasing levels of hCS.

Human chorionic somatomammotropin (hCS)

↑ Lipolysis ← (hCS)
↓ Glucose uptake

↑ Estrogen
↑ Progesterone

↑ Blood pressure

Maternal complications.
Ketoacidosis, glycosuria, hyperglycemia, preterm labor, ↑BP, UTI, uterine atony, polyhydramnios, retinopathy.

Fetal complications.
Spontaneous abortion, fetal demise, cardiac defects, neural tube defects, limb defects, hypocalcemia, hypoglycemia, macrosomia, hyperbilirubinemia, polycythemia, prematurity, respiratory distress syndrome.

Urinary glucose is useless to screen or monitor diabetes during pregnancy.

Physiologic glycosuria

Screening for gestational diabetes is accomplished via measurement of serum glucose after challenge followed by 3-hour glucose tolerance test for those with positive test results.

Diabetes is monitored by using a glucose reflectance meter or continuous glucose monitoring.

Management objectives involve efforts to return glucose levels to as close to normal as possible through a combination of diet, exercise, insulin (as indicated), and tight control in patients with pregestational diabetes.

Insulin doses should be titrated based on findings on blood glucose self-monitoring. Fetal growth and development should be monitored by ultrasonography.

Diabetes comorbidities, including hypertension (increased BP), retinopathy in patients with pregestational diabetes, ketoacidosis, and UTIs, should be monitored and treated during pregnancy as indicated.

In most females with GDM, the blood glucose concentrations return to normal postpartum; however, there is a 60% risk of recurrent GDM with future pregnancies. In addition, females who are diagnosed with GDM are at a 50% risk of developing permanent diabetes over the subsequent 10 years.

There are also long-term effects on children whose mothers had diabetes in pregnancy. In utero exposure to maternal hyperglycemia promotes fetal hyperinsulinemia and an increase in fetal fat cells, changes that have been linked to obesity and insulin resistance in children and impaired glucose tolerance and diabetes in adults.

Plate 5.21

Endocrine System: VOLUME 2

TREATMENT OF TYPE 2 DIABETES MELLITUS

Improved glycemic control in individuals with type 2 diabetes mellitus is associated with decreased rates of microvascular complications (retinopathy, nephropathy, and neuropathy). The treatment goal should be to maintain the hemoglobin A_{1c} (HbA$_{1c}$) at a level less than 7%, recognizing that HbA$_{1c}$ values in the normal range (<6%) are optimal. Additional glycemic targets include fasting and premeal plasma glucose of 70 to 130 mg/dL and 2-hour postprandial glucose <180 mg/dL.

NONPHARMACOLOGIC THERAPY

The key to successful implementation of lifestyle interventions is comprehensive diabetes education with emphasis on self-management. Interventions include dietary modification based on nutrition counseling, regular isotonic exercise, weight reduction, behavior modification, and SMBG. Exercise improves glycemic control, insulin sensitivity, and cardiovascular fitness. The frequency and timing of SMBG depend on the type of pharmacologic therapy.

PHARMACOTHERAPY

Pharmacotherapeutic options for the management of type 2 diabetes include eight broad classes of drugs that are targeted at different pathophysiologic mechanisms that contribute to hyperglycemia.

Insulin Sensitizers With Primary Action in the Liver—Biguanides

Metformin is a biguanide that activates adenosine monophosphate–activated protein kinase. Metformin reduces hepatic insulin resistance, resulting in decreased hepatic gluconeogenesis. There is no risk for hypoglycemia, and this agent should be considered in all patients with type 2 diabetes. The main side effect is gastrointestinal intolerance. Because of the risk of lactic acidosis, metformin should not be used in patients with advanced chronic kidney disease.

Insulin Sensitizers With Primary Action on Peripheral Tissues—Thiazolidinediones

Pioglitazone and rosiglitazone are thiazolidinediones (TZDs) that modulate peroxisome proliferator–activated receptors. TZDs decrease peripheral insulin resistance and lower serum triglyceride levels.

Insulin Secretagogues—Sulfonylurea Receptor Agonists

The sulfonylurea receptor (SUR2) is a subunit of the ATP-sensitive potassium channel on the plasma membrane of the β-cell, where it functions as a glucose sensor to trigger insulin secretion. Sulfonylureas include first-generation agents (acetohexamide, chlorpropamide, tolazamide, and tolbutamide) and second-generation agents (glipizide, glyburide, gliclazide, and glimepiride). Long-acting forms of sulfonylureas facilitate once-daily dosing. Repaglinide and nateglinide are agents in the meglitinide family of insulin secretagogues, which activate a distinct SUR1 binding site. Because of their short half-lives, repaglinide and nateglinide are administered with each meal. Insulin secretagogues can cause hypoglycemia.

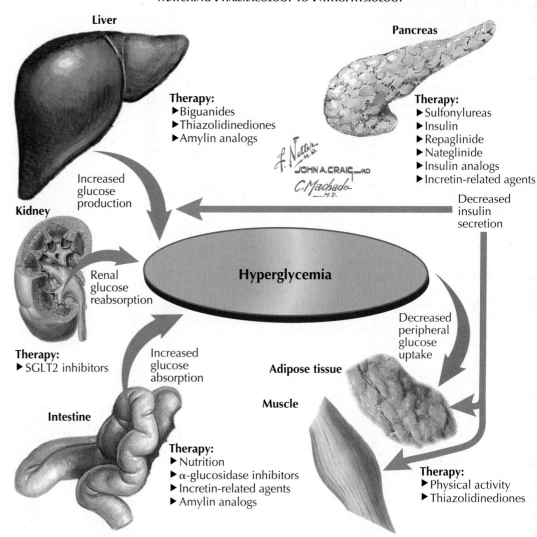

Liver

Therapy:
▶ Biguanides
▶ Thiazolidinediones
▶ Amylin analogs

Pancreas

Therapy:
▶ Sulfonylureas
▶ Insulin
▶ Repaglinide
▶ Nateglinide
▶ Insulin analogs
▶ Incretin-related agents

Increased glucose production

Decreased insulin secretion

Kidney

Renal glucose reabsorption

Hyperglycemia

Decreased peripheral glucose uptake

Therapy:
▶ SGLT2 inhibitors

Increased glucose absorption

Adipose tissue

Muscle

Intestine

Therapy:
▶ Nutrition
▶ α-glucosidase inhibitors
▶ Incretin-related agents
▶ Amylin analogs

Therapy:
▶ Physical activity
▶ Thiazolidinediones

Agents that Slow Enteric Carbohydrate Absorption—α-Glucosidase Inhibitors

α-Glucosidase inhibitors (acarbose, miglitol) inhibit the terminal step of carbohydrate digestion at the intestinal epithelium and delay carbohydrate absorption. They must be administered at the beginning of each meal.

Incretin-Related Agents

The finding that orally administered glucose has a greater stimulatory effect on insulin secretion than intravenously administered glucose is called the *incretin effect*. GLP-1 and GIP mediate the incretin effect. GLP-1 stimulates insulin secretion, slows gastric emptying, and reduces appetite. GLP-1 has a short plasma half-life because of rapid degradation by dipeptidyl peptidase IV (DPP-IV). DPP-IV–resistant GLP-1 receptor agonists include exenatide, liraglutide, lixisenatide, exenatide extended-release, albiglutide, semaglutide, and dulaglutide. Tirzepatide is a dual-acting GLP-1 and GIP receptor agonist. Sitagliptin, saxagliptin, alogliptin, and vildagliptin are orally administered DPP-IV inhibitors that result in mild increases in endogenous GLP-1 and GIP.

Sodium-Glucose Cotransporter 2 Inhibitors

Sodium-glucose cotransporter 2 (SGLT2) inhibitors (canagliflozin, dapagliflozin, empagliflozin, ertugliflozin) reduce blood glucose by increasing urinary glucose excretion. SGLT2 is expressed in the proximal tubule and mediates reabsorption of approximately 90% of the filtered glucose load. SGLT2 inhibitors promote renal

excretion of glucose and lower elevated blood glucose levels in patients with poorly controlled type 2 diabetes.

Amylin Analogs

Amylin is cosecreted with insulin by the β-cell and has complementary actions to insulin by delaying gastric emptying, reducing appetite, and suppressing glucagon secretion. Pramlintide is an amylin analog that is administered subcutaneously at each meal.

Insulin

Subcutaneous administration of insulin serves to supplement endogenous insulin production. The types of insulin include rapid-acting insulin analogs (lispro, aspart, glulisine), short-acting analogs (regular insulin), intermediate-acting analogs (neutral protamine Hagedorn [NPH]), and long-acting analogs (glargine, detemir).

INITIAL APPROACH TO MEDICAL MANAGEMENT

In general, metformin along with diet and exercise should be the initial therapy for patients with type 2 diabetes. For patients with newly diagnosed diabetes who have fasting glucose concentration >250 mg/dL, more than one pharmacologic agent is usually needed (e.g., metformin and a sulfonylurea or insulin). For established patients with suboptimal glycemic control, the addition of rapid-acting insulin, GLP-1 receptor agonist, or SGLT2 inhibitor should be considered.

Plate 5.22

Pancreas

INTENSIVE DIABETES THERAPY OF TYPE 1 DIABETES MELLITUS

It has been clearly demonstrated that optimizing glycemic control (goal $HbA_{1c} \leq 7\%$) with intensive diabetes therapy in patients with type 1 diabetes mellitus leads to clinically significant decreased risks for retinopathy, nephropathy, neuropathy, and cardiovascular disease. Intensive diabetes therapy includes the coordination of meals and activity with insulin replacement, which involves the frequent SMBG or continuous glucose monitoring (CGM) of interstitial glucose levels every 1 to 5 minutes. Interstitial glucose concentrations correlate well with blood glucose results. CGM metrics are being increasingly used to assess glycemic control. In general, the target glucose range is 70 to 180 mg/dL while minimizing time in hypoglycemia (<70 mg/dL) and hyperglycemia (>180 mg/dL) and avoiding glucose readings of <54 mg/dL and >250 mg/dL. Two methods of insulin delivery that can be used to achieve these glycemic targets are continuous subcutaneous insulin infusion (CSII; insulin pump) and multiple daily injections (MDIs) of insulin.

The types of insulin currently available include rapid-acting insulin analogs (lispro, aspart, glulisine) with an onset of action at 15 minutes and peak effect at 1 hour; short-acting (regular insulin) analogs with an onset of action at 30 to 60 minutes and peak effect at 2 to 4 hours; intermediate-acting analogs (NPH) with an onset of action at 1 to 3 hours and a peak effect at 6 to 8 hours; and long-acting analogs (glargine, detemir) with an onset of action at 1 hour, peak effect at 9 or more hours, and duration of effect for 24 hours.

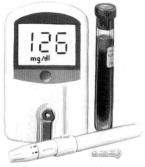

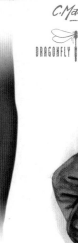

Intensive insulin therapy should be started as soon as possible after the diagnosis of type 1 diabetes mellitus.

The MDI and CSII methods to deliver insulin are designed to replicate normal physiology.

CSII and MDI require self-monitoring of blood glucose and then adjusting and/or supplementing the premeal insulin doses.

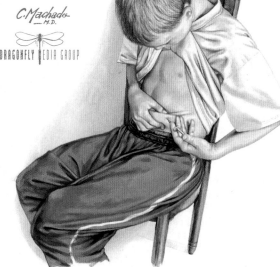

Continuous glucose monitor (CGM)

MONOMERIC INSULIN ANALOGS

Modifications of the human insulin molecule can change its kinetics. For example, rapid-acting insulin analogs are made with recombinant DNA technology by modifying insulin structure to decrease the ability of insulin to self-aggregate after subcutaneous injection, leading to rapid absorption and action. Insulin lispro is synthesized by reversing the amino acids at positions 28 and 29 in the β-chain of human insulin (lysine at β-28 and proline at β-29). Aspartic acid is substituted for proline at β-28 to form insulin aspart. Insulin glulisine is produced by substituting lysine for asparagine at β-3 and substituting glutamic acid for lysine at β-29.

LONG-ACTING INSULIN ANALOGS

Insulin glargine is modified from human insulin by replacing asparagine at α-21 with glycine and by adding two arginine amino acids to the C-terminus of the β-chain. Insulin glargine is solubilized in an acidic solution, and after it has been administered subcutaneously, it microprecipitates and is slowly absorbed over 24 hours to simulate basal production of insulin. Insulin detemir is modified from human insulin by removing the

threonine at β-30, and a C14 fatty acid is attached to the amino acid at β-29. Insulin detemir remains soluble after subcutaneous injection; the long duration of action relates to the molecular modifications.

CONTINUOUS SUBCUTANEOUS INSULIN INFUSION AND MULTIPLE DAILY INJECTIONS

Intensive insulin therapy should be started as soon as possible after the diagnosis of type 1 diabetes. Intensive insulin therapy programs require a team approach that includes the patient, diabetes nurse educators, registered dietitians, medical social workers, and physicians with an interest in diabetes management. Thus CSII and MDI require SMBG or CGM and adjusting and/or supplementing the premeal insulin treatment. The dose of the premeal bolus is determined by the ambient blood glucose level before the meal, the size and composition of the meal, anticipated activity levels, and trending glucose levels from CGM. With MDI, a long-acting insulin analog is administered at bedtime, and rapid-acting analogs are administered before meals. With CSII, an external mechanical pump continuously

administers rapid-acting insulin analogs through a catheter that is inserted into the abdominal wall subcutaneous fat. The pump delivers preprogrammed basal insulin (e.g., 1 unit per hour), and the patient directs the pump to administer boluses premeal. The basal rate can be programmed to change over 24 hours (e.g., an increased basal rate may be needed in the early morning hours). Real-time CGM devices measure and transmit glucose values automatically every 5 minutes to a receiver and can alert for hypoglycemia and hyperglycemia. CGM devices provide feedback to insulin pumps, allowing automatic adjustments of basal rate infusions for low glucose values or trends and high or rising glucose levels.

Hypoglycemia is the most serious complication of both forms of intensive insulin programs. Hypoglycemia can result in falls, motor vehicle accidents, and seizures. Autonomic neuropathy may mask the usual adrenergic-type symptoms (e.g., tremor, tachycardia, sweat) to alert the patient to hypoglycemia; this is termed *hypoglycemic unawareness*. All patients should have readily available carbohydrate (e.g., glucose tablets) and injectable glucagon kits.

Plate 5.23

Endocrine System: VOLUME 2

INSULINOMA

Hypoglycemia due to excess endogenous insulin production is usually caused by a neoplasm of the pancreatic β-cells, termed *insulinoma.* Insulinomas are rare (4 cases per million people per year), usually benign (~95%), and sporadic (~95%). Approximately 5% of patients with insulinomas have multiple endocrine neoplasia type 1 (MEN 1) (see Plate 8.1). Insulinomas are usually solitary (~85%) but may be multiple (~10%) (especially in MEN 1) or malignant (~5%). Pancreatic β-cell hyperplasia can also cause hypoglycemia (see Plate 5.24). In patients with insulinomas, insulin secretion fails to decrease normally as plasma glucose concentrations decrease.

Patients with insulinomas typically note discrete episodes of neuroglycopenia (visual change, confusion, and unusual behavior) and sympathoadrenal symptoms (tremulousness, sweating, and palpitations). Less commonly, patients with insulinoma have episodes of unconsciousness and rarely hypoglycemia-induced seizures. Whipple triad—neuroglycopenia and sympathoadrenal symptoms consistent with hypoglycemia, documented low plasma glucose concentration at the time of symptoms, and relief of symptoms with caloric ingestion—should be documented in all patients with suspected hypoglycemia. The hypoglycemia in patients with insulinoma is caused primarily by an insulin-induced decrease in hepatic glucose output in the fasting state.

Confirmation of endogenous hyperinsulinemic hypoglycemia requires the documentation of hypoglycemia (laboratory-based measurement of venous plasma glucose <45 mg/dL) with inappropriate levels of plasma insulin, C-peptide, and proinsulin. These findings can usually be obtained with fasting—either a short overnight fast in a supervised outpatient setting or a 72-hour fast in a hospital setting—or after a mixed-meal test (for the minority of patients with insulinoma who have primarily postprandial symptoms). Most patients with insulinoma become hypoglycemic within 48 hours of fasting. Laboratory values, obtained when the patient becomes symptomatic during a fast, that are consistent with insulinoma include plasma glucose level below 45 mg/dL, plasma insulin above 3 μU/mL, plasma C-peptide above 200 pmol/L, proinsulin above 5 pmol/L, and β-hydroxybutyrate below 2.7 mmol/L. At the time of documented hypoglycemia, a drug screen should be obtained for sulfonylureas and other insulin secretagogues (e.g., nateglinide, repaglinide). In addition, at the end of the fast, 1 mg of glucagon should be administered intravenously. Insulin is antiglycogenolytic, and hyperinsulinemia permits retention of glycogen within the liver. Whereas normal individuals have released virtually all glucose from the liver at the end of a 72-hour fast and do not have a glucose response glucagon, patients with insulinoma have an increase in plasma glucose of more than 25 mg/dL within 30 minutes of glucagon administration.

The differential diagnosis of disorders that can cause hypoglycemia is broad and includes insulinoma, nesidioblastosis, insulin-autoimmune hypoglycemia, drugs (e.g., sulfonylurea, insulin, or alcohol), critical illness (e.g., hepatic failure, renal failure, or sepsis), counterregulatory hormone deficiency (e.g., Addison disease), and large mesenchymal tumors.

Preoperative localization of an insulinoma is important for operative planning. Localization of the insulinoma within the pancreas may be difficult because they are usually small (40% are <1.0 cm in largest lesional diameter). Approximately 75% of insulinomas can be detected on contrast-enhanced

computed tomography (CT). Transabdominal and endoscopic ultrasonography can usually localize 90% of these tumors. In selected patients, additional localization tests may be needed. Gallium-68 DOTATATE PET/CT can be considered when conventional imaging studies do not identify an insulinoma. In addition, the selective arterial calcium stimulation with hepatic venous sampling can regionalize the insulinoma within the pancreas (see Plate 5.24). Intraoperative pancreatic ultrasonography provides confirmatory localization.

The treatment of choice for insulinoma is complete surgical resection; it may be possible to enucleate the

tumor and spare normal pancreas tissue, or a partial pancreatectomy may be required. When the insulinoma is located in the pancreatic head and enucleation is not possible, a Whipple procedure (resection of the head of the pancreas, duodenectomy, gastrectomy, and splenectomy) may be required. Malignant insulinomas should be removed if possible. When metastatic, the liver is the most common site. Additional treatment approaches for metastatic and unresectable insulin-secreting neoplasms include embolization, thermal ablation, endoscopic ultrasound-guided ethanol ablation, radiotherapy, diazoxide, octreotide, lanreotide, or chemotherapy.

Microscopic view showing nests of islet cells separated by delicate fibrous strands and capillaries

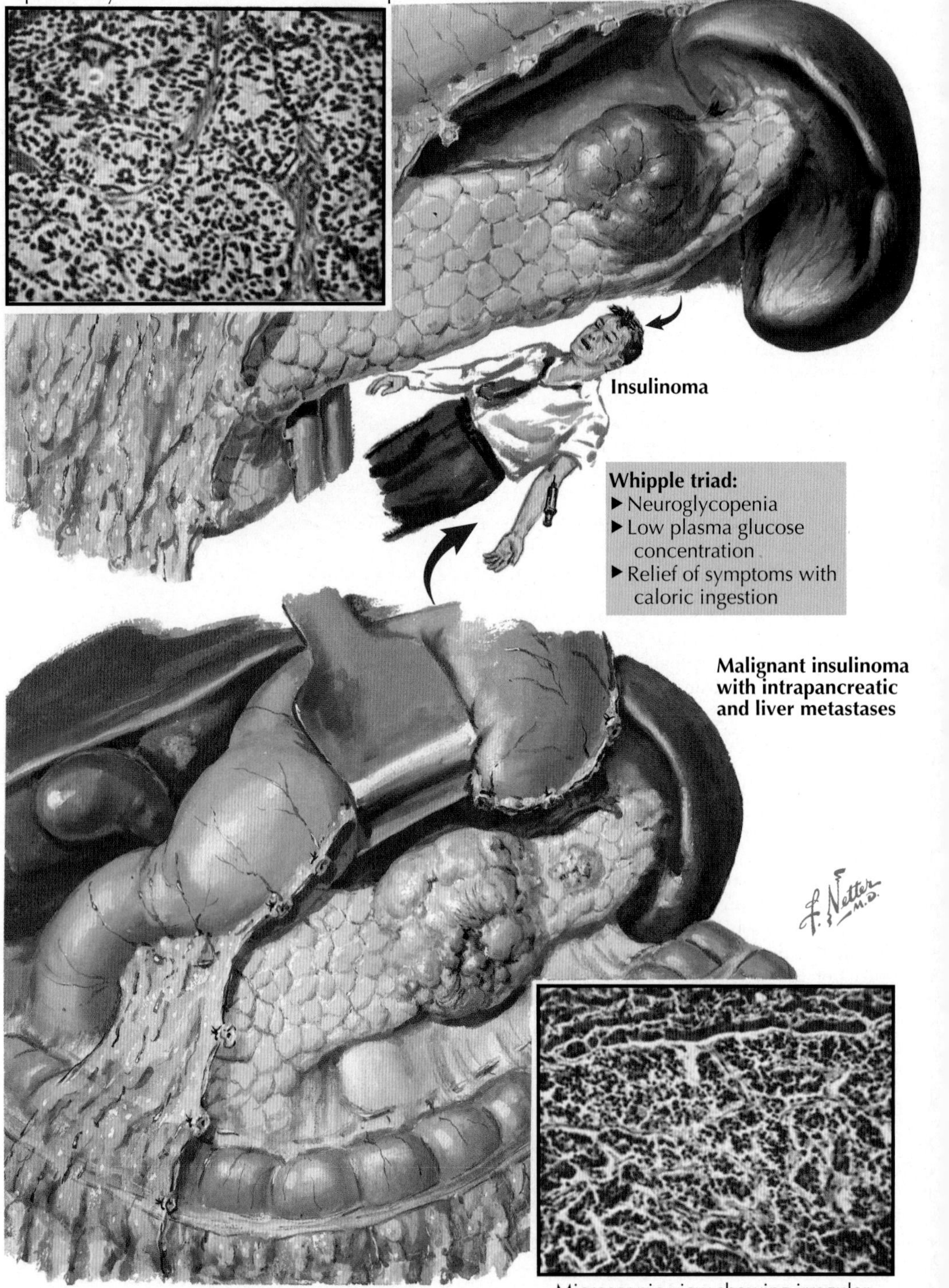

Insulinoma

Whipple triad:
▶ Neuroglycopenia
▶ Low plasma glucose concentration
▶ Relief of symptoms with caloric ingestion

Malignant insulinoma with intrapancreatic and liver metastases

Microscopic view showing irregular nests of more polymorphic, partly atypical islet cells

Plate 5.24

Pancreas

PRIMARY PANCREATIC β-CELL HYPERPLASIA

Primary pancreatic β-cell hyperplasia is a rare cause of hypoglycemia in children and adults. The hyperplastic process may be focal or diffuse. Nesidioblastosis, the neoformation of islets of Langerhans from pancreatic duct epithelium, is present in some patients with pancreatic β-cell hyperplasia.

CONGENITAL HYPERINSULINISM

Congenital hyperinsulinism is a rare (1 in 50,000 live births) autosomal dominant or autosomal recessive disorder usually caused by pathogenic variants in the genes that encode the ATP-sensitive potassium channels (e.g., SUR1, potassium channel subunit [Kir6.2]). These loss-of-function pathogenic variants result in closure of the potassium channel and persistent β-cell membrane depolarization and insulin release despite the prevailing hypoglycemia. Diffuse β-cell hyperplasia and intractable hypoglycemia result. Congenital hyperinsulinism may also be caused by activating pathogenic variants in the genes that encode glutamate dehydrogenase or glucokinase.

Focal adenomatous islet-cell hyperplasia may result from focal loss of the normal maternally inherited allele and somatic expression of the paternally inherited abnormal genes encoding SUR1 or Kir6.2 (*ABCC8* and *KCNJ11*, respectively), which cause β-cell hyperplasia only in the involved cells. Whereas focal islet-cell hyperplasia can be cured by resection of the focally hyperplastic areas of the pancreas, diffuse hyperplasia may require more extensive pancreatic resections.

Signs of hypoglycemia in neonates include changes in level of consciousness, tremor, hypotonia, seizures, apnea, and cyanotic spells. Symptoms are usually evident in the first days after birth. Detection may be delayed until later in childhood in those with partial or mild defects in the *ABCC8* or *KCNJ11* genes. Early diagnosis can prevent neurologic damage from recurrent episodes of hypoglycemia. Macrosomia is common in newborns with congenital hyperinsulinism.

The differential diagnosis of hypoglycemia in infancy and childhood includes hyperinsulinism (congenital hyperinsulinism, nesidioblastosis, insulinoma, infant of a diabetic mother, maternal drugs [e.g., sulfonylurea]); drugs; severe illness; transient intolerance of fasting; lack of counterregulatory hormones (e.g., hypopituitarism); Beckwith-Wiedemann syndrome; or enzymatic defects in the metabolism of carbohydrate (e.g., glycogen storage diseases, glycogen synthase deficiency), protein (e.g., branched-chain α-keto acid dehydrogenase complex deficiency), or fat (e.g., defects in fatty acid oxidation). Transient intolerance of fasting is seen in premature infants and relates to incomplete development of glycogen stores and gluconeogenic mechanisms.

NONINSULINOMA PANCREATOGENOUS HYPOGLYCEMIA SYNDROME AND POST–GASTRIC BYPASS HYPOGLYCEMIA

Noninsulinoma pancreatogenous hypoglycemia syndrome is a form of islet-cell hyperplasia that presents with postprandial symptoms caused by hyperinsulinemic hypoglycemia. The signs and symptoms are cured with partial pancreatectomy. Pathologic examination shows β-cell hypertrophy with or without hyperplasia. Nesidioblastosis is usually present. Similar presentation and pathologic findings have been found after Roux-en-Y

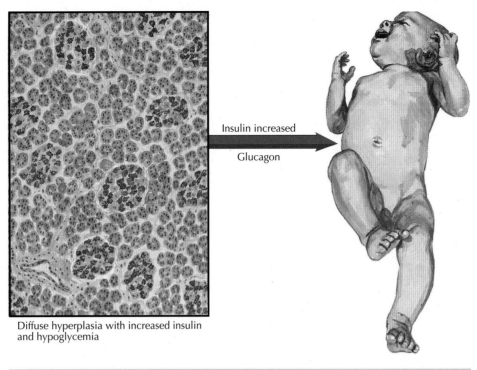

Insulin increased

Glucagon

Diffuse hyperplasia with increased insulin and hypoglycemia

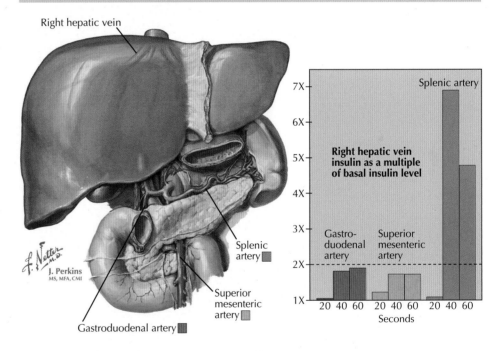

Selective arterial calcium stimulation test

Right hepatic vein

Right hepatic vein insulin as a multiple of basal insulin level

Splenic artery

Gastroduodenal artery

Superior mesenteric artery

Splenic artery ▬

Superior mesenteric artery ▬

Gastroduodenal artery ▬

Seconds

gastric bypass surgery for obesity, in which symptomatic postprandial hypoglycemia can develop 6 months to 8 years after surgery. The underlying pathophysiology is uncertain but may relate to decreased ghrelin, unidentified small intestine factors, or an inability to reset from the preoperative state of insulin-resistant hyperinsulinemia.

EVALUATION

Islet-cell hyperplasia may predispose to hypoglycemia, primarily in the postprandial state rather than in the fasting state as is seen with insulinoma. With the exception of the timing of hypoglycemia, the laboratory abnormalities are identical to those of patients with insulinomas (see Plate 5.23). The diagnosis of postprandial hypoglycemia should not be based on results of oral

glucose tolerance testing but rather on results after a mixed meal.

β-Cell hyperplasia may be diffuse, asymmetric, or focal. Imaging studies are usually not helpful in localizing β-cell hyperplasia. Selective arterial calcium stimulation with hepatic venous sampling can regionalize the dysfunctional β-cells to arterial distributions within the pancreas. Calcium gluconate is selectively injected into the gastroduodenal, splenic, and superior mesenteric arteries, with timed hepatic venous sampling for measurement of insulin. Calcium stimulates the release of insulin from abnormal β-cells but not from normal β-cells. An abnormal result is defined as more than a two- to threefold increase from baseline in hepatic venous insulin concentrations. The selective arterial calcium stimulation test can lead to a gradient-guided partial pancreatectomy.

BONE AND CALCIUM

Plate 6.1

Endocrine System: VOLUME 2

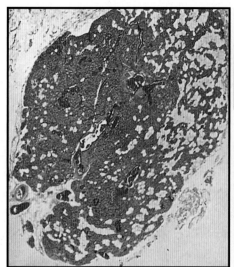

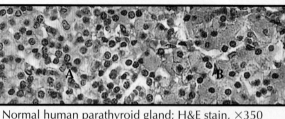

Normal human parathyroid gland; H&E stain, ×350
A=light and dark chief cells; B=oxyphil cells

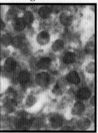 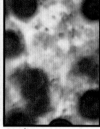 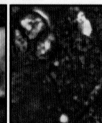

Normal human parathyroid gland; H&E stain, ×17.5

PAS stain, ×675 Glycogen in chief cells

Bodian stain, ×1800 Secretory granules in chief cells

BAAF stain, ×1350 Mitochondria in oxyphil cells

HISTOLOGY OF THE NORMAL PARATHYROID GLANDS

The parathyroid glands are derived from branchial pouches III and IV and number between two and six, although four is the usual number. In adults, each of these ovoid (bean-shaped) glands measures 4 to 6 mm × 2 to 4 mm × 0.5 to 2 mm and weighs approximately 30 mg (the lower parathyroid glands are generally larger than the upper glands). They vary in color from yellow to tan, depending on vascularity and percentage of oxyphil cells and stromal fat.

In infants and children, the glands are composed of sheets of closely packed chief cells, with little intervening stroma. Oxyphil (or oncocytic) cells first make their appearance at the time of puberty. Fat cells begin to appear in the stroma in late childhood. Both the oxyphil cells and the fat cells increase in number until they may occupy more than 50% of the volume of the glands during the fifth and sixth decades of life.

In adults, the glands are composed of cords, sheets, and acini of chief cells in a loose areolar stroma containing numerous mature fat cells. Chief cells appear in an active synthetic phase ("dark chief cell") with well-formed endoplasmic reticulum and prominent Golgi apparatus or in a resting phase ("light chief cell") with less well-developed endoplasmic reticulum. Scattered individually or in groups among these chief cells are the oxyphil cells. The chief cell measures approximately 8 μm in diameter. It has a well-defined cell membrane and a 4- to 5-μm centrally located nucleus. The chromatin is densely packed, appearing almost pyknotic, or it is finely fibrillar with peripheral margination. Nucleoli are rare. The cell cytoplasm is clear and amphophilic in hematoxylin-eosin (H&E) preparations. The periodic acid-Schiff (PAS) reaction reveals abundant glycogen in these cells. Chief cells also contain abundant intracytoplasmic neutral lipid droplets demonstrated with azure B or Erie garnet A procedures or with oil red O or Sudan IV stains. Immunohistochemical studies show stronger staining for parathyroid hormone (PTH) in chief cells than in oxyphilic cells.

The oxyphilic cells are larger than chief cells (12–20 μm in diameter) and are polygonal in shape. The cell membranes are usually clear, and the nucleus is identical to that of the chief cell. The cytoplasm is composed of highly eosinophilic fine granules, which stain carmine with Bensley acid aniline fuchsin (BAAF) and dark blue with phosphotungstic acid hematoxylin. These cells contain tightly packed mitochondria filling the cytoplasm and have high levels of oxidative enzymes. Unlike chief cells, the oxyphilic cells have very little intracytoplasmic lipid or glycogen. Variants of the oxyphilic cells include transitional oxyphilic cells, which are smaller and contain less eosinophilic cytoplasm.

Ultrastructure of parathyroid gland

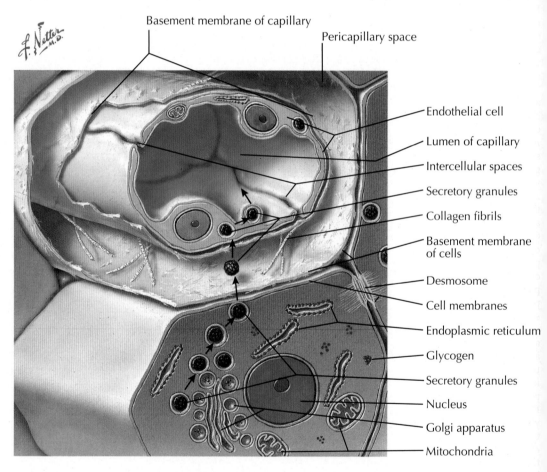

Basement membrane of capillary

Pericapillary space

Endothelial cell

Lumen of capillary

Intercellular spaces

Secretory granules

Collagen fibrils

Basement membrane of cells

Desmosome

Cell membranes

Endoplasmic reticulum

Glycogen

Secretory granules

Nucleus

Golgi apparatus

Mitochondria

The ultrastructure of the active form of the chief cell and the mode of secretion are schematized in the illustration. The chief cells are arranged in cords and nests and separated from the interstitium by basal laminae. The chief cells have straight plasma membranes and are attached to other cells by desmosomes. During the active phase, in addition to the usual organelles, the Golgi apparatus enlarges, numerous vacuoles and vesicles appear in the Golgi apparatus, and many mature secretory granules (50–300 nm in diameter) appear in the cell. The mature secretory granule is oval to dumbbell-shaped and has a single membrane surrounding a thin clear space inside of which is a dense area composed of short rod-like profiles. The granule migrates out of the cell through the basement membrane into the wide pericapillary space. It then goes through the capillary basement membrane and into the fenestrated endothelial cells that line the capillaries, from which PTH is liberated into the bloodstream.

Plate 6.2

Bone and Calcium

PHYSIOLOGY OF THE PARATHYROID GLANDS

Secretion of PTH from the four parathyroid glands is regulated by the blood level of ionized calcium (Ca^{2+}). Serum ionized calcium concentrations below the reference range stimulate PTH secretion, and levels above the reference range inhibit PTH secretion. The principal action of PTH is the regulation and maintenance of a normal serum total calcium level between 8.9 and 10.1 mg/dL. The calcium-sensing receptors (CaSRs) in the parathyroid glands are responsible for maintaining this calcium-dependent regulation of PTH secretion. The CaSRs in the kidneys serve to adjust tubular calcium reabsorption independent of PTH.

A normal serum concentration of ionized calcium is critical for many extracellular and cellular functions, and it is normally maintained in the very narrow range through a tightly regulated calcium-PTH homeostatic system. Neuromuscular activity is just one function that is dependent on calcium homeostasis; cytosolic free calcium serves as a key second messenger. Thus disturbances in extracellular calcium concentration result in symptoms of abnormal neuromuscular activity. For example, hypercalcemia may cause muscle weakness and areflexia, anorexia, constipation, vomiting, drowsiness, depression, confusion, or coma. Hypocalcemia may result in anxiety, muscle twitching, Chvostek and Trousseau signs, carpal or pedal spasm, seizures, stridor, bronchospasm, or intestinal cramps.

The daily dietary calcium intake ranges between 300 and 1500 mg/d; total net gastrointestinal (GI) calcium absorption averages 200 mg/d. The urinary calcium excretion averages 200 mg/d (2% of the filtered load). Although the urinary calcium excretion is rather constant, the excretion of calcium in the stool depends greatly on the body's need and the dietary intake; normally, 500 to 700 mg of calcium is excreted per 24 hours (100–200 mg/d is endogenous fecal calcium that is unaffected by dietary or serum calcium). The average dietary intake of phosphate is 800 to 900 mg/d. GI tract phosphate absorption is enhanced by 1,25-dihydroxyvitamin D (1,25[OH]$_2$D; calcitriol). Phosphate absorption is impaired by increasing dietary calcium. Whereas the fecal excretion of inorganic phosphate (P_i) is roughly 30% of dietary intake, the urinary phosphate excretion varies widely with intake and serum PTH concentration.

If dietary calcium is restricted in healthy individuals, a decrease in the blood calcium concentration leads to a compensatory increase in intestinal calcium absorption. This occurs because a small decrease in serum ionized calcium triggers the CaSR, and there is a prompt increase in PTH secretion. The increased blood PTH concentration leads to increased renal 1α hydroxylation of 25-hydroxyvitamin D (25[OH]D; calcidiol) to the more potent calcitriol. Calcitriol acts on enterocytes to increase active transport of calcium. In addition, renal tubular calcium reabsorption is increased both by PTH and by a direct effect of hypocalcemia via the CaSRs in the loop of Henle. The direct actions of PTH and calcitriol at bone increase bone resorption and calcium release. Because of these three mechanisms of action, the serum ionized calcium concentration increases, and the serum PTH concentration decreases.

With increased dietary calcium exposure, there is suppression of PTH secretion, inhibition of the 1α hydroxylation of calcidiol, decreased intestinal absorption of calcium, increased renal excretion of calcium,

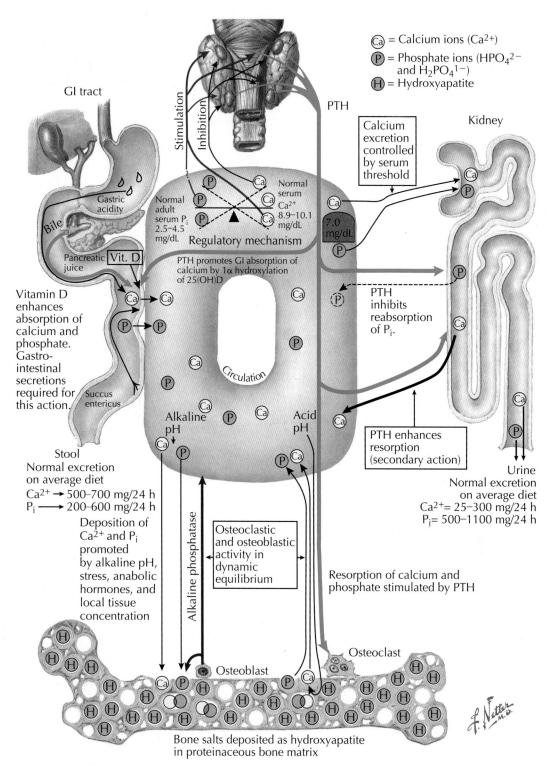

= Calcium ions (Ca^{2+})

= Phosphate ions (HPO_4^{2-} and $H_2PO_4^{1-}$)

= Hydroxyapatite

GI tract

Stimulation

Inhibition

PTH

Kidney

Calcium excretion controlled by serum threshold

Gastric acidity

Bile

Normal adult serum P_i 2.5–4.5 mg/dL

Normal serum Ca^{2+} 8.9–10.1 mg/dL

Regulatory mechanism

7.0 mg/dL

Pancreatic juice

Vit. D

PTH promotes GI absorption of calcium by 1α hydroxylation of 25(OH)D

PTH inhibits reabsorption of P_i.

Vitamin D enhances absorption of calcium and phosphate. Gastrointestinal secretions required for this action.

Succus entericus

Circulation

Alkaline pH

Acid pH

PTH enhances resorption (secondary action)

Urine
Normal excretion on average diet
Ca^{2+} = 25–300 mg/24 h
P_i = 500–1100 mg/24 h

Stool
Normal excretion on average diet
Ca^{2+} → 500–700 mg/24 h
P_i → 200–600 mg/24 h

Deposition of Ca^{2+} and P_i promoted by alkaline pH, stress, anabolic hormones, and local tissue concentration

Alkaline phosphatase

Osteoclastic and osteoblastic activity in dynamic equilibrium

Resorption of calcium and phosphate stimulated by PTH

Osteoblast

Osteoclast

Bone salts deposited as hydroxyapatite in proteinaceous bone matrix

Matrix growth requires protein, vitamin C, anabolic hormones (androgens, estrogen, IGF-1) + stress of mobility. Matrix resorption favored by catabolic hormones (11-oxysteroids [cortisol], thyroid), parathyroid hormone + immobilization.

decreased renal excretion of phosphate, and decreased bone resorption.

If the parathyroid glands are not functioning properly or are absent, the serum calcium level decreases, usually below the renal threshold of 7 mg/dL, and urinary calcium is absent. The presence of a large reservoir of calcium in the skeleton (~1000 g) as hydroxyapatite ($Ca_{10}[PO_4]_6[OH]_2$), however, prevents the serum calcium from falling below 5 mg/dL even in the absence of the parathyroid glands.

In states of excessive PTH secretion, resorption of calcium and phosphate from bone matrix occurs through stimulation of the osteoclasts. The osteoclastic overresponse then evokes a tendency for the osteoblasts to become overactive and leads to bone repair, with the subsequent rise of the alkaline phosphatase level in the serum. Bone repair is promoted by enhanced absorption of calcium and phosphate from the GI tract facilitated in part by the increased serum concentration of calcitriol.

Plate 6.3

Endocrine System: VOLUME 2

BONE REMODELING UNIT

Bone is composed of a collagen matrix, distributed in a lamellar pattern and strengthened by pyridinoline crosslinks between the triple-helical collagen molecules, on which calcium and phosphorus are deposited to form hydroxyapatite. The bone matrix also includes calcium-binding proteins such as osteocalcin. The resulting bone mineral is complex crystals of hydroxyapatite that contain fluoride and carbonate.

Bone modeling is the process of change in bone size and shape in childhood, where linear growth is the result of cartilaginous growth at the epiphyses, and bone width enlargement results from endosteal resorption and periosteal apposition. During puberty and early adulthood, endosteal apposition occurs, and peak bone mass is achieved.

Bone remodeling is the lifelong process of bone repair, which has three phases: resorption, reversal, and formation. The bone remodeling unit (osteon) involves a cycle of coupled osteoclastic and osteoblastic activities.

Osteoblasts develop from determined osteoblast progenitor cells that originate from mesenchymal stem cells. The osteoblast progenitor cells are localized to the periosteum and bone marrow. Osteoblasts have receptors for PTH, calcitriol, testosterone, estrogen, glucocorticoids, growth hormone, thyroid hormone, and insulinlike growth factors. After osteoblasts lay down collagen and noncollagen proteins, some of the osteoblasts become osteocytes that are buried in the bone matrix. The remaining osteoblasts either become the less metabolically active, flattened lining cells or undergo apoptosis.

Osteoclasts, derived from monocytes and macrophages, are multinucleated, large cells that dissolve bone mineral and degrade matrix. Osteoclast progenitors can be found in the bone marrow and the spleen. Osteoclastic differentiation is triggered by the production of macrophage colony-stimulation factor. Excessive osteoclastic activity is associated with Paget disease, hyperparathyroidism (HPT), and a subset of osteoporosis.

RESORPTION

The bone remodeling cycle is activated by osteoblast cells that release collagenase, macrophage colony-stimulating factor, and receptor activator of NF-κB (RANK) ligand. RANK ligand interacts with the RANK receptor and activates osteoclast formation and the initiation of bone resorption. RANK ligand also binds to osteoprotegerin, which is an osteoclastogenesis inhibitory factor. Macrophage colony-stimulating factor is also required for normal osteoclast activation. This initial osteoblast activation of osteoclasts can be affected by multiple hormones and factors. For example, PTH induces the osteoblastic production of RANK ligand and inhibits production of osteoprotegerin. Vitamin D also increases the production of RANK ligand.

Osteoclasts enzymatically degrade bone matrix protein and remove mineral within cortical bone or on the trabecular surfaces. This process is self-limited—perhaps by high local concentrations of calcium or bone matrix substances—and is completed over 2 weeks.

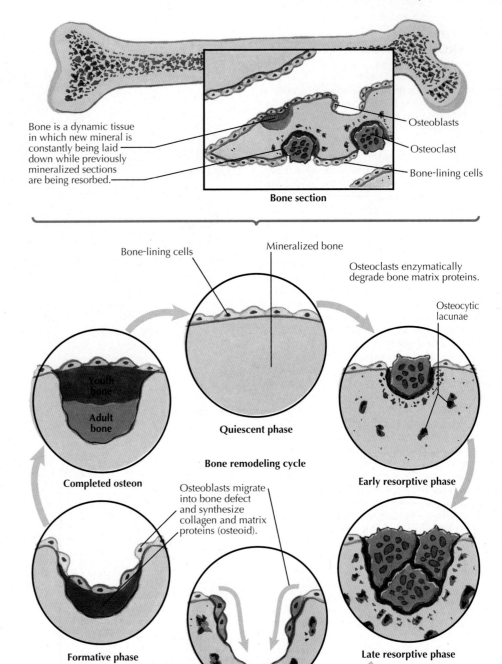

Bone is a dynamic tissue in which new mineral is constantly being laid down while previously mineralized sections are being resorbed.

Osteoblasts
Osteoclast
Bone-lining cells

Bone section

Bone-lining cells
Mineralized bone
Osteoclasts enzymatically degrade bone matrix proteins.
Osteocytic lacunae

Quiescent phase

Bone remodeling cycle

Completed osteon

Early resorptive phase

Osteoblasts migrate into bone defect and synthesize collagen and matrix proteins (osteoid).

Formative phase

Reversal phase

Late resorptive phase

REVERSAL

After osteoclastic resorption, the reversal phase is initiated by mononuclear cells that lay down a glycoprotein-rich material (cement) on the resorbed surface and signal for osteoblast differentiation. The new osteoblasts adhere to this material. The reversal phase is approximately 4 weeks in duration.

FORMATION

During the formation phase, osteoblasts lay down osteoid (collagen and matrix proteins) until the resorbed bone is completely replaced. The formation phase takes approximately 16 weeks to complete. Normally, the new bone formed is equivalent to what was resorbed. When the formation phase is complete, the bone surface is covered with bone-lining cells, and very little cellular

activity occurs until another bone remodeling cycle begins.

DEFECTIVE BONE REMODELING

In a normal bone remodeling unit, resorption and formation are tightly coupled. However, a mismatch between resorption and formation can lead to abnormally thin or dense bones. For example, if the osteoclastic resorption depth is excessive, it can perforate and weaken trabecular structure; if the osteoblasts do not completely fill the deep resorption cavity, bone density and quality decline. If the resorptive process is incomplete because the osteoclasts are not fully activated (e.g., with macrophage colony-stimulating factor deficiency) or if they are dysfunctional, excessively dense bones may result (osteopetrosis).

Plate 6.4

Bone and Calcium

PATHOPHYSIOLOGY OF PRIMARY HYPERPARATHYROIDISM

The annual incidence of primary HPT is approximately 4 in 100,000. HPT is twice as common in females, and most patients are diagnosed after age 45 years. Primary HPT is caused by a single parathyroid adenoma (89%), multiple ("double") parathyroid adenomas (4%), multi-gland parathyroid hyperplasia (6%), or parathyroid carcinoma (1%). The distinction between these forms of primary HPT directs the surgical approach.

Most parathyroid adenomas are encapsulated and arise from chief cells; the others are composed of oxyphilic cells. Parathyroid adenomas are usually localized to the neck, but ectopic parathyroid tumors may arise anywhere in the anterior mediastinum or even in the posterior mediastinum. The cells in the adenomas are monoclonal and are a result of somatic mutations in genes that control growth. For example, the cyclin D1 protooncogene (*CCND1*) encodes a major regulator of the cell cycle. Overexpression of cyclin D1 is found in approximately 30% of parathyroid adenomas. Multiple endocrine neoplasia (MEN) type 1 (see Plate 8.1) is caused by germline pathogenic variants in *MEN1*, a tumor suppressor gene, and somatic mutations are found in approximately 15% of sporadic parathyroid adenomas.

Multiple-gland hyperplasia, characterized by enlargement of all four glands, is occasionally mistaken for multiple adenomas. Chief cell hyperplasia is much more common than clear cell hyperplasia (the latter is associated with hyperplasia primarily of the superior parathyroid glands). Parathyroid hyperplasia may be sporadic or associated with a familial syndrome (e.g., MEN 1, MEN 2A, HPT-jaw tumor syndrome, or familial isolated HPT). Distinguishing between parathyroid gland hyperplasia and normal parathyroid tissue can be difficult for the pathologist. In general, abnormal parathyroid glands are increased in size and contain less fat. Primary HPT affects almost all patients with MEN 1, and the hypercalcemia is typically present by the third decade of life, but primary HPT affects only 10% of patients with MEN 2A and tends to occur later in life. Parathyroid adenomas and hyperplasia are multiple and cystic in patients with HPT-jaw tumor syndrome. The jaw tumor is usually fibrous in nature.

The diagnosis of parathyroid carcinoma is based on local invasion of contiguous tissues or metastases (lymph node or distant). Both sporadic and germline inactivating pathogenic variants in *CDC73* (previously known as *HRPT2*) are responsible for HPT-jaw tumor syndrome, which is associated with an increased risk for parathyroid carcinoma.

A normal serum concentration of ionized calcium is critical for many extracellular and cellular functions, and it is normally maintained in the very narrow range through a tightly regulated calcium-PTH homeostatic system. In healthy individuals, a small decrease in serum ionized calcium triggers the CaSR, and there is a prompt increase in PTH secretion. The increased blood PTH concentration leads to an immediate increase in bone resorption and renal 1α-hydroxylation of calcidiol to the more potent calcitriol. Calcitriol leads to increased intestinal calcium absorption over several days. Finally, PTH leads to an immediate decrease in urinary calcium excretion by stimulating calcium reabsorption at the distal renal tubule. Because of these three mechanisms of action, the serum ionized calcium concentration increases, and the serum PTH concentration decreases.

Patients with primary HPT have abnormal regulation of PTH secretion by calcium, a finding partly caused by an elevation in the set point. The set point for calcium-dependent feedback suppression of PTH release is 15% to 30% above normal. It is important to note that PTH secretion in primary HPT is not completely autonomous and can usually be partially inhibited by a further rise in serum calcium. The excessive production of PTH leads to hypercalcemia by increased stimulation of the osteoclastic activity of bone (with the release of calcium and phosphate), increased absorption of calcium from the gut, and increased reabsorption of calcium by the renal tubules. In addition, PTH inhibits the tubular reabsorption of inorganic phosphate (P_i), causing an excessive loss of phosphate. The net effect of these chemical changes is an increase in serum calcium and a decrease in serum phosphate, with increasing amounts of both calcium and phosphate being excreted in the urine. This predisposes to the formation of calcium phosphate and calcium oxalate renal stones. At times, there may be precipitation of calcium in the soft tissues of the kidneys, producing nephrocalcinosis.

Roughly 25% of patients with primary HPT have evidence of bone disease, with marked bone resorption and a compensatory increase in osteoblastic activity. Bone mineral is formed by small hydroxyapatite crystals that contain carbonate, magnesium, sodium, and potassium.

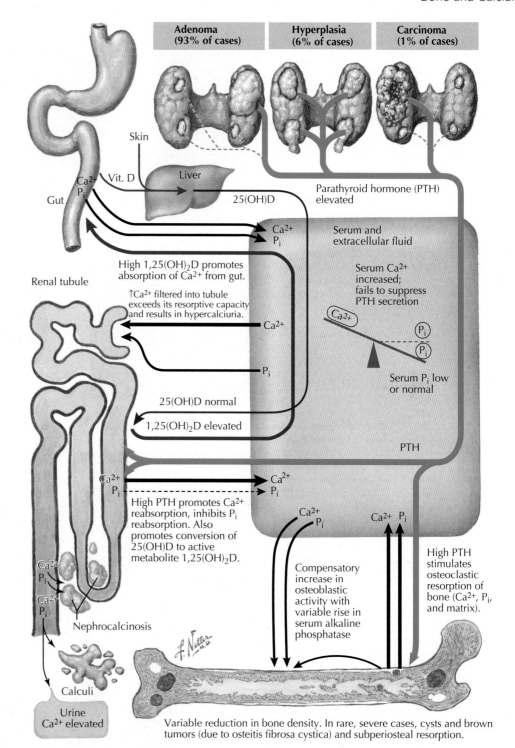

Adenoma (93% of cases) · Hyperplasia (6% of cases) · Carcinoma (1% of cases)

Skin

Vit. D

Liver

25(OH)D

Gut

Ca^{2+}
P_i

Renal tubule

High 1,25(OH)$_2$D promotes absorption of Ca^{2+} from gut.

↑Ca^{2+} filtered into tubule exceeds its resorptive capacity and results in hypercalciuria.

Ca^{2+}

P_i

25(OH)D normal

1,25(OH)$_2$D elevated

Ca^{2+}
P_i

High PTH promotes Ca^{2+} reabsorption, inhibits P_i reabsorption. Also promotes conversion of 25(OH)D to active metabolite 1,25(OH)$_2$D.

Ca^{2+}
P_i

Ca^{2+}
P_i

Nephrocalcinosis

Calculi

Urine Ca^{2+} elevated

Parathyroid hormone (PTH) elevated

Ca^{2+}
P_i

Serum and extracellular fluid

Serum Ca^{2+} increased; fails to suppress PTH secretion

Ca^{2+}

P_i
P_i

Serum P_i low or normal

PTH

Ca^{2+}
P_i

Ca^{2+} P_i

Compensatory increase in osteoblastic activity with variable rise in serum alkaline phosphatase

High PTH stimulates osteoclastic resorption of bone (Ca^{2+}, P_i, and matrix).

Variable reduction in bone density. In rare, severe cases, cysts and brown tumors (due to osteitis fibrosa cystica) and subperiosteal resorption.

Plate 6.5

Endocrine System: VOLUME 2

PATHOLOGY AND CLINICAL MANIFESTATIONS OF PRIMARY HYPERPARATHYROIDISM

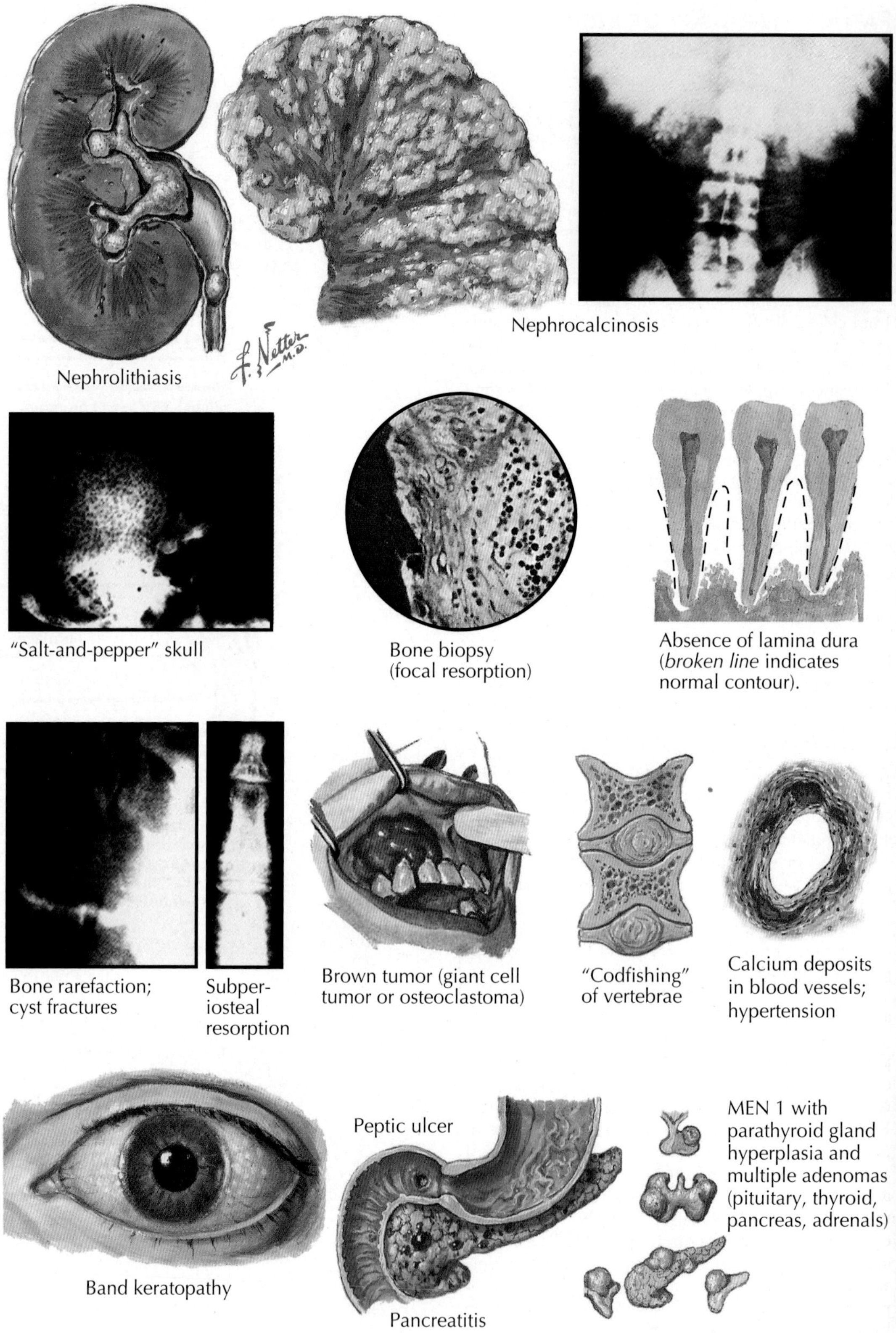

Approximately 80% of patients with primary HPT are asymptomatic, and hypercalcemia is detected by routine biochemical testing. Less commonly, primary HPT is diagnosed during the evaluation of symptomatic hypercalcemia, renal lithiasis, osteoporosis, or osteitis fibrosa cystica. Although most patients with primary HPT do not have overt symptoms, it may be responsible for more subtle symptomatology (e.g., weakness, fatigue, depressed mood, or mild cognitive dysfunction).

The more overt signs and symptoms of long-standing, untreated primary HPT have been referred to as *bones, stones, abdominal moans, and groans*. The "stones" refer to nephrolithiasis, which occurs in 20% of patients with primary HPT. The nephrolithiasis is caused by the hypercalciuria (a result of increased filtered calcium in the setting of hypercalcemia) that predisposes to the development of calcium oxalate stones. The most common effect on bones is osteopenia and osteoporosis. Less common bone-related sequelae of severe, long-standing primary HPT include absence of the lamina dura around the teeth; subperiosteal resorption of the bone, especially around the radial margins of the phalanges, around the sternal end of the clavicle, and along the margins of other bones; diffuse "salt-and-pepper" decalcification of the skull, resembling multiple myeloma; fractures of the terminal phalanges with telescoping, giving the appearance of pseudoclubbing (the phalangeal joints may show increased flexibility); large bone cysts (osteitis fibrosa cystica) in various locations (fractures through these cysts or fractures through rarefied bone may occur); diffuse demineralization of the skeleton, especially of the spine, with "codfishing" of the vertebral bodies; and brown tumors (also known as *giant cell tumors*, *osteoclastoma*, or *epulis*), which are radiolucent bone tumors that may develop in the jaw and other bones.

Hypercalcemia may also cause nausea, anorexia, constipation, nephrogenic diabetes insipidus (polyuria and polydipsia), glucose intolerance, peptic ulcer disease, pancreatitis, and hypertension. Parathyroid crisis occurs with severe hypercalcemia (calcium >15 mg/dL), and patients who are affected present with central nervous system dysfunction (e.g., confusion, coma). Parathyroid crisis—typically precipitated by volume depletion—is treated with volume repletion with isotonic saline and an agent to decrease bone resorption (e.g., a bisphosphonate).

Physical examination typically reveals no specific findings for primary HPT. Parathyroid adenomas are not palpable; when a parathyroid tumor is palpable, it is usually parathyroid carcinoma. With a slit-lamp examination of the eyes, calcium phosphate deposition may be seen in a semicircular form around the limbus of the cornea and is termed *band keratopathy*.

Laboratory abnormalities in patients with primary HPT include increased serum total and ionized calcium concentrations, decreased serum phosphorus concentration (PTH inhibits the proximal renal

Nephrolithiasis

Nephrocalcinosis

"Salt-and-pepper" skull

Bone biopsy (focal resorption)

Absence of lamina dura (*broken line* indicates normal contour).

Bone rarefaction; cyst fractures

Subperiosteal resorption

Brown tumor (giant cell tumor or osteoclastoma)

"Codfishing" of vertebrae

Calcium deposits in blood vessels; hypertension

Band keratopathy

Peptic ulcer

Pancreatitis

MEN 1 with parathyroid gland hyperplasia and multiple adenomas (pituitary, thyroid, pancreas, adrenals)

tubular reabsorption of phosphate), serum PTH concentration that is either above the reference range or inappropriately (in the setting of hypercalcemia) within the reference range, and increased serum calcitriol concentration (a result of PTH-stimulated renal hydroxylation of calcidiol). Serum creatinine concentrations can be increased in patients with marked and long-standing primary HPT and can be associated with nephrocalcinosis. Patients with severe primary HPT may also have a normochromic normocytic anemia.

Vitamin D deficiency is frequently present in patients with primary HPT, a state that can attenuate the degree of hypercalcemia. Treating the vitamin D deficiency in this setting can aggravate the hypercalcemia and hypercalciuria.

The treatment of primary HPT rests on the surgical removal of the parathyroid adenoma (for single-gland disease) or, rarely, of 3.5 hyperplastic parathyroid glands in the setting of diffuse parathyroid hyperplasia (e.g., with MEN type 1).

Plate 6.6

Bone and Calcium

DIFFERENTIAL DIAGNOSIS OF HYPERCALCEMIC STATES

Condition	Serum Ca²⁺	Serum Pi	Serum PTH	Serum 25(OH)D	Serum 1,25(OH)₂D	Associated findings
Primary hyperparathyroidism	↑	N or ↓	High N or ↑	N	N or ↑	80% Asymptomatic Nephrolithiasis Osteoporosis Hypercalcemic symptoms
Cancer with extensive bone metastases	↑	N or ↑	↓	N	↓ or N	History of primary tumor, destructive lesions on radiograph, bone scan
Multiple myeloma and lymphoma	↑	N or ↑	↓	N	↓ or N	Abnormal serum or urine protein electrophoresis, abnormal bone radiographs
Humoral hypercalcemia of malignancy	↑	N or ↓	↓	N	↓ or N	↑PTHrP Solid malignancy usually evident
Sarcoidosis and other granulomatous diseases	↑	N or ↑	↓	N	↑	Hilar adenopathy interstitial lung disease, elevated angiotensin-converting enzyme
Hyperthyroidism	↑	N	↓	N	N	Symptoms of hyperthyroidism, elevated serum thyroxine
Vitamin D intoxication	↑	N or ↑	↓	Very ↑	N or ↑	History of excessive vitamin D intake
Milk-alkali syndrome	↑	N or ↑	↓	N	N or ↓	History of excessive calcium and alkali ingestion, heavy use of over-the-counter calcium-containing antacids
Total body immobilization	↑	N or ↑	↓	N	↓ or N	Multiple fractures, paralysis (children, adolescents, patients with Paget disease of bone)

N = Normal.

TESTS FOR THE DIFFERENTIAL DIAGNOSIS OF THE CAUSES OF HYPERCALCEMIA

The most common causes of hypercalcemia are primary HPT and malignancy. The first question the clinician should ask is whether the hypercalcemia is a persistent finding; thus a serum calcium concentration should be remeasured. If levels of serum calcium have been measured in the past, they should be reviewed. Whereas long-standing mild hypercalcemia (<11 mg/dL) is typical of primary HPT, an abrupt onset of severe hypercalcemia (>13 mg/dL) is more typical of hypercalcemia of malignancy. The patient's diet and medications should be reviewed for clues suggestive of milk-alkali syndrome and medication-related hypercalcemia.

For patients with persistent hypercalcemia, the first step is to determine whether it is PTH mediated. Whereas PTH-mediated hypercalcemia is primary HPT, non-PTH-mediated hypercalcemia is usually caused by underlying malignancy, granulomatous disease, or vitamin D intoxication.

PTH-MEDIATED HYPERCALCEMIA

Most patients with primary HPT have serum PTH concentrations above the reference range. However, 20% of patients with primary HPT have serum PTH concentrations in the upper portion of the reference range, but they are inappropriately in the reference range for the setting of hypercalcemia. Measurement of serum inorganic phosphate concentration and 24-hour urinary excretion of calcium are usually helpful in confirming PTH-mediated disease. Hypophosphatemia results from the PTH-related inhibition of renal proximal tubular phosphate reabsorption. Although hypophosphatemia may also be seen with PTH-related protein (PTHrP)-mediated hypercalcemia, it is not seen with the other forms of non-PTH-mediated hypercalcemia. The 24-hour urinary excretion of calcium is either at the high end of the reference range or above the reference range in most patients with primary HPT. However, this finding is not specific to primary HPT and is seen with most other causes of hypercalcemia. The 24-hour urinary excretion of calcium is typically less than 100 mg in patients with milk-alkali syndrome or familial hypocalciuric hypercalcemia (FHH) or in patients treated with thiazide diuretics. Serum calcitriol concentrations are usually increased in patients with primary HPT because PTH increases the 1α-hydroxylation of calcidiol in the kidney.

NON-PTH-MEDIATED HYPERCALCEMIA

When the serum PTH concentration is low in a patient with hypercalcemia, additional stepwise testing to consider includes measurement of calcidiol, calcitriol, PTHrP, serum thyrotropin (TSH) (for hyperthyroidism), and vitamin A and performance of serum protein electrophoresis (for multiple myeloma).

PTHrP—the hormone responsible for humoral hypercalcemia of malignancy—is an agonist at the PTH receptor and may be hypersecreted by solid malignancies. However, unlike PTH, PTHrP does not induce renal conversion of calcidiol to calcitriol.

If the serum concentration of PTHrP is low, serum concentrations of calcidiol and calcitriol should be measured. Whereas a markedly increased serum concentration of calcidiol is consistent with vitamin D intoxication, increased serum concentrations of calcitriol may be seen with the enhanced extrarenal 1α-hydroxylation of calcidiol that occurs in granulomatous disorders and lymphoma. In this setting, sarcoidosis is usually evident on a plain chest radiograph or computed tomography (CT); these images usually demonstrate bilateral hilar adenopathy and reticular pulmonary opacities.

If vitamin D and PTHrP levels are low in a patient with non-PTH-mediated hypercalcemia, then serum protein electrophoresis should be performed, and serum TSH and vitamin A concentrations should be measured. In this setting, hypercalcemia is usually associated with stimulation of bone resorption (e.g., multiple myeloma, hyperthyroidism, vitamin A intoxication, or immobilization) or increased calcium intake in the setting of renal insufficiency (milk-alkali syndrome).

OTHER CAUSES OF APPARENT HYPERCALCEMIA

Increased serum total calcium concentration is usually the result of an increased amount of free (ionized) calcium—the physiologically relevant fraction. Rarely, an increased measured amount of total blood calcium may be attributable to increased amounts of calcium bound to protein (e.g., in multiple myeloma with increased calcium-binding paraprotein) and the ionized fraction is normal; this is termed *pseudohypercalcemia*.

FHH is a rare autosomal dominant disorder associated with an inactivating pathogenic variant in the gene encoding the CaSR. Typically identified because of incidental discovery of hypercalcemia, these patients have hypocalciuria with the fractional urinary excretion of calcium less than 1%. Patients with FHH have mild hypercalcemia with either normal or slightly increased concentrations of serum PTH. The pathogenic variant responsible for FHH makes the CaSR less sensitive to calcium. Thus a higher-than-normal serum calcium concentration is required to reduce PTH release; an increase in tubular calcium and magnesium reabsorption in the kidney results in hypercalcemia, hypocalciuria, and hypermagnesemia. These patients are asymptomatic; FHH has a benign natural history, and no treatment is required. All first-degree relatives should be tested for hypercalcemia and alerted that it is not primary HPT and that no surgery is needed.

Plate 6.7

Endocrine System: VOLUME 2

RENAL OSTEODYSTROPHY

The kidneys have a central role in regulating mineral metabolism. *Renal osteodystrophy* refers to the bone morphology alterations found in patients with chronic kidney disease. Common forms of renal osteodystrophy in patients with progressive renal failure include high bone turnover with secondary or tertiary HPT and the associated osteitis fibrosa cystica, low bone turnover with adynamic bone disease, low bone turnover combined with increased amounts of unmineralized bone (osteomalacia), bone cysts related to β2-microglobulin-associated amyloid deposits, and mixed osteodystrophy in which components of high and low bone turnover are found. The two key factors in renal osteodystrophy are decreased renal conversion of calcidiol to calcitriol and decreased ability to excrete inorganic phosphate.

As renal failure progresses, the glomerular filtration rate (GFR) decreases, resulting in a decreased filtered load of phosphate. As the serum phosphate concentration rises, the serum calcium concentration decreases, and the serum PTH secretion increases. The secondary HPT state is also a result of decreased blood concentration of calcitriol; when GFR decreases below 30 mL/min, the decreased renal mass leads to decreased renal 1α-hydroxylation of calcidiol. Over the short term, the increased serum PTH concentrations provide a temporary and partial correction in the biochemical abnormalities by decreasing renal tubule reabsorption of filtered phosphate, increasing bone reabsorption of calcium and stimulating the renal 1α-hydroxylation of calcidiol. However, over the long term, these effects are pathologic as renal failure progresses, and PTH effects have no influence on the failed kidneys. This maladaptive situation is made worse by the renal failure–associated hyperphosphatemia directly decreasing the renal conversion of calcidiol to calcitriol, leading to less calcitriol inhibition on PTH secretion.

Tertiary HPT results when there is refractory hypersecretion of PTH associated with severe parathyroid gland hyperplasia and neoplastic transformation with monoclonal parathyroid adenomas. Because of the limited effect of PTH on enhancing phosphate excretion in failing kidneys and the continued effect on reabsorption of calcium and phosphate from bone, hypercalcemia develops. The increased calcium-phosphate product leads to metastatic calcification with calcium-phosphate precipitation into soft tissues, joints, viscera, and arteries. Blood vessel involvement can lead to ischemia and gangrene. Tertiary HPT results in subperiosteal resorption, cyst formation, variably diminished bone density, osteitis fibrosa cystica with brown tumors, and fractures. Spine radiographs may show banded sclerosis of the upper and lower margins of the vertebral bodies with rarefaction between them. Skull radiographs may show spotty decalcification ("salt-and-pepper" skull).

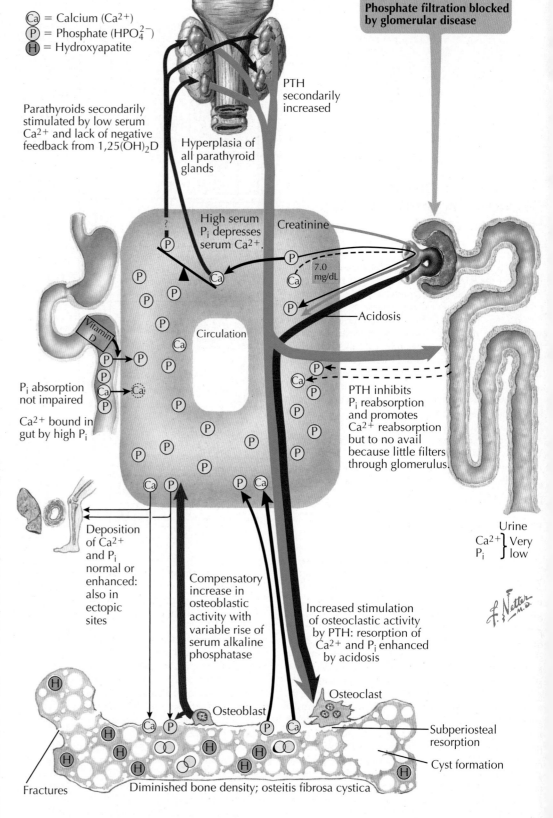

Plate 6.8

Bone and Calcium

BONY MANIFESTATION OF RENAL OSTEODYSTROPHY

Secondary hyperparathyroidism

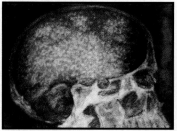

Radiograph shows spotty decalcification of skull ("salt-and-pepper" skull).

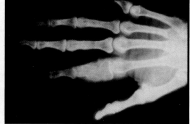

Brown tumor of proximal phalanx

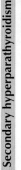

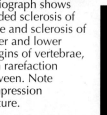

Radiograph shows banded sclerosis of spine and sclerosis of upper and lower margins of vertebrae, with rarefaction between. Note compression fracture.

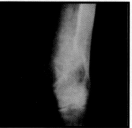

Osteitis fibrosa cystica of distal femur

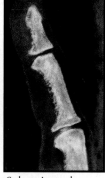

Subperiosteal resorption of phalanges (chiefly on palmar aspect of middle phalanx)

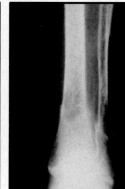

Osteitis fibrosa cystica of tibia with brown tumor

Loss of lamina dura of teeth (*broken lines* indicate normal contours).

RENAL OSTEODYSTROPHY (Continued)

Subperiosteal resorption of the phalanges may be evident—primarily on the palmar aspect of the middle phalanx. In children, renal osteodystrophy results in growth retardation and skeletal deformities.

The most common bony abnormality in patients treated with peritoneal dialysis or hemodialysis is adynamic bone disease—bone turnover does not occur, and bone cell activity is absent. Unlike what is observed with osteomalacia, osteoid formation does not increase. Adynamic bone disease is, in part, a result of excess PTH suppression with calcium-based phosphate binders and vitamin D analogs. Adynamic bone disease predisposes to bone fractures (e.g., hip fracture). This disorder can be confirmed by bone biopsy or by a serum PTH concentration less than 100 pg/mL. The key to treatment is to allow PTH to increase by decreasing or discontinuing calcium-based phosphate binders and vitamin D analogs.

Osteomalacia is the result of decreased bone turnover and an increase in unmineralized bone caused by either vitamin D deficiency or aluminum intoxication (the latter from aluminum-containing antacids). There is decreased bone density with thinning of the cortex. Looser zones are a characteristic radiologic finding in osteomalacia (also see Plate 6.22). Looser zones are pseudofractures or narrow radiolucent lines (2–5 mm in width) with sclerotic borders that lie perpendicular to the cortical margin. Frequently bilateral and symmetric, they are located in the scapula, femoral neck, medial part of the femoral shaft, ribs, pubic and ischial rami, and clavicle. Bone resorption may be seen at the lateral ends of the clavicles. Milkman syndrome refers to the findings of bilateral and symmetric pseudofractures in a patient with osteomalacia. Fractures may occur with minimal or no trauma and usually involve the long bones (e.g., hip), ribs, and vertebral bodies. A bone biopsy—usually obtained from the iliac crest after the administration of

tetracycline markers to determine the rate of new bone formation (see Plate 6.22)—may be needed to determine the pathogenesis of renal osteodystrophy.

Other contributing factors to bone disease in patients with renal failure include vitamin K deficiency (required for carboxylation of bone matrix proteins) and bone morphogenetic protein-7 (required for normal osteoblast differentiation and produced in the normal kidney).

The goals of treatment should be to maintain normal serum calcium and phosphorus concentrations while minimizing the exposure to aluminum. These targets are achieved by a low-phosphate diet, addition of phosphate binders when GFR is below 25% of normal, and vitamin D supplementation to maintain a normal blood concentration of calcitriol. With advanced renal failure and tertiary HPT, parathyroidectomy may be indicated.

Osteomalacia

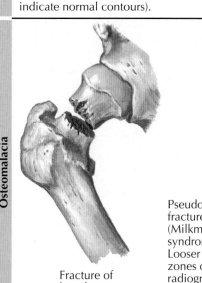

Fracture of long bones

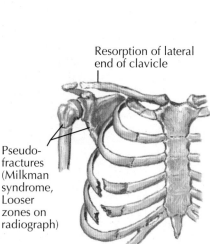

Resorption of lateral end of clavicle

Pseudo-fractures (Milkman syndrome, Looser zones on radiograph)

Fractured ribs

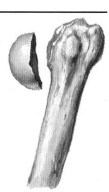

Slipped capital femoral epiphysis

Plate 6.9

Endocrine System: VOLUME 2

HISTOLOGY OF THE PARATHYROID GLANDS IN HYPERPARATHYROIDISM

Primary HPT is caused by a single parathyroid adenoma (89%), multiple ("double") parathyroid adenomas (4%), multigland parathyroid hyperplasia (6%), or parathyroid carcinoma (1%).

PARATHYROID ADENOMA

Most parathyroid adenomas are encapsulated and arise from chief cells; the others are composed of oxyphilic cells. The adenoma is composed of tightly packed sheets, cords, and acini of predominantly chief cells. Clear cells and oxyphilic cells, singly and in groups, are often present, and some adenomas may be composed entirely of oxyphilic cells. The tumor may be homogeneous or nodular. The chief cell of an adenoma is usually somewhat larger than a normal chief cell. The nuclei are variable in size, and mononuclear giant cells with hyperchromatic nuclei, not indicative of malignancy, are often present. Multinuclear giant cells are frequently seen in adenomas. Immunohistochemical staining is typically positive for PTH and chromogranin A. The most important criterion for differentiating an adenoma from chief cell hyperplasia is the identification of normal parathyroid tissue in a patient with an adenoma; this may occur either as a rim outside the capsule of the adenoma or in another gland. This "normal" parathyroid in the presence of an adenoma is composed almost entirely of large, light, inactive chief cells, with abundant glycogen, small Golgi apparatuses, and rare secretory granules. The cells in the adenomas are monoclonal and result from somatic mutations in genes that control growth. For example, the cyclin D1 protooncogene (*CCND1*) encodes a major regulator of the cell cycle. Overexpression of cyclin D1 is found in approximately 30% of parathyroid adenomas. MEN type 1 is caused by germline pathogenic variants in *MEN1*, a tumor suppressor gene, and somatic mutations are found in approximately 15% of sporadic parathyroid adenomas.

PRIMARY CHIEF CELL HYPERPLASIA

Chief cell hyperplasia is much more common than clear cell hyperplasia (the latter is associated with hyperplasia primarily of the superior parathyroid glands). In hyperplasia, all four glands are invariably involved. Each gland is composed of cords, sheets, and acini of tightly packed chief, oxyphilic, and clear cells. The cells are similar in size to or slightly more enlarged than normal cells. The gland is often nodular, owing to separation of the cells by stroma or to aggregation of cell types. In primary chief cell hyperplasia, the appearance of each gland may be identical to that of an adenoma except for the absence of normal parathyroid tissue. Immunohistochemical studies show diffuse staining for PTH and chromogranin A. Parathyroid hyperplasia may be sporadic or associated with a familial syndrome (e.g., MEN 1, MEN 2A, HPT-jaw tumor syndrome, or familial isolated HPT).

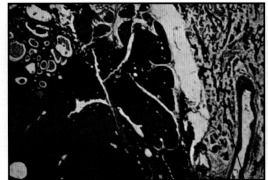

Adenoma. Rim of relatively normal parathyroid tissue about compact adenoma (H&E stain, ×11.5).

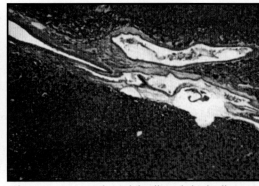

Adenoma. Mixture of oxyphil cells and chief cells in adenoma (H&E stain, ×35).

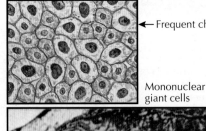

← Frequent characteristics of chief cells in adenomas →

Mononuclear giant cells

Multinuclear giant cells and acinar structures

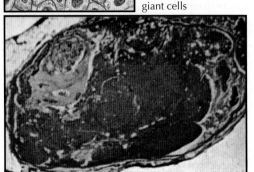

Primary hyperplasia: chief cell

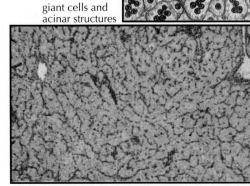

Primary hyperplasia: clear cell

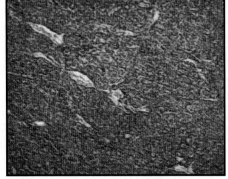

Secondary hyperplasia

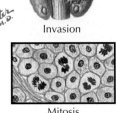

Invasion

Mitosis

Metastases (to lymph nodes, liver, elsewhere)

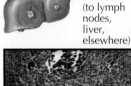

Fibrous bands and hyperchromicity

Carcinoma

PRIMARY CLEAR CELL HYPERPLASIA

The four glands are composed of sheets, cords, and acini of uniform, large (10–40 μm) cells, with distinct cell membranes and empty-appearing cytoplasm (wasserhelle cells). The nuclei are small and densely stained. There is a tendency for nuclear palisading, generally at the pole of the cell adjacent to the stroma and vessel, giving a "bunch of berries" appearance. Immunohistochemical staining is usually weak for PTH and strong for chromogranin A.

SECONDARY PARATHYROID GLAND HYPERPLASIA

Secondary parathyroid gland hyperplasia is often indistinguishable from primary chief cell hyperplasia, although nodularity is somewhat less common in secondary hyperplasia, and each gland is often composed of uniform sheets of small, dark chief cells. Oxyphilic cells and clear cells are occasionally seen. Immunohistochemical staining is typically positive for PTH and chromogranin A.

CARCINOMA

The diagnosis of parathyroid carcinoma is based on local invasion of contiguous tissues or metastases (lymph node or distant). A large, dense, fibrous capsule (with invasion of the capsule) and broad, dense, fibrous bands traversing the tumor are present. The cells are large and uniform and have distinct cell membranes. The nuclei are large, regular, and hyperchromatic. Mitotic figures are almost invariably seen. A rim of normal parathyroid tissue may rarely be noted. Both somatic and germline inactivating pathogenic variants in *CDC73* (formerly *HRPT2*) are responsible for HPT-jaw tumor syndrome, which is associated with an increased risk for parathyroid carcinoma.

Plate 6.10

Bone and Calcium

PATHOPHYSIOLOGY OF HYPOPARATHYROIDISM

The chemical picture of hypoparathyroidism is a low serum calcium concentration (usually <7 mg/dL), a high serum inorganic phosphate (P_i) concentration (typically >5 mg/dL), and decreased excretion of calcium and phosphorus in the urine. These chemical features can be explained by the absence of the major actions of PTH. The calcium level is low because of the following: (1) decreased PTH-dependent stimulation of the osteoclastic activity of bone, causing little resorption of calcium and (2) decreased PTH-dependent stimulation of the renal conversion of calcidiol to the more potent calcitriol, with resultant diminished absorption of calcium from the GI tract. Because the serum calcium level is usually below the kidney threshold of 7 mg/dL, little urinary calcium is found. By contrast, the serum phosphorus concentration is elevated because there is excessive reabsorption of phosphate by the renal tubules, which is not blocked by PTH. The high serum phosphorus level has the additional effect of depressing the serum calcium level. A great deal of calcium is "bound" in the GI tract by the high phosphate concentration, and the action of vitamin D on calcium absorption is less effective in the presence of high phosphate concentrations. The combination of a low serum calcium concentration, a high serum phosphorus level, and a normal alkaline phosphatase concentration in the absence of renal failure or malabsorption is pathognomonic of a state of hypoparathyroidism.

PTH deficiency is most commonly seen as a complication after neck surgery (e.g., subtotal or total thyroidectomy, parathyroid gland surgery, or neck cancer surgery). Surgery-induced hypoparathyroidism may be transient (if viable parathyroid tissue persists) or permanent. Transient hypoparathyroidism may complicate as many as 20% of operations for thyroid cancer that require total or near-total thyroidectomy. Transient hypoparathyroidism is also seen in patients after resection of a parathyroid adenoma associated with severe and long-standing hypercalcemia. In this setting, the normal parathyroid glands are suppressed, and calcium is avidly taken up by the bones ("hungry bone syndrome"). Less commonly, the cause of hypoparathyroidism may relate to autoimmune destruction; abnormal parathyroid gland development; or abnormal regulation of PTH production, secretion, or action.

When hypoparathyroidism is acquired in a patient who has not had neck surgery, it most commonly results from autoimmune destruction of the parathyroid glands. Autoimmune hypoparathyroidism usually occurs as part of the polyglandular autoimmune syndrome type 1; these patients are also at increased risk for primary adrenal insufficiency and chronic mucocutaneous candidiasis (see Plate 8.6). A rarer cause of acquired primary hypoparathyroidism is the development of activating autoantibodies to the CaSR.

GENETIC CAUSES OF HYPOPARATHYROIDISM

Congenital hypoparathyroidism is associated with abnormal parathyroid development or PTH synthesis. Abnormal parathyroid gland development may be

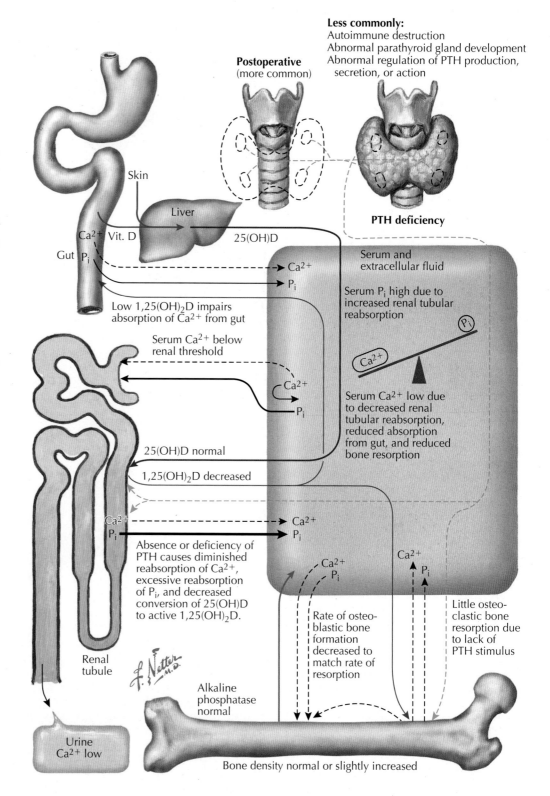

Less commonly:
Autoimmune destruction
Abnormal parathyroid gland development
Abnormal regulation of PTH production, secretion, or action

Postoperative (more common)

PTH deficiency

Skin

Liver

Gut

Ca^{2+} Vit. D
P_i

$25(OH)D$

Low $1,25(OH)_2D$ impairs absorption of Ca^{2+} from gut

Ca^{2+}
P_i

Serum and extracellular fluid

Serum P_i high due to increased renal tubular reabsorption

P_i

Ca^{2+}

Serum Ca²⁺ below renal threshold

Ca^{2+}
P_i

Ca^{2+}

P_i

Serum Ca^{2+} low due to decreased renal tubular reabsorption, reduced absorption from gut, and reduced bone resorption

25(OH)D normal

$1,25(OH)_2D$ decreased

Ca^{2+}
P_i

Ca^{2+}
P_i

Absence or deficiency of PTH causes diminished reabsorption of Ca^{2+}, excessive reabsorption of P_i, and decreased conversion of 25(OH)D to active $1,25(OH)_2D$.

Ca^{2+}

Ca^{2+}
P_i

P_i

Rate of osteoblastic bone formation decreased to match rate of resorption

Little osteoclastic bone resorption due to lack of PTH stimulus

Renal tubule

Alkaline phosphatase normal

Urine Ca^{2+} low

Bone density normal or slightly increased

caused by X-linked or autosomal recessive mutations (e.g., pathogenic variants in *GCM2*, a gene encoding a transcription factor). Pathogenic variants in the gene responsible for the synthesis of preproPTH may result in defects of the production of biologically active PTH. In addition, autosomal dominant activating pathogenic variants in the gene encoding the CaSR decrease the set point for calcium feedback; thus PTH secretion is not triggered until the patient is markedly hypocalcemic. Because of the activated CaSR at the kidney, the urinary calcium excretion is high (unlike what is observed in all other forms of hypoparathyroidism).

PSEUDOHYPOPARATHYROIDISM: HYPOCALCEMIA DESPITE A HIGH SERUM PTH CONCENTRATION

In patients with pseudohypoparathyroidism (PHP), the hypocalcemia stimulates release of PTH from the parathyroid glands. However, because PTH is ineffective in mobilizing calcium from bone or in increasing the renal conversion of calcidiol to calcitriol, hypocalcemia persists. The causes of this clinical scenario include PTH resistance and vitamin D deficiency (see Plates 6.12 and 6.13).

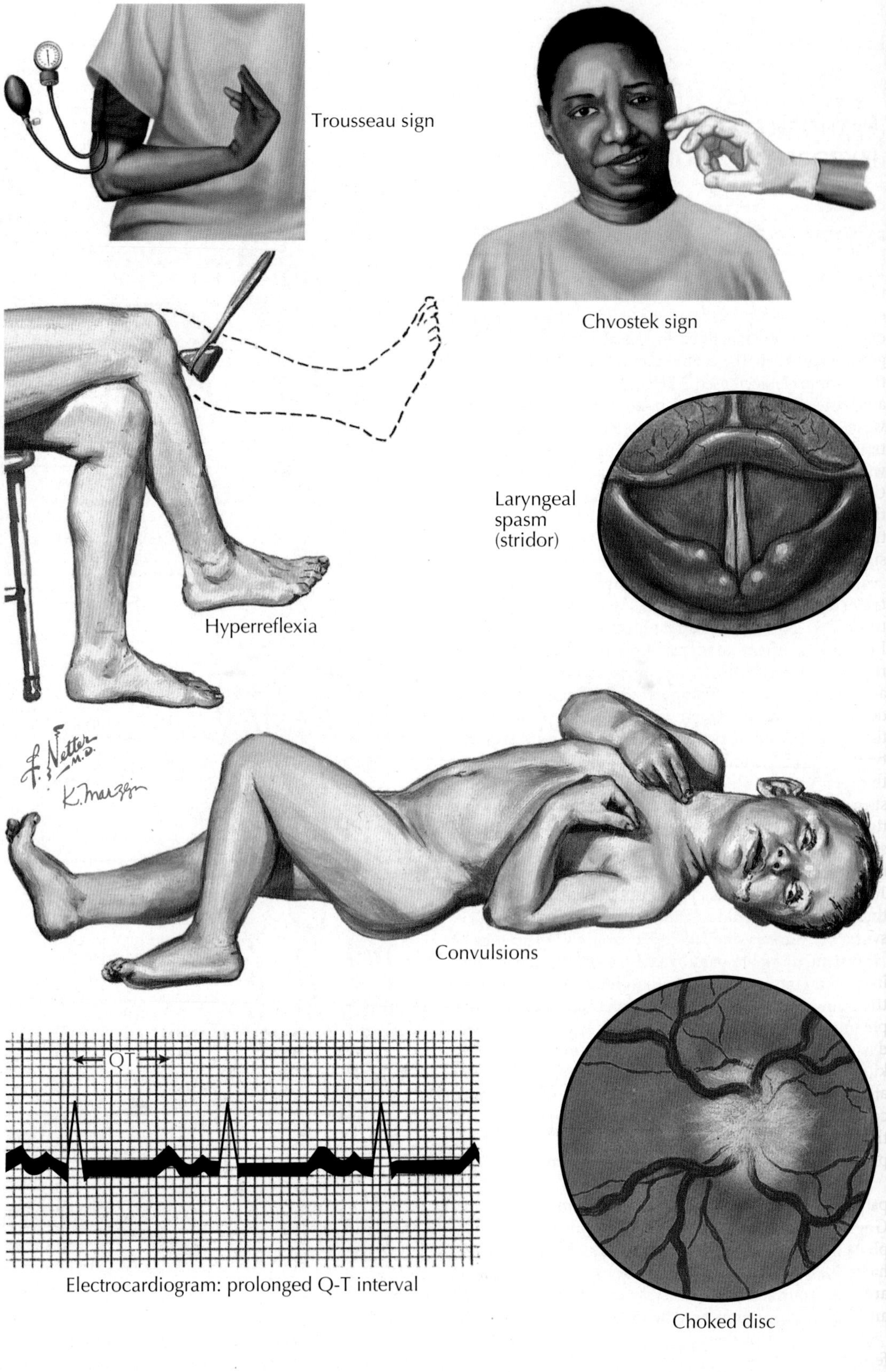

Plate 6.11

Endocrine System: VOLUME 2

Trousseau sign

Chvostek sign

Hyperreflexia

Laryngeal spasm (stridor)

Convulsions

CLINICAL MANIFESTATIONS OF ACUTE HYPOCALCEMIA

The classic manifestations of acute hypocalcemia vary from minor to severe symptoms with tetany, seizures, laryngospasm, papilledema (choked disc), or heart failure. The degree of symptoms relates not only to the severity of hypocalcemia but also to the rapidity of onset. The dominant clinical features of chronic hypocalcemia are cataracts, basal ganglia calcification, extrapyramidal disorders, and changes in dentition.

Tetany is the result of acute increased peripheral neuromuscular irritability; early and mild symptoms include anxiety, muscle spasms and cramps, hyperreflexia, photophobia, diplopia, perioral and acral paresthesias, and hyperirritability. Advanced and more severe symptoms of tetany include carpopedal spasm (the forced adduction of the thumb, extension of the fingers, and flexion of the wrist and metacarpophalangeal joints), laryngospasm and stridor (caused by muscular spasm of the glottis), and seizures (grand mal, petit mal, or focal). Tetany usually does not occur unless the serum total calcium concentration falls below 7.0 mg/dL. However, tetany may be aggravated by alkalosis, hypomagnesemia, and hypokalemia. Patient anxiety related to the perioral and acral paresthesias may lead to hyperventilation, resulting in respiratory alkalosis that further aggravates tetany. Acidosis can completely suppress the clinical manifestations of hypocalcemia.

The Trousseau sign is the induction of carpopedal spasm by inflating a sphygmomanometer cuff above the systolic blood pressure for 3 minutes. For example, if the systolic blood pressure is 120 mm Hg, the sphygmomanometer cuff should be inflated to 140 mm Hg and kept at that pressure for 3 minutes. The ischemia induced by the Trousseau maneuver increases the excitability of the forearm nerve trunks. With a positive Trousseau sign, patients are unable to open the hand.

The Chvostek sign is the demonstration of ipsilateral facial muscle contraction by tapping the facial nerve just anterior to the ear and below the zygoma. In severe hypocalcemic states, contracture of the orbicularis oculi and even contraction of the contralateral facial muscles may be seen. Both the Trousseau and Chvostek signs are not specific for hypocalcemia; they can also be elicited in alkalotic states (e.g., hyperventilation, primary aldosteronism with severe hypokalemia).

Dental anomalies (e.g., defective enamel, dental hypoplasia) can occur if hypocalcemia is present in early

Electrocardiogram: prolonged Q-T interval

Choked disc

development. Chronic hypocalcemia usually results in dry and coarse skin. The fingernails may become brittle and have transverse grooves. Scalp hair can be sparse, coarse, and brittle.

In addition to hypocalcemia-related heart failure, the Q-T interval on electrocardiography may be prolonged. QRS and ST changes may mimic acute myocardial infarction. Hypocalcemia can trigger torsades de pointes.

The most common cause of severe hypocalcemia is acute hypoparathyroidism related to the removal of a parathyroid neoplasm or accidental removal of the parathyroid glands at the time of thyroid surgery.

The diagnosis of severe and symptomatic hypocalcemia is an endocrine emergency, and immediate treatment is indicated to prevent seizures, laryngospasm, cardiac events, and death. Correction of the hypocalcemia reverses the signs and symptoms.

Plate 6.12

Bone and Calcium

PATHOPHYSIOLOGY OF PSEUDOHYPOPARATHYROIDISM

PHP is the result of end-organ resistance to PTH. The key laboratory findings are hypocalcemia, hyperphosphatemia, and increased blood PTH concentration. There are two forms of PHP, known as *type 1* and *type 2*.

PSEUDOHYPOPARATHYROIDISM TYPE 1

PHP type 1 is characterized by decreased renal production of cyclic adenosine monophosphate (cAMP) when exogenous PTH is administered. The pathophysiology of this type of PHP relates to pathogenic variants in the gene encoding the α-subunit of the G protein (*GNAS*) that is coupled to the PTH receptor. Pathogenic variants in *GNAS* lead to lack of adenyl cyclase activation when PTH binds to its receptor. This lack of signal transduction prevents PTH activity. *GNAS* is associated with tissue-specific parental imprinting. For example, *GNAS* expression in the kidney, pituitary, gonads, and thyroid is determined by the maternal allele. This tissue-specific parental imprinting has led to a subclassification of PHP type 1 into three subtypes.

PHP type 1a, also known as *Albright hereditary osteodystrophy*, is caused by an autosomal dominant, maternally transmitted pathogenic variant in *GNAS*. PHP type 1a has a unique phenotype with short stature, a rounded face, obesity, ocular abnormalities, short fourth and fifth metacarpals, dental hypoplasia, developmental delay, intellectual disability, and subcutaneous calcifications (see Plate 6.13). The secondary HPT found in PHP type 1a is ineffective in producing phosphaturia because the renal tubule is relatively unresponsive, but in some instances, the other end organ, bone, can show overstimulation of the osteoclasts, and bone resorptive changes may be seen. PTH is also ineffective in converting calcidiol to the more potent calcitriol. Because individuals with PHP type 1a also have resistance to other G-coupled hormones (at the thyroid, pituitary, and gonads), they may have signs and symptoms of thyroid and gonadal dysfunction.

Pseudopseudohypoparathyroidism occurs when the inactivating *GNAS* pathogenic variant is paternally transmitted. Individuals who are affected have the body phenotype characteristic of Albright hereditary osteodystrophy but without resistance to PTH action at the kidney because of the presence of the normal maternal allele. Thus these individuals have normal blood concentrations of calcium, phosphate, and PTH. However, they can have excessive dermal ossification caused by progressive osseous heteroplasia.

PHP type 1b is caused by maternal transmission of pathogenic variants in the regulatory elements for *GNAS*. These individuals lack the characteristic body phenotype of Albright hereditary osteodystrophy but have PTH resistance at the kidney. Thus patients who are affected have hypocalcemia, hyperphosphatemia, and increased blood PTH concentrations.

PHP type 1c is caused by pathogenic variants that affect the coupling of the G protein to the PTH receptor. Thus the adenyl cyclase system is intact, but it is not coupled to the binding of PTH to its receptor. These patients have the body phenotype characteristic of Albright hereditary osteodystrophy, hypocalcemia, hyperphosphatemia, and increased blood PTH concentrations.

PSEUDOHYPOPARATHYROIDISM TYPE 2

Individuals with PHP type 2 have the same biochemical profile as those with PHP type 1, which includes

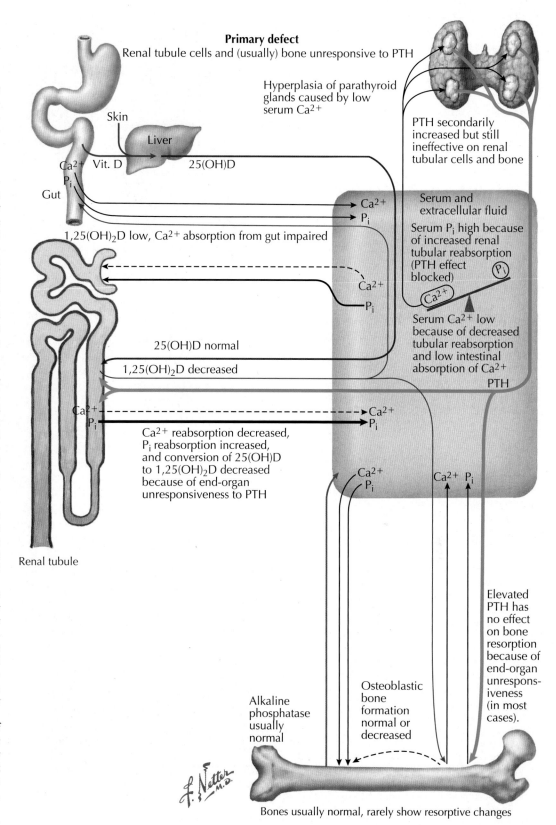

Primary defect
Renal tubule cells and (usually) bone unresponsive to PTH

Hyperplasia of parathyroid glands caused by low serum Ca^{2+}

Skin

Liver

PTH secondarily increased but still ineffective on renal tubular cells and bone

Ca^{2+} Vit. D   25(OH)D
P_i

Gut

Ca^{2+}
P_i

Serum and extracellular fluid

Serum P_i high because of increased renal tubular reabsorption (PTH effect blocked) P_i

Ca^{2+}

1,25(OH)$_2$D low, Ca^{2+} absorption from gut impaired

Ca^{2+}
P_i

Serum Ca^{2+} low because of decreased tubular reabsorption and low intestinal absorption of Ca^{2+}

25(OH)D normal

1,25(OH)$_2$D decreased

PTH

Ca^{2+}
P_i

Ca^{2+}
P_i

Ca^{2+} reabsorption decreased, P_i reabsorption increased, and conversion of 25(OH)D to 1,25(OH)$_2$D decreased because of end-organ unresponsiveness to PTH

Renal tubule

Ca^{2+}
P_i

Ca^{2+} P_i

Elevated PTH has no effect on bone resorption because of end-organ unresponsiveness (in most cases).

Alkaline phosphatase usually normal

Osteoblastic bone formation normal or decreased

Bones usually normal, rarely show resorptive changes

hypocalcemia, hyperphosphatemia, and increased blood concentrations of PTH. Individuals with PHP type 2 do not have the body phenotype characteristic of Albright hereditary osteodystrophy and do not have resistance to other hormones. In addition, they have a normal renal cAMP response to exogenous PTH administration. However, PTH does not lead to phosphaturia. Thus the PTH receptor–adenyl cyclase complex functions normally, but the resistance is at the level of activity of cAMP, suggesting a defect in cAMP-dependent protein kinase A. PHP type 2 is not familial, and the age of onset ranges from infancy to senescence. In most cases the underlying pathogenesis is unknown. However, pathogenic variants in the *PRKAR1A* gene (protein kinase, cAMP-dependent, regulatory, type 1, alpha), which encodes the catalytic subunit of adenylate cyclase, have been found in some cases.

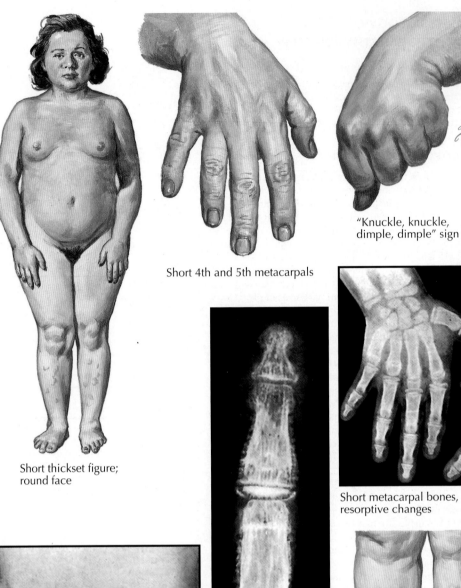

"Knuckle, knuckle, dimple, dimple" sign

Short 4th and 5th metacarpals

Plate 6.13

CLINICAL MANIFESTATIONS OF PSEUDOHYPOPARATHYROIDISM TYPE 1A

PHP is a congenital disorder associated with end-organ resistance to PTH. PHP type 1a, also known as *Albright hereditary osteodystrophy*, is caused by an autosomal dominant, maternally transmitted loss-of-function pathogenic variant in *GNAS* (see Plate 6.12). Children who are affected usually develop symptomatic hypocalcemia between ages 3 and 8 years as serum phosphate and PTH concentrations rise. PHP type 1a has a unique phenotype with short stature, a rounded face, a short neck, obesity, a flattened nose bridge, ocular abnormalities, short fourth and fifth metacarpals, dental hypoplasia, developmental delay, mental retardation, and subcutaneous calcifications. The most outstanding distinguishing feature is brachydactyly with shortening of the fourth and fifth (and sometimes the third) metacarpal and metatarsal bones. This can be demonstrated not only on radiographs but also by having the patient make a fist, which demonstrates the so-called *knuckle, knuckle, dimple, dimple sign*, first described by Albright. Instead of a proper knuckle appearing, the short metacarpal leads to a depression. The short metacarpals result from premature fusion of the epiphyses and failure of the proper appearance of some of the epiphyses, not only of the metacarpals but also of the phalanges, which, therefore, are short. The distal phalanx of the thumb is typically short ("potter's thumb"). Other long bones also can be short (e.g., ulna) or deformed (e.g., bowed radius). The skull can show hyperostosis frontalis interna. In addition to these features, there may be multiple exostoses, resembling a dyschondroplasia, and striking subcutaneous calcification and ossification, at times in the form of osseous plaques or nodules, which may be seen and felt in soft tissues or skin (osteoma cutis). Stone-hard papular or nodular lesions occur at sites of minor trauma (e.g., over the anterior surface of the lower legs). Ocular abnormalities include microphthalmia, strabismus, hypertelorism, diplopia, nystagmus, optic atrophy, and macular degeneration.

Because the *GNAS* gene has a role in many functions throughout the body, patients with PHP type 1a can also have clinical presentations dominated by resistance to other hormones (e.g., TSH, gonadotropins, or growth hormone-releasing hormone). Hypothyroidism is common in individuals with PHP type 1a; serum

Short thickset figure; round face

Short metacarpal bones, resorptive changes

Subperiosteal resorption

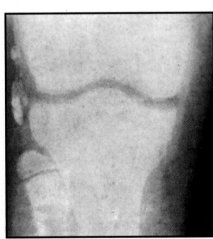

Subcutaneous osseous plaques

Nodules in soft tissue with ulceration

Short metatarsals; deformity of toes

TSH concentrations are above the reference range, and free thyroxine concentrations are below the reference range. Females with PHP type 1a can have delayed puberty, oligomenorrhea, and infertility. Males with PHP type 1a frequently have low serum testosterone concentrations and infertility. Most patients with PHP type 1a have growth hormone deficiency. G proteins are also associated with signal transduction pathways for vision, olfaction, and taste. Thus patients with PHP type 1a may have symptoms related to olfactory, gustatory, and

auditory dysfunction. Mild to moderate intellectual disability is common and presumably related to the effect of the *GNAS* pathogenic variant on brain tissue.

Although PTH can lack activity at the renal tubule, it can be functional at the bone. Therefore all of the manifestations of secondary HPT may be seen at times, especially if the skeleton responds to this stimulation. Subperiosteal resorptive changes in the digits and changes in the epiphyses, which are indistinguishable from renal osteitis fibrosa, can be seen.

Plate 6.14

Bone and Calcium

PATHOGENESIS OF OSTEOPOROSIS

Osteoporosis is a common structural skeletal disorder characterized by low bone mass and bone fragility that increase the risk of bone fracture (see Plates 6.15 to 6.17). Bone structural integrity is jeopardized as the bony microarchitecture is disrupted (e.g., the trabecular plates become perforated and discontinuities develop in the trabecular struts). The cause of low bone mass in patients with osteoporosis is usually a combination of factors that include low peak bone mass, increased bone resorption, and decreased bone formation. High-turnover osteoporosis occurs when increased bone resorption is dominant, and low-turnover osteoporosis occurs when decreased bone formation predominates. Approximately 50% of peak bone mass is genetically determined, and 50% is determined by environmental factors (e.g., physical activity and calcium intake).

The main contributor to osteoporosis in postmenopausal females is estrogen deficiency. When present, estrogen inhibits bone resorption by affecting osteoclast function. Prolonged estrogen deficiency in premenopausal females (e.g., hypogonadotropic hypogonadism that may occur with eating disorders, low body fat, excessive exercise, hypopituitarism, or hyperprolactinemia) also results in decreased bone mass. Estrogen also has a role in maintaining bone density in males; osteoporosis occurs in males who lack estrogen (e.g., aromatase deficiency). Testosterone deficiency in males predisposes them to osteoporosis.

Advancing age, a history of fragility (low-impact trauma) fracture, glucocorticoid therapy, low body mass index, family history of hip fracture, cigarette smoking, excessive alcohol use, and low bone mineral density (BMD) are the most consistent and strongest predictors of bone fracture risk.

Additional risk factors for osteoporosis include dietary deficiency in calcium and vitamin D, medications (e.g., anticonvulsants, heparin, methotrexate), frailty and recurrent falls, prolonged bed rest or general inactivity, neurologic disorders that limit mobility (e.g., paralysis), and weightlessness (e.g., space travel).

Glucocorticoid excess inhibits bone formation by negatively affecting the differentiation and life span of osteoblasts. A dosage-dependent relationship exists between chronic glucocorticoid therapy and fracture risk. Although excess glucocorticoid exposure is most commonly caused by medical therapy for an underlying inflammatory disorder (e.g., asthma, arthritis), it may also result from endogenous Cushing syndrome (pituitary or adrenal dependent).

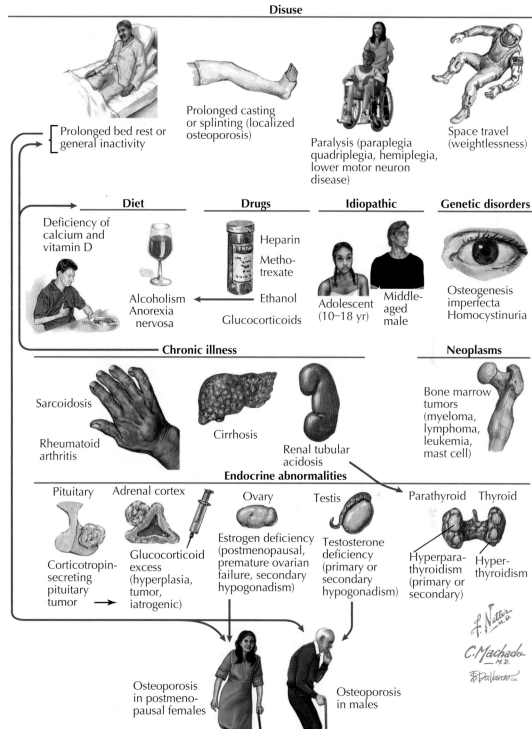

RISK FACTORS FOR OSTEOPOROSIS

Disuse

Prolonged bed rest or general inactivity

Prolonged casting or splinting (localized osteoporosis)

Paralysis (paraplegia quadriplegia, hemiplegia, lower motor neuron disease)

Space travel (weightlessness)

Diet

Deficiency of calcium and vitamin D

Alcoholism
Anorexia nervosa

Drugs

Heparin
Methotrexate
Ethanol
Glucocorticoids

Idiopathic

Adolescent (10–18 yr)

Middle-aged male

Genetic disorders

Osteogenesis imperfecta
Homocystinuria

Chronic illness

Sarcoidosis

Rheumatoid arthritis

Cirrhosis

Renal tubular acidosis

Neoplasms

Bone marrow tumors (myeloma, lymphoma, leukemia, mast cell)

Endocrine abnormalities

Pituitary — Corticotropin-secreting pituitary tumor

Adrenal cortex — Glucocorticoid excess (hyperplasia, tumor, iatrogenic)

Ovary — Estrogen deficiency (postmenopausal, premature ovarian failure, secondary hypogonadism)

Testis — Testosterone deficiency (primary or secondary hypogonadism)

Parathyroid — Hyperparathyroidism (primary or secondary)

Thyroid — Hyperthyroidism

Osteoporosis in postmenopausal females

Osteoporosis in males

HPT (primary or secondary) results in decreasing bone mass and, if untreated, in osteoporosis.

The prevalence of osteoporosis is increased in patients affected by medical disorders that are associated with inflammation (e.g., rheumatoid arthritis, inflammatory bowel disease, sarcoidosis), malabsorption (e.g., celiac disease, cystic fibrosis), renal excretion of calcium (e.g., renal tubular acidosis), thyroid hormone excess (endogenous or exogenous), or direct bone involvement (e.g., multiple myeloma, leukemia, systemic mastocytosis, lymphoma).

The osteoporosis that occurs in females with anorexia nervosa results not only from dietary insufficiencies of calcium and vitamin D but also from estrogen deficiency with secondary hypogonadism.

Genetic disorders that cause osteoporosis include osteogenesis imperfecta (OI) (see Plates 6.25 and 6.26) and homocystinuria.

Plate 6.15

Endocrine System: VOLUME 2

OSTEOPOROSIS IN POSTMENOPAUSAL FEMALES

Osteoporosis in postmenopausal females refers to markedly low bone mass that can occur with estrogen deficiency and aging. Osteoporosis is usually clinically silent until a bone fracture occurs; even then, most vertebral fractures are asymptomatic. The most common sites of bone fracture in postmenopausal females with osteoporosis are vertebral, hip, rib, and distal radius (Colles fracture). Multiple vertebral fractures lead to progressive thoracic kyphosis (dowager's hump), loss of height, and abdominal protrusion. Osteoporosis also predisposes to appendicular fractures (e.g., proximal femur, distal radius, and proximal humerus) that may occur with minor trauma.

Bone strength is derived from bone mass (size, shape, and microarchitecture) and bone turnover status (rates of formation and resorption). Bone mass can be estimated by measuring BMD with dual energy-x-ray absorptiometry (DXA) at the hip and lumbar spine. The risk of fracture is inversely proportional to BMD. The BMD T score is the standard deviation (SD) difference between a patient's BMD and that of a young adult reference population. Normal bone density is defined as a BMD value within 1 SD of the mean in a young adult reference group. Based on increased risk of fracture, osteoporosis is defined as a BMD T score that is −2.5 SD or more below the mean of the young adult reference population. The value obtained when a patient's BMD is compared with that of an age-matched population is termed the *Z score*. A Z score less than −2.0 SD is considered low.

BMD may be low because the individual's peak bone mass reached as a young adult was low, bone formation is decreased, bone resorption is increased, or a combination of all three of these factors. Excessive bone resorption is a major contributor to osteoporosis in postmenopausal females.

Secondary osteoporosis should be considered in all patients with low BMD, and evaluation for the following disorders should be considered: vitamin D deficiency, osteomalacia, hyperthyroidism, HPT, celiac disease, mast cell disease, and hypercortisolism. The first step of evaluation is a thorough interview and physical examination. Laboratory evaluation should include complete blood cell count and measurement of blood concentrations of calcium, phosphorus, liver enzymes, creatinine, TSH, and calcidiol. The role of additional laboratory testing is based on the findings from the history and physical examination. Bone turnover markers may be helpful for some patients in assessing fracture risk, selecting treatment, and monitoring response to therapy.

TREATMENT

Nonpharmacologic treatment—diet, exercise, smoking cessation, fall prevention, and avoidance of medications that increase bone loss (e.g., glucocorticoids)—is key to the successful management of osteoporosis. The daily intake of calcium and vitamin D should average 1500 mg and 800 IU, respectively. Regular weight-bearing exercise (e.g., walking) helps maintain BMD and reduce the risk of hip fracture (the latter is likely because of improved muscular strength).

The decision of when to institute pharmacologic therapy can be guided by fracture risk assessment. A fracture risk assessment tool (FRAX), available from the World Health Organization's website, provides

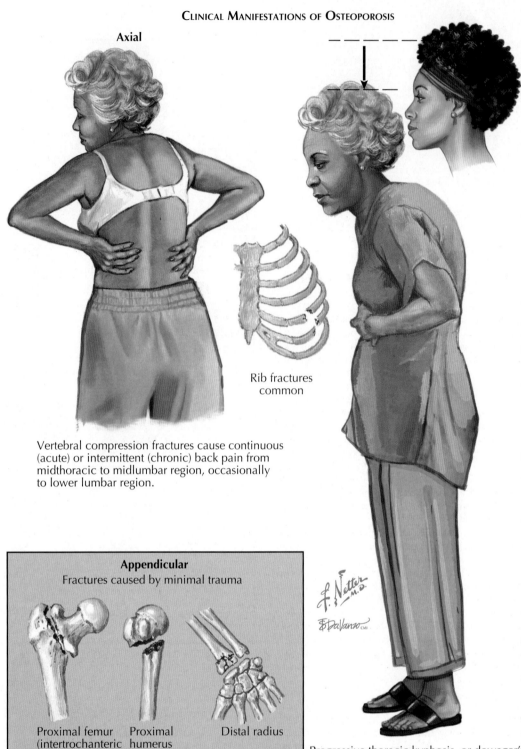

CLINICAL MANIFESTATIONS OF OSTEOPOROSIS

Axial

Rib fractures common

Vertebral compression fractures cause continuous (acute) or intermittent (chronic) back pain from midthoracic to midlumbar region, occasionally to lower lumbar region.

Appendicular
Fractures caused by minimal trauma

Proximal femur (intertrochanteric or femoral neck)

Proximal humerus

Distal radius

Most common types

Progressive thoracic kyphosis, or dowager's hump, with loss of height and abdominal protrusion

personalized data on 10-year probabilities of hip fracture and osteoporotic fractures.

Pharmacologic treatment options include antiresorptive agents and anabolic agents. Antiresorptive medications include estrogen, selective estrogen receptor modulators, bisphosphonates (e.g., orally administered alendronate or risedronate or intravenously administered zoledronic acid), calcitonin, and denosumab, which is a fully human monoclonal antibody to the receptor activator of RANK ligand. The main anabolic agent is PTH 1-34 (teriparatide). Additional anabolic options include abaloparatide and sclerostin inhibitors (e.g., romosozumab).

Treatment effectiveness can be monitored with bone markers at baseline and 3 to 6 months after initiation of treatment. DXA of the lumbar spine and hip should be performed 1 year after treatment initiation and periodically (e.g., every 2–3 years) thereafter.

Plate 6.16

Bone and Calcium

PROGRESSIVE SPINAL DEFORMITY IN OSTEOPOROSIS

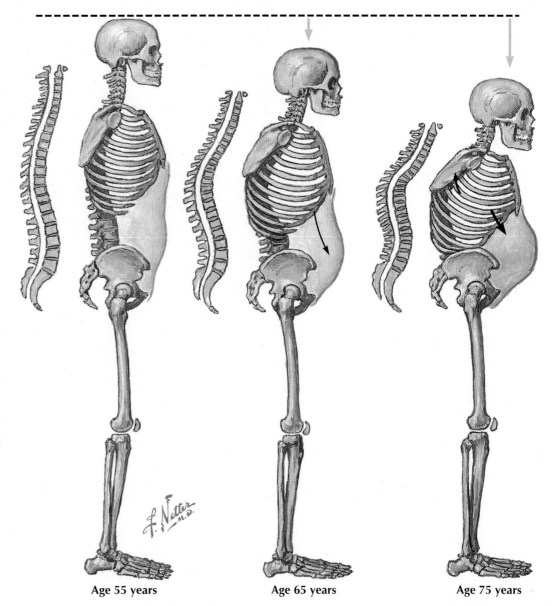

Age 55 years   Age 65 years   Age 75 years

Compression fractures of thoracic vertebrae lead to loss of height and progressive thoracic kyphosis (dowager's hump). Lower ribs eventually rest on iliac crests, and downward pressure on viscera causes abdominal distension.

OSTEOPOROSIS IN MALES

Although BMD is routinely measured in postmenopausal females, it is not often measured in males. Thus osteoporosis in males is diagnosed after low-impact trauma fractures or incidental finding of osteopenia on radiographs performed for other reasons. Osteoporosis may also be found in males because of purposeful case-detection testing in high-risk groups (e.g., those taking glucocorticoid therapy and those with long-standing hypogonadism, HPT, or malabsorption). Compression fractures of the thoracic vertebral bodies lead to loss of height and progressive thoracic kyphosis. With multiple vertebral compression fractures, the lower ribs may reach the iliac crests, and abdominal distension becomes more evident.

Osteoporosis occurs when there is low bone mass and skeletal fragility, leading to an increased risk of fracture (e.g., vertebral bodies, hips, and ribs). Measurement of BMD is a key tool to assess the risk of bone fracture. BMD measurement with DXA at the lumbar spine and hip should be considered in males in the following clinical settings: low-trauma fractures, incidental finding of apparent osteopenia on plain radiographs, loss of more than 4 cm of height, or presence of a known risk factor for osteoporosis (e.g., glucocorticoid therapy, long-standing hypogonadism, HPT, malabsorption). A DXA T score less than or equal to −2.5 is consistent with osteoporosis. A DXA T score between −1.0 and −2.5 is consistent with osteopenia.

A secondary osteoporosis evaluation is indicated in males with low-impact fractures or a DXA bone mass T score less than −2.5. These males should be evaluated for underlying malabsorption (e.g., celiac disease), hypogonadism, Cushing syndrome, hepatic and renal disorders, hypercalciuria, HPT, genetic disorders (e.g., OI), and bone marrow tumors (e.g., multiple myeloma, mastocytosis). Many of these diagnoses may be evident on a thorough interview and physical examination. Initial laboratory testing should include complete blood cell count, serum protein electrophoresis, and measurement of blood concentrations of testosterone, calcium, phosphorus, PTH, calcidiol, tissue transglutaminase antibodies, hepatic enzymes, creatinine, and tryptase. A 24-hour urine collection should be completed to measure cortisol, calcium, and creatinine. Findings on these tests may lead to further case-directed testing (e.g., dexamethasone suppression testing for suspected Cushing syndrome). Measurement of markers of bone formation and resorption may be helpful in selected cases.

TREATMENT

The treatment of osteoporosis in males includes lifestyle measures and pharmacologic therapy.

Lifestyle measures include weight-bearing exercise (e.g., walking), smoking cessation, and avoidance of excessive alcohol use. These patients should be advised to take calcium (1500 mg/d) and vitamin D (800 IU/d) supplementation. If the patient has secondary osteoporosis, treatment of the underlying disorder is the mainstay of therapy (e.g., testosterone replacement in males with long-standing hypogonadism).

Pharmacologic therapy is indicated in males age 50 years or older who have a history of hip or vertebral fracture or who have been diagnosed with osteoporosis on the basis of BMD (DXA T score of −2.5 or less). Pharmacologic treatment for these patients with osteopenia determined by BMD (DXA T score between −1.0 and −2.5) should be considered when the 10-year probability of hip fracture reaches 3% or when the 10-year probability of osteoporotic fractures combined reaches 20%. These 10-year fracture probabilities can be calculated with a FRAX available from the World Health Organization's website. FRAX provides personalized data on 10-year probabilities of hip fracture and osteoporotic fractures. In addition, pharmacologic treatment should be considered for males who do not meet these FRAX risk cutoffs but are at high risk for progressive bone loss (e.g., chronic high-dose glucocorticoid therapy).

Bisphosphonates are the primary form of pharmacologic therapy for osteoporosis in males. Anabolic agents are reserved for patients with progressive bone loss despite secondary factors being addressed and treatment with a bisphosphonate.

Plate 6.17

Endocrine System: VOLUME 2

CLINICAL MANIFESTATIONS OF OSTEOPOROTIC VERTEBRAL COMPRESSION FRACTURES

Compression fractures of the thoracic and lumbar vertebral bodies are the most common type of fracture in patients with osteoporosis. Because of less resistance to anteroposterior displacement, the most common location for vertebral fractures is in the region of the thoracolumbar junction (thoracic vertebrae 11 and 12 and lumbar vertebrae 1 and 2). Vertebral compression fractures may be asymptomatic and detected incidentally on chest radiographs. In patients with osteoporosis, vertebral compression fractures may occur spontaneously or with low-impact trauma. When present, the pain—dull or sharp in character and aggravated by movement—related to a compression fracture may be severe and radiate around the flanks to the anterior abdomen. The severe pain related to vertebral compression fractures usually resolves over 4 to 8 weeks; however, chronic back discomfort may be permanent.

Kyphosis results from multiple thoracic vertebral compression fractures. Both the kyphosis and the loss of vertical vertebral body height lead to loss of total body height. Patients with thoracic kyphosis may present with multiple symptoms. For example, neck discomfort may result from the persistent neck extension required to keep the head vertical. Also, with height loss, compression of the abdominal organs causes increased abdominal prominence and restrictive pulmonary physiology. The lowest rib may contact the iliac crest and cause pain near the 12th thoracic vertebral body and at the iliac crest.

The occurrence of a vertebral fracture is highly predictive of future vertebral fractures; approximately 20% of these patients experience a second fracture within 1 year of their first one.

The types of vertebral fractures include anterior wedge, biconcave ("codfish") deformity, and compression. Fractures can be graded as grade 1, 20% to 25% deformity; grade 2, 26% to 40% deformity; and grade 3, more than 40% deformity.

EVALUATION AND TREATMENT

Patients with symptoms consistent with acute vertebral fracture should be evaluated with plain spine films. If radicular symptoms are present, magnetic resonance imaging (MRI) of the spine may be needed. BMD testing

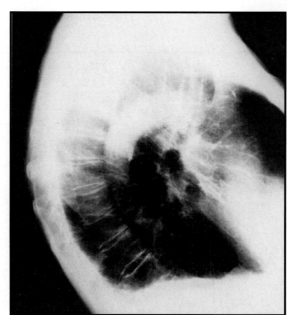
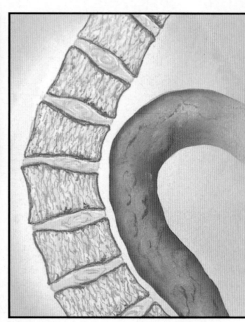

Marked kyphosis is evident. Anterior wedge and biconcave (codfish) deformities are present.

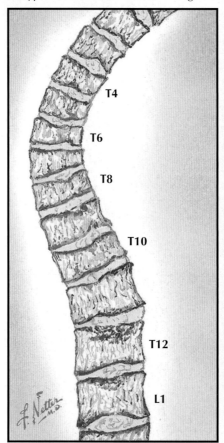
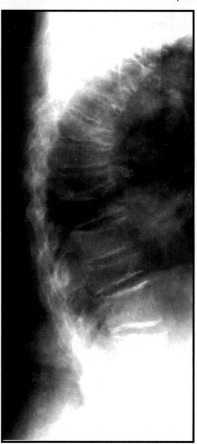

Multiple grade 3 compression fractures are evident in the thoracic vertebral bodies, resulting in marked kyphosis.

is indicated in all patients with vertebral compression fractures. The underlying cause of the vertebral fracture should be determined to direct disease-specific therapy to prevent future fractures. For example, if postmenopausal osteoporosis is the underlying cause predisposing the patient to vertebral fractures, treatment with an antiresorptive agent (e.g., bisphosphonates) should be considered.

Pain control, with nonopioid medications if possible, is important to allow normal physical activity. For patients with severe or persistent pain, vertebroplasty or kyphoplasty should be considered. These interventions involve the percutaneous injection of polymethylmethacrylate bone cement into the collapsed vertebral body, which resolves the acute pain and prevents long-term pain and height loss.

Plate 6.18

Bone and Calcium

NUTRITIONAL-DEFICIENCY RICKETS AND OSTEOMALACIA

Calcium and phosphate—the two main mineral components of bone—are required for normal bone growth and mineralization. Rickets occurs in children with deficient mineralization at the growth plate and causes widened and irregular epiphyseal plates. Osteomalacia refers to deficient mineralization of bone matrix, resulting in uncalcified osteoid seams, soft bones with bowing, and pseudofractures. Nutritional-deficiency rickets and osteomalacia may result from deficiencies in calcium, phosphate, or both.

Calcipenic rickets and osteomalacia are caused by decreased intestinal absorption of calcium, either because of lack of dietary calcium or decreased absorption of intestinal calcium. Decreased absorption of intestinal calcium occurs with malabsorption (e.g., celiac disease) and with decreased action of vitamin D at its receptor—a result of vitamin D deficiency, a defect in the 1α-hydroxylation of vitamin D, or an abnormality at the vitamin D receptor. The hypocalcemia of calcipenic rickets and osteomalacia leads to secondary HPT, which may partially correct the hypocalcemia, but because of increased urinary inorganic phosphate excretion, it also results in hypophosphatemia. Thus with nutritional-deficiency rickets and osteomalacia, the serum phosphorus concentration is below the lower limit of the reference range, and the serum calcium concentration is in the low-normal range or below the lower limit of the reference range. In addition, secondary HPT leads to increased osteoclastic reabsorption of bone. Increased osteoblastic activity with deposition of bone matrix occurs in response to the osteoclast activation. However, the bone matrix cannot be mineralized because of low blood levels of calcium and phosphorus, leading to rickets in children and osteomalacia in adults.

Vitamin D (calciferol) is a fat-soluble compound with a four-ringed cholesterol structure. The synthesis of vitamin D_3 (cholecalciferol) from 7-dehydrocholesterol occurs in the skin with exposure to ultraviolet rays in sunlight (photoisomerization). Vitamin D in the form of ergocalciferol (vitamin D_2) is ingested in the diet, primarily from plants, fish, eggs, and fortified products (e.g., milk and cereals). Vitamins D_3 and D_2 are hydroxylated in the liver by 25-vitamin D hydroxylase to form calcidiol. Calcidiol is 1α-hydroxylated in the proximal convoluted tubule cells of the kidney to form to the more potent calcitriol. Vitamin D deficiency can occur at multiple levels—decreased exposure to sunlight; decreased dietary intake of vitamin D; decreased GI absorption of vitamin D (e.g., after gastric surgery or with long-term, high-dose glucocorticoid therapy); decreased hepatic 25-hydroxylation of vitamin D (e.g., in premature infants, in patients with advanced liver disease) or renal 1α-hydroxylation of vitamin D; accelerated breakdown of vitamin D at the liver (e.g., with medications that induce P450 enzyme activity such as anticonvulsants); renal loss of vitamin D (e.g., nephrotic syndrome); or end-organ insensitivity to vitamin D (see Plate 6.19).

Vitamin D–deficient rickets usually presents in the first 3 years of life, when bone growth is high and exposure to sunlight may be limited. Vitamin D in fetuses is dependent on placental transfer of maternal calcidiol. Adequate vitamin D in infants is dependent on dietary intake and exposure to sunlight. Infants and children require approximately 400 IU of vitamin D per day. Whereas breast milk contains 25 IU of vitamin D per liter, infant formulas contain at least 400 IU of vitamin D per liter. Thus breastfed infants are at increased risk for vitamin D deficiency and should be supplemented with 400 IU vitamin D daily.

TREATMENT

Effective treatment of vitamin D–deficient rickets and osteomalacia can usually be accomplished with vitamin D_2. The treatment dosage of vitamin D_2 is adjusted based on patient age and clinical response. Optimizing calcium intake is also important (≥1000 mg/d of total dietary calcium). Treatment effectiveness should be monitored by measurement of serum calcium, phosphorus, calcidiol, and alkaline phosphatase. Urinary calcium excretion can also be monitored to document recovery. Radiographs should be obtained to document bone healing.

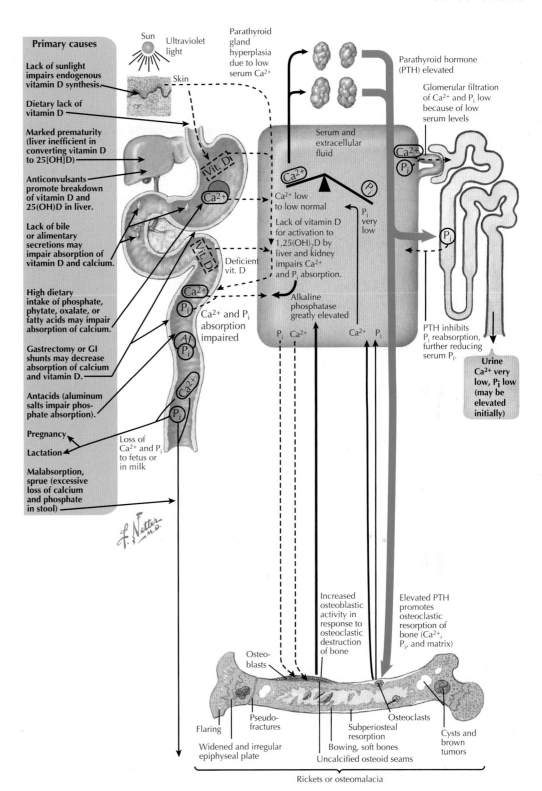

Primary causes

Lack of sunlight impairs endogenous vitamin D synthesis.

Dietary lack of vitamin D

Marked prematurity (liver inefficient in converting vitamin D to 25[OH]D)

Anticonvulsants promote breakdown of vitamin D and 25(OH)D in liver.

Lack of bile or alimentary secretions may impair absorption of vitamin D and calcium.

High dietary intake of phosphate, phytate, oxalate, or fatty acids may impair absorption of calcium.

Gastrectomy or GI shunts may decrease absorption of calcium and vitamin D.

Antacids (aluminum salts impair phosphate absorption).

Pregnancy

Lactation

Malabsorption, sprue (excessive loss of calcium and phosphate in stool)

Sun Ultraviolet light

Parathyroid gland hyperplasia due to low serum Ca^{2+}

Skin

Parathyroid hormone (PTH) elevated

Glomerular filtration of Ca^{2+} and P_i low because of low serum levels

Serum and extracellular fluid

Ca^{2+} low to low normal

Lack of vitamin D for activation to 1,25(OH)$_2$D by liver and kidney impairs Ca^{2+} and P_i absorption.

Alkaline phosphatase greatly elevated

P_i very low

PTH inhibits P_i reabsorption, further reducing serum P_i.

Urine Ca^{2+} very low, P_i low (may be elevated initially)

Deficient vit. D

Ca^{2+} and P_i absorption impaired

Loss of Ca^{2+} and P_i to fetus or in milk

Increased osteoblastic activity in response to osteoclastic destruction of bone

Elevated PTH promotes osteoclastic resorption of bone (Ca^{2+}, P_i, and matrix)

Osteoblasts

Osteoclasts

Cysts and brown tumors

Flaring

Pseudofractures

Subperiosteal resorption

Widened and irregular epiphyseal plate

Bowing, soft bones

Uncalcified osteoid seams

Rickets or osteomalacia

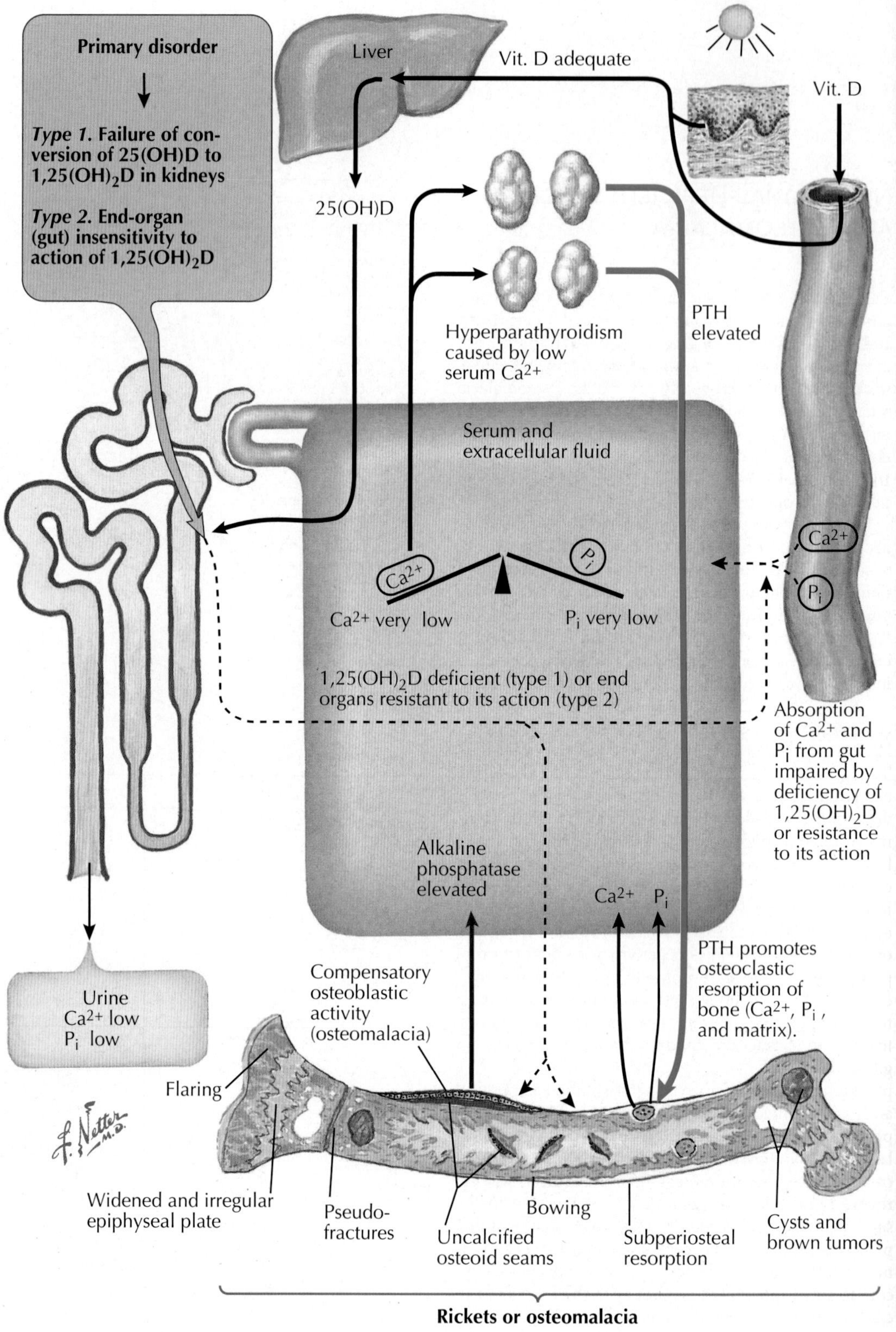

Plate 6.19

Endocrine System: VOLUME 2

PSEUDOVITAMIN D–DEFICIENT RICKETS AND OSTEOMALACIA

Pseudovitamin D–deficient rickets is caused either by lack of calcitriol or by target-organ resistance to the actions of calcitriol. Type 1 pseudovitamin D–deficient rickets occurs when renal 1α-hydroxylase deficiency results in insufficient conversion of calcidiol to the more potent calcitriol. Type 2 pseudovitamin D–deficient rickets results from end-organ resistance to the action of calcitriol and is also referred to as *hereditary vitamin D-resistant rickets*.

TYPE 1 PSEUDOVITAMIN D–DEFICIENT RICKETS: RENAL 1α-HYDROXYLASE DEFICIENCY

Type 1 pseudovitamin D–deficient rickets is an autosomal recessive disorder caused by inactivating pathogenic variants in the gene encoding the 1α-hydroxylase enzyme that leads to no or minimal conversion of calcidiol to calcitriol. Children who are affected usually present in the first year of life with hypocalcemia, hypophosphatemia, phosphaturia, normal or increased blood concentrations of calcidiol, decreased blood concentrations of calcitriol, elevated blood concentrations of alkaline phosphatase, increased blood concentrations of PTH, and the typical signs and symptoms of rickets and osteomalacia (see Plates 6.18 and 6.21). Additional presenting symptoms include motor retardation, muscle weakness, and growth failure.

The mainstay of therapy for patients with renal 1α-hydroxylase deficiency is lifelong administration of calcitriol in physiologic doses (e.g., 1 μg/d) with treatment goals of healing the bones and maintaining normal blood concentrations of calcium, phosphorus, PTH, creatinine, and alkaline phosphatase. Adequate calcium supplementation is important, especially during the bone-healing phase. Overtreatment with calcitriol—resulting in hypercalcemia, hypercalciuria, and nephrocalcinosis—should be avoided.

TYPE 2 PSEUDOVITAMIN D–DEFICIENT RICKETS: HEREDITARY VITAMIN D-RESISTANT RICKETS

Hereditary vitamin D-resistant rickets is an autosomal recessive disorder resulting from pathogenic variants in the gene encoding the vitamin D receptor, which lead to decreased target-organ responsiveness to calcitriol. The clinical presentation depends on the pathogenic

variant and the amount of residual vitamin D-receptor activity. Children who are affected usually present in the first 2 years of life with hypocalcemia, hypophosphatemia, phosphaturia, blood concentrations of calcitriol increased three- to fivefold above the upper limit of the reference range, elevated blood concentrations of alkaline phosphatase, increased blood concentrations of PTH, and the typical signs and symptoms of rickets and osteomalacia (see Plates 6.18 and 6.21). The lack of vitamin D-receptor activation in keratinocytes causes alopecia totalis in some kindreds.

In addition to oral calcium supplementation, administration of high-dose calcitriol (e.g., 5–60 μg/d) in an attempt to overcome the receptor resistance should be tried in these patients. If high-dose calcitriol is ineffective, long-term, intravenously administered calcium infusions should be considered. Treatment effectiveness should be monitored with bone radiographs and measurement of blood levels of calcium, phosphorus, PTH, creatinine, and alkaline phosphatase. The correct calcitriol dosage is the dosage that heals the rachitic bone and normalizes the laboratory parameters.

Primary disorder

Type 1. Failure of conversion of 25(OH)D to 1,25(OH)$_2$D in kidneys

Type 2. End-organ (gut) insensitivity to action of 1,25(OH)$_2$D

Liver

Vit. D adequate

Vit. D

25(OH)D

Hyperparathyroidism caused by low serum Ca^{2+}

PTH elevated

Serum and extracellular fluid

Ca^{2+}

P$_i$

Ca^{2+} very low

P$_i$ very low

1,25(OH)$_2$D deficient (type 1) or end organs resistant to its action (type 2)

Ca^{2+}

P$_i$

Absorption of Ca^{2+} and P$_i$ from gut impaired by deficiency of 1,25(OH)$_2$D or resistance to its action

Alkaline phosphatase elevated

Ca^{2+} P$_i$

PTH promotes osteoclastic resorption of bone (Ca^{2+}, P$_i$, and matrix).

Urine
Ca^{2+} low
P$_i$ low

Compensatory osteoblastic activity (osteomalacia)

Flaring

Widened and irregular epiphyseal plate

Pseudo-fractures

Uncalcified osteoid seams

Bowing

Subperiosteal resorption

Cysts and brown tumors

Rickets or osteomalacia

Plate 6.20

Bone and Calcium

HYPOPHOSPHATEMIC RICKETS

Hypophosphatemic rickets is caused by renal inorganic phosphate wasting, either in isolation or as a component of a more generalized renal disorder (e.g., Fanconi syndrome). The usual biochemical profile includes hypophosphatemia, normal serum calcium concentration, normal serum PTH concentration, and increased blood concentration of fibroblast growth factor 23 (FGF23). The most common hereditary form of hypophosphatemic rickets is X-linked followed by autosomal dominant forms (associated with activating pathogenic variants in the *FGF23* gene), autosomal recessive forms, and forms associated with hypercalciuria (e.g., Dent disease). Several forms of autosomal recessive hypophosphatemic rickets have been described and include inactivating pathogenic variants in the dentin matrix protein 1 gene [*DMP1*] that result in increased *FGF23* expression; inactivating pathogenic variants in the ectonucleotide pyrophosphatase/phosphodiesterase 1 gene [*ENPP1*], which encodes the enzyme critical for the generation of the mineralization inhibitor, pyrophosphate; and pathogenic variants in the *FAM20C* gene that encodes a protein kinase that phosphorylates FGF23. If the onset of hypophosphatemia is delayed until adolescence, the differential diagnosis should include tumor-induced osteomalacia (see later).

X-LINKED HYPOPHOSPHATEMIC RICKETS

The incidence of X-linked hypophosphatemic rickets is approximately 1 case per 20,000 live births. Pathogenic variants in the phosphate-regulating endopeptidase homolog on the X chromosome gene (*PHEX*) are responsible for this disorder. Although penetrance is 100%, the expression is variable, even in individuals who are affected from the same kindred. *PHEX* regulates the degradation and production of FGF23. Excess circulating levels of FGF23 mediate renal phosphate wasting by inhibiting phosphate reabsorption by the renal sodium-phosphate cotransporter. Children with X-linked hypophosphatemic rickets usually present with typical signs and symptoms of osteomalacia (see Plate 6.21) and retarded linear growth. Additional findings unique to X-linked hypophosphatemic rickets include calcification of ligaments and tendons (enthesopathy) and abnormal dentin predisposing to early tooth decay and tooth abscesses. Typical laboratory findings include low serum concentrations of phosphorus and calcitriol (the effects of FGF23 at the renal tubule also impair calcitriol synthesis), increased serum FGF23 concentration and 24-hour urinary phosphate excretion, normal to increased blood concentrations of PTH and alkaline phosphatase, and normal blood concentrations of calcium and calcidiol. The diagnosis can be confirmed with molecular genetic testing for germline pathogenic variants in *PHEX*.

In the past, treatment in children included orally administered phosphate (sodium phosphate or potassium phosphate) and calcitriol. The treatment goals include decreasing the severity of the bony abnormalities, optimizing normal growth, and reducing joint and bone pain. Unfortunately, treatment with phosphate and calcitriol frequently did not meet these objectives. In 2018 the US Food and Drug Administration (FDA) approved a human anti-FGF23 monoclonal antibody (burosumab), and it has proven to be a more effective therapeutic option. Burosumab is administered every 2 weeks by subcutaneous injection.

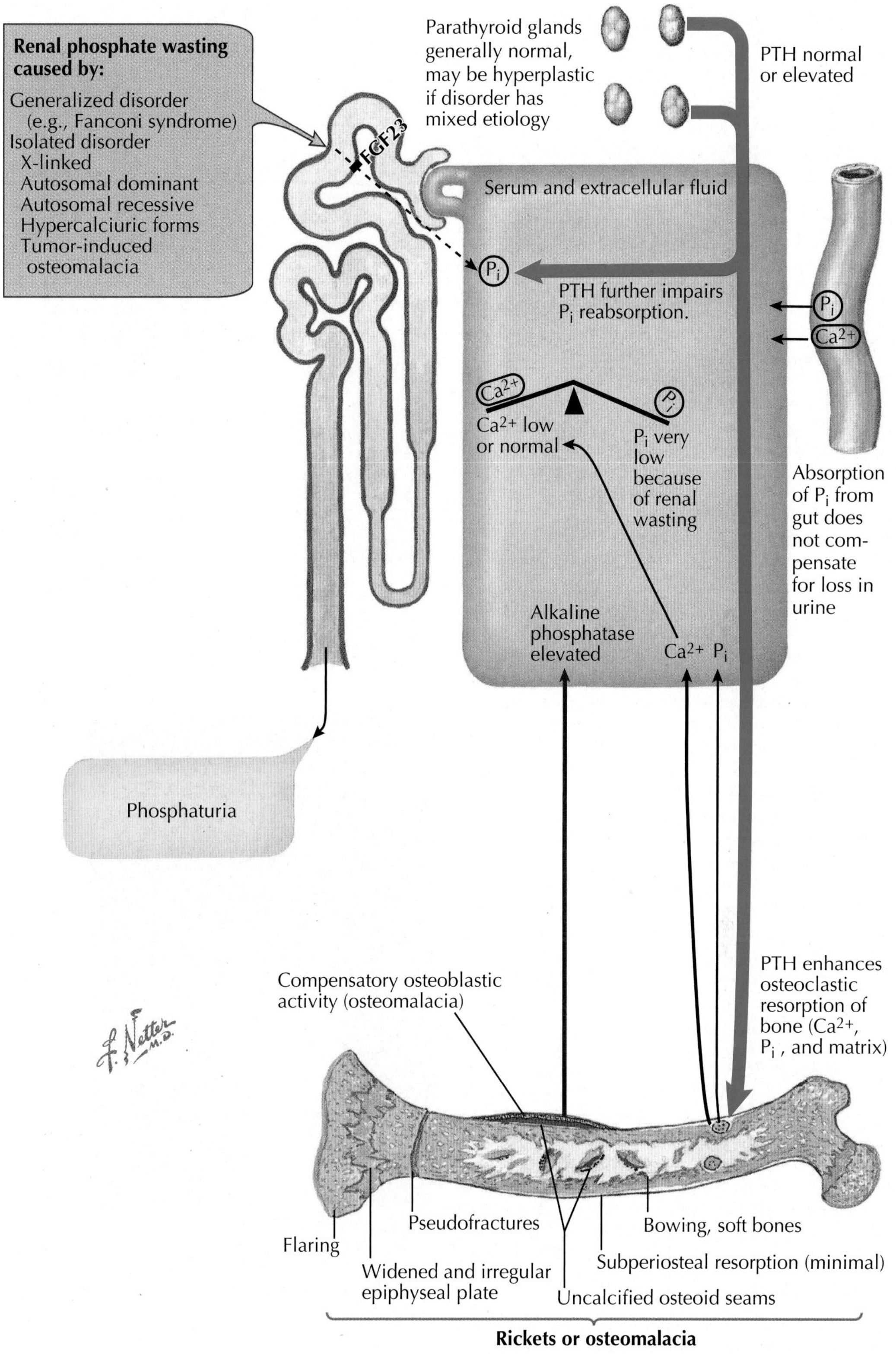

Renal phosphate wasting caused by:

Generalized disorder
  (e.g., Fanconi syndrome)
Isolated disorder
  X-linked
  Autosomal dominant
  Autosomal recessive
  Hypercalciuric forms
  Tumor-induced
    osteomalacia

Parathyroid glands generally normal, may be hyperplastic if disorder has mixed etiology

PTH normal or elevated

FGF23

Serum and extracellular fluid

P_i

PTH further impairs P_i reabsorption.

Ca^{2+}

Ca^{2+} low or normal

P_i

P_i very low because of renal wasting

P_i

Ca^{2+}

Absorption of P_i from gut does not compensate for loss in urine

Alkaline phosphatase elevated

Ca^{2+} P_i

Phosphaturia

Compensatory osteoblastic activity (osteomalacia)

PTH enhances osteoclastic resorption of bone (Ca^{2+}, P_i, and matrix)

Flaring

Pseudofractures

Bowing, soft bones

Widened and irregular epiphyseal plate

Subperiosteal resorption (minimal)

Uncalcified osteoid seams

Rickets or osteomalacia

TUMOR-INDUCED OSTEOMALACIA

Tumor-induced osteomalacia is an acquired disorder caused by small, benign mesenchymal tumors (e.g., sclerosing type of hemangiopericytoma) that hypersecrete FGF23. The clinician should suspect tumor-induced osteomalacia in patients who present with signs, symptoms, and laboratory profiles identical to those observed in patients with X-linked hypophosphatemic rickets but who do not have a personal or family history of the genetic disorder. The main challenge is to localize the small tumor; it may be a small subcutaneous lesion on an extremity or more centrally located. Careful total body palpation can be a key part of the physical examination. Localization studies usually include somatostatin receptor imaging with indium-111-diethylenetriamine pentaacetic acid-pentetreotide or gallium-68 (68-Ga) 1,4,7,10-tetraazacyclododecane-1,4,7,10-tetraacetic acid (DOTA)-octreotate (DOTATATE) positron emission tomography. An apparent tumor found on nuclear imaging should be colocalized with cross-sectional imaging (e.g., MRI or CT). In addition, when nuclear imaging is negative, total body MRI may be helpful. Tumor resection corrects all biochemical abnormalities.

Plate 6.21

Endocrine System: VOLUME 2

CLINICAL MANIFESTATIONS OF RICKETS IN CHILDHOOD

Rickets, a result of chronic hypocalcemia or hypophosphatemia, occurs before closure of the epiphyses and is usually most evident at sites of rapid bone growth (e.g., knees, costochondral junctions, distal forearm). Enlargement of the costochondral junctions results in visible nodules—the "rachitic rosary"—and chest wall deformities (e.g., tunnel chest). The wrist enlarges, and there is bowing of the distal ulna and radius. Impaired mineralization causes weak long bones, leading to weight-bearing-dependent skeletal deformities. For example, whereas an infant who is affected may have posterior bowing of the distal tibia, children who can walk may have lateral bowing of the femur and tibia (genu varum). In infants, the closure of the fontanelles may be delayed, and parietal and frontal bossing and evidence of soft skull bones (craniotabes) may be present. The "Harrison groove" refers to the indentation that results from the muscular pull of the diaphragmatic attachments to the lower ribs.

The clinical presentation of rickets is dominated by skeletal pain, skeletal deformity, fracture, slippage of epiphyses, and retarded growth. Hip pain and deformity may result in a waddling or antalgic gait. In patients with hypocalcemic rickets, extraskeletal symptoms may include decreased muscle tone, proximal myopathy, hypocalcemic seizures, hyperhidrosis, and predisposition to infections.

A uniform component of the laboratory profile in patients with rickets is a marked increase in the blood concentration of alkaline phosphatase. The serum calcium concentration is low in patients with hypocalcemic rickets and is either normal or slightly depressed in those with hypophosphatemic rickets; serum phosphorus is low in both hypocalcemic and hypophosphatemic rickets. The serum PTH concentration is above the reference range in patients with hypocalcemic rickets and is normal in those with hypophosphatemic rickets.

Radiographs of the distal ulna usually show findings of impaired mineralization, widening of the epiphyseal plates, irregular trabeculation, thin cortices, subperiosteal erosions (caused by the marked secondary HPT), and increased axial width of the epiphyseal line. Similar findings are evident in radiographs of the knees, which show flaring of the metaphyseal ends of the tibia and femur and thick and irregular growth plates. The zones of provisional calcification at the epiphyseal-metaphyseal interface are fuzzy and indistinct. With advanced rickets, the epiphyseal plates become more irregular and cupped. Osteopenia is evident in the long bones. Pelvic radiographs may disclose variegated rarefaction of the pelvic bones, coxa vara (where the angle between the ball and the shaft of the femur is reduced to <120 degrees, resulting in a shortened leg), deepened acetabula, pathologic fractures, and pseudofractures (Looser zones). Pseudofractures are narrow (2–4 mm) radiolucent lines with sclerotic borders that are perpendicular to the cortical bone margin and a few millimeters to several centimeters in length. Pseudofractures are frequently bilateral and symmetric and can be seen in the pubic rami, ischial rami, medial part of the femoral shaft, femoral neck, outer edge of the scapula, clavicle, ulna, and ribs. Pseudofractures appear at sites where major arteries cross the bone and may be caused by the mechanical forces of normal arterial pulsation on poorly mineralized bone (see Plate 6.22).

In children with suspected rickets, obtaining thorough dietary (e.g., calcium and vitamin D) and

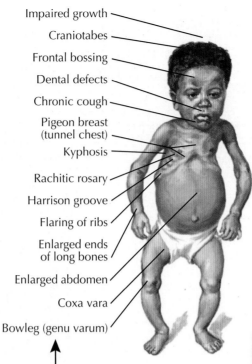

Impaired growth
Craniotabes
Frontal bossing
Dental defects
Chronic cough
Pigeon breast (tunnel chest)
Kyphosis
Rachitic rosary
Harrison groove
Flaring of ribs
Enlarged ends of long bones
Enlarged abdomen
Coxa vara
Bowleg (genu varum)

Clinical findings (all or some present in variable degree)

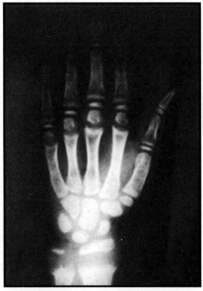

Radiograph of rachitic hand shows decreased bone density, irregular trabeculation, and thin cortices of metacarpal and proximal phalanges. Note increased axial width of epiphyseal line, especially in radius and ulna.

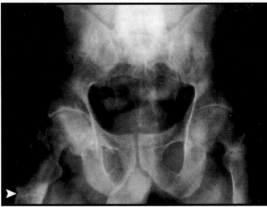

Flaring of metaphyseal ends of tibia and femur. Growth plates thickened, irregular, cupped, and axially widened. Zones of provisional calcification fuzzy and indistinct. Bone cortices thinned and medullae rarefied.

Radiographic findings

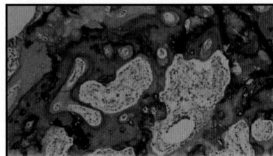

Radiograph shows variegated rarefaction of pelvic bones, coxa vara, deepened acetabula, and subtrochanteric pseudofracture of right femur.

Section of rachitic bone shows sparse, thin trabeculae surrounded by much uncalcified osteoid (osteoid seams) and cavities caused by increased resorption.

medication histories is key. Initial laboratory studies should exclude renal failure and hepatic disease. Laboratory testing should include measurement of blood concentrations of calcium, phosphorus, PTH, and calcidiol. For a description of the typical laboratory findings in patients with nutritional-deficiency rickets, pseudovitamin D–deficient rickets, and hypophosphatemic rickets, see Plates 6.18 to 6.20. Although bone biopsies are usually not needed to

confirm rickets, they show sparse, thin trabeculae; thick layers of uncalcified osteoid (osteoid seams); and large bone resorption cavities.

Effective treatment of patients with rickets is determined by the underlying cause. Deformities that occur before age 4 years usually slowly correct themselves with effective therapy. When deformities occur after age 4 years (e.g., bowleg, knock-knee), they may be permanent.

Plate 6.22

Bone and Calcium

CLINICAL MANIFESTATIONS OF OSTEOMALACIA IN ADULTS

Osteomalacia is a disorder of impaired mineralization of newly formed osteoid in adults. Bone is composed of a collagen matrix (osteoid) distributed in a lamellar pattern and strengthened by pyridinoline crosslinks between the triple-helical collagen molecules, on which alkaline phosphate facilitates the deposition of calcium and phosphorus to form hydroxyapatite (see Plate 6.3). Bone remodeling is a continuous process, and new bone formation requires osteoid production from osteoblasts followed by mineralization of the osteoid. The mineralization step requires an adequate supply of calcium and phosphorus in extracellular fluid and normal bioactivity of alkaline phosphatase. Hypophosphatemia is the most common cause of osteomalacia (see Plate 6.20). Hypophosphatasia, a rare inherited disorder, is associated with low concentrations of alkaline phosphatase in serum and bone that cause defective bone and tooth mineralization, resulting in osteomalacia and severe periodontal disease (see Plate 6.27).

The clinical presentation of osteomalacia ranges from incidental detection of osteopenia on radiographs to markedly symptomatic patients with diffuse bone pain (most prominent in the pelvis, lower extremities, and lower spine), proximal muscle weakness, muscle wasting, hypotonia, and waddling gait. Low-impact fractures of the ribs and vertebral bodies may also be the initial presentation.

Radiographs typically show osteopenia with thinning of the cortex and loss of vertebral body trabeculae. With advanced vertebral body softening, end-plate concavities develop ("codfish" deformities) (see Plate 6.17). Looser zones (pseudofractures) are narrow (2- to 4-mm) radiolucent lines with sclerotic borders that are perpendicular to the cortical bone margin and a few millimeters to several centimeters in length. Pseudofractures are frequently bilateral and symmetric and can be seen in the pubic rami, ischial rami, medial part of the femoral shaft, femoral neck, outer edge of the scapula, clavicle, ulna, and ribs. Pseudofractures appear at sites where major arteries cross the bone and may be caused by the mechanical forces of normal arterial pulsation on poorly mineralized bone. Pseudofractures appear as hot spots on bone scintigraphy. Because Milkman initially recognized pseudofractures in 1930, the term *Milkman syndrome* has been used when a patient with osteomalacia has multiple, bilateral, symmetric pseudofractures. If secondary HPT is present, additional radiographic findings may be evident (e.g., subperiosteal resorption, bone cysts). With severe and long-standing osteomalacia, bowing of the tibia, radius, and ulna, as well as coxa profunda hip deformities, may occur.

The findings on laboratory testing in adults with osteomalacia depend on the underlying pathophysiology. For example, the typical laboratory profile in patients with osteomalacia caused by nutritional vitamin D deficiency includes hypocalcemia, hypophosphatemia, low blood concentration of calcidiol, and increased blood concentration of PTH (see Plate 6.18).

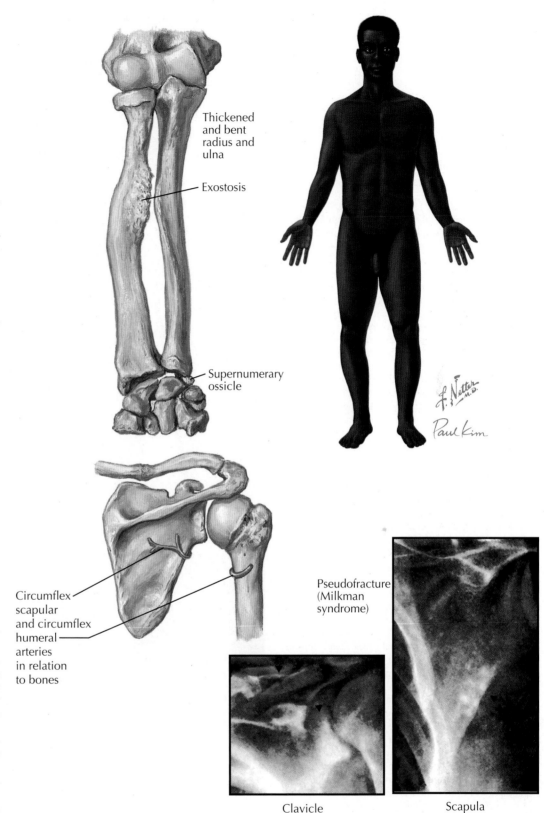

Thickened and bent radius and ulna

Exostosis

Supernumerary ossicle

Circumflex scapular and circumflex humeral arteries in relation to bones

Pseudofracture (Milkman syndrome)

Clavicle

Scapula

If there is doubt about the diagnosis of osteomalacia, a bone biopsy using double labeling with tetracycline can be performed. Tetracyclines are fluorescent; they are deposited in a band at the mineralization front and are easily seen with a fluorescence microscope. A tetracycline is administered for 3 days, and the dosing is repeated 11 to 14 days later. An iliac crest bone biopsy is performed 3 to 5 days after the second tetracycline course is completed. The bone growth rate can be estimated on the basis of the distance between the two bands of deposited tetracycline. Normal bone growth rate is 1 µm per day. In patients with osteomalacia, the bone growth rate is slow, and there are large amounts of unmineralized osteoid.

The treatment of osteomalacia is guided by the underlying cause. For example, patients with vitamin D deficiency should be treated with vitamin D and calcium supplementation.

Plate 6.23

Endocrine System: VOLUME 2

PAGET DISEASE OF THE BONE

Paget disease of the bone (osteitis deformans) is a localized skeletal disorder of uncontrolled, highly active, large osteoclasts that results in increased bone resorption, which triggers intense and chaotic osteoblastic bone formation. Increased local bone blood flow is observed, and fibrous tissue develops in the adjacent bone marrow. The new bone lacks the usual lamellar structure and is disorganized. This disorder affects approximately 3% of adults older than 40 years; it is usually asymptomatic and evolves slowly.

Although the prevalence of Paget disease is the same in males and females, it is more commonly symptomatic in males. The typical age at the time of detection is in the sixth decade of life. The method of detection is frequently incidental (e.g., increased serum alkaline phosphatase observed on routine blood testing or evidence seen on a radiograph done for other reasons). When symptomatic, the primary symptom is pain caused by periosteal stretching or microfractures. The bone pain is aggravated by weight-bearing. The skin may be warm over pagetic bone because of the increased blood flow. Paget disease can affect one bone (monostotic) or multiple bones (polyostotic). The most common bones to be involved are the pelvis, spine, femur, skull, and tibia. With femur or tibia involvement, bowing of the legs is common. The bowing deformities in the bones of the lower extremities lead to gait changes. Transverse traumatic and pathologic bone fractures are common complications.

Spine involvement can lead to kyphosis and symptoms related to spinal cord compression. Hearing loss (caused by compression of the eighth cranial nerve or pagetic involvement of the middle ear ossicles) and skull deformities (frontal and occipital areas) are common when the skull is involved. Compression of the second, fifth, and seventh cranial nerves in the skull may result in visual symptoms and facial palsy. Skull base involvement predisposes to platybasia (invagination of the skull by cervical vertebral bodies) and hydrocephalus by compression of the cerebral aqueduct.

Other complications of Paget disease may develop over time. Bony neoplasia (giant cell tumors [osteoclastomas], fibrosarcomas, chondrosarcomas, and osteosarcoma) occurs more frequently in patients with Paget disease. Primary HPT is also more common. The increased blood flow to bone (when more than 20% of the skeleton is involved) can lead to high-output heart failure.

EVALUATION

A thorough history and physical examination are important. A radionuclide bone scan can be helpful in identifying the sites of involved bone; areas of pagetic bone appear as focal areas of increased uptake. Plain radiographs should be obtained of all the sites identified on the bone scan to confirm Paget disease and its extent. For patients with skull involvement, baseline and annual

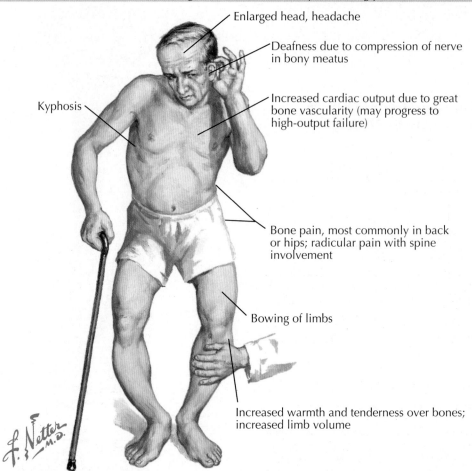

Manifestations of advanced, diffuse Paget disease of bone (may occur singly or in combination)

Enlarged head, headache

Deafness due to compression of nerve in bony meatus

Increased cardiac output due to great bone vascularity (may progress to high-output failure)

Kyphosis

Bone pain, most commonly in back or hips; radicular pain with spine involvement

Bowing of limbs

Increased warmth and tenderness over bones; increased limb volume

Mild cases often asymptomatic (may be discovered incidentally on radiographs taken for other reasons)

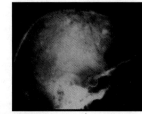

Lateral radiograph shows patchy density of skull, with areas of osteopenia (osteoporosis circumscripta cranii)

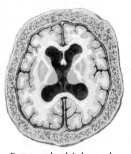

Extremely thickened skull bones, which may encroach on nerve foramina or brainstem and cause hydrocephalus (shown) by compressing cerebral aqueduct.

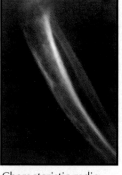

Characteristic radiographic findings in tibia include thickening, bowing, and coarse trabeculation, with advancing radiolucent wedge.

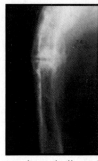

Healing chalk-stick fracture

audiograms should be performed. Because of the increased risk of primary HPT, serum calcium should be measured. If the imaging studies cannot distinguish between Paget disease and metastatic neoplasm, a bone biopsy may be needed. On bone biopsy, an irregular marble bone-type pattern and giant osteoclasts are seen. Measurement of bone markers at baseline and with treatment is useful. Markers of bone formation include blood concentrations of bone-specific alkaline phosphatase (BSAP; reflecting cellular activity of osteoblasts),

osteocalcin (an estimate of the rate of synthesis of osteocalcin by osteoblasts), and C-terminal and N-terminal propeptides of type I collagen (reflecting changes in synthesis of new collagen). Bone resorption can be followed by measuring urinary excretion of hydroxyproline (reflecting breakdown of collagen in bone) and the collagen N-telopeptide crosslinks (NTX) and C-telopeptide crosslinks (CTX). Both the resorption and synthetic markers are increased in patients with untreated Paget disease and normalize with effective treatment.

Plate 6.24

Bone and Calcium

PATHOGENESIS AND TREATMENT OF PAGET DISEASE OF THE BONE

The cause of Paget disease may be a viral trigger superimposed on a genetic predisposition. Viral inclusions are common in the pagetic osteoclasts and are absent in normal osteoclasts. Approximately 30% of patients with Paget disease have a family history of this disorder. The understanding of this genetic predisposition is evolving; pathogenic variants in the ubiquitin-associated domain of the gene encoding sequestosome 1 (SQSTM1) have been found in patients with familial and sporadic Paget disease. Likely a consequence of Paget disease, primary HPT is also more common in patients who are affected.

Most patients with Paget disease are asymptomatic and do not require treatment. The main indications for treatment are to ameliorate symptoms (e.g., bone pain, nerve compression) and to prevent complications. Treatment should be considered in asymptomatic patients who have moderately active disease (e.g., serum alkaline phosphatase concentration higher than threefold above the upper limit of the reference range), sites of disease that can predispose to complications (e.g., major weight-bearing bones, joints), or extensive skull involvement. Also, early treatment in young patients should be considered with a goal of preventing more advanced disease.

The key to treatment is to suppress osteoclastic activity. In the past, the cornerstones of pharmacologic therapy were calcitonin and plicamycin. However, bisphosphonates specifically inhibit osteoclast activity and are the treatment of choice. Bisphosphonates (e.g., etidronate, pamidronate, alendronate, tiludronate, risedronate, and zoledronic acid) are long-acting pyrophosphate analogs that are poorly absorbed from the GI tract. They are given either in large oral doses or intravenously. For example, in patients with mild disease, a single dose of intravenous pamidronate or zoledronic acid may maintain a biochemical remission for 12 to 18 months. The main adverse effect of intravenous bisphosphonates is a flu-like symptom complex in 20% of patients that lasts for 1 or 2 days after the infusion. With oral bisphosphonates, the main adverse effect is esophageal irritation; thus they should be taken in the fasting state with 240 mL of water, and patients should remain in the upright position for at least 30 minutes. Oral bisphosphonates are administered for 4 to 6 months or until the bone markers normalize. Because bisphosphonates can lower the serum calcium level and cause secondary HPT, all patients should take optimal oral calcium and vitamin D supplementation. Adequate vitamin D repletion should be documented with measurement of the serum calcidiol concentration.

Measurement of bone resorption and formation markers at baseline and with treatment is useful. With bisphosphonate treatment, resorption markers decrease first followed by bone formation markers. Markers of bone formation include blood concentrations of BSAP (reflecting cellular activity of osteoblasts and the single best marker of treatment efficacy), osteocalcin

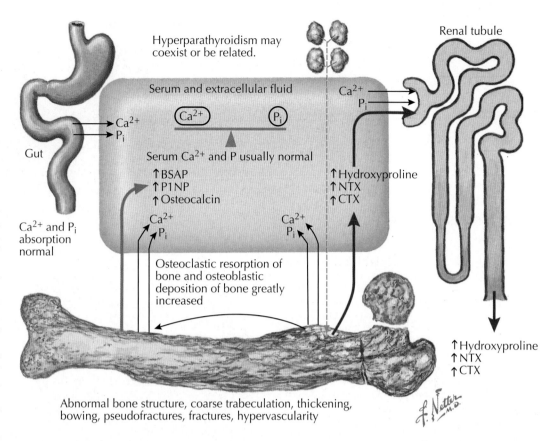

Serum and extracellular fluid

Ca^{2+} and P_i absorption normal

Serum Ca^{2+} and P usually normal

↑BSAP
↑P1NP
↑Osteocalcin

Hyperparathyroidism may coexist or be related.

Renal tubule

↑Hydroxyproline
↑NTX
↑CTX

Osteoclastic resorption of bone and osteoblastic deposition of bone greatly increased

↑Hydroxyproline
↑NTX
↑CTX

Abnormal bone structure, coarse trabeculation, thickening, bowing, pseudofractures, fractures, hypervascularity

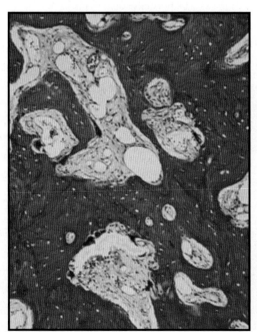

Section of bone shows intense osteoclastic and osteoblastic activity and mosaic of lamellar bone.

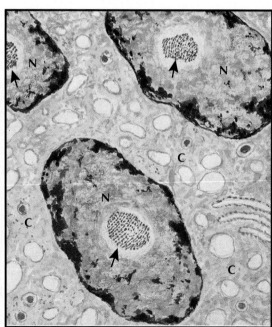

Electron-microscopic view of multinucleated osteoclast with nuclear inclusions that may be viruses (*arrows*). C = cytoplasm; N = nuclei.

(an estimate of the rate of synthesis of osteocalcin by osteoblasts), and N-terminal propeptides of type I collagen (reflecting changes in synthesis of new collagen). Bone resorption can be followed by measuring urinary excretion of hydroxyproline (reflecting breakdown of collagen in bone) and the collagen NTX and CTX. Both the resorption and synthetic markers are increased in patients with untreated Paget disease and normalize with effective treatment. Many clinicians simply follow BSAP and consider measurement of

other bone formation or resorption markers if the clinical course is atypical.

BSAP can be periodically measured every 2 to 6 months after a single intravenous infusion of a bisphosphonate, and when they start to rise above the reference range, an additional infusion can be considered. A similar strategy with oral bisphosphonates can be used: treatment with an oral agent for 4 to 6 months or until the bone markers normalize, then treatment reinitiation when the bone markers become abnormal again.

Plate 6.25

Endocrine System: VOLUME 2

MODERATE TO SEVERE OSTEOGENESIS IMPERFECTA TYPES III, IV, V, VI, VII, AND VIII

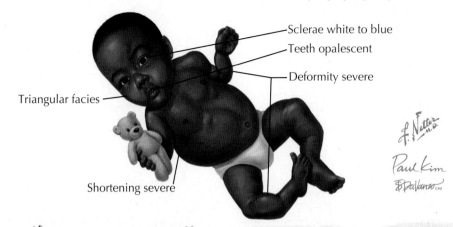

Triangular facies

Sclerae white to blue
Teeth opalescent
Deformity severe

Shortening severe

OSTEOGENESIS IMPERFECTA

OI, frequently referred to as *brittle bone disease*, is a rare (1 per 200,000 live births) hereditary connective tissue disorder with a variable clinical presentation. Moderate to severe OI is evident in infancy with bone fractures associated with little or no trauma; mild OI may not become clinically evident until adulthood when individuals who are affected present with premature osteoporosis.

Approximately 90% of individuals with OI have autosomal dominant germline pathogenic variants in the genes encoding the proteins that form type I collagen (*COL1A1* and *COL1A2*). Both normal structure and normal amount of type I collagen are necessary for normal bones, sclerae, tendons, ligaments, teeth, and skin. Although there are 16 subtypes of OI, it is more practical to classify OI into three groups based on severity of disease and genetic testing.

- **Mild OI:** OI type I is caused by autosomal dominant pathogenic variants in *COL1A1* or *COL1A2* and is the least severe type of OI. Type I OI is associated with mild manifestations, including infrequent bone fractures (primarily long bones and ribs), normal stature, premature osteoporosis, mild scoliosis, blue sclerae, teeth that appear normal or opalescent, and premature hearing loss. Locomotion is usually normal.
- **Moderate to severe OI:** Moderate-to-severe forms of OI include types III (autosomal dominant *COL1A1* or *COL1A2* pathogenic variants), IX (autosomal recessive pathogenic variants in peptidyl-prolyl isomerase B [*PPIB*]), XV (homozygous or compound heterozygous pathogenic variants in *WNT1*), and XVI (homozygous pathogenic variants in the cAMP-responsive element binding protein 3-like 1 [*CREB3L1*]). Children present with frequent fractures and severe limb deformities. Fractures can even include the ossicles of the ear, resulting in conductive hearing loss. Kyphoscoliosis and short stature are typical of moderate-to-severe OI. Locomotion is usually severely limited. Hypermobility of the joints at the wrists, hands, and feet may be evident. Patients with OI types IV (autosomal dominant *COL1A1* or *COL1A2* pathogenic variants), V (autosomal dominant pathogenic variants in interferon-induced transmembrane protein 5 [*IFITM5*]), VI (pathogenic variants in FK506-binding protein 10 [*FKBP10*]), VII (recessive pathogenic variants in cartilage-associated protein [*CRTAP*]), or VIII (recessive pathogenic variants in leprecan-like 1 [*LEPRE1*]) can have normal sclerae. Type III is a progressive deforming form of OI that eventuates in the use of a wheelchair. Type IV OI is associated with less growth retardation than type III. Type V

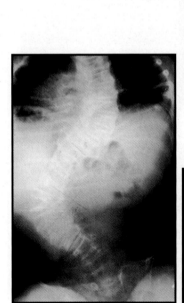

Teeth usually opalescent

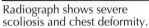

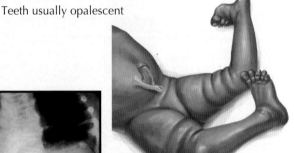

Sclerae normal to blue

Limb deformity severe

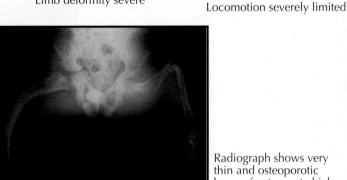

Locomotion severely limited

Radiograph shows severe scoliosis and chest deformity.

Radiograph shows very thin and osteoporotic bones; fracture rate high.

OI, previously termed "congenital brittle bones with redundant callus formation," is not associated with dentinogenesis imperfecta. Type VI OI, previously termed "congenital brittle bones with mineralization defect," is associated with an accumulation of osteoid in bone tissue and a fish-scale pattern of bone lamellation.

- **Lethal perinatal:** OI type II is caused by pathogenic variants that disrupt the formation of the normal type I collagen triple helix (type IIA) and

pathogenic variants in cartilage-associated protein (*CRTAP*) (type IIB). Type II OI is characterized by multiple severe fractures and respiratory failure, leading to death in utero or shortly after birth. Individuals who are affected in the same family may have markedly different disease severity, implicating other genetic or environmental factors that affect the pathogenesis of OI. The key clinical features of OI include recurrent bone fractures, blue sclerae, opalescent teeth (dentinogenesis imperfecta with fragile and

Plate 6.26

Bone and Calcium

MILD OSTEOGENESIS IMPERFECTA TYPE I

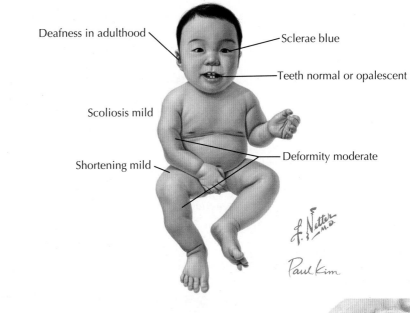

Deafness in adulthood

Sclerae blue

Teeth normal or opalescent

Scoliosis mild

Shortening mild

Deformity moderate

OSTEOGENESIS IMPERFECTA (Continued)

discolored teeth), easy bruising, basilar skull deformities, hearing loss, and increased ligament laxity.

All laboratory parameters can be normal in patients with OI. Hypercalciuria may be present, and it correlates with the severity of bone disease (increased lifelong risk of fractures and shorter stature). In patients with more severe disease, bone marker measurement may be abnormal. Decreased levels of bone formation markers may be found. For example, the blood concentrations of the following bone formation markers may be low: BSAP (reflecting cellular activity of osteoblasts), osteocalcin (an estimate of the rate of synthesis of osteocalcin by osteoblasts), and the C-terminal and N-terminal propeptides of type I collagen (reflecting changes in synthesis of new collagen). Bone resorption markers that may be increased above the upper limit of the reference range are urinary excretion of hydroxyproline (reflecting breakdown of collagen in bone) and collagen crosslinks (NTX and CTX).

A bone biopsy is usually not needed to confirm the diagnosis. However, if performed, bone histology shows disorganized bone, increased bone turnover, decreased cortical width, decreased trabecular number and width, and decreased cancellous bone volume.

The diagnosis of OI is based on the presentation of increased bone fragility, positive family history of bone fragility, blue sclerae, dentinogenesis imperfecta, hearing loss, and molecular genetic testing for pathogenic variants in *COL1A1* and *COL1A2*. In addition to OI, the differential diagnosis of frequent bone fractures in childhood includes rickets and child abuse. Less common disorders to consider include idiopathic juvenile osteoporosis (nonhereditary form of isolated and transient childhood osteoporosis), hypophosphatasia (autosomal recessive disorder caused by a deficiency of tissue nonspecific alkaline phosphatase; see Plate 6.27), juvenile Paget disease (autosomal recessive disorder), polyostotic fibrous dysplasia (McCune-Albright syndrome) with bony cystic or ground-glass lesions, Ehlers-Danlos syndrome (caused by a deficiency in the collagen crosslinking enzyme lysyl oxidase), Menkes disease (copper deficiency that impairs the function of the collagen crosslinking enzyme lysyl oxidase), and Cole-Carpenter syndrome (osteoporosis, craniosynostosis, hydrocephalus, proptosis, and short stature).

TREATMENT

A multidisciplinary team—including specialists in genetics, orthopedics, neurology, physical therapy, occupational therapy, dental care, otolaryngology, psychology, and endocrinology—is needed for

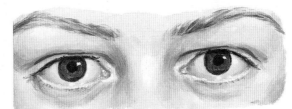

Sclerae usually blue

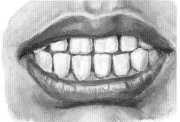

Teeth normal or opalescent

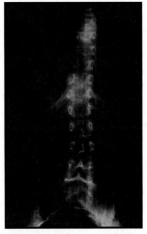

Radiograph shows thin and osteoporotic bones (variable). Fracture rate moderate; deformity mild, often amenable to intramedullary fixation.

Radiograph shows mild scoliosis.

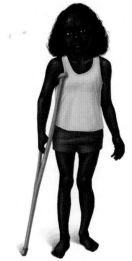

Locomotion normal or with crutch

effective treatment of symptoms and complications related to OI. Treatment goals include decreasing bone fracture incidence, enhancing mobility, preventing bone deformities and scoliosis, and managing pain effectively.

Patients with OI should be evaluated regularly for BMD, fractures detected on skeletal radiographs, pulmonary function, and hearing loss. Patients with OI type III should also have periodic echocardiograms to assess for aortic valve insufficiency caused by aortic root dilation. Nerve compression syndromes may develop with basilar skull deformities.

Pharmacologic therapy with a bisphosphonate agent should be considered in patients with any form of OI unless there is a mineralization defect (e.g., type VI OI). Bisphosphonate therapy inhibits bone resorption and bone turnover and results in improved BMD, decreased number of fractures, and improved mobility. Treatment options under investigation include growth hormone, bone marrow transplantation, and gene therapy.

Individuals with type I OI have a normal life expectancy. Individuals with moderately severe OI may have a shortened life span related to thoracic deformities and immobility.

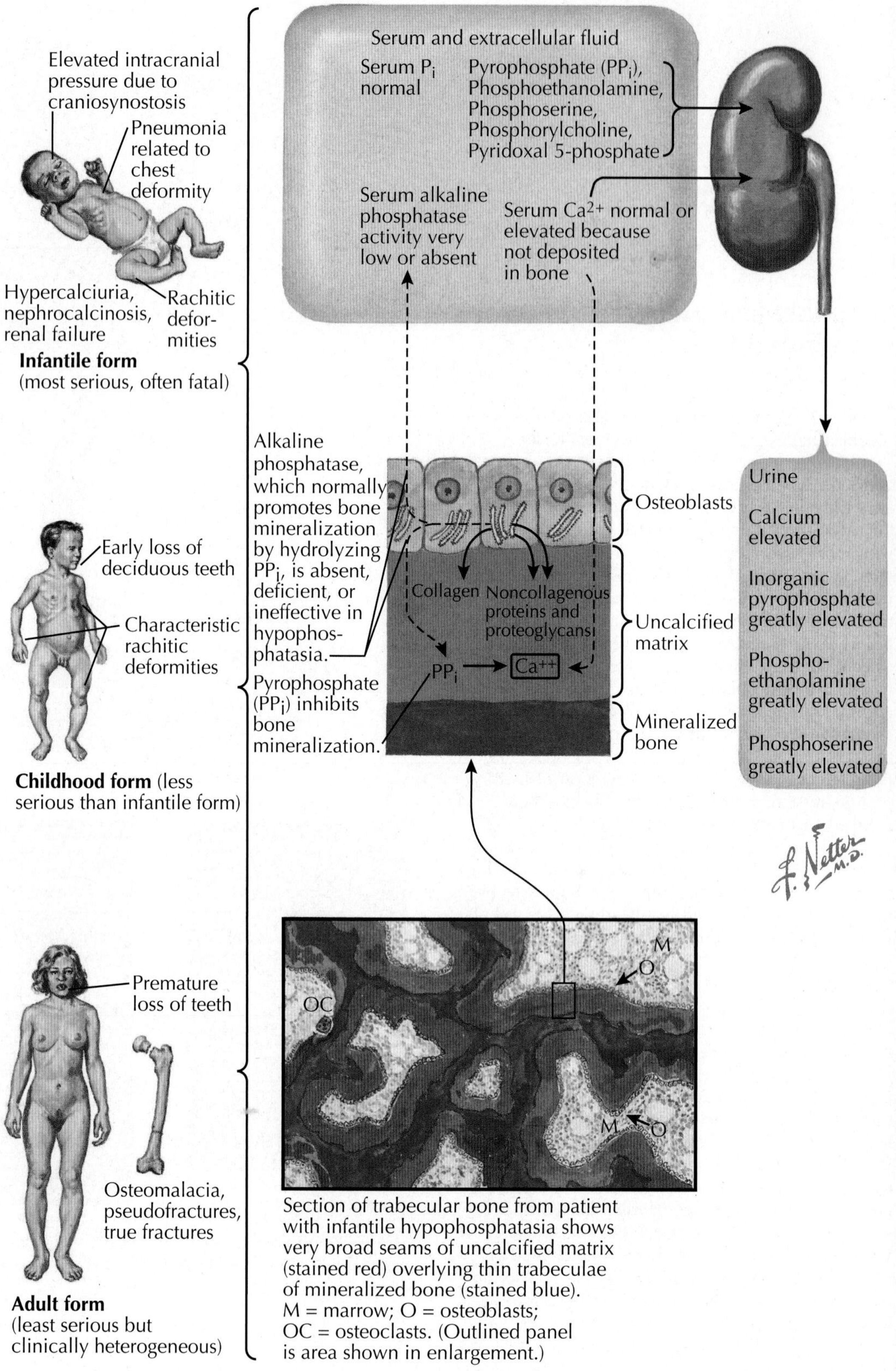

Plate 6.27

Endocrine System: VOLUME 2

HYPOPHOSPHATASIA

Hypophosphatasia, a rare inherited disorder, is associated with low concentrations of alkaline phosphatase in serum and bone that cause defective bone and tooth mineralization, resulting in osteomalacia and severe periodontal disease. Hypophosphatasia results from pathogenic variants in the tissue-nonspecific alkaline phosphatase (*TNSALP*) gene that encodes the tissue-nonspecific isoenzyme of alkaline phosphatase. Perinatal and infantile forms are inherited in an autosomal recessive manner, and milder forms that present later in life can be either autosomal dominant or autosomal recessive, depending on the specific gene pathogenic variant(s).

The perinatal lethal form, with an estimated prevalence of 1 in 100,000, results from complete absence of alkaline phosphatase. Perinatal lethal hypophosphatasia causes lack of mineralized bone in utero, severe deformities with skin-covered osteochondral spurs protruding from the legs and forearms, rachitic deformities of the chest, hypoplastic lungs, premature craniosynostosis with secondary increased intracranial pressure, seizures, hypercalcemia, nephrocalcinosis, and renal failure.

Milder *TNSALP* pathogenic variants, characterized by autosomal dominant transmission and variable expressivity, are associated with presentation during childhood or in adulthood with early loss of teeth and osteomalacia. Childhood hypophosphatasia presents with skeletal deformities (e.g., enlarged joints), focal defects at the end of long bones, short stature, and premature loss of teeth. The bone disease may seem to spontaneously resolve, only to reappear in adulthood. Individuals with the adult form of hypophosphatasia usually become symptomatic in the fourth or fifth decades of life. Presenting symptoms include thigh pain caused by femoral pseudofractures, metatarsal stress fractures, chondrocalcinosis, and odontohypophosphatasia (severe dental caries, loose teeth on dental examination, and premature exfoliation of primary teeth [especially incisors]).

Alkaline phosphatases catalyze the hydrolysis of phosphomonoesters with release of P_i. At the osteoblast cell surface, tissue-nonspecific isoenzyme of alkaline phosphatase generates inorganic phosphate that is needed for hydroxyapatite crystallization. In addition, the buildup of pyrophosphate inhibits bone mineralization.

Hypophosphatasia should be suspected when the blood concentration of total alkaline phosphatase is below the reference range. Blood total alkaline phosphatase concentrations may be decreased in other settings (e.g., early pregnancy, anemia, or hypothyroidism). Hypophosphatasia can be confirmed by finding increased blood and urine concentrations of organic phosphate compounds (e.g., phosphoethanolamine, phosphorylcholine, and pyridoxal 5-phosphate). Findings on bone biopsy are indistinguishable from findings of other forms of rickets. In adults, blood concentrations of calcium and phosphorus are normal.

Genetic testing is a key step to confirm the diagnosis of hypophosphatasia. Most pathogenic variants in the *TNSALP* gene are missense mutations; the rest are

deletions, splice site mutations, nonsense mutations, or small insertions. The array of different pathogenic variants is responsible in part for the variable clinical expression; in other words, patients with severe disease have *TNSALP* pathogenic variants that result in no enzyme activity, and patients with mild disease have *TNSALP* pathogenic variants that result in some tissue-nonspecific isoenzyme of alkaline phosphatase activity.

In 2015, the FDA approved a recombinant human tissue-nonspecific isoenzyme of alkaline phosphatase (asfotase alfa) for perinatal, infantile, and juvenile-onset hypophosphatasia. In infants and young children, asfotase alfa infusions result in improvement in skeletal radiographs and in pulmonary and physical function as well as improved overall survival, ventilator-free survival, growth, and bone mineralization.

Elevated intracranial pressure due to craniosynostosis

Pneumonia related to chest deformity

Hypercalciuria, nephrocalcinosis, renal failure

Rachitic deformities

Infantile form (most serious, often fatal)

Serum and extracellular fluid

Serum P_i normal

Pyrophosphate (PP_i), Phosphoethanolamine, Phosphoserine, Phosphorylcholine, Pyridoxal 5-phosphate

Serum alkaline phosphatase activity very low or absent

Serum Ca^{2+} normal or elevated because not deposited in bone

Early loss of deciduous teeth

Characteristic rachitic deformities

Childhood form (less serious than infantile form)

Alkaline phosphatase, which normally promotes bone mineralization by hydrolyzing PP_i, is absent, deficient, or ineffective in hypophosphatasia.

Pyrophosphate (PP_i) inhibits bone mineralization.

Osteoblasts

Collagen Noncollagenous proteins and proteoglycans

$PP_i \rightarrow Ca^{++}$

Uncalcified matrix

Mineralized bone

Urine

Calcium elevated

Inorganic pyrophosphate greatly elevated

Phospho-ethanolamine greatly elevated

Phosphoserine greatly elevated

Premature loss of teeth

Osteomalacia, pseudofractures, true fractures

Adult form (least serious but clinically heterogeneous)

Section of trabecular bone from patient with infantile hypophosphatasia shows very broad seams of uncalcified matrix (stained red) overlying thin trabeculae of mineralized bone (stained blue). M = marrow; O = osteoblasts; OC = osteoclasts. (Outlined panel is area shown in enlargement.)

LIPIDS AND NUTRITION

Plate 7.1

Endocrine System: VOLUME 2

CHOLESTEROL SYNTHESIS AND METABOLISM

Cholesterol is a four-ring hydrocarbon structure with an eight-carbon side chain. Cholesterol serves as a key component of cell membranes, and it is the substrate for synthesis of steroid hormones and bile acids. Cholesterol is either synthesized endogenously or obtained exogenously by ingestion of animal fats (e.g., meat, eggs, and dairy products). The biosynthesis of cholesterol starts with three molecules of acetate that are condensed to form 3-hydroxy-3-methylglutaryl coenzyme A (HMG-CoA). HMG-CoA is then converted to mevalonic acid by HMG-CoA reductase—the rate-limiting step in cholesterol biosynthesis—and mevalonic acid is converted to cholesterol. Competitive inhibitors of HMG-CoA reductase (statins) are used clinically to decrease cholesterol biosynthesis and to lower serum cholesterol concentrations.

Cholesterol is metabolized by the biliary excretion of free cholesterol or by conversion to bile acids that are secreted into the intestine. Approximately 50% of biliary cholesterol and 97% of bile acids are reabsorbed in the small intestine and recirculate to the liver (enterohepatic circulation); the remaining biliary cholesterol and bile acids are excreted in the feces.

Lipoproteins, which are composed of protein, triglycerides, cholesterol esters, and free cholesterol, are macromolecules that transport cholesterol and triglycerides in the blood to target tissues (for bile acid formation, adrenal and gonadal steroidogenesis, energy production). The 12 proteins in the lipoproteins are termed *apolipoproteins* (apo), are given letter designations, and act as ligands for receptors and as cofactors for enzymes. The lipoproteins have a nonpolar lipid core surrounded by a polar monolayer of phospholipids and the polar portions of cholesterol and apolipoproteins. Specific lipoproteins differ in the lipid core content, the proportion of lipids in the core, and the protein on the surface. Lipoproteins are classified on the basis of density as chylomicrons, very-low-density lipoprotein (VLDL), low-density lipoprotein (LDL), and high-density lipoprotein (HDL).

- Chylomicrons are large, low-density particles that transport dietary lipid (see Plate 7.2). The associated apolipoproteins include apo A (I, II, IV); apo B_{48}; apo C (I, II, III); and apo E.
- VLDL transports primarily triglycerides. The associated apolipoproteins include apo B_{100}, apo C (I, II, III), and apo E.
- LDL transports primarily cholesterol esters and is associated with apo B_{100}.
- HDL also transports cholesterol esters. HDL is associated with apo A (I, II), apo C (I, II, III), and apo E.

How lipids are transported and metabolized is determined in large part by the apolipoproteins. For example, apo AI is not only a structural protein in HDL, but it also activates lecithin-cholesterol acyltransferase (LCAT). Apo AII is a structural protein of HDL and activates hepatic lipase. Apo AIV is an activator for

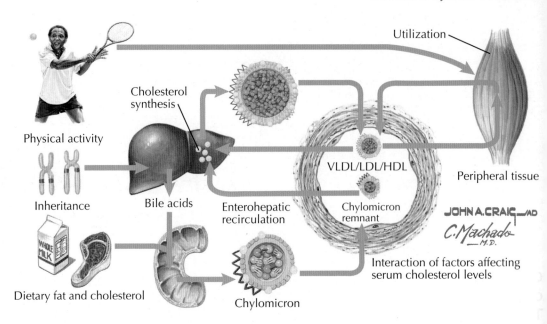

Utilization

Cholesterol synthesis

Physical activity

Inheritance

Bile acids

VLDL/LDL/HDL

Enterohepatic recirculation

Chylomicron remnant

Peripheral tissue

JOHN A. CRAIG—MD
C. Machado—M.D.

Dietary fat and cholesterol

Chylomicron

Interaction of factors affecting serum cholesterol levels

Lipoprotein structure

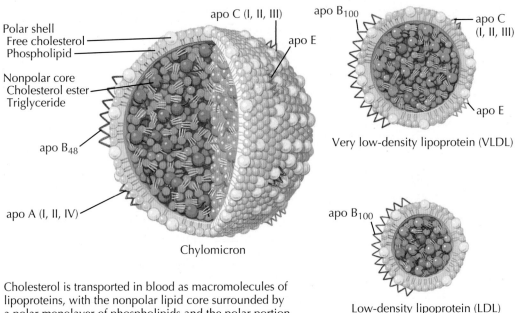

Polar shell
Free cholesterol
Phospholipid

Nonpolar core
Cholesterol ester
Triglyceride

apo B_{48}

apo A (I, II, IV)

apo C (I, II, III)

apo E

apo B_{100}

apo C (I, II, III)

apo E

Very low-density lipoprotein (VLDL)

Chylomicron

apo B_{100}

Low-density lipoprotein (LDL)

apo A (I, II)

apo E

apo C (I, II, III)

High-density lipoprotein (HDL)

Cholesterol is transported in blood as macromolecules of lipoproteins, with the nonpolar lipid core surrounded by a polar monolayer of phospholipids and the polar portion of cholesterol and apolipoproteins. Specific lipoproteins differ in lipid core content, proportion of lipids in the core, and proteins on the surface. Lipoproteins are classified by density as chylomicrons, VLDLs, LDLs, and HDLs.

lipoprotein lipase (LPL) and LCAT. Apo B_{100} is a structural protein for VLDL and LDL and serves as a ligand for the LDL receptor. Apo B_{48} is critical for the formation and secretion of chylomicrons. Apo CI serves to activate LCAT. Apo CII is a key cofactor for LPL. Apo CIII inhibits the hydrolysis of triglycerides by LPL. The three genetically determined isoforms of apo E clear lipoproteins (VLDL and chylomicrons) from the circulation by serving as ligands for the VLDL remnant receptor. The presence of two copies of the apo E2

isoform (homozygous) results in less efficient clearance of chylomicrons and VLDL and is clinically referred to as *familial dysbetalipoproteinemia* (see Plate 7.9).

The cholesterol concentration in the blood is controlled by the LDL receptor. The LDL receptor mediates the endocytosis of apo B– and apo E–containing lipoproteins (LDL, chylomicron remnants, VLDL, and VLDL remnants) into cells. The number of LDL receptors on the cell surface is regulated to maintain normal intracellular cholesterol content.

Plate 7.2

Lipids and Nutrition

Gastrointestinal Absorption of Cholesterol and Triglycerides

Dietary fat digestion starts in the stomach and is completed in the small intestine. Most dietary lipid is in the form of long-chain triglycerides (three fatty acids [with at least 12 carbon atoms each] that are esterified to glycerol). Other dietary lipids include phospholipids, plant sterols, cholesterol, and fat-soluble vitamins (vitamins A, D, E, and K). Gastric peristalsis and mixing serve to disperse dietary triglycerides and phospholipids into an emulsion. Intestinal (gastric) lipase acts on the oil droplets in the emulsion to generate free fatty acids and diglycerides. The presence of fatty acids in the small intestine leads to the secretion of cholecystokinin. Cholecystokinin promotes the secretion and release of pancreatic enzymes into the intestinal lumen (see Plate 5.2); it also promotes contraction of the gallbladder, leading to release of concentrated bile. The pancreatic lipase metabolizes triglycerides to fatty acids and monoglycerides. Another pancreatic enzyme is phospholipase A_2, which breaks down dietary phospholipids.

By partially solubilizing water-insoluble lipids, bile salt micelles facilitate intestinal transport of lipids to the intestinal epithelial cells (enterocytes) for absorption. Specific carrier proteins facilitate diffusion of lipids across the brush border membrane. In addition, enterocytes in the duodenum and proximal jejunum directly take up long-chain fatty acids by passive transfer. Medium-chain fatty acids (6–12 carbon atoms) are not esterified, and the enterocytes release these directly into the portal venous system along with other absorbed nutrients. Long-chain fatty acids and monoglycerides are reesterified into triglyceride in the smooth endoplasmic reticulum of the enterocyte. In addition, cholesterol is esterified by cholesterol acyltransferase. The reassembled lipids are coated with apolipoproteins (apo) (see Plate 7.1) to produce chylomicrons in the Golgi apparatus. The primary intestinal apolipoproteins are apo B_{48}, apo AI, and apo AIV. Chylomicrons acquire apo C and apo E during transit in the lymph and blood. Approximately 85% of the chylomicron is composed of triglyceride. The chylomicrons are too large to cross intercellular junctions linking to capillary epithelial cells. Thus chylomicrons are transported across the basolateral membrane by exocytosis into the mesenteric lymphatic system that flows to the thoracic duct, where they enter the systemic circulation. Chylomicrons are therefore present in postprandial plasma but are absent with

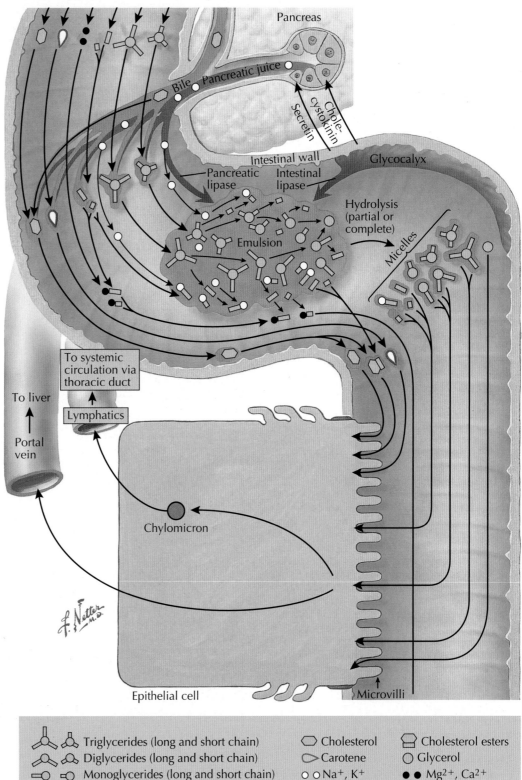

fasting. Apo CII is a cofactor for LPL, the enzyme that hydrolyzes the core triglycerides of the chylomicron and releases free fatty acids. LPL is bound to the capillary endothelial cells in muscle, adipose, and breast tissues. The activity of LPL is regulated based on energy needs. For example, in the fasting state, LPL activity increases in heart muscle and decreases in adipose tissue. In addition, in the postpartum state, breast LPL activity increases 10-fold to promote milk production. Because of the action of LPL, the circulating chylomicrons become progressively smaller, and triglyceride-poor chylomicron remnants are removed from the circulation in the liver, where apo E is the ligand for the hepatic LDL receptor-related protein.

Plate 7.3

Endocrine System: VOLUME 2

Regulation of Low-Density Lipoprotein Receptor and Cholesterol Content

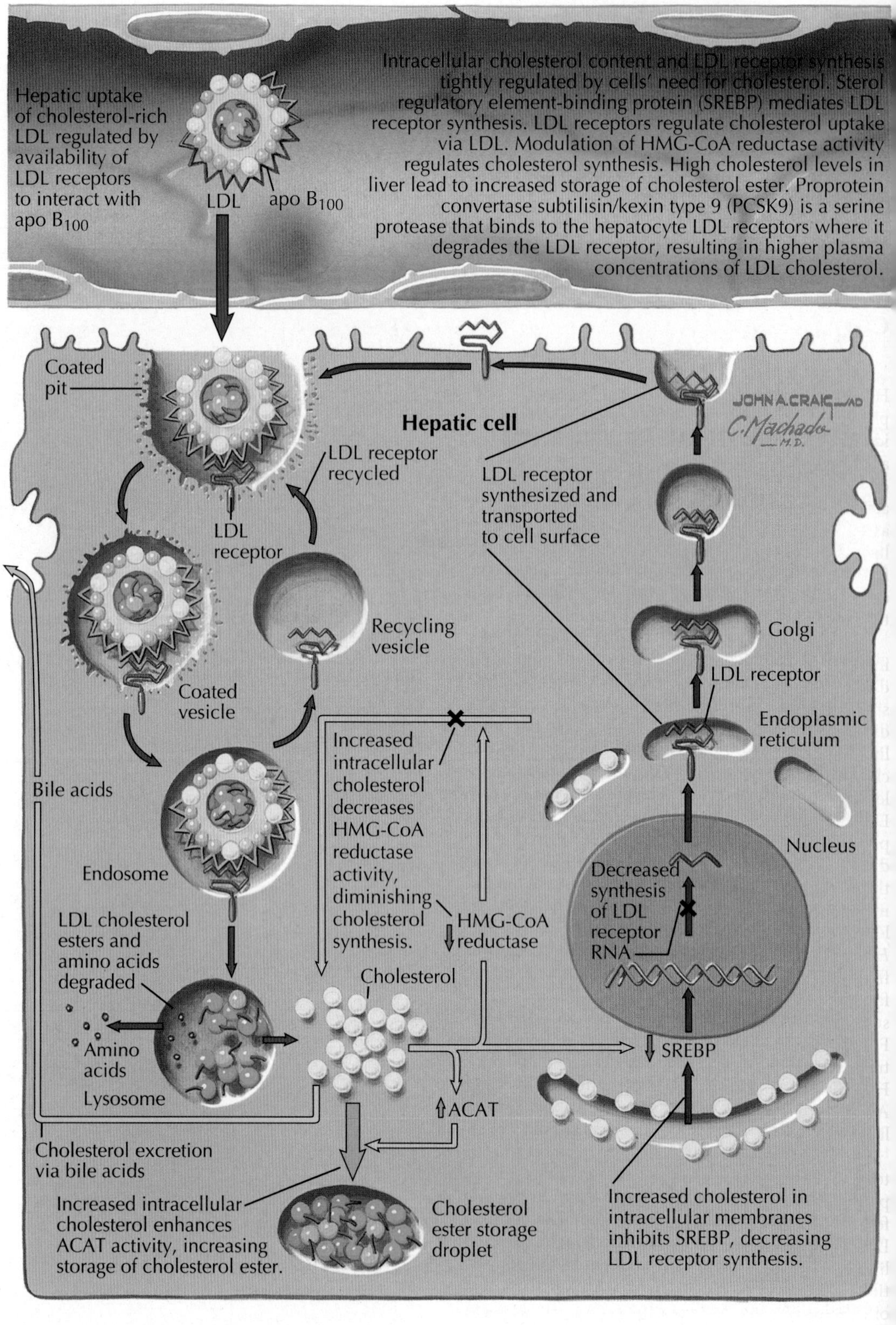

The cholesterol concentration in the blood is controlled primarily by the LDL pathway. Approximately 70% of total plasma cholesterol is LDL. The LDL receptor—located on the surface of all cells—facilitates the internalization of lipoproteins. Approximately 75% of LDL is taken up by hepatocytes. The number of LDL receptors on each cell is in flux and is tightly regulated to keep the intracellular cholesterol concentration constant. Sterol regulatory element-binding protein (SREBP) mediates LDL receptor synthesis. Thus, when a cell's cholesterol content is in positive balance, LDL receptor expression is downregulated by decreased expression of SREBP. In addition, with increased cellular cholesterol, the cholesterol synthetic enzyme HMG-CoA reductase is also downregulated. When a cell's cholesterol content is in negative balance, increased expression of SREBP leads to increased numbers of LDL receptors and enhanced cholesterol uptake from the circulation.

The LDL receptor binds lipoproteins that contain apo B_{100} and apo E (e.g., LDL, chylomicron remnants, VLDL, and VLDL remnants). The lipoprotein-LDL receptor complex localizes to an area of the cell membrane referred to as the *coated pit*. The coated pit contains clathrin that facilitates the clustering of LDL receptors to an area of the cell membrane that can invaginate to form an intracellular vesicle (endosome). As the endosome becomes more acidic, the LDL receptor and lipoprotein dissociate and the lipoproteins are degraded in lysosomes. The free LDL receptor returns to the cell surface in a recycling vesicle. The intracellular pool of cholesterol and cholesterol esters in the hepatocyte is dynamic. Increased intracellular cholesterol enhances acyl-CoA:cholesterol acyltransferase (ACAT) activity, increasing the esterification and storage of cholesterol. In turn, cholesterol ester hydrolase can generate free cholesterol.

The guidelines from the 2002 National Cholesterol Education Program suggest the following cutoffs for plasma total cholesterol concentrations: less than 200 mg/dL, desirable; between 200 and 240 mg/dL, borderline high; and greater than 240 mg/dL, high. Increased blood concentrations of cholesterol are related to increased production or secretion into the circulation or to decreased clearance or removal from the circulation (or both).

Familial hypercholesterolemia (FH) is an autosomal dominant disorder that increases susceptibility to atherosclerotic cardiovascular disease (ASCVD). FH is caused by pathogenic variants in the gene encoding the LDL receptor, leading to two- to threefold increased plasma cholesterol concentrations in individuals who are heterozygous (prevalence of 1 in 500) and a three- to sixfold increase above the upper limit of the reference range in individuals who are homozygous. These patients may have characteristic physical findings (see Plates 7.6 and 7.7). Familial defective apo B_{100} is a disorder caused by pathogenic variants in the gene

encoding apo B_{100}. Defective apo B_{100} binding to the LDL receptor results in a high plasma LDL concentration and an increased ASCVD risk.

Type III hyperlipoproteinemia (familial dysbetalipoproteinemia) is an autosomal recessive disorder characterized by moderate to severe hypercholesterolemia and hypertriglyceridemia and is the result of pathogenic variants in the gene encoding apo E, with resultant defective lipoprotein binding to the LDL receptor (see Plate 7.9).

Elevated plasma lipoprotein(a) (Lp[a]) is a disorder characterized by increased concentrations of modified LDL particles in the plasma, in which the apo B_{100} protein of LDL is covalently bonded to Lp(a). Lp(a) has structural similarity to plasminogen and can interfere with fibrinolysis. Increased plasma Lp(a) is associated with increased ASCVD risk.

Polygenic hypercholesterolemia refers to combinations of multiple genetic and environmental factors that contribute to hypercholesterolemia. Polygenic hypercholesterolemia is diagnosed by exclusion of other primary genetic causes, absence of tendon xanthomas, and documentation that hypercholesterolemia is present in fewer than 10% of first-degree relatives.

Plate 7.4

Lipids and Nutrition

HIGH-DENSITY LIPOPROTEIN METABOLISM AND REVERSE CHOLESTEROL TRANSPORT

HDLs are small particles that contain 50% lipid (phospholipid, cholesteryl esters, free cholesterol, triglyceride) and 50% protein. The main apolipoproteins (apo) are apo AI (65%), apo AII (25%), and smaller amounts of apo C and apo E. The two major subclasses of HDL are HDL_2 and HDL_3. HDL_1 is a minor subclass and is associated with apo E. HDLs function to redistribute lipids among cells and lipoproteins by a process referred to as *reverse cholesterol transport*, in which HDL acquires cholesterol from cells and transports it either to other cells or to the liver.

The steps in the formation and metabolism of HDL include the following: small nascent or precursor HDL disks composed of apo AI and phospholipid are synthesized in the liver and small intestine; precursor HDL disks accept free cholesterol from cells or from other lipoproteins (triglyceride-rich lipoproteins [TGRL] and chylomicron and VLDL remnants); and HDL free cholesterol is esterified by the apo AI–activated enzyme, LCAT. The esterified cholesterol increases its hydrophobicity, and it moves away from the surface of the disk to form a cholesteryl ester-rich core and changes the HDL shape from a disk to a sphere. The spherical, mature HDL_2 particles function to remove excess cholesterol, and as they enlarge, the particle is termed HDL_3. HDL acquires cholesterol by aqueous transfer from cells (passive desorption) or by transport that is facilitated by cell surface-binding proteins. Several cell surface proteins facilitate the efflux of free cholesterol. For example, ABCA1 binds apo AI and facilitates the transfer of free cholesterol and phospholipids onto HDL. Pathogenic variants in the gene that encodes ABCA1 can prevent this transfer process, resulting in a lipid disorder called *Tangier disease* (see Plate 7.8).

Because of its apo E, HDL_1 is taken up by LDL receptors in the liver. In addition, cholesteryl ester transfer protein (CETP) transfers cholesteryl esters (in exchange for triglycerides) from HDL_2 to TGRL (e.g., VLDL, LDL, and remnants), which are then delivered to the liver. An additional pathway of cholesterol redistribution from HDL is via scavenger receptor B1 facilitation of selective uptake of cholesteryl esters by the adrenal glands, gonads, and liver. The HDL_2 particles that have been partially depleted of cholesteryl esters and enriched with triglycerides by CETP can be converted back to HDL_3 by the action of hepatic lipase that hydrolyzes the triglycerides.

Reverse cholesterol transport—with a redistribution of cholesterol from cells with excess (e.g., arterial walls) to cells requiring cholesterol or to the liver for excretion—is antiatherogenic. There is an inverse relationship between plasma HDL concentration and cardiovascular risk. In addition to reverse cholesterol transport, HDL has other antiatherogenic properties. For example, the HDL-associated enzyme paraoxonase

Reverse cholesterol transport
Cholesterol from peripheral tissues returned to liver

Direct mechanism. Because of its apo E, HDL_1 is taken up by LDL receptors in the liver.

Indirect mechanism. Cholesterol-rich form of apo B_{100} lipoproteins (LDL, VLDL remnants) taken up by liver.

JOHN A. CRAIG—AD
C. Machado —M.D.

Nascent HDL synthesized and secreted into circulation by liver and gut

LPL
apo C
apo E
apo A

TGRLP (apo B_{100} lipoproteins)

apo B_{100}

TGRLP

apo A, C, E
Phospholipids
Cholesterol

Acquisition and esterification of free cholesterol by nascent HDL mediated by LCAT. HDL_3 formed.

apo A, E
apo C II, III

CETP
Cholesterol esters

apo E
apo C II, III

Triglycerides

Exchange of cholesterol esters in HDL_{2a} for triglycerides in TGRLP mediated by CETP. HDL_{2b} formed, and cholesterol-rich form of apo B_{100} lipoprotein provided for uptake by liver.

LCAT

HDL_{2a}

CETP

apo A

LCAT
apo E

HDL cycle

apo C

Hepatic lipase

Nascent HDL
HDL cholesterol mobilized from peripheral tissues

Free cholesterol

HDL_3

HDL_{2b}

HDL_{2b} hydrolyzed by hepatic lipase to yield HDL_3 and fatty acids

Free fatty acids

Free cholesterol

Peripheral (extrahepatic) tissues

Free fatty acids

Adipose tissue

Energy utilization

Triglycerides

Fatty acids

Muscle

serves to inhibit oxidation of LDL. In addition, HDL and apo AI stabilize the erythrocyte cell membrane and prevent transbilayer diffusion of anionic lipids, a step that is required for prothrombin activation and thrombus formation.

Several alterations in the HDL pathway can result in low or high plasma HDL concentrations. For example, pathogenic variants in the gene encoding apo AI can decrease HDL formation because of lack of LCAT

activation; resultant plasma concentrations are less than 10 mg/dL (reference ranges: low, less than 40 mg/dL; normal, 40–60 mg/dL; desirable, greater than 60 mg/dL). Increased plasma HDL concentrations are found in individuals with CETP deficiency because of the decreased transfer of cholesteryl esters from HDL to apo B–containing lipoproteins. CETP deficiency homozygotes have HDL concentrations greater than 100 mg/dL.

Plate 7.5

Endocrine System: VOLUME 2

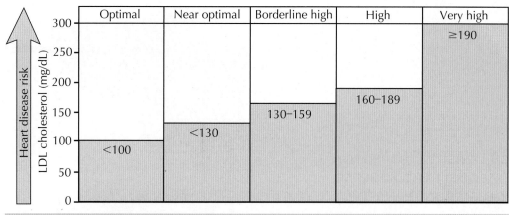

Hypercholesterolemia

Cholesterol has a chief role in the function of cell membranes and serves as a precursor of steroid hormones. However, when blood concentrations of LDL cholesterol exceed certain levels, it is termed *hypercholesterolemia*. Hypercholesterolemia can predispose to atherosclerosis and increase the risk for vascular disease (e.g., ASCVD, cerebrovascular disease, and peripheral vascular disease).

Many factors contribute to high plasma LDL concentrations. For example, diets high in saturated fats and cholesterol lead to increased blood cholesterol concentrations. Although the level of cholesterol in the blood is controlled at multiple sites, the primary regulator is the LDL receptor pathway. LDL receptors are present on the cell surface of most cells and mediate the uptake of lipoproteins that contain apo B_{100} and apo E (e.g., LDL, chylomicron remnants, VLDL, VLDL remnants, and HDL_1).

FH is a relatively common disorder caused by pathogenic variants in the gene that encodes the LDL receptor. Decreased synthesis or synthesis of defective LDL receptors leads to increased plasma concentrations of LDL cholesterol (three- and sixfold increase above the reference range in heterozygotes and homozygotes, respectively; see Plates 7.6 and 7.7).

Pathogenic variants in the gene that encodes apo B_{100} are relatively common and lead to defective binding of LDL cholesterol to the LDL receptor. The clinical findings and the blood lipid profile are similar to those of FH (see Plates 7.6 and 7.7).

Familial hyperapobetalipoproteinemia (with overproduction of apo B_{100}) and familial combined hyperlipidemia are both inherited in an autosomal dominant fashion. Although the genetic defects underlying these conditions have yet to be identified (probably multiple genetic defects), they are relatively common disorders and are associated with elevations of plasma LDL cholesterol and triglyceride concentrations and increased susceptibility to ASCVD. Other associations include moderate decrease in plasma HDL cholesterol concentrations, fasting hyperglycemia, obesity, and hyperuricemia. Familial combined hyperlipidemia should be suspected in individuals with moderate hypercholesterolemia in combination with moderate hypertriglyceridemia in the setting of a family history of premature ASCVD. Xanthomas are not seen in individuals with familial hyperapobetalipoproteinemia or with familial combined hyperlipidemia. In 2018 the American Heart Association and American College of Cardiology (AHA/ACC) released a new clinical practice guideline on cholesterol management. It was accompanied by a risk assessment

report on primary prevention of ASCVD. The guideline gives more attention to percentage reduction in LDL cholesterol as a treatment goal and to long-term monitoring of therapeutic efficacy. All individuals with high LDL cholesterol should pursue lifestyle modifications of aerobic exercise and consuming a healthy diet. Whether to lower LDL cholesterol with pharmacotherapy incorporates both the level of LDL cholesterol level and a patient's estimated 10-year ASCVD risk. ASCVD risk refers to fatal or nonfatal myocardial infarction, acute coronary

syndrome, sudden cardiac death, coronary artery revascularization, stroke, and peripheral vascular arterial disease. The AHA/ACC risk calculator triages patients into four risk categories. Based on the estimated 10-year cardiovascular disease risk, shared decision-making discussions between patients and their providers help determine whether a 30% relative risk reduction with a medication results in an absolute risk reduction large enough to be worth the cost and potential side effects of daily therapy (see Plate 7.17).

Plate 7.6   Lipids and Nutrition

HYPERCHOLESTEROLEMIC XANTHOMATOSIS

Severe hypercholesterolemia can lead to cutaneous and tendinous xanthomas. These cutaneous protuberances represent the accumulation of large (10–20 μm in diameter), cholesterol-filled macrophages. The high concentrations of LDL cholesterol in the blood are taken up by the nonsaturable scavenger receptors on macrophages. Xanthelasma of the eyelids is frequently accompanied by premature arcus corneae (i.e., in persons younger than 40 years). Plain and tuberous xanthomas are most frequently found over the elbows, knees, and buttocks, possibly related to continuous irritation by garments. Tuberous xanthomas are seen most frequently in individuals with homozygous pathogenic variants in the gene that encodes the LDL receptor (see later).

The characteristic lesions of tendinous xanthoma are actually part of the tendon, from which they cannot be mechanically separated. The nodules are found in the extensor tendons of the hands, Achilles tendons, and patellar tendons. This type of nodular lesion may be easily confused with the nodules of rheumatoid arthritis, but it can readily be distinguished because a xanthoma is not painful, and patients with rheumatoid arthritis lack the marked increased in blood LDL cholesterol concentrations that are seen in patients with xanthomas.

In the first phase, atherosclerotic lesions consist of cushion-like elevations of lipid-filled macrophages (foam cells) beneath the intima. Later, they become sclerotic (see Plates 7.12 and 7.13). The atheroma of the arterial intima is the most dangerous feature of familial hypercholesterolemic xanthomatosis because of its frequent occurrence in the coronary vessels, which may cause angina and myocardial infarction at an early age.

Hypercholesterolemic xanthomatosis is a manifestation of either FH (an autosomal dominant disorder caused by pathogenic variants in the gene that encodes the LDL receptor) or familial defective apo B_{100} (caused by pathogenic variants in the gene that encodes apo B_{100}).

FAMILIAL HYPERCHOLESTEROLEMIA: LOW-DENSITY LIPOPROTEIN RECEPTOR MUTATIONS

FH is a monogenic disorder caused by pathogenic variants in the gene that encodes the LDL receptor. Thus LDL cholesterol is not effectively cleared from the circulation, and plasma concentrations of LDL cholesterol are increased. There is increased uptake of LDL cholesterol by the macrophage scavenger receptors, with marked lipid accumulation in the macrophages (foam cells). More than 900 different pathogenic variants in the LDL receptor have been identified to cause FH. The types of pathogenic variants in the gene that encodes the LDL receptor include pathogenic variants that cause decreased LDL receptor synthesis, decreased intracellular transport of the LDL receptor from the endoplasmic reticulum to the Golgi apparatus, defective binding of LDL cholesterol to the LDL receptor, and a defect in the internalization of the LDL receptor after binding LDL cholesterol. Thus the effect of the LDL

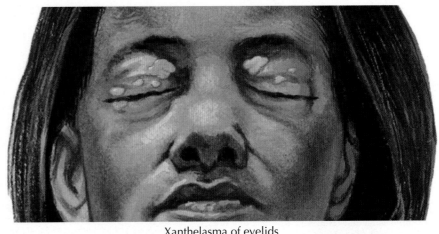

Xanthelasma of eyelids

Clear serum

Plain and tuberous xanthomas of elbows and knees

Plain and tuberous xanthomas of buttocks

receptor mutation on plasma LDL cholesterol concentrations and ASCVD risk is very dependent on the specific pathogenic variant. In addition, individuals with homozygous LDL receptor pathogenic variants are much more severely affected than individuals who are heterozygous.

Heterozygous FH is a relatively common disorder, affecting 1 in 500 persons, and its manifestations are present from birth. In individuals with heterozygous FH, the plasma total cholesterol concentrations are typically more than 300 mg/dL, and the LDL cholesterol concentrations are more than 250 mg/dL. Plasma triglycerides are not elevated in this condition. Approximately 75% of patients with heterozygous FH have

xanthelasma and tendon xanthomas. Also, premature ASCVD and heart valvular disease occurring before age 45 years are common. Heterozygous FH should be suspected in individuals with high plasma concentrations of LDL cholesterol, normal plasma triglyceride concentrations, tendon xanthomas, and a family history of premature ASCVD. The diagnosis of heterozygous FH is made on clinical grounds. Because of the large number of potential mutations, germline genetic testing for abnormalities in the gene that encodes the LDL receptor is not routinely done.

Fortunately, homozygous FH is rare. These individuals come to clinical attention either because of a family history of premature ASCVD or the appearance of

Plate 7.7

Endocrine System: VOLUME 2

HYPERCHOLESTEROLEMIC XANTHOMATOSIS (Continued)

xanthomas at a young age (i.e., younger than 10 years). Typical plasma total cholesterol concentrations range from 600 to 1000 mg/dL; plasma LDL cholesterol concentrations range from 550 to 950 mg/dL. Tuberous xanthomas usually develop before age 6 years and are unique to homozygous FH; these individuals also develop the xanthelasma and tendon xanthomas that are common in individuals who are heterozygous for pathogenic variants in the LDL receptor gene. Symptomatic ASCVD can occur before age 10 years, and fatal myocardial infarction usually occurs before age 20 years if the hypercholesterolemia is not treated. Aortic valvular disease (e.g., aortic stenosis) is more common (occurring in ~50% of individuals who are affected) and is more severe in homozygous FH than in heterozygous FH. The diagnosis of homozygous FH should be suspected when the plasma LDL cholesterol concentration is more than 500 mg/dL.

Treatment of individuals with heterozygous FH includes a low-cholesterol diet and pharmacologic therapy with an HMG-CoA reductase inhibitor (statin). Some patients may require the addition of a bile acid sequestrant or an intestinal cholesterol absorption inhibitor.

Treatment of individuals with homozygous FH is problematic. Children and adolescents with homozygous FH should receive prompt and aggressive lipid-lowering therapy with a goal LDL cholesterol of <135 mg/dL. High-potency statin therapy should be initiated along with lifestyle modification. Intestinal cholesterol absorption inhibitors and additional treatments are invariably required. These include anti-PCSK9 therapy, LDL apheresis, and lomitapide (a microsomal triglyceride transfer protein inhibitor). Liver transplant is a last resort intervention.

FAMILIAL DEFECTIVE APOLIPOPROTEIN B$_{100}$

Familial defective apo B$_{100}$ is relatively common disorder affecting 1 in 500 persons that is caused by a pathogenic variant in the gene encoding apo B$_{100}$. To date, most patients who are affected have the same single point pathogenic variant at nucleotide number 3500. Apo B$_{100}$ is the ligand that binds LDL cholesterol to the LDL receptor; thus biochemical and clinical phenotypes are very similar to those in individuals with LDL receptor pathogenic variants. These individuals have isolated elevations in plasma LDL cholesterol concentrations, xanthelasma, tendon xanthomas, and premature ASCVD. In general, the clinical presentations of heterozygous and homozygous familial defective apo B$_{100}$ are less severe than those of the heterozygous and homozygous forms of FH, respectively. Clinically, familial defective apo B$_{100}$ cannot be distinguished from FH; germline genetic testing is the only method currently available to make this distinction.

Treatment of familial defective apo B$_{100}$ is similar to that of heterozygous FH, with emphasis on a low-cholesterol diet and pharmacologic therapy with statins, bile acid sequestrants, and intestinal cholesterol absorption inhibitors.

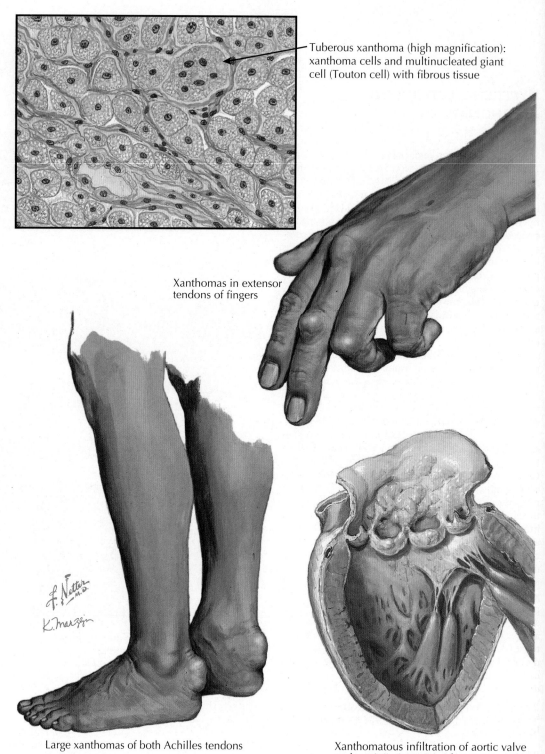

Tuberous xanthoma (high magnification): xanthoma cells and multinucleated giant cell (Touton cell) with fibrous tissue

Xanthomas in extensor tendons of fingers

Large xanthomas of both Achilles tendons

Xanthomatous infiltration of aortic valve and aortic intima around coronary orifice

SITOSTEROLEMIA AND CEREBROTENDINOUS XANTHOMATOSIS

Tendon xanthomas and premature ASCVD can also occur independently of an abnormality in LDL cholesterol metabolism. Sitosterolemia is an autosomal recessive disorder resulting from pathogenic variants in the genes encoding the adenosine triphosphate (ATP)-binding cassettes G5 and G8 that normally limit plant sterol absorption. There is a resultant increase in gastrointestinal absorption of cholesterol and plant sterols. The plant sterols and LDL cholesterol accumulate in the plasma and peripheral tissues, leading to premature ASCVD and tendon xanthomas. Plasma levels of LDL cholesterol are high. Gas-liquid chromatography shows high levels of plant sterols.

Cerebrotendinous xanthomatosis (CTX) is an autosomal recessive lipid storage disease and a form of leukodystrophy. CTX is caused by a block in bile acid synthesis because of absent 27-hydroxylase (caused by pathogenic variants in *CYP27A1*), resulting in an accumulation of cholesterol and cholestanol in all tissues. The plasma lipid levels in individuals with CTX are normal. Xanthomas develop in the central nervous system (CNS), tendons, skin, bones, and lungs. Because of the associated defects in synthesis and maintenance of the myelin sheath of nerves, CTX has dominant effects on the CNS with resultant cerebellar ataxia and pyramidal tract signs.

Plate 7.8

Lipids and Nutrition

ABETALIPOPROTEINEMIA AND TANGIER DISEASE

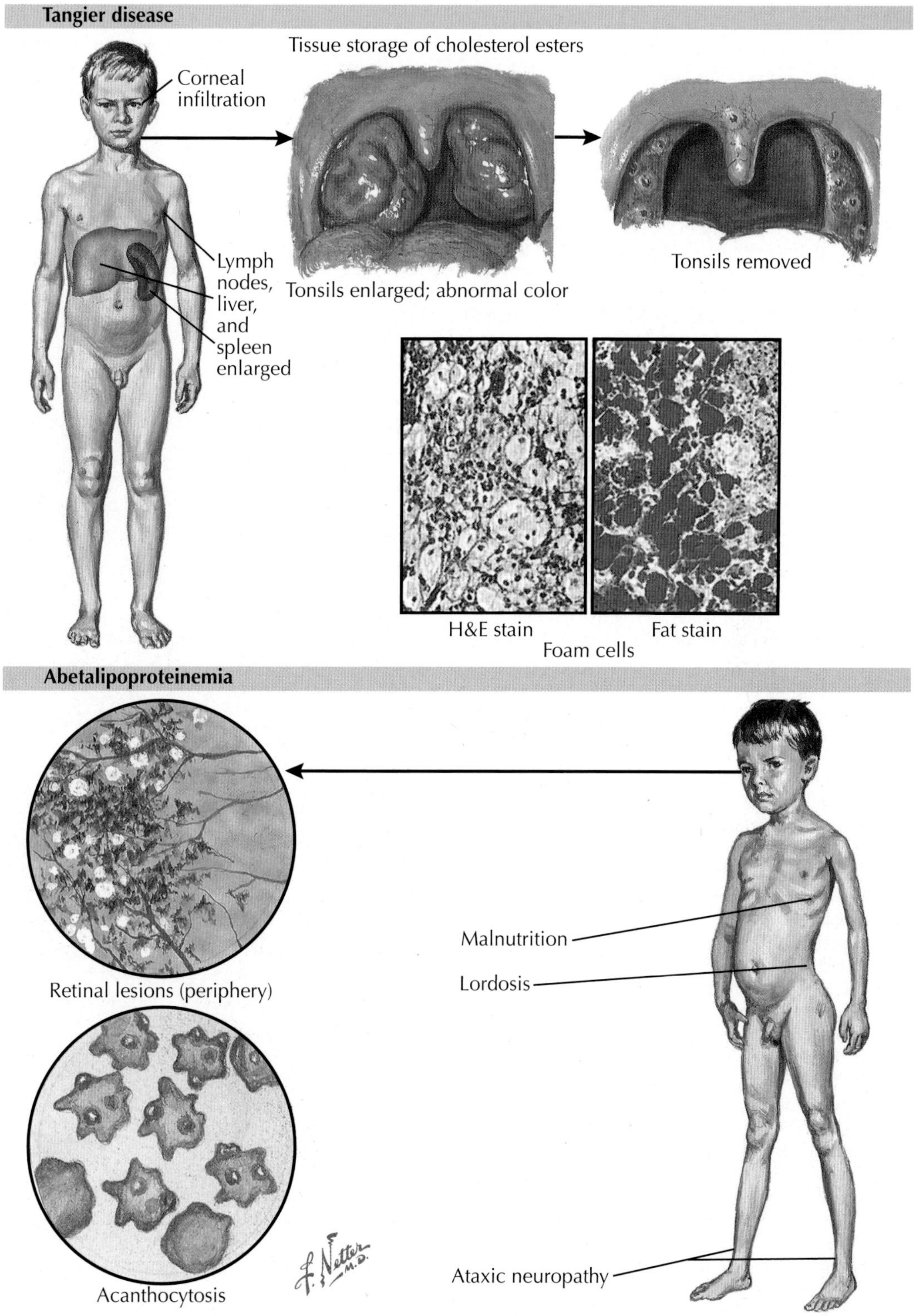

Two familial syndromes are characterized by severe deficiency or absence of specific lipoproteins: abetalipoproteinemia and Tangier disease.

ABETALIPOPROTEINEMIA

Abetalipoproteinemia (OMIM 200100) is a rare autosomal recessive disorder that usually presents in infancy with fat malabsorption, hypocholesterolemia, and acanthocytosis. Later in life, deficiencies in fat-soluble vitamins result in atypical retinitis pigmentosa, posterior column neuropathy, and myopathy. Abetalipoproteinemia is caused by pathogenic variants in the gene encoding the large subunit of microsomal triglyceride transfer protein, resulting in abnormal production and secretion of apo B and apo B–containing lipoproteins. Microsomal triglyceride transfer protein is key in the transfer of triglycerides and phospholipids into the lumen of the endoplasmic reticulum of the enterocyte for the assembly of VLDL, a step required for normal hepatic secretion of apo B_{100}. Insufficient lipidation of these nascent particles prevents synthesis and secretion of chylomicrons and VLDL by the intestine and liver. This defect results in gastrointestinal fat malabsorption and extremely low plasma concentrations of cholesterol and VLDL triglycerides and absent betalipoprotein.

The absence of apo B results in steatorrhea, symptoms associated with deficiency of fat-soluble vitamins (vitamins A, D, E, and K), neurologic manifestations (e.g., retinitis pigmentosa, peripheral neuropathy, ataxia, lordosis caused by muscular weakness, sensory motor neuropathy, intellectual disabillity), and acanthocytosis (crenated appearance of erythrocytes). In individuals who are homozygous for pathogenic variants in the disease-causing gene, there may be deficient adrenocortical glucocorticoid production. The neurologic manifestations may dominate the clinical presentation with early onset (e.g., age 1–2 years) of generalized weakness, distal muscular atrophy, loss of proprioception, posterior column degeneration with sensory neuropathy, and cerebellar atrophy with ataxia and nystagmus. Children with abetalipoproteinemia appear malnourished and have growth retardation. Some patients may have hepatic steatosis and cirrhosis, which can result from treatment with medium-chain triglycerides. In one patient who underwent liver transplantation for hepatic cirrhosis, the serum lipoprotein profile normalized but gastrointestinal fat malabsorption persisted.

Laboratory studies show the absence of plasma apo B–containing proteins and extremely low levels of total cholesterol (<50 mg/dL). Early diagnosis and treatment are key to avoid growth retardation and neuroretinal complications. Treatment includes a lipid-poor diet (e.g., 5 g/d in children) to treat digestive intolerance and allow normal absorption of carbohydrates and proteins, provision of dietary essential fatty acids in the form of vegetable oils, and high doses of fat-soluble vitamins (vitamins A, D, E, and K).

TANGIER DISEASE

Tangier disease (OMIM 205400) is an autosomal dominant disorder that results in low serum concentrations of HDL cholesterol. Tangier disease was originally described and named on the basis of a kindred living on Tangier Island in Chesapeake Bay. Tangier disease is caused by pathogenic variants in the ATP-binding cassette transporter-1 gene (*ABCA1*), which encodes the cholesterol efflux regulatory protein. *ABCA1* is critical for intracellular cholesterol transport, the impairment of which results in decreased cholesterol efflux onto nascent HDL particles, leading to lipid-depleted particles that are then rapidly catabolized. Thus the inability of newly synthesized apolipoproteins to acquire cellular lipids by the *ABCA1* pathway leads to their rapid degradation and an overaccumulation of cholesterol in macrophages. *ABCA1* has a critical role in modulating flux of tissue cholesterol and phospholipids into the reverse cholesterol transport pathway. The impaired HDL-mediated cholesterol efflux from macrophages leads to massive accumulation of cholesteryl esters (foam cells) throughout the body and resultant hepatosplenomegaly. These individuals frequently develop premature coronary disease. Individuals with homozygous pathogenic variants in *ABCA1* have absent plasma HDL, and heterozygotes have HDL concentrations about 50% of those in individuals with two normal alleles.

Findings on physical examination include orange tonsils (caused by cholesterol deposits), corneal opacities, hepatosplenomegaly, and peripheral neuropathy. Findings from laboratory studies show absent HDL cholesterol and low total cholesterol concentrations. Currently, there is no disease-specific treatment for Tangier disease.

Tangier disease

Corneal infiltration

Lymph nodes, liver, and spleen enlarged

Tissue storage of cholesterol esters

Tonsils enlarged; abnormal color

Tonsils removed

H&E stain   Fat stain
Foam cells

Abetalipoproteinemia

Retinal lesions (periphery)

Acanthocytosis

Malnutrition

Lordosis

Ataxic neuropathy

Plate 7.9

Endocrine System: VOLUME 2

HYPERTRIGLYCERIDEMIA

Based on coronary risk, serum triglyceride concentrations can be stratified as follows: normal, less than 150 mg/dL; borderline high, 150 to 199 mg/dL; high, 200 to 499 mg/dL; and very high, 500 mg/dL or greater. Serum triglyceride concentrations greater than 199 mg/dL are termed *hypertriglyceridemia* and are associated with an increased risk of cardiovascular disease. Hypertriglyceridemia can be caused by or exacerbated by obesity, poorly controlled diabetes mellitus, nephrotic syndrome, hypothyroidism, and orally administered estrogen therapy.

Hypertriglyceridemia results from the accumulation of TGRL (e.g., VLDL, VLDL remnants, and chylomicrons) in blood. Hypertriglyceridemia is associated with variable degrees of hypercholesterolemia because the TGRL also transport cholesterol. Triglycerides in chylomicrons and VLDL are hydrolyzed by LPL, and the free fatty acid molecules are used as an energy source. LPL also facilitates the transfer of cholesterol to HDL cholesterol. Thus, when LPL activity is deficient, hypertriglyceridemia and low blood HDL cholesterol concentrations occur.

Disorders in lipid metabolism can be categorized by the Fredrickson hyperlipoproteinemia phenotype classification, which is based on the pattern of lipoproteins on electrophoresis or ultracentrifugation:

- Phenotype I (LPL deficiency): increased serum chylomicron concentration and markedly increased serum triglyceride concentration. The serum has a creamy top layer.
- Phenotype IIa (FH): increased serum LDL cholesterol and total cholesterol concentrations. The serum is clear.
- Phenotype IIb: increased serum concentrations of LDL and VLDL cholesterol. The serum is clear.
- Phenotype III (familial dysbetalipoproteinemia): increased serum concentrations of VLDL remnants and chylomicrons. The serum is turbid.
- Phenotype IV (familial hypertriglyceridemia): increased serum concentrations of VLDL. The serum is turbid.
- Phenotype V (mixed hypertriglyceridemia): increased serum concentrations of chylomicrons and VLDL. The serum has a creamy top layer and a turbid bottom layer.

The type I hyperlipoproteinemia phenotype is caused by rare recessive disorders and is associated with complete absence of either LPL activity or apo CII (the ligand for LPL on chylomicrons and VLDL). Severe hypertriglyceridemia results because the clearance of TGRL from plasma is blocked. Chylomicronemia syndrome is a frequent finding in patients with type I hyperlipoproteinemia (see Plates 7.10 and 7.11).

Type IIa hyperlipoproteinemia is FH and is associated with LDL receptor deficiency, resulting in markedly increased serum concentrations of LDL (see Plates 7.6 and 7.7). Type IIb hyperlipoproteinemia is combined hyperlipidemia caused by decreased LDL receptor availability or function and increased apo B, resulting in increased blood levels of LDL cholesterol and VLDL (see Plate 7.5).

Familial dysbetalipoproteinemia, also termed *type III hyperlipoproteinemia,* is associated with specific isoforms of the *APOE* gene; however, other genetic and

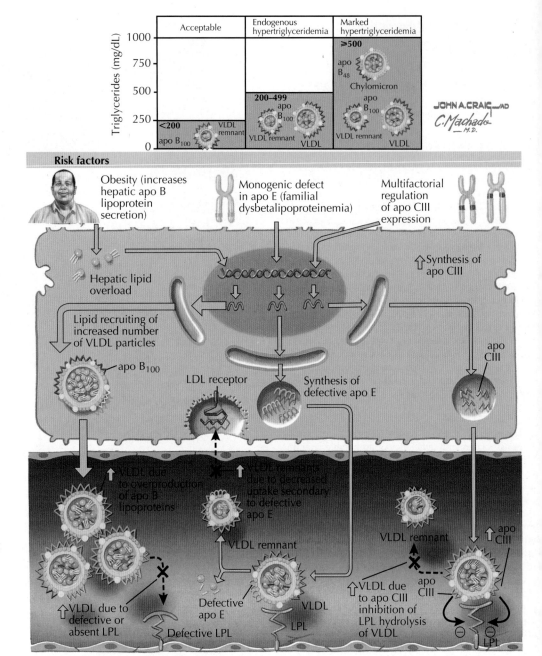

environmental factors probably contribute to disease development and severity. Apo E is required for receptor-mediated clearance of chylomicron and VLDL remnants. The most common *APOE* genotype is *APOE*E3/APOE*E3.* The E2 isoform has lower affinity for the LDL receptor than the E3 isoform, which leads to poor clearance of VLDL and chylomicron remnants that contain the E2 isoform. Familial dysbetalipoproteinemia occurs when individuals are homozygous for the E2 allele. This defect leads to premature chronic heart disease and peripheral vascular disease. Tuberoeruptive xanthomas may be evident on physical examination (see Plates 7.6 and 7.7).

Familial hypertriglyceridemia (type IV hyperlipoproteinemia phenotype) is an autosomal dominant disorder caused by inactivating pathogenic variants in the gene encoding LPL and is associated with moderately increased serum triglyceride concentrations (200–500 mg/dL), normal serum LDL cholesterol concentrations, and low serum HDL cholesterol concentrations. The degree of hypertriglyceridemia can be

aggravated by exogenous agents (e.g., orally administered estrogen replacement therapy). Familial hypertriglyceridemia is usually associated with obesity, insulin resistance, hyperglycemia, and hypertension.

Mixed hypertriglyceridemia (type V hyperlipoproteinemia phenotype) is characterized by triglyceride levels above the 99th percentile of normal. The plasma supernatant is creamy, and there are increased concentrations of chylomicrons and VLDL. The clinical manifestations include hepatosplenomegaly and eruptive xanthomas.

Familial combined hyperlipidemia is a genetically heterogenous disorder caused by overproduction of hepatically derived apo B_{100} associated with VLDL. Patients who are affected typically present with hypercholesterolemia and hypertriglyceridemia.

The C apolipoproteins also regulate triglyceride metabolism. Apo CI and apo CIII modulate the uptake of TGRL (chylomicron remnants, VLDL) by interfering with the ability of apo E to mediate binding to lipoprotein receptor pathways.

Plate 7.10

Lipids and Nutrition

CLINICAL MANIFESTATIONS OF HYPERTRIGLYCERIDEMIA

Hypertriglyceridemia is usually asymptomatic. However, serum triglyceride concentrations higher than 1000 mg/dL may result in chylomicronemia syndrome. Signs and symptoms associated with chylomicronemia syndrome include abdominal pain, pancreatitis, eruptive xanthoma, flushing with alcohol intake, memory loss, and lipemia retinalis. The acute pancreatitis can be life threatening, and the patients most commonly affected are those with poorly controlled diabetes mellitus or alcoholism. Serum triglyceride values higher than 1000 mg/dL result in opalescent serum caused by an increase in VLDL. At markedly increased levels, the serum may be milky because of hyperchylomicronemia.

Triglycerides in chylomicrons and VLDL are hydrolyzed by LPL, and the free fatty acid molecules are used as an energy source in muscle for triglyceride synthesis or for storage in adipocytes or formation of hepatic VLDL. LPL is synthesized by adipocytes, myocytes, and macrophages. LPL attaches to heparan sulfate proteoglycans on the surface of capillary endothelial cells, where it interacts with circulating chylomicrons and VLDL. Apo CII is a cofactor for LPL. Mutations that inactivate LPL or apo CII result in severe hypertriglyceridemia (see later).

Hepatic lipase is synthesized by hepatocytes and is found in capillary endothelial cells of the liver, adrenals, and gonads. Hepatic lipase—activated by androgens and suppressed by estrogens—functions to release lipids from lipoproteins by hydrolyzing triglycerides in the processing of chylomicron remnants and also to convert HDL cholesterol from HDL_2 to HDL_3 by removing phospholipid and triglyceride from HDL_2. Thus, when the hepatic lipase activity is high, serum concentrations of total HDL cholesterol levels are low. Unlike LPL, apo CII is not a cofactor for hepatic lipase. Defects or deficiencies in hepatic lipase result in an accumulation of remnant lipoproteins and HDL_2.

LIPOPROTEIN LIPASE DEFICIENCY

Pathogenic variants in the gene encoding LPL can result in deficient LPL activity, a rare autosomal recessive disorder that manifests with severe hypertriglyceridemia because the clearance of TGRL from the plasma is blocked. Individuals heterozygous for a pathogenic variant in the *LPL* gene (approximate frequency of 1 in 500) may have LPL activity that is 50% of normal, leading to mild hypertriglyceridemia.

Normally, chylomicrons are cleared from plasma within 8 hours of eating. In persons with complete LPL deficiency, the chylomicrons can take days to be cleared after a single meal. Chylomicronemia syndrome results when there are massive accumulations of these lipoproteins in the blood. LPL deficiency is usually diagnosed in infancy or childhood when individuals present with chylomicronemia syndrome. Manifestations of chylomicronemia syndrome include recurrent abdominal pain, pancreatitis, hepatosplenomegaly caused by the accumulation of triglycerides in reticuloendothelial cells, eruptive xanthomas, lipemia retinalis, lipemic plasma, neurologic manifestations, dyspnea, and severe hypertriglyceridemia (>2000 mg/

dL). The pancreatitis resulting from chemical irritation by fatty acids and lysolecithin can be life threatening. Chylomicrons are usually present whenever the triglyceride concentration is higher than 1000 mg/dL in a fasting blood sample. The serum appears creamy. Because of the effect on blood volume, severe hypertriglyceridemia can lead to measurement errors in serum electrolytes. For example, if serum is not cleared of TGRL by centrifugation, serum sodium may appear low (pseudohyponatremia).

LPL deficiency should be suspected in infants and children with recurrent abdominal pain and pancreatitis. Eruptive xanthomas are usually present in this setting, especially when serum triglyceride concentrations are higher than 2000 mg/dL. LPL deficiency can be confirmed with the heparin infusion test. Heparin displaces LPL from heparan sulfate proteoglycans on the surface of capillary endothelial cells, and LPL activity can be assayed in plasma.

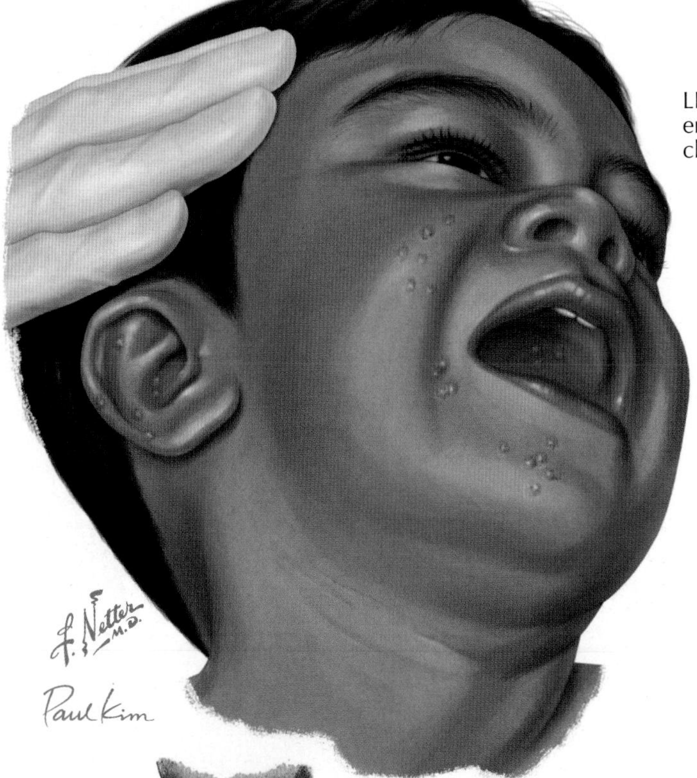

LPL or apo CII deficiency: eruptive xanthomas of cheek, chin, ear, and palate

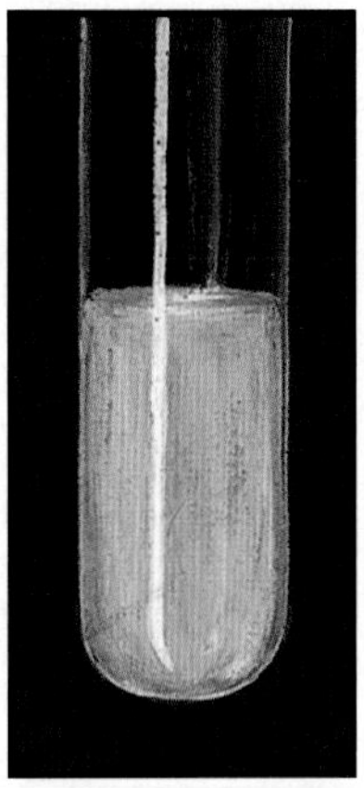

Creamy serum

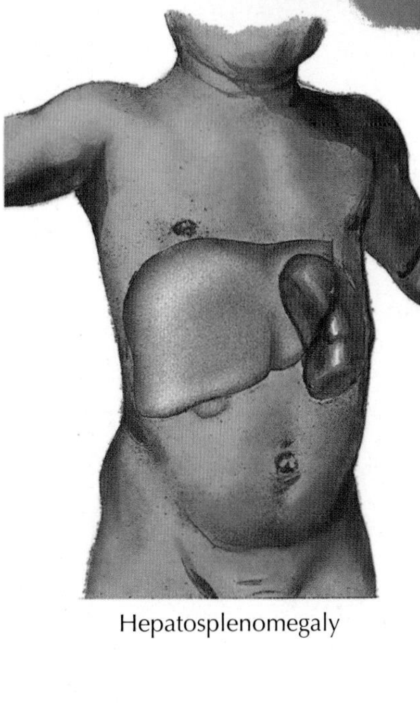

Hepatosplenomegaly

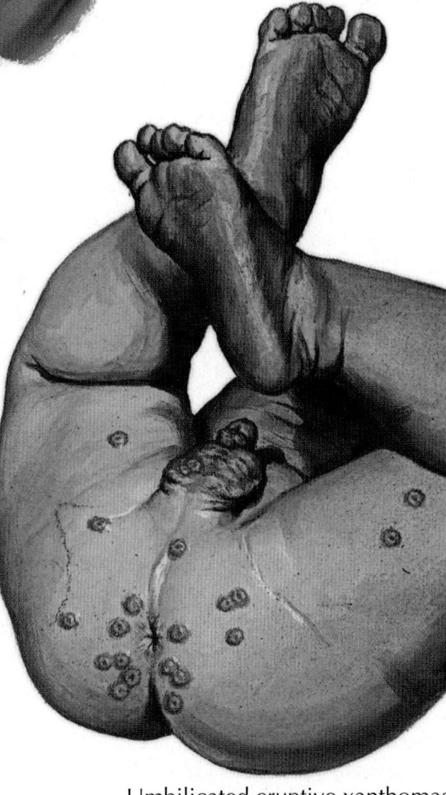

Umbilicated eruptive xanthomas of buttocks, thighs, and scrotum

Plate 7.11

Endocrine System: VOLUME 2

CLINICAL MANIFESTATIONS OF HYPERTRIGLYCERIDEMIA (Continued)

When patients with LPL deficiency present with pancreatitis, the initial treatment should include a fat-free diet. Long term, patients with LPL deficiency should be treated with a fat-restricted diet, with fat accounting for less than 10% of total calories. The therapeutic goal is to maintain serum triglyceride concentrations at less than 1000 mg/dL. Pharmacologic options are limited for patients with LPL deficiency (see later).

APOLIPOPROTEIN CII DEFICIENCY

Apo CII deficiency is another rare autosomal recessive disorder that can cause chylomicronemia syndrome. The clinical presentation is identical to that of LPL deficiency. The lack of apo CII, an activating cofactor for LPL, results in a functional LDL deficiency. Apo CII deficiency can be confirmed by the absence of apo CII on electrophoresis of plasma apolipoproteins. The treatment of apo CII deficiency is identical to that of LPL deficiency.

FAMILIAL HYPERTRIGLYCERIDEMIA

Individuals with familial hypertriglyceridemia overproduce VLDL triglycerides, resulting in serum triglyceride concentrations in the range of 200 to 500 mg/dL and normal LDL cholesterol concentrations. The hypertriglyceridemia typically occurs in concert with low serum HDL cholesterol levels and obesity. Because of the relative mild degree of hypertriglyceridemia and the lack of associated symptomatology, most patients who are affected are not diagnosed until adulthood. The degree of hypertriglyceridemia is usually less than 1000 mg/dL unless aggravated by alcohol use, orally administered estrogen, or hypothyroidism. Treatment of individuals with familial hypertriglyceridemia includes avoidance of alcohol and orally administered estrogens as well as implementation of some of the nonpharmacologic and pharmacologic approaches outlined next.

TREATMENT

Hypertriglyceridemia promotes atherosclerosis, and treatment should be considered when serum triglyceride concentrations are higher than 200 mg/dL. Nonpharmacologic treatment options include weight loss in patients with obesity, a regular isotonic exercise program, improved glycemic control in patients with diabetes mellitus, limitation of alcohol intake, and avoidance of free carbohydrates in the diet. Pharmacologic therapy is indicated when hypertriglyceridemia persists despite nonpharmacologic interventions.

When serum LDL cholesterol concentrations are elevated in concert with serum triglycerides, a HMG-CoA reductase inhibitor (statin) may lower the blood triglyceride concentration as well as the LDL cholesterol concentration. When the main lipid profile anomaly is hypertriglyceridemia, it can be treated with a fibric acid derivative (i.e., fenofibrate or gemfibrozil), nicotinic acid, or omega-3 fatty acids (e.g., fish oil

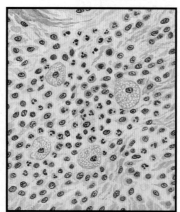

Hyperlipemia retinalis

Chylomicronemia syndrome:
▶ Recurrent abdominal pain
▶ Pancreatitis
▶ Hepatosplenomegaly
▶ Eruptive xanthomas
▶ Lipemia retinalis
▶ Lipemic plasma
▶ Severe hypertriglyceridemia (e.g., >2000 mg/dL)

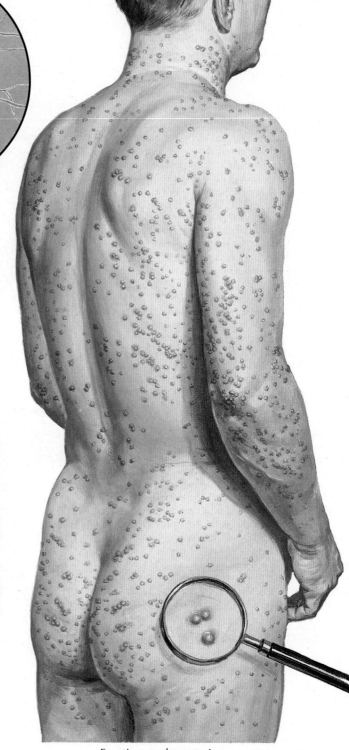

Hyperlipemic xanthomatous nodule (high magnification): few foam cells amid inflammatory exudate

Eruptive xanthomatosis

at doses >3 g/d). Fish oil decreases VLDL production and can lower serum triglyceride concentrations by as much as 50%. Nicotinic acid may cause hyperglycemia and should be avoided in patients with hyperglycemia or impaired glucose tolerance. Gemfibrozil may increase the risk for statin-related myositis and should be avoided in these patients. Orlistat may be helpful in patients with type V hyperlipoproteinemia and very high serum triglyceride levels that are refractory to the

aforementioned therapies because it inhibits gastrointestinal fat absorption and decreases intestinal chylomicron synthesis.

When the serum triglyceride concentration is very high (≥500 mg/dL), the first goal is to avoid pancreatitis. Prompt institution of pharmacologic therapy with nicotinic acid or a fibrate is indicated. For example, gemfibrozil can lower serum triglyceride concentrations in this setting by as much as 70%.

Plate 7.12

Lipids and Nutrition

ATHEROGENESIS: FATTY STREAK FORMATION

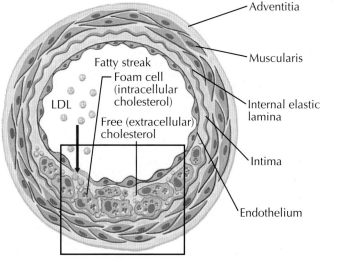

Adventitia

Muscularis

Fatty streak

Foam cell (intracellular cholesterol)

LDL

Internal elastic lamina

Free (extracellular) cholesterol

Intima

Endothelium

Extracellular cholesterol and cholesterol-filled macrophages (foam cells) accumulate in subendothelial space. Subsequent structural modifications of LDL particles render them more atherogenic. Oxidation of subendothelial LDL attracts monocytes, which enter subendothelium and change into macrophages. Macrophages may take up oxidized LDL to form foam cells.

JOHN A.CRAIG—MD
C.Machado—M.D.

ATHEROSCLEROSIS

Atherogenesis starts in the arterial wall and eventually may lead to ASCVD, peripheral vascular disease, or cerebrovascular disease. Occlusive arterial disease resulting from atherosclerosis is a leading cause of disability and death. Atherosclerosis, a result of a chronic inflammatory response to vascular injury, is the buildup of plaque in the walls of arteries that is composed of lipoproteins, inflammatory cells, extracellular matrix, vascular smooth muscle cells, and calcium. The sites of atherosclerosis are typically those parts of the arterial vascular tree associated with increased turbulent blood flow (bifurcations and curvatures). Typical locations for symptomatic atherosclerotic lesions are the proximal left anterior descending coronary artery, proximal renal arteries, and carotid bifurcations. These sites have an upregulation of proinflammatory adhesion molecules for inflammatory cells (e.g., monocytes and T cells). Risk factors for endothelial dysfunction and injury include increased serum concentrations of LDL cholesterol, decreased serum concentrations of HDL cholesterol, increased oxidant stress (e.g., cigarette smoking, hypertension, diabetes mellitus), and aging. The serum concentration of LDL cholesterol is a strong predictor of ASCVD and atherosclerosis; more than 70% of individuals with premature ASCVD have hyperlipidemia. Total serum cholesterol concentrations less than 160 mg/dL markedly decrease ASCVD risk.

Atherogenesis is a slow process that occurs over years. The clinical manifestations of atherosclerosis may be chronic (e.g., stable angina pectoris or intermittent claudication) or acute (e.g., myocardial infarction, stroke). However, most atheromata produce no symptoms. The normal arterial wall is composed of the endothelial cell layer, intima and subendothelial space, internal elastic lamina, media (muscularis layer formed by smooth muscle cells), and adventitia (loose connective tissue). The initial events in atherosclerosis involve movement of electronegative LDL cholesterol and other apo B_{100}–containing lipoproteins (e.g., VLDL, Lp[a]) from the blood into the subendothelial space where they are retained because of a charge-mediated interaction with the positively charged proteoglycans. Small LDL particles penetrate the endothelial barrier more effectively than large LDL particles. LDL cholesterol in the subendothelial space becomes oxidized. The presence of oxidized LDL promotes synthesis of monocyte chemoattractant protein 1 and other chemoattractants by endothelial and smooth muscle cells.

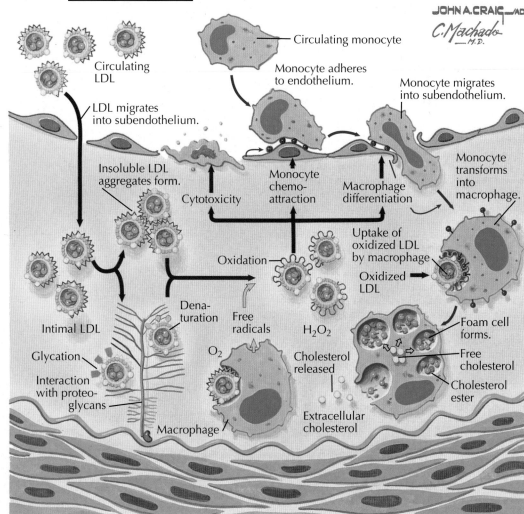

Circulating monocyte

Circulating LDL

Monocyte adheres to endothelium.

Monocyte migrates into subendothelium.

LDL migrates into subendothelium.

Insoluble LDL aggregates form.

Monocyte chemoattraction

Macrophage differentiation

Monocyte transforms into macrophage.

Cytotoxicity

Uptake of oxidized LDL by macrophage

Oxidation

Oxidized LDL

Intimal LDL

Denaturation

Free radicals

H_2O_2

Glycation

O_2

Cholesterol released

Foam cell forms.

Interaction with proteoglycans

Free cholesterol

Macrophage

Extracellular cholesterol

Cholesterol ester

Circulating monocytes then attach to the surface of endothelial cells and subsequently migrate between these cells to enter the subendothelial space, where they differentiate into macrophages. The activated macrophage releases mitogens and chemoattractants, which recruit more macrophages and smooth muscle cells. The macrophages take up the oxidized LDL cholesterol in an unregulated fashion by scavenger receptors. The internalization of oxidized LDL cholesterol leads to formation of lipid peroxides and facilitates the accumulation of cholesterol esters, resulting in foam cell formation. As foam cells accumulate, they form a visible atherosclerotic lesion—the fatty streak. Fatty streaks, the initial lesion of atherosclerosis, can be seen in infants and young children. The fatty streak may resolve (based on HDL cholesterol reverse cholesterol

Plate 7.13

Endocrine System: VOLUME 2

ATHEROGENESIS: FIBROUS PLAQUE FORMATION

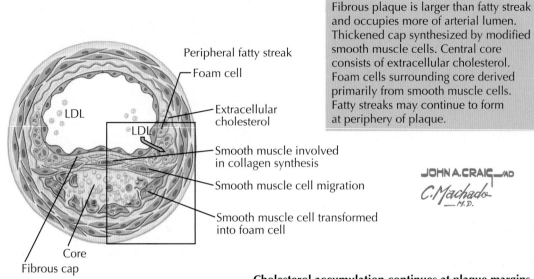

> Fibrous plaque is larger than fatty streak and occupies more of arterial lumen. Thickened cap synthesized by modified smooth muscle cells. Central core consists of extracellular cholesterol. Foam cells surrounding core derived primarily from smooth muscle cells. Fatty streaks may continue to form at periphery of plaque.

Peripheral fatty streak

Foam cell

LDL

LDL

Extracellular cholesterol

Smooth muscle involved in collagen synthesis

Smooth muscle cell migration

Smooth muscle cell transformed into foam cell

Core

Fibrous cap

JOHN A. CRAIG—MD

C. Machado —M.D.

ATHEROSCLEROSIS (Continued)

transport) or may mature into a fibrous plaque that extends into the vessel lumen.

As fibrous plaques enlarge and age, foam cells necrose and release oxidized LDL, intracellular enzymes, and oxygen free radicals that can damage the vessel wall. Oxidized LDL induces apoptosis of endothelial cells and vascular smooth muscle cells. The extracellular cholesterol deposition and continued inflammatory response promote smooth muscle cell proliferation and migration and collagen synthesis. Smooth muscle cells become the main cell type, lying in parallel layers with proteoglycan and basement membrane in between them. Continued inflammation results in the recruitment of increased numbers of macrophages and lymphocytes that release proteolytic enzymes, cytokines, chemokines, and growth factors. Focal necrosis develops, and free cholesterol forms the central lipid core of the fibrous plaque. Some smooth muscle cells accumulate lipid to become foam cells. Cycles of accumulation of mononuclear cells, migration and proliferation of smooth muscle cells, and formation of fibrous tissue lead to a continuous restructuring of the atherosclerotic lesion. A fibrous cap develops that overlies the core of lipid and necrotic tissue.

With progression of an atherosclerotic lesion, new microvessels arise from the arterial vasa vasorum. The microvessels provide a portal of entry for monocytes and lymphocytes into the developing plaque. The microvessels are fragile and are prone to rupture, resulting in small focal hemorrhages within the plaque. Calcification may occur as a late event in fibrous plaques, and the elasticity of the arterial wall becomes limited. Bone-related proteins (e.g., osteopontin and osteocalcin) can be found in atherosclerotic plaques. Coronary calcification is a marker of atherosclerosis that can be quantified with the use of cardiac computed tomography (CT), and it is proportional to the extent and severity of atherosclerotic disease. Cardiac CT is a noninvasive tool to assess the presence of coronary artery disease. Increased cardiac CT calcium scores indicate higher risk for ASCVD in both asymptomatic and symptomatic individuals and can be used to guide management decisions. For example, aggressive preventive medical therapy (see Plate 7.17) and risk factor modification (see Plate 7.14) should be considered for asymptomatic individuals with high cardiac CT calcium scores.

The plaque can progress to a complicated lesion, where the surface endothelial cells may be lost, and

Cholesterol accumulation continues at plaque margins

Fibrous cap forms over core

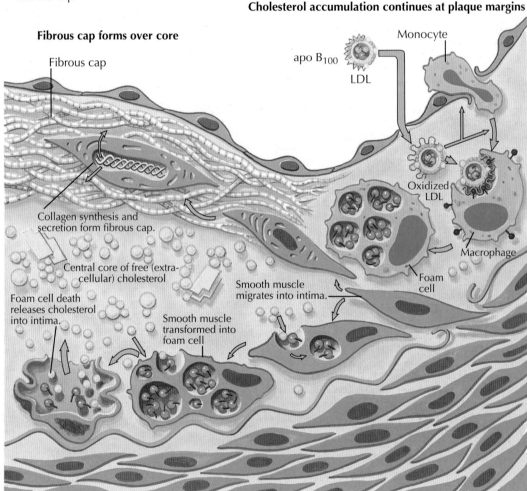

Fibrous cap

apo B$_{100}$

Monocyte

LDL

Oxidized LDL

Macrophage

Collagen synthesis and secretion form fibrous cap.

Foam cell

Central core of free (extra-cellular) cholesterol

Smooth muscle migrates into intima.

Foam cell death releases cholesterol into intima.

Smooth muscle transformed into foam cell

the fibrous cap ruptures to expose the subendothelial space. Platelets adhere to the exposed surface, and thrombus formation is initiated. Platelets release their granules, which contain cytokines, growth factors, and thrombin, resulting in further proliferation and migration of smooth muscle cells and monocytes. A large thrombus may form in unstable ruptured plaques where blood dissects into the artery wall. The plaque rupture and thrombosis can lead to acute ischemic syndromes and sudden cardiac death. Plaque rupture is responsible for approximately 75% of fatal coronary thrombi; these plaques tend to have thin fibrous caps, increased macrophage content, and large lipid cores.

Plate 7.14

Lipids and Nutrition

ATHEROSCLEROSIS RISK FACTORS

The main modifiable cardiovascular risk factors are hypercholesterolemia with hyperlipidemia, hypertension, cigarette smoking, and diabetes mellitus.

HYPERLIPIDEMIA

In 2018 the AHA/ACC released a new clinical practice guideline on cholesterol management. The guideline included a risk assessment report on primary prevention of ASCVD, and it gave more attention to percentage reduction in LDL cholesterol as a treatment goal and to long-term monitoring of therapeutic efficacy. All individuals with high LDL cholesterol should pursue lifestyle modifications of aerobic exercise and consuming a healthy diet. Whether to lower LDL cholesterol with pharmacotherapy should incorporate both the level of LDL cholesterol level and a patient's estimated 10-year ASCVD risk. ASCVD risk refers to fatal or nonfatal myocardial infarction, acute coronary syndrome, sudden cardiac death, coronary artery revascularization, stroke, and peripheral vascular arterial disease. The AHA/ACC risk calculator triages patients into four risk categories. Based on the estimated 10-year ASCVD risk, shared decision-making discussions between patients and their providers can help determine whether a 30% relative risk reduction with a medication results in an absolute risk reduction large enough to be worth the cost and potential side effects of daily therapy.

The risk factors included in the AHA/ACC heart risk calculator are age, sex, race, total cholesterol, HDL cholesterol, systolic blood pressure (SBP), diastolic blood pressure (DBP), treatment of hypertension, treatment for diabetes, and cigarette smoking. The intensity of treatment of hypercholesterolemia should be personalized on the basis of ASCVD risk. As plasma LDL cholesterol levels increase, cardiovascular risk increases.

Although LDL-lowering treatments do not markedly regress known obstructing coronary artery lesions, they do markedly decrease coronary events. Thus the benefit of lipid lowering in patients with known ASCVD may not be plaque regression but rather plaque stabilization. In addition, the consistent benefit of LDL lowering by HMG-CoA reductase inhibitors (statins) may depend not only on their effects on LDL cholesterol but also on their direct influence on plaque biology.

HYPERTENSION

Observational studies have shown graded associations between higher SBP and DBP and increased ASCVD risk. In a metaanalysis of 61 prospective studies, the risk of ASCVD increased in a log-linear fashion from SBP levels <115 mm Hg to >180 mm Hg and from DBP levels <75 mm Hg to >105 mm Hg. In that analysis, 20 mm Hg higher SBP and 10 mm Hg higher DBP were each associated with a doubling in the risk of death from stroke, heart disease, or other vascular disease. The 2017 AHA/ACC blood pressure (BP) guideline provided the following definitions: *normal BP* = SBP <120 mm Hg and DBP <80 mm Hg; **elevated BP** = SBP 120 to 139 mm Hg and DBP <80 mm Hg; *stage 1 hypertension* = SBP 130 to 139 mm Hg or DBP 80 to

RISK FACTORS IN CHRONIC HEART DISEASE

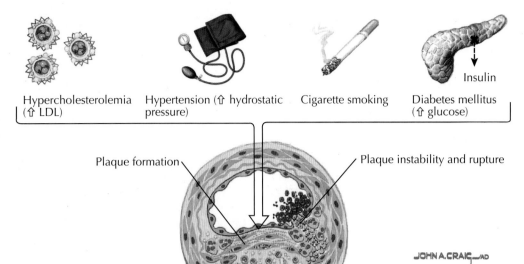

Hypercholesterolemia (⇧ LDL) — Hypertension (⇧ hydrostatic pressure) — Cigarette smoking — Diabetes mellitus (⇧ glucose) — Insulin

Plaque formation — Plaque instability and rupture

JOHN A. CRAIG—MD
C. Machado—M.D.
K. Marzzn

Interaction of risk factors in atherogenesis

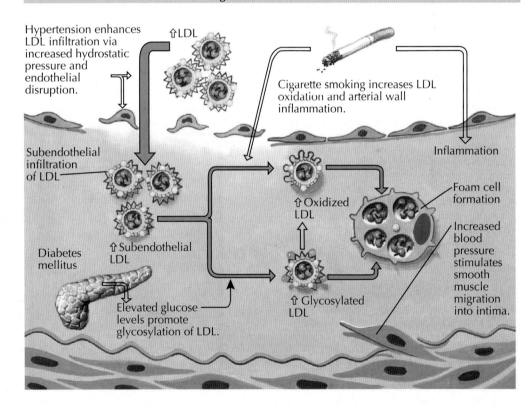

Hypertension enhances LDL infiltration via increased hydrostatic pressure and endothelial disruption.

⇧LDL

Cigarette smoking increases LDL oxidation and arterial wall inflammation.

Subendothelial infiltration of LDL

Inflammation

⇧Oxidized LDL

Foam cell formation

Diabetes mellitus

⇧Subendothelial LDL

Elevated glucose levels promote glycosylation of LDL.

⇧Glycosylated LDL

Increased blood pressure stimulates smooth muscle migration into intima.

89 mm Hg; *stage 2 hypertension* = SBP ≥140 mm Hg or DBP ≥90 mm Hg. Normalization of BP by nonpharmacologic measures (e.g., weight reduction, sodium-restricted diet, regular isotonic exercise) and pharmacologic measures reduces the risk of stroke, heart failure, and ASCVD events.

DIABETES MELLITUS

Most individuals with diabetes mellitus die of atherosclerosis complications. The increased prevalence of atherosclerosis in individuals with diabetes is partly caused by the presence of small and dense LDL

cholesterol, low serum HDL cholesterol concentrations, and increased serum triglyceride concentrations. Increased blood glucose levels also promote glycosylation of LDL cholesterol.

CIGARETTE SMOKING

The understanding of the mechanisms involved in cigarette smoking–related atherosclerosis is not complete. However, cigarette smoking clearly increases inflammation, thrombosis, and oxidation of LDL cholesterol, leading to increased oxidative stress and arterial wall inflammation.

Plate 7.15

Endocrine System: VOLUME 2

METABOLIC SYNDROME

The metabolic syndrome is characterized by insulin resistance, hyperinsulinemia, predisposition to diabetes mellitus, dyslipidemia, atherosclerotic vascular disease, and hypertension. Most individuals with the components of the metabolic syndrome are overweight (body mass index [BMI], 25 to 29 kg/m²) or obese (BMI ≥30 kg/m²). Excess abdominal visceral fat is very characteristic. Based on the Third Report of the Expert Panel on Detection, Evaluation, and Treatment of High Blood Cholesterol in Adults (Adult Treatment Panel III [ATP III]) guidelines, approximately 50 million people in the United States have the metabolic syndrome. Individuals with this diagnosis have a two- to fourfold increase in subsequent cardiovascular events. It is debated whether the metabolic syndrome is truly a unique entity and whether it confers risk beyond its individual components. However, identifying and treating components of the metabolic syndrome are important to decrease morbidity and mortality related to cardiovascular disease and diabetes.

Insulin resistance occurs when more than normal amounts of insulin are required to elicit a normal biologic response, a situation inferred by high fasting levels of blood insulin. Insulin resistance affects muscle, liver, and adipose tissues and results in decreased peripheral glucose and fatty acid use. Biomarkers consistent with the concept that the metabolic syndrome is a prothrombotic and proinflammatory state include increased serum levels of C-reactive protein, plasminogen activator inhibitor 1, interleukin 6, and adipocyte cytokines (e.g., adiponectin).

No single test is available to diagnose the metabolic syndrome. The ATP III diagnostic criteria include the presence of any three of the following five traits: (1) abdominal obesity defined as a waist circumference larger than 102 cm in males or larger than 88 cm in females; (2) serum triglyceride concentration above 150 mg/dL or medication therapy for hypertriglyceridemia; (3) serum HDL cholesterol concentration below 40 mg/dL in males or below 50 mg/dL in females or medication therapy for low HDL cholesterol; (4) BP above 130/80 mm Hg or medication therapy for hypertension; and (5) fasting plasma glucose concentration 100 mg/dL or above or medication therapy for hyperglycemia. The diagnostic criteria from the World Health Organization include insulin resistance (identified by type 2 diabetes mellitus, impaired fasting glucose, or impaired glucose tolerance) plus any two of the following five traits: (1) antihypertensive medication use or high BP (i.e., ≥140/90 mm Hg); (2) serum triglyceride concentration 150 mg/dL or above; (3) serum HDL cholesterol concentration below 35 mg/dL in males or below 39 mg/dL in females; (4) BMI above 30 kg/m² or a waist-to-hip ratio above 0.9 in males or above 0.85 in females; and (5) urinary albumin excretion rate of 20 μg/min or above or albumin-to-creatinine ratio of 30 mg/g or above.

Clinical assessment of patients with one or more risk factors for the metabolic syndrome should include a

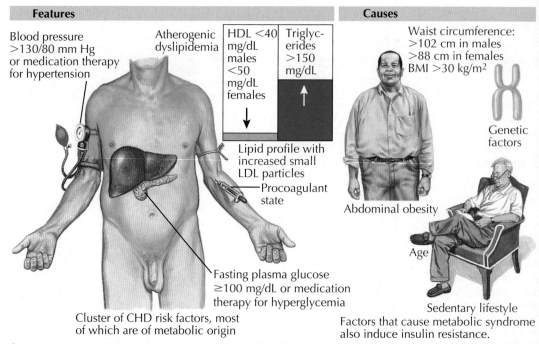

Features

Blood pressure >130/80 mm Hg or medication therapy for hypertension

Atherogenic dyslipidemia

HDL <40 mg/dL males <50 mg/dL females

Triglycerides >150 mg/dL

Lipid profile with increased small LDL particles

Procoagulant state

Fasting plasma glucose ≥100 mg/dL or medication therapy for hyperglycemia

Cluster of CHD risk factors, most of which are of metabolic origin

Causes

Waist circumference: >102 cm in males >88 cm in females BMI >30 kg/m²

Genetic factors

Abdominal obesity

Age

Sedentary lifestyle

Factors that cause metabolic syndrome also induce insulin resistance.

Insulin resistance (biochemical basis of metabolic syndrome)

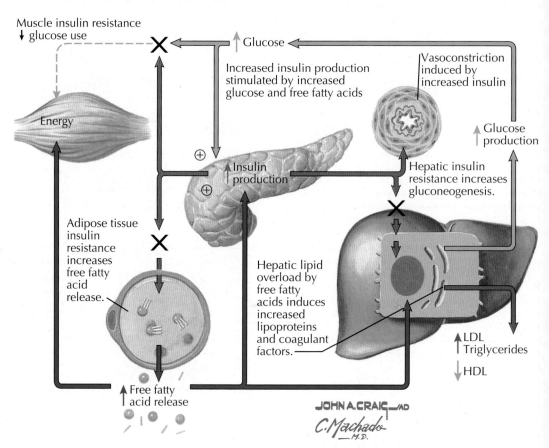

Muscle insulin resistance ↓ glucose use

↑ Glucose

Increased insulin production stimulated by increased glucose and free fatty acids

Vasoconstriction induced by increased insulin

↑ Glucose production

Energy

↑ Insulin production

Hepatic insulin resistance increases gluconeogenesis.

Adipose tissue insulin resistance increases free fatty acid release.

Hepatic lipid overload by free fatty acids induces increased lipoproteins and coagulant factors.

↑ LDL ↑ Triglycerides

↓ HDL

Free fatty acid release

JOHN A. CRAIG—MD
C. Machado—M.D.

history, physical examination (including BP measurement, determination of BMI, and waist circumference measurement), fasting lipid profile, and fasting plasma glucose.

The cornerstone of treatment of the metabolic syndrome is lifestyle modification with weight loss and increased physical activity. Diet and exercise can delay the onset of diabetes in patients with impaired glucose tolerance. Exercise (e.g., ≥30 minutes of moderate-intensity physical activity daily) has the potential to

decrease abdominal fat. Cigarette smoking should be discouraged. In patients with impaired fasting glucose or type 2 diabetes, the addition of metformin can very effectively improve glycemic control because it enhances insulin action. The overall management of diabetes in patients with the metabolic syndrome should follow clinical guidelines for diabetes (see Plate 5.21). The metabolic syndrome is a coronary risk equivalent, and serum cholesterol targets should follow clinical guidelines (see Plates 7.5 and 7.17).

Plate 7.16

Lipids and Nutrition

MECHANISMS OF ACTION OF LIPID-LOWERING AGENTS

CHOLESTEROL ABSORPTION INHIBITORS

Ezetimibe is a cholesterol absorption inhibitor that impairs cholesterol absorption at the brush border of the intestine. Its mechanism of action involves Niemann-Pick C1-like 1 proteins that have a role in intestinal cholesterol transport. At a dose of 10 mg/d, ezetimibe lowers the serum LDL cholesterol concentration by an average of 17%. The effect of ezetimibe is additive to that of statins.

STATINS

Statins are competitive inhibitors of HMG-CoA reductase—the rate-limiting step in cholesterol biosynthesis. The statin-induced decrease in hepatocyte cholesterol content results in increased LDL-receptor turnover and LDL-receptor cycling. Statins lower serum LDL cholesterol concentrations by 30% to 60%. In addition, statins modify the atherogenic lipoprotein phenotype by decreasing the serum concentration of small, dense LDL cholesterol. Most statins lower triglyceride concentrations by 20% to 40% and increase HDL cholesterol by 5% to 10%. Currently available statins include lovastatin, simvastatin, pravastatin, fluvastatin, atorvastatin, pitavastatin, and rosuvastatin.

PCSK9 INHIBITORS

PCSK9 is a serine protease that binds to the hepatocyte LDL receptors where it degrades the LDL receptor, resulting in higher plasma concentrations of LDL cholesterol. Antibodies to PCSK9 are approved for use in individuals with inadequately treated levels of LDL cholesterol. PCSK9 inhibitors can lower LDL cholesterol by as much as 60% in patients on statin therapy. Alirocumab and evolocumab are fully humanized monoclonal antibodies that bind free plasma PCSK9 and result in degradation of this enzyme. Another method of interfering with PCSK9 is to block its synthesis with inclisiran, which is an antisense small interfering mRNA.

BILE ACID SEQUESTRANTS

Bile acid sequestrants bind bile acids in the intestine and interrupt the usually efficient (90%) reabsorption of bile acids. The resultant reduction in intrahepatic cholesterol promotes the synthesis of LDL receptors. The increased numbers of hepatocyte LDL receptors bind LDL cholesterol from the plasma and thus reduce the serum LDL cholesterol concentration by 10% to 24%. The cholesterol-lowering effect of bile acid sequestrants is additive to that of statins. Currently available bile acid sequestrants include cholestyramine, colestipol, and colesevelam.

NICOTINIC ACID

Nicotinic acid inhibits the hepatic production of VLDL, which results in reduced lipolysis to LDL cholesterol. Nicotinic acid also increases serum HDL cholesterol concentrations by up to 35% by decreasing lipid transfer of cholesterol from HDL to VLDL and by inhibiting HDL clearance.

FIBRIC ACIDS

Fibric acids lower serum triglyceride concentrations and increase serum HDL cholesterol concentrations by

Ezetimibe.
Localizes at intestinal brush border of small intestine. Blocks absorption of intestinal cholesterol.

Statins (HMG-CoA reductase inhibitors).
Reduce cholesterol synthesis, lowering intracellular cholesterol, which stimulates LDL receptor synthesis.

Bile acid sequestrants.
Bind bile acids in gut, decreasing intracellular cholesterol content, which stimulates LDL receptor synthesis.

Nicotinic acid.
Decreases hepatic production of VLDL.

PCSK9 inhibitors.
PCSK9 degrades LDL receptors. PCSK9 inhibitors either decrease availability of this enzyme (e.g., with monoclonal antibodies [mAb]) or block its synthesis with a small interfering mRNA.

JOHN A. CRAIG—MD

C. Machado—M.D.

J. Perkins
CMI, FAMI

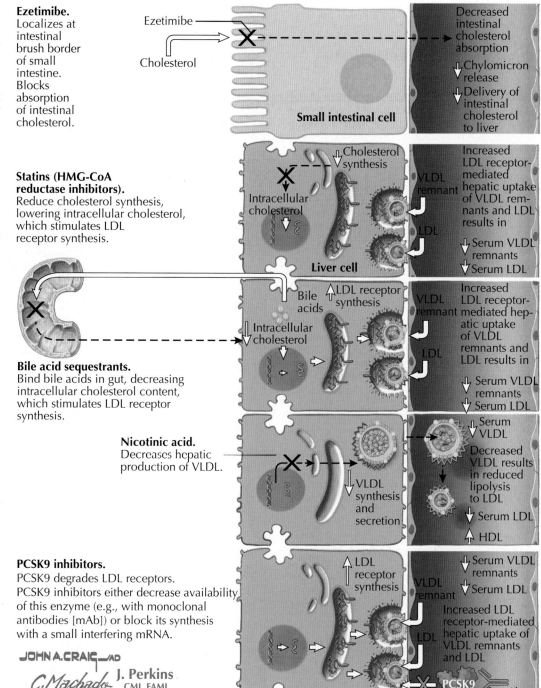

activation of peroxisome proliferator-activated receptor-α. Fibric acids reduce serum triglyceride concentrations by reducing hepatic secretion of VLDL and by stimulating LPL activity that increases the clearance of triglyceride-enriched lipoproteins. These effects are also mediated by downregulation of apo CIII gene expression. Fibric acids increase serum HDL cholesterol concentrations by stimulating synthesis of apo AI and apo AII. Fibric acid administration lowers serum triglyceride concentrations by 35% to 50%, increases serum HDL cholesterol concentrations by 15% to 25%, and lowers serum Lp(a) concentrations to a variable degree. Currently available fibric acids are gemfibrozil and fenofibrate.

FISH OIL

The active components in fish oil are the long-chain omega-3 fatty acids, eicosapentaenoic acid (EPA; 20:5n-3) and docosahexaenoic acid (DHA; 22:6n-3). EPA and DHA are absorbed in the small intestine and transported to the liver as triglycerides in chylomicron particles. The liver releases EPA and DHA into the circulation as triglycerides in lipoprotein particles (e.g., LDL cholesterol and HDL cholesterol). EPA and DHA decrease the hepatic secretion of TGRL. Daily intake of 3 to 4 g of EPA and DHA lowers serum triglyceride concentrations by 20% to 50%. Fish oil supplementation also increases serum HDL cholesterol concentrations by 3% and lowers the proportion of small, dense LDL cholesterol.

Plate 7.17

Endocrine System: VOLUME 2

TREATMENT OF HYPERLIPIDEMIA

All patients with elevated serum concentrations of LDL cholesterol should engage in lifestyle modifications such as regular aerobic exercise, a prudent diet that is low in saturated fat and high in fiber, and weight loss if overweight. The impact of lifestyle measures on serum LDL cholesterol concentrations is quite variable and depends in part on baseline dietary habits. The treatment of hyperlipidemia is influenced by the absence (primary prevention) or the presence (secondary prevention) of ASCVD.

PRIMARY PREVENTION

The decision about whether to lower LDL cholesterol with pharmacotherapy should be based on the LDL cholesterol level and a patient's estimated 10-year ASCVD risk. However, an ASCVD risk calculation is not needed for individuals with an LDL cholesterol >190 mg/dL where high-intensity statin (atorvastatin 40–80 mg/d or rosuvastatin 20–40 mg/d), therapy is indicated. Treatment with a statin results in a 30% relative risk reduction regardless of the baseline LDL cholesterol level. Based on the estimated 10-year ASCVD risk, the patient and clinician can decide whether a 30% relative risk reduction results in an absolute risk reduction large enough to be worth the cost and potential side effects of statin therapy. If the predicted 10-year ASCVD risk is 10%, most clinicians recommend treatment with a moderate-dose statin (e.g., 20 mg of atorvastatin or 10 mg of rosuvastatin). However, if the 10-year ASCVD risk is 20% or higher, a high-intensity statin (e.g., atorvastatin 40–80 mg/d or rosuvastatin 20–40 mg/d) is indicated. Elevation in hepatic enzymes and diffuse myalgias are unusual but potentially serious adverse effects. Very rarely (one case per 15 million prescriptions), statins cause rhabdomyolysis, a serious adverse effect that is more common in patients also treated with a fibrate (the risk is much greater with gemfibrozil than with fenofibrate) or cyclosporine.

SECONDARY PREVENTION

The risk of a future myocardial infarction is 20 times higher in individuals with ASCVD than in those without ASCVD. Large trials have shown that cholesterol lowering in individuals with ASCVD is associated with a 13% to 16% reduction in mortality. In addition, serial angiographic studies have shown that cholesterol lowering can slow the progression and induce regression of coronary atherosclerosis, a finding most evident when LDL cholesterol concentrations are reduced below 100 mg/dL. In patients with stable ASCVD or an ASCVD equivalent (e.g., diabetes mellitus), the statin dosage can be titrated upward every 6 weeks to achieve the LDL cholesterol target (usually <100 mg/dL). In patients who present with an acute myocardial infarction, it is reasonable to start a high-intensity statin in the hospital (e.g., atorvastatin 40–80 mg/d or rosuvastatin 20–40 mg/d), which will result in a >50% reduction in LDL cholesterol levels. If the serum LDL cholesterol concentration does not drop more than 50% or if it is >70 mg/dL, the clinician should first ensure compliance. If the patient is compliant, then ezetimibe should be added. If LDL cholesterol remains >70 mcg/dL

despite high-intensity statin and ezetimibe, treatment with a PCSK9 inhibitor should be considered.

RAISING HIGH-DENSITY LIPOPROTEIN CHOLESTEROL

Low serum concentrations of HDL cholesterol are common in individuals with premature ASCVD. Exercise, weight loss in individuals with obesity, and smoking cessation can all increase serum HDL cholesterol concentrations. However, studies have failed to show evidence of benefit from medication-related attempts (e.g., with nicotinic acid or gemfibrozil) to raise HDL cholesterol. A better approach is to pursue lowering LDL cholesterol more vigorously in those patients with low levels of HDL cholesterol.

HYPERTRIGLYCERIDEMIA

Treatment directed at hypertriglyceridemia (see Plates 7.10 and 7.11) should be considered in patients who also have hypercholesterolemia. Triglyceride-rich lipoproteins (VLDL) also transport cholesterol, and the hypercholesterolemia is partly caused by the hypertriglyceridemia.

MONITORING

Monitoring the fasting lipid panel every 6 to 8 weeks until the serum LDL cholesterol target is achieved is reasonable. Thereafter, rechecks every 6 to 12 months are indicated. With each dose change, liver function tests should be performed at the time of blood sampling.

Dietary management

Weight control

Increase exercise.

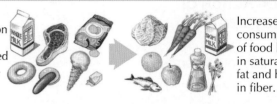

Reduce consumption of foods high in cholesterol, saturated fat, trans fatty acids, and salt. Decrease total caloric intake.

Increase consumption of food low in saturated fat and high in fiber.

Appropriate diet and exercise are cornerstones of cholesterol management. Dietary counseling and reinforcement and a planned program of physical activity are recommended.

Fish oil supplements

Actions of lipid-lowering medications

Statins.
Statins (HMG-CoA reductase inhibitors) inhibit cholesterol synthesis and increase LDL receptor uptake of LDL.

Increased LDL receptor-mediated hepatic uptake of VLDL remnants and LDL

Bile acid sequestrants.
Bind bile acids in the intestine, and the resultant reduction in intrahepatic cholesterol promotes the increased synthesis of LDL receptors that clear more VLDL and LDL cholesterol from plasma.

Increased LDL receptor-mediated hepatic uptake of VLDL remnants and LDL

PCSK9 inhibitors.
PCSK9 degrades LDL receptors. PCSK9 inhibitors either decrease availability of this enzyme (e.g., with monoclonal antibodies [mAb]) or block its synthesis with a small interfering mRNA.

Increased LDL receptor-mediated hepatic uptake of VLDL remnants and LDL

Fibric acid derivatives.
Interact with peroxisome proliferator-activated receptor α (PPAR-α) to reduce serum triglyceride concentrations by reducing hepatic secretion VLDL and by stimulating LPL activity that increases the clearance of triglyceride-enriched lipoproteins.

Increased LPL and decreased apo CIII stimulate lipolysis and lower VLDL levels.

Plate 7.18

Lipids and Nutrition

ABSORPTION OF ESSENTIAL VITAMINS

Vitamins are organic substances that cannot be synthesized by humans; they must be ingested in the diet. They are divided into water-soluble and fat-soluble vitamins.

WATER-SOLUBLE VITAMINS

All water-soluble vitamins (with the exception of vitamin B_{12}; see later discussion) are absorbed in the jejunum and ileum by passive diffusion and by a sodium (Na^+)-coupled active transport pump. The water-soluble vitamins leave the enterocyte to the portal circulation by a Na^+-coupled adenosine-5'-triphosphate (ATP)-dependent pump.

Vitamin B_1 (thiamine) has limited tissue storage, and its biologic half-life is 10 to 20 days. Thiamine is a key cofactor for enzymes involved in amino acid and carbohydrate metabolism. The main food sources of thiamine are yeast, brown rice, whole-grain cereals, legumes, and pork.

Vitamin B_2 (riboflavin) is a flavin and is incorporated as a component of flavin-adenine dinucleotide. Flavoproteins serve as catalysts in a number of mitochondrial oxidative and reductive reactions and function as electron transporters. The dietary sources of riboflavin include meats, fish, milk, eggs, yeast, green vegetables, and enriched foods.

Vitamin B_3 (niacin) is nicotinic acid and nicotinamide. Through a series of biochemical reactions in the mitochondria, niacin, nicotinamide, and tryptophan form nicotinamide adenine dinucleotide (NAD) and NAD phosphate (NADP). As essential components of redox reactions and hydrogen transport, NAD and NADP are crucial in the synthesis and metabolism of carbohydrates, fatty acids, and proteins. Food sources of niacin include meats (especially liver), yeasts, cereals, legumes, and seeds.

Vitamin B_5 (pantothenic acid) is an essential cofactor in many acetylation reactions, including the tricarboxylic acid cycle. After ATP-dependent phosphorylation, pantothenic acid becomes coenzyme A. The main dietary sources of pantothenic acid are egg yolk, liver, broccoli, milk, chicken, beef, potatoes, and whole grains.

Vitamin B_6 (pyridoxine) is absorbed by passive diffusion in the jejunum and ileum. Pyridoxine is involved in many metabolic steps, including decarboxylation of amino acids and gluconeogenesis. Pyridoxine and pyridoxamine are found in meats, whole grains, vegetables, and nuts.

Biotin functions as a cofactor to the carboxylase enzyme. Biotin is an essential component of several enzyme complexes in carbohydrate and lipid metabolism, where it acts as a carbon dioxide carrier on the surface of each enzyme. Biotin is found in liver, egg yolk, soybean products, and yeast.

Vitamin C (ascorbic acid) functions as a cofactor and cosubstrate in providing reducing equivalents for a number of biochemical reactions involving iron and copper. Ascorbic acid provides electrons needed to reduce molecular oxygen. Food sources of vitamin C include citrus fruits, tomatoes, Brussels sprouts, potatoes, cauliflower, broccoli, strawberries, cabbage, and spinach.

Vitamin B_{12} (cobalamin) binds to gastric-derived intrinsic factor (IF) in the small intestine. The IF–vitamin B_{12} complex binds to a specific ileal receptor, cubilin, from which it is absorbed into the enterocyte in an energy-requiring process. Vitamin B_{12} then enters the plasma and is bound to transcobalamin (TC); the

Water-soluble vitamins		
Vitamin C	Ileum	Na^+-coupled/2° active
Thiamine (B_1)	Jejunum	Na^+-coupled/2° active
Riboflavin (B_2)	Jejunum	Na^+-coupled/2° active
Biotin	Jejunum	Na^+-coupled/2° active
Vitamin B_{12}	Ileum	Facilitated diffusion
Pyridoxine (B_6)	Jejunum and ileum	Passive diffusion
Fat-soluble vitamins		
Vitamin A	Jejunum and ileum	Passive diffusion
Vitamin D	Jejunum and ileum	Passive diffusion
Vitamin E	Jejunum and ileum	Passive diffusion
Vitamin K	Jejunum and ileum	Passive diffusion

Water-soluble vitamins

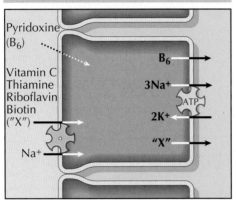

Fat-soluble vitamins

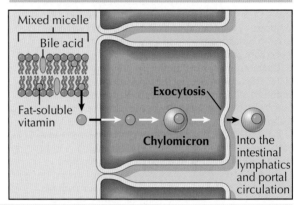

Vitamin B_{12}

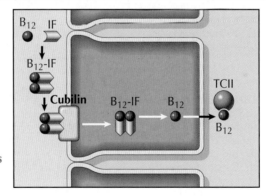

J. Perkins
MS, MFA

vitamin B_{12}-TCII complex is the most physiologically important one. Vitamin B_{12} is required for DNA synthesis in cells undergoing rapid turnover. Meat and dairy products are the only dietary sources of vitamin B_{12}.

FAT-SOLUBLE VITAMINS

Fat-soluble vitamins are released from dietary proteins via proteolysis in the stomach and by the proteolytic action of pancreatic enzymes in the small intestine. Bile salts then solubilize the vitamins into micelles for absorption into enterocytes, where they are incorporated into chylomicrons, thereby facilitating absorption into the intestinal lymphatics and portal circulation for transport to the liver.

Vitamin A is part of a family of lipid-soluble compounds (retinols, β-carotenes, and carotenoids) referred to as *retinoic acids*. Vitamin A has a major role in phototransduction and cellular differentiations in the eyes. The best food sources of retinols are liver, egg yolk, and butter. β-Carotene is found in green leafy vegetables.

Vitamin D (calciferol) includes a group of lipid-soluble compounds with a four-ringed cholesterol backbone. Vitamin D is critical for normal calcium absorption and bone metabolism. Sunlight and ultraviolet light photoisomerize provitamin D to vitamin D_3 (cholecalciferol) in the skin. Intestinal absorption is the other major source of vitamin D. The main dietary sources of vitamin D are fortified milk, fatty fish, cod liver oil, and eggs.

Vitamin E functions as a free radical scavenger and protects polyunsaturated fatty acids (that serve as structural components of cell membranes) from peroxidation. Vitamin E is found in a variety of foods, including oils, meat, eggs, and leafy vegetables.

Vitamin K is a cofactor required for the activity of several key proteins in the coagulation pathway. For example, vitamin K is necessary for activation of coagulation factors VII, IX, X, and prothrombin. Dietary vitamin K_1 (phylloquinone) is found in green leafy vegetables. In addition, gut microflora synthesize vitamin K_2 (menaquinone), which provides a portion of the dietary requirement of vitamin K.

Plate 7.19

Endocrine System: VOLUME 2

VITAMIN B₁ DEFICIENCY: BERIBERI

Vitamin B₁ (thiamine) deficiency (beriberi) was first described in Chinese medical texts as early as 2697 BC. Thiamine is a water-soluble vitamin that consists of a pyrimidine and a thiazole moiety. Dietary thiamine is obtained primarily from whole-grain cereals, whole-wheat bread, brown rice, legumes, yeast, and fresh meats. The thiamine molecule is denatured at high temperatures or at an alkaline pH; thus cooking, baking, pasteurization, and canning can destroy the bioactivity of thiamine.

Thiamine is absorbed in the jejunum and ileum (see Plate 7.18). Upon entering the bloodstream, thiamine is bound to albumin, and it enters cells by passive diffusion and active transport. Thiamine is localized primarily to the heart, skeletal muscles, brain, liver, and kidneys. Because thiamine does not have large functional tissue depots, its biologic half-life is only 10 to 20 days. Thus continuous dietary intake is required.

Thiamine serves as a cofactor for enzymes involved in carbohydrate and amino acid metabolism. For example, thiamine catalyzes the conversion of pyruvate to acetyl coenzyme A (see Plates 5.6 and 5.7). Thiamine also has a key role in the pentose phosphate pathway (see Plate 5.8). Normal nerve impulse propagation is dependent on thiamine. The main disorders associated with thiamine deficiency are beriberi and Wernicke-Korsakoff syndrome.

BERIBERI

Beriberi results from nutritional deficiency in thiamine. Beriberi can occur in infants who are breastfed by mothers who are deficient in thiamine. More often it occurs in children and adults whose diets are deficient in thiamine (e.g., diets in which the primary caloric source is polished rice or alcohol). The clinical manifestations of thiamine deficiency are variable and depend on the severity and duration of deprivation. Muscle and nerve tissue symptoms predominate. Infantile beriberi usually becomes apparent by 2 months with CNS disability (vomiting, nystagmus, purposeless movements, or seizures), cardiac disease (cardiomegaly, tachycardia, or cyanosis), and sudden death. In adults, the manifestations are primarily those of peripheral neuropathy and muscular disease affecting function of skeletal and cardiac muscles. "Dry beriberi" refers to a primarily neurologic presentation, with gradual onset of symmetric peripheral neuropathy (e.g., distal paresthesias); myalgias; and weakness that may advance to foot drop, wrist drop, flaccid paralysis, muscle wasting, aphonia, and emaciation. "Wet beriberi" refers to a primarily cardiac presentation with signs (e.g., cardiomegaly) and symptoms (e.g., dyspnea, orthopnea, peripheral edema, or tachycardia) of congestive heart failure.

In addition to supportive care, patients with beriberi should be treated with thiamine that is initially administered intravenously or intramuscularly. The daily dose for the first 2 weeks should be 50 to 100 mg. Thereafter, an oral dosage of 10 mg/d can be given until full recovery is achieved. All patients with thiamine deficiency should also be assessed for other potential vitamin deficiencies.

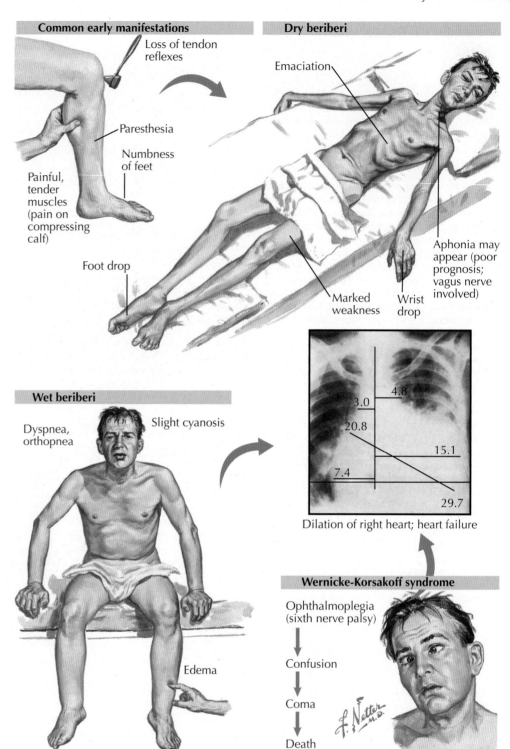

Common early manifestations
Loss of tendon reflexes
Paresthesia
Numbness of feet
Painful, tender muscles (pain on compressing calf)
Foot drop

Dry beriberi
Emaciation
Aphonia may appear (poor prognosis; vagus nerve involved)
Marked weakness
Wrist drop

Wet beriberi
Dyspnea, orthopnea
Slight cyanosis
Edema

3.0
4.8
20.8
15.1
7.4
29.7
Dilation of right heart; heart failure

Wernicke-Korsakoff syndrome
Ophthalmoplegia (sixth nerve palsy)
↓
Confusion
↓
Coma
↓
Death

WERNICKE-KORSAKOFF SYNDROME

Wernicke-Korsakoff syndrome is the most serious form of thiamine deficiency in adults. The Wernicke encephalopathy phase is characterized by ophthalmoplegia (sixth cranial nerve palsy), nystagmus, ataxia, and confusion that may progress to coma. Survival requires prompt recognition and treatment with 50 mg of intravenously administered thiamine daily until the same dosage can be given orally. Wernicke encephalopathy is seen primarily in individuals with alcoholism who deplete thiamine stores through prolonged bouts of alcohol use. The Korsakoff phase is the chronic neurologic condition of impaired short-term memory and confabulation—the end result of the Wernicke encephalopathy phase.

DIAGNOSIS

When thiamine deficiency is suspected, it can be confirmed by measuring the blood thiamine concentration (reference range, 80–150 nmol/L).

PREVENTION

The recommended daily allowance for thiamine in the United States is 0.5 to 0.9 mg for children, 1.2 mg for males, and 1.1 mg for nonpregnant females (1.4 mg during pregnancy and lactation). These amounts of thiamine are easily obtained from a nutritious diet that is rich in whole-grain cereals, whole-wheat bread, brown rice, legumes, yeast, and fresh meats.

Plate 7.20

Lipids and Nutrition

VITAMIN B₃ DEFICIENCY: PELLAGRA

Pellagra ("raw skin") is a nutritional deficiency disorder caused by insufficient intake of vitamin B_3 (niacin). Pellagra was first described by Casál in 1735 in Spanish peasants eating maize-based diets. Subsequently, it was found worldwide where maize and corn were the principal foodstuffs. Although still a problem in some areas of India, China, and Africa, pellagra is only seen in the United States as a complication of gastrointestinal malabsorptive disorders, anorexia nervosa, and alcoholism. Food sources of niacin include meats (especially liver), yeasts, whole-grain cereals, legumes, and seeds.

Nicotinic acid and nicotinamide are the principal forms of vitamin B_3. Mitochondria transform niacin, nicotinamide, and tryptophan to form NAD and NADP. Many enzymatic reactions depend on NAD and NADP. As essential components of redox reactions and hydrogen transport, NAD and NADP are crucial in the synthesis and metabolism of carbohydrates, fatty acids, and proteins (see Plates 5.6 and 5.7). Niacin is absorbed in the jejunum and ileum (see Plate 7.18). Upon entering the bloodstream, niacin is rapidly taken up by the liver, kidneys, and erythrocytes. Intracellular nicotinamide and nicotinic acid are converted to the coenzyme forms NAD and NADP, which are used and stored in tissues with high metabolic activities (e.g., liver and muscle).

Pellagra is characterized by dermatitis, stomatitis, gastritis, diarrhea, encephalopathy, anemia, and peripheral neuropathy. The "3 Ds" (dermatitis, diarrhea, and dementia) describe most cases. The dermatitis is characterized by photosensitivity with symmetric lesions with a sharp line of demarcation between involved and uninvolved skin. These lesions are typically located on the extensor surfaces of the hands, arms, and feet; they may have a "glove-and-stocking" distribution. Another prominent site is the exposed area of the neck, where the circumferential lesion is termed *Casál necklace*. The facial lesions tend to be distributed over the alae of the nose and on the forehead. Intertriginous folds and areas of skin such as the perineum and under the breasts are other typical sites of involvement. The dermatitis begins with an erythema resembling sunburn, which then becomes reddish-brown, roughened, and scaly. Desquamation usually starts in the center of the lesion and reveals underlying skin, which is red and thickened. The skin becomes permanently roughened and pigmented. Patients typically describe a sore mouth, angular cheilitis, and indigestion. The tongue is bright red, with flattened papillae. The diarrhea is watery and may contain blood and pus. The encephalopathy of pellagra may mimic

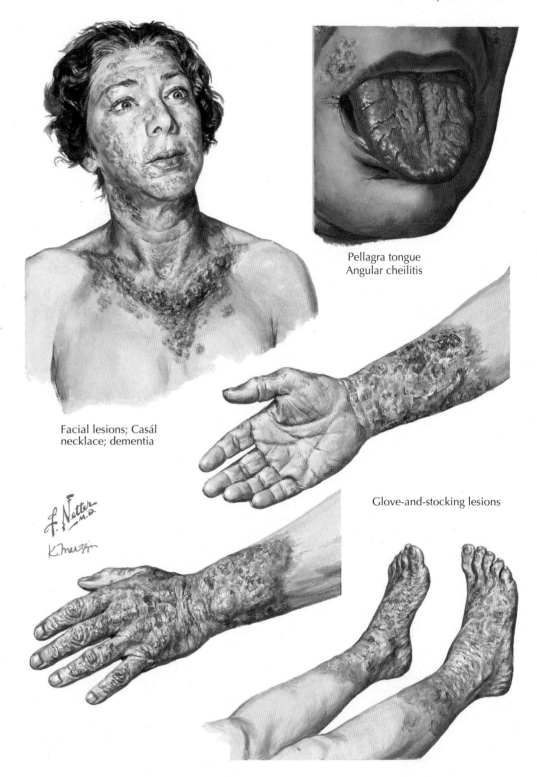

Pellagra tongue
Angular cheilitis

Facial lesions; Casál necklace; dementia

Glove-and-stocking lesions

mental disease with depression and suicidal behavior predominating. Other signs of pellagra encephalopathy are anxiety, disorientation, hallucinations, confusion, delirium, dementia, and coma.

Diagnosis. The clinical features of this diagnosis are quite recognizable. However, because of its rare occurrence in the United States, clinicians may not be very familiar with the signs and symptoms. When niacin deficiency is suspected, it can be confirmed by measuring the blood niacin concentration (reference ranges, 0.50–8.45 µg/mL if >10 years; 0.50–8.91 µg/mL if ≤10 years).

Prevention. Niacin is dosed as a "niacin equivalent." One niacin equivalent = 1 mg of niacin or 60 mg of dietary tryptophan. The US Recommended Dietary Allowance (RDA) for niacin is 6 to 12 niacin equivalents per day in children, 16 per day for males, and 14 for females (18 niacin equivalents during pregnancy and 17 niacin equivalents daily during lactation). Increased supplementation may be needed for those who have had a malabsorptive procedure to treat obesity (see Plate 7.27) or for individuals treated with renal dialysis. Balanced diets that include meat, yeasts, whole-grain cereals, legumes, and seeds provide sufficient niacin.

Plate 7.21

Endocrine System: VOLUME 2

VITAMIN C DEFICIENCY: SCURVY

Scurvy is a nutritional deficiency disorder resulting from a lack of vitamin C (ascorbic acid). Known since antiquity, during the 15th and 16th centuries scurvy became well recognized as an important disorder of seafaring men and was related to lack of fresh foods on prolonged journeys. In 1754 a British naval surgeon Dr. James Lind noted that consumption of oranges or lemons could prevent scurvy. Humans cannot synthesize ascorbic acid, and it is an essential dietary nutrient. Food sources high in ascorbic acid content include citrus fruits, tomatoes, potatoes, cabbage, spinach, Brussels sprouts, cauliflower, broccoli, and strawberries. Scurvy can occur as early as 3 months of being on an ascorbic acid–free diet.

Ascorbic acid is the enolic form of α-ketolactone and functions as a cofactor and cosubstrate in providing reducing equivalents for a number of biochemical reactions involving iron and copper. Ascorbic acid provides electrons needed to reduce molecular oxygen. For example, ascorbic acid serves as an enzymatic cofactor for carnitine synthesis. Ascorbic acid is necessary for normal collagen synthesis, where it is a cofactor for the enzymatic hydroxylation of proline and lysine. Deficiency in this hydroxylation step results in impaired wound healing, defective tooth formation, and impaired osteoblast function. Ascorbic acid is also a cofactor for dopamine β-hydroxylase that converts dopamine to norepinephrine (see Plate 3.26). Absorbed in the jejunum and ileum (see Plate 7.18), blood levels of ascorbic acid are regulated by renal excretion.

Scurvy usually develops with an insidious onset of weakness, malaise, shortness of breath, bone pain, myalgias, arthralgias, edema, neuropathy, and vasomotor instability. Impaired collagen and connective tissue functions result in dry, rough skin with impaired wound healing, hyperkeratotic papules, perifollicular hemorrhages, and follicular hyperkeratosis (hair follicles may be coiled and fragmented). Petechial hemorrhages occur in the lower extremities initially and then may involve the skin around the joints or along other irritated areas. Patients who are affected have positive test results for the Rumpel-Leede test for abnormal capillary fragility; after inflating the BP cuff between the SBP and DBP for 1 minute, numerous petechial hemorrhages occur. Massive hemorrhages with ecchymoses and proptosis caused by retrobulbar hemorrhage may occur. Hemorrhages into joints result in marked pain, swelling, and immobility. Subungual "splinter" hemorrhages may be seen. Gingival tissues may become swollen, reddish-blue in color, spongy, and friable, and teeth may loosen and fall out.

Subperiosteal hemorrhages in infants with scurvy prompt a less painful "frog leg" position, and infants may have "pseudoparalysis" caused by pain. Radiographs show large periosteal calcium deposits and central epiphyseal lucency. Also in infants, the costochondral junctions may be prominent, which is termed the *scorbutic rosary*. Children who are affected have impaired growth because of osteoblast dysfunction.

Death may occur in individuals with scurvy because of widespread cerebral petechial hemorrhages with associated hyperpyrexia, tachycardia, cyanosis, hypotension, and Cheyne-Stokes respirations.

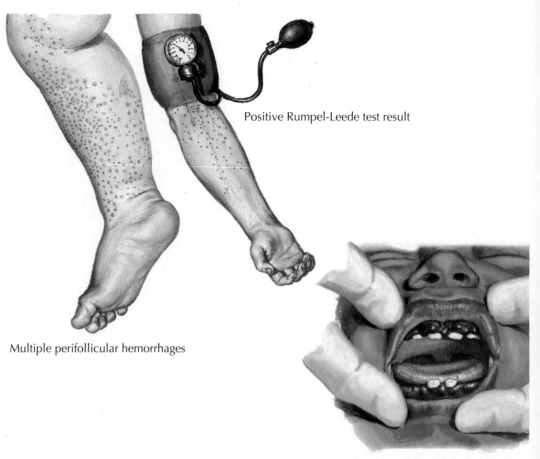

Positive Rumpel-Leede test result

Multiple perifollicular hemorrhages

Swollen, congested, bleeding gums

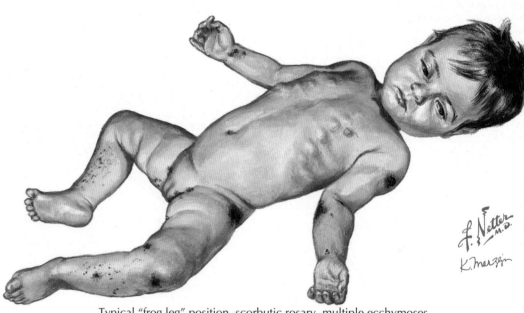

Typical "frog leg" position, scorbutic rosary, multiple ecchymoses

Diagnosis. In the United States, scurvy may be seen in individuals who are severely malnourished. If vitamin C deficiency is suspected, a blood test for ascorbic acid may be performed (reference range, 0.6–2.0 mg/dL; values <0.3 mg/dL indicate significant deficiency).

Treatment. Scurvy is treated by the administration of 500 mg daily of ascorbic acid until all signs and symptoms resolve. Also, the factors that predisposed to the dietary deficiency must be addressed.

Prevention. The recommended daily dietary allowance of ascorbic acid is 15 to 45 mg daily for children, 90 mg daily for adult males, and 75 mg daily for females (120 mg daily for pregnant or lactating females). These amounts of ascorbic acid are easily achieved with a balanced diet that includes citrus fruits and vegetables.

Plate 7.22

Lipids and Nutrition

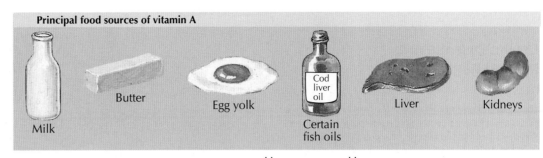

Principal food sources of vitamin A

Milk   Butter   Egg yolk   Certain fish oils   Liver   Kidneys

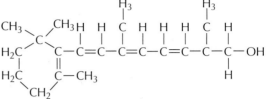

Vitamin A

VITAMIN A DEFICIENCY

Vitamin A is part of a family of lipid-soluble compounds (retinols, β-carotenes [provitamin A], and carotenoids) referred to as *retinoic acids*. Vitamin A has a major role in phototransduction and cellular differentiation of the eyes, which was recognized by the ancient Egyptians who used liver ingestion to treat poor vision in dim light (referred to as *night blindness* [nyctalopia]). The best food sources of vitamin A are liver, egg yolk, kidneys, fish oils, and butter. β-Carotene is found in green leafy vegetables, carrots, sweet potatoes, apricots, tomatoes, and pimentos.

β-Carotene is hydrolyzed in the gastrointestinal tract to two molecules of vitamin A. Vitamin A is absorbed in the jejunum and ileum (see Plate 7.18). The enterocytes form retinyl-esters that are incorporated into chylomicrons and released into lymph and plasma. The chylomicrons are then broken down into multiple remnants, including apo B and apo E, which contain retinol esters. Apo B and apo E are then taken up by the liver; the retinol esters are freed and combine with retinol-binding proteins (RBP) and are stored in vitamin A–containing lipid globules within the hepatic stellate cells. The liver stores 50% to 85% of the total body vitamin A. When released from the liver, vitamin A circulates bound to RBP.

Vitamin A plays a key role in the function of the retina, growth and differentiation of epithelial tissue, bone growth, and immune function. The two types of retinal photoreceptor cells are cone and rod cells. The rod cells are responsible for night vision and motion detection. The cone cells are responsible for color vision in bright light. Deficiency in vitamin A leads to a deficiency in retinal 11-cis-retinol and rhodopsin, which affects rod vision more than cone vision. Xerophthalmia (keratinization of ocular tissue) is a progressive vitamin A deficiency disorder of night blindness, xerosis (dryness), and keratomalacia (corneal thinning). The xerosis is caused by both poor lacrimal gland function and the conversion of secretory epithelium (goblet mucous cells) to keratinized epithelium (basal cells). Bitot spots are distinctive triangular white patches on the sclera that represent areas of abnormal conjunctival squamous cell proliferation and keratinization. The corneal thinning can lead to perforation of the cornea and permanent blindness. Vitamin A deficiency is also associated with poor bone growth and follicular hyperkeratosis.

Diagnosis. Vitamin A deficiency can occur from inadequate vitamin A ingestion or from malabsorption. When vitamin A deficiency is suspected, it can be confirmed by measuring a serum vitamin A (retinol) level (adult reference range, 325–780 μg/L; severe deficiency <100 μg/L).

Treatment. Patients with xerophthalmia should be treated with 60 mg of vitamin A and repeated 1 and

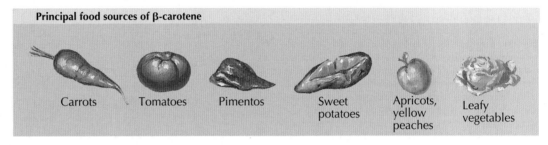

Principal food sources of β-carotene

Carrots   Tomatoes   Pimentos   Sweet potatoes   Apricots, yellow peaches   Leafy vegetables

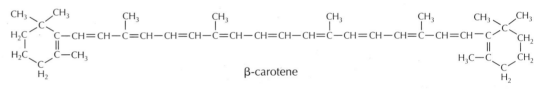

β-carotene

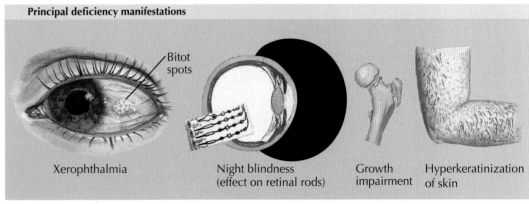

Principal deficiency manifestations

Bitot spots

Xerophthalmia   Night blindness (effect on retinal rods)   Growth impairment   Hyperkeratinization of skin

14 days later. If the deficiency is not as severe and the presentation is limited (e.g., night blindness and Bitot spots), it may be treated with lower doses of vitamin A (e.g., 3 mg daily for 3 months). In both settings, the cause of the deficiency must be addressed.

Prevention. The RDA for vitamin A is given as retinol activity equivalents (RAE), where 1 RAE = 1 microgram retinol or 3.3 international units.

The RDA for retinol in the United States is 900 μg/d for adult males and 700 μg/d females (1.4 mg/d during pregnancy and lactation). One μg of retinol is equivalent to 12 μg of β-carotene. The recommended daily amounts of retinol and β-carotene equivalents are easily obtained with a nutritious diet that is rich in milk, eggs, fish, butter, and yellow and dark green vegetables.

Plate 7.23

Endocrine System: VOLUME 2

Celiac Disease and Malabsorption

The signs and symptoms of celiac disease—also known as *gluten-sensitive enteropathy* and *nontropical sprue*—were first described by Aretaeus in the second century AD.

In the 1940s, it was recognized that the ingestion of foods that contained wheat, barley, and rye caused malabsorption, which resolved when these food sources were eliminated from the diet. Eventually, the source of this sensitivity was identified as the gliadin component of gluten. Celiac disease is a small bowel disorder associated with mucosal inflammation, villous atrophy, and crypt hyperplasia. The clinical presentations of celiac disease are those of malabsorption (e.g., steatorrhea, weight loss) and vitamin and nutrient deficiencies.

Celiac disease is relatively common with a prevalence of approximately 1 in 300 individuals. However, it is less common in individuals of Chinese, Japanese, or African descent. Celiac disease is a genetically determined immune disorder that becomes evident with the environmental exposure to gluten. The presence of immunoglobulin (Ig)A antibodies to endomysium (located in connective tissue surrounding smooth muscle cells) and to the autoantigen tissue transglutaminase are sensitive and specific for celiac disease. Tissue transglutaminase is an intracellular enzyme that is released by inflamed endothelial cells and fibroblasts. When released by small bowel enterocytes, tissue transglutaminase deamidates glutamine residues in gliadin to glutamic acid, creating a more immunogenic peptide.

The classic clinical presentation of celiac disease includes diarrhea with steatorrhea (foul-smelling, floating stools); abdominal pain; weight loss; growth failure in children; microcytic (iron deficiency) or macrocytic (vitamin B_{12} deficiency) anemia; vitamin B deficiency signs and symptoms (e.g., glossitis, peripheral neuropathy, myalgias, weakness); ecchymoses (vitamin K malabsorption); dental enamel defects; edema; and osteopenia, osteoporosis, or osteomalacia associated with deficiencies in vitamin D and calcium. Mild forms of celiac disease may go undetected (subclinical) because of limited signs and symptoms.

Disorders associated with celiac disease include Down syndrome, dermatitis herpetiformis, type 1 diabetes mellitus, autoimmune thyroid disease, IgA deficiency, and liver disease. Dermatitis herpetiformis is caused by autoantibodies to epidermal transglutaminase, and patients present with pruritic papulovesicles on the trunk and extremities. Approximately 5% of individuals with type 1 diabetes and 16% of those with Down syndrome have celiac disease.

DIAGNOSTIC EVALUATION

Celiac disease should be suspected when initial investigations are unrevealing in patients with gastrointestinal symptoms (e.g., diarrhea, malabsorption, abdominal distension, weight loss), abnormal liver function test results, iron-deficiency anemia, vitamin deficiencies, osteoporosis, osteomalacia, infertility, short stature, or delayed puberty. Testing should be completed while individuals are on a gluten-containing diet. An assessment of the presence and degree of steatorrhea can be determined with a 72-hour stool fat measurement. Excretion of more than 7 g of fat per 24 hours, when on a diet of 100 g to 150 g of fat, is suggestive of a malabsorption defect. The evaluation for possible celiac disease should start with serologic

testing for the presence of IgA tissue transglutaminase antibody and IgA endomysial antibody. If the antibody test results are negative, it is extremely unlikely that celiac disease is present. When the clinical suspicion for celiac disease is high but the IgA tissue transglutaminase and endomysial antibodies are absent, IgA deficiency should be considered. In the setting of IgA deficiency, the IgG-antitissue transglutaminase test should be obtained. If the IgA or IgG tissue transglutaminase or IgA endomysial antibody test results are positive, then a small bowel biopsy is indicated for histopathologic confirmation. Findings on small bowel biopsy that are consistent with celiac disease include increased intraepithelial lymphocytes, flat mucosa with mucosal atrophy, complete loss of villi, and crypt hyperplasia.

TREATMENT

The small intestine mucosa improves morphologically when individuals with celiac disease are treated with a gluten-free diet. Thus the treatment of choice is a lifelong gluten-free diet. The primary sources of gluten are wheat, rye, and barley. Individuals should be counseled by a dietitian and must carefully read labels on prepared foods to determine whether gluten is present. In addition, any identified nutritional deficiencies (e.g., vitamin D and other fat-soluble vitamins, water-soluble vitamins, calcium, and iron) should be addressed. Most patients have symptomatic improvement in their malabsorption symptoms within 2 weeks of initiating a gluten-free diet. The most common reason for lack of symptomatic response is lack of compliance with a true gluten-free diet.

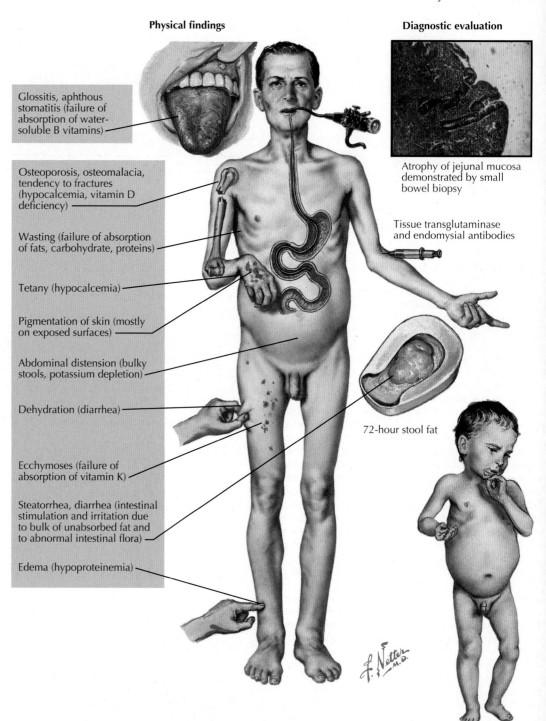

Physical findings

Glossitis, aphthous stomatitis (failure of absorption of water-soluble B vitamins)

Osteoporosis, osteomalacia, tendency to fractures (hypocalcemia, vitamin D deficiency)

Wasting (failure of absorption of fats, carbohydrate, proteins)

Tetany (hypocalcemia)

Pigmentation of skin (mostly on exposed surfaces)

Abdominal distension (bulky stools, potassium depletion)

Dehydration (diarrhea)

Ecchymoses (failure of absorption of vitamin K)

Steatorrhea, diarrhea (intestinal stimulation and irritation due to bulk of unabsorbed fat and to abnormal intestinal flora)

Edema (hypoproteinemia)

Diagnostic evaluation

Atrophy of jejunal mucosa demonstrated by small bowel biopsy

Tissue transglutaminase and endomysial antibodies

72-hour stool fat

Infantile celiac disease

Plate 7.24

Lipids and Nutrition

LYSOSOMAL STORAGE DISORDERS: SPHINGOLIPIDOSES

Lysosomes are membrane-bound, cytoplasmic organelles that contain enzymes responsible for the degradation of sphingolipids, mucopolysaccharides, and glycoproteins. Lysosomal enzyme deficiencies lead to the accumulation of partially degraded substrate, cell distension, and disruption of cellular function. The clinical presentation of lysosomal storage disorders depends on the site(s) and extent of abnormal substrate accumulation. The general categories of lysosomal storage disorders include the following:

- Sphingolipidoses
- Mucopolysaccharidoses (e.g., Hurler syndrome)
- Glycoproteinoses (e.g., sialidosis, mannosidosis)
- Mucolipidoses (disorders of lysosomal enzyme transport)
- Lysosomal membrane transport disorders (e.g., sialic acid storage disease, cystinosis)

The heritable disorders characterized by the accumulation of sphingolipids include Tay-Sachs disease, Niemann-Pick disease (NPD), Gaucher disease (GD), metachromatic leukodystrophy (MLD), Fabry disease, GM1 gangliosidosis, Krabbe disease, and multiple sulfatase deficiency. Sphingolipids contain sphingosine, an 18-carbon amino alcohol synthesized in the body from palmitic acid and serine. A long-chain fatty acid is bound in peptide linkage to the amide group of sphingosine to form ceramide. The sphingolipids are distinguished by the polar group linked to the C_1 hydroxyl of their ceramide moiety (R). Some are concentrated in nervous tissue, either in ganglion cells (gangliosides) or in myelin (cerebrosides, cerebroside sulfatides); others are distributed more widely in cell membranes (globosides, various glycolipids). Sphingomyelin, the phosphorylcholine ester of ceramide, is found in almost every cell type.

TAY-SACHS DISEASE

Tay-Sachs disease (gangliosidosis), characterized by the accumulation of excessive amounts of gangliosides, is caused by a deficiency in the lysosomal enzyme β-hexosaminidase A (Hex A). This is an inherited autosomal recessive disease with a carrier frequency of 1 in 25 in the Ashkenazi Jewish population, resulting in a disease incidence of 1 in 3600 in this ethnic group (compared with 1 in 360,000 in the non-Jewish population). It is usually detected by 6 months of age, with progressive neurologic deficits such as hypotonia, hyperreflexia, weakness, spasticity, seizures, blindness, and loss of motor function. Destructive swelling of ganglion cells and gliosis are so widespread that the cranium becomes abnormally enlarged. Cherry-red spots may be seen on the macula. Tay-Sachs is a progressive disease with a life expectancy of 2 to 5 years. Testing includes DNA mutation analysis and enzyme assays to measure leukocyte Hex A activity.

NIEMANN-PICK DISEASE

NPD (sphingomyelin-cholesterol lipidosis) is a rare autosomal recessive disorder that results in lysosomal accumulation of sphingomyelin. NPD has three clinical forms. NPD disease types A and B are caused by pathogenic variants in the gene encoding sphingomyelin phosphodiesterase-1 that result in a deficiency of acid sphingomyelinase activity. NPD type A, because of a complete absence of acid sphingomyelinase activity, is an early-onset neuropathic form that presents with

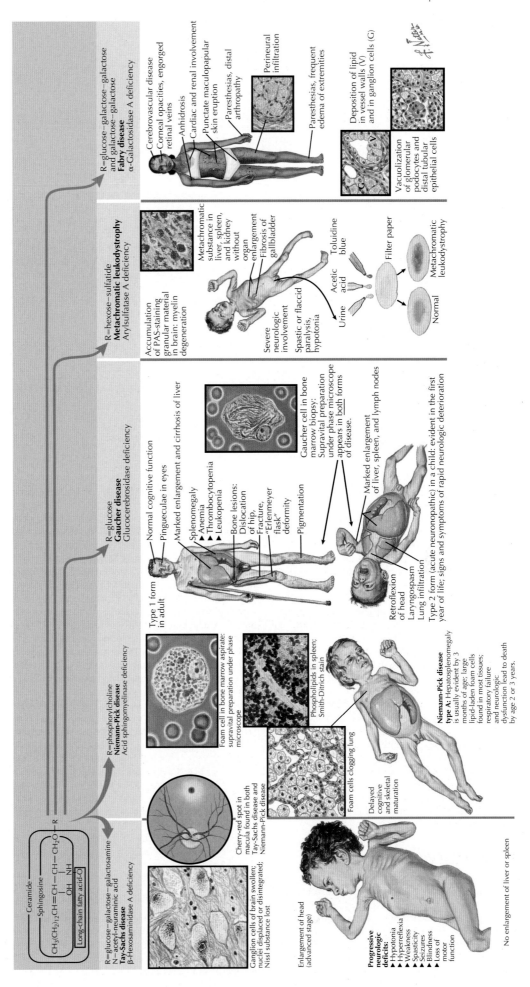

Plate 7.24

Endocrine System: VOLUME 2

LYSOSOMAL STORAGE DISORDERS: SPHINGOLIPIDOSES (Continued)

hepatosplenomegaly (evident at 3 months of age), respiratory failure, and neurologic dysfunction that leads to death by age 2 or 3 years. Macular cherry-red spots are found in most patients by 1 year of age. Large lipid-laden foam cells are found in most tissues. NPD type B is characterized by a partial deficiency in acid sphingomyelinase (5% of normal) and has a later onset than NPD type A. Hepatosplenomegaly and secondary thrombocytopenia are evident in early childhood. Most children who are affected have delayed skeletal maturation, short stature, interstitial lung involvement, and macular cherry-red spots. However, neurologic abnormalities are absent or delayed in onset in NPD type B. NPD types A and B can be detected by biochemical testing for acid sphingomyelinase activity and confirmed with molecular genetic testing.

NPD type C is caused by pathogenic variants in either the *NPC1* or *NPC2* gene and may become clinically evident at any age with cerebellar signs (e.g., ataxia), impaired vertical gaze, cognitive dysfunction, dysphagia, and hepatosplenomegaly. *NPC1* and *NPC2* encode proteins that have key roles in intracellular cholesterol transport, and when defective, lipid accumulation and neuronal degeneration occur. NPD type C can be detected with biochemical tests on cultured fibroblasts and confirmed with molecular genetic testing.

GAUCHER DISEASE

GD is caused by a deficiency in glucocerebrosidase due to autosomal recessive pathogenic variants in the gene encoding this protein. Glucocerebrosides accumulate in macrophages (Gaucher cells with a wrinkled tissue paper appearance) throughout the liver, spleen, bone marrow, and lungs. The cerebroside in visceral tissues is ceramide-glucose instead of the normal ceramide-galactose. GD is the most common lysosomal storage

disorder (1 in 75,000 births). There are three clinical types of GD.

Type 1 GD—the chronic adult form—is most common and accounts for 90% of cases, with an increased prevalence in the Ashkenazi Jewish population. The clinical presentation is variable and clinically evident anywhere from 1 year of age to adulthood. The presentation of GD type 1 is dominated by visceral involvement (e.g., massive splenomegaly, hepatomegaly), bone disease (e.g., osteoporosis, avascular necrosis, bone pain), and bleeding caused by thrombocytopenia. Abnormal bone remodeling of the metaphysis results in an Erlenmeyer flask deformity of the distal femur. Pingueculae (single yellow nodules that may occur on either side of the cornea but more commonly on the nasal aspect) are found frequently on the conjunctiva.

GD types 2 and 3 are associated with neurologic involvement in addition to visceral involvement. Type 2 GD (acute neuronopathic) is the rarest form and is usually fatal by age 2 years. Type 2 GD becomes evident in the first year of life with signs and symptoms of rapid neurologic deterioration such as oculomotor dysfunction, hypertonia, arching, retroflexion of the head, rigidity, laryngospasm, and seizures. Type 3 GD (chronic neuronopathic) is later in onset and is not as severe as type 2 GD.

Testing includes DNA mutation analysis and enzyme assays to measure leukocyte glucocerebrosidase activity.

METACHROMATIC LEUKODYSTROPHY

MLD (sulfatidosis) is caused by a deficiency in arylsulfatase A due to autosomal recessive pathogenic variants in the gene encoding this enzyme. Because of defective desulfation, cerebroside sulfate accumulates in the CNS and peripheral nerves, leading to central and peripheral

demyelination. MLD may present at different ages. The late infantile form presents between age 6 months and 2 years with ataxia, hypotonia, regression of motor skills, and optic atrophy. There are also juvenile and adult-onset forms of MLD. Visceral involvement is not prominent, but excess sulfatides are found in the liver, kidney, and spleen. Biliary excretion of sulfatides results in fibrosis and gallbladder dysfunction. Electromyography shows decreased nerve conduction velocities, and cerebrospinal fluid examination shows increased protein concentration. Testing includes enzyme assays to measure arylsulfatase A activity in leukocytes. Similar to other acidic polysaccharides, certain dyes may be used to detect the sulfatides by the metachromasia they produce.

FABRY DISEASE

Fabry disease, caused by a deficiency in α-galactosidase A, is the second most common lysosomal storage disorder. The gene that encodes α-galactosidase A is located on the X chromosome, and the disease is inherited in an X-linked recessive manner. α-Galactosidase A cleaves the terminal galactose from globotriaosylceramide (Gb3). In individuals with Fabry disease, Gb3 accumulates in the vascular endothelium, glomeruli, and distal renal tubules. Clinical manifestations typically start in the second decade of life and include neuropathic pain in the extremities; diffuse angiokeratomas located primarily in the periumbilical, groin, and hip regions; corneal opacities (cornea verticillata); anhidrosis; coronary artery disease; cerebrovascular disease; peripheral vascular disease; proteinuria; edema; and renal failure. The diagnosis can be confirmed by documenting low leukocyte α-galactosidase A activity. Molecular genetic testing is also available.

Plate 7.25

Lipids and Nutrition

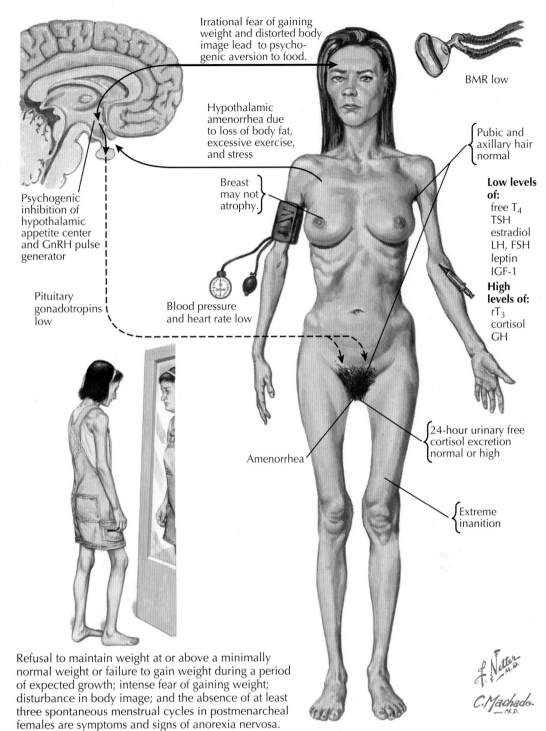

Irrational fear of gaining weight and distorted body image lead to psychogenic aversion to food.

BMR low

Hypothalamic amenorrhea due to loss of body fat, excessive exercise, and stress

Pubic and axillary hair normal

Low levels of:
free T_4
TSH
estradiol
LH, FSH
leptin
IGF-1

High levels of:
rT_3
cortisol
GH

Psychogenic inhibition of hypothalamic appetite center and GnRH pulse generator

Breast may not atrophy.

Pituitary gonadotropins low

Blood pressure and heart rate low

24-hour urinary free cortisol excretion normal or high

Amenorrhea

Extreme inanition

Refusal to maintain weight at or above a minimally normal weight or failure to gain weight during a period of expected growth; intense fear of gaining weight; disturbance in body image; and the absence of at least three spontaneous menstrual cycles in postmenarcheal females are symptoms and signs of anorexia nervosa.

ANOREXIA NERVOSA

The diagnosis of anorexia nervosa includes four criteria: (1) refusal to maintain weight within a normal range for height and age (i.e., >15% below ideal body weight, which equates to a BMI of approximately ≤ 18.5 kg/m^2); (2) fear of weight gain; (3) severe body image disturbance with the body image becoming a predominant measure of self-worth; and (4) amenorrhea in females. Although rare in males, the lifetime prevalence of anorexia nervosa among females is 1%. "Restricting" anorexia nervosa occurs when weight loss is maintained primarily by caloric restriction and exercise. "Binge eating/purging" anorexia nervosa is characterized by binge eating and self-induced vomiting (usually supplemented by laxative and diuretic abuse).

Although the cause is unknown, anorexia nervosa is associated with cultural, biologic, and psychologic risk factors. In general, individuals who develop anorexia nervosa are perfectionists. Although the concordance is higher in monozygotic twins than in dizygotic twins, specific genes that contribute to anorexia nervosa have not been identified. Most of the neurochemical, metabolic, and hormonal changes seen in individuals with anorexia nervosa are a result of weight loss and are not a cause of the disorder.

The signs and symptoms of anorexia nervosa usually begin in middle to late adolescence; the disorder rarely develops after age 40 years. The onset of anorexia nervosa may be triggered by a stressful life event. Individuals with anorexia nervosa, despite being underweight, are irrationally afraid of gaining weight. In addition, they have a distorted body image and think they are "too fat." Weight loss provides a sense of accomplishment, and weight gain a sense of failure. Individuals who are affected tend to become socially withdrawn and focus on dieting, exercise, and work or study.

Individuals with anorexia nervosa usually have very few physical complaints. They may have cold intolerance and constipation. On physical examination, they may be hypothermic, hypotensive, and bradycardic. Lanugo hair may be evident on the cheeks of females. Enlargement of the salivary glands is common and associated with starvation and then binge eating and emesis. A diet of predominantly yellow and orange vegetables, which have a high β-carotene content, results in a yellow tint to the skin, especially evident on the palms.

Typical laboratory findings include normochromic normocytic anemia, mild leukopenia, increased serum creatinine concentration caused by dehydration, increased hepatic enzymes, low-normal fasting plasma glucose concentration, and moderately increased total serum cholesterol concentration. Recurrent emesis or diuretic abuse may result in hypokalemic alkalosis. Other causes of weight loss should be excluded (e.g., human immunodeficiency virus, inflammatory bowel disease, diabetes mellitus, or CNS neoplasm).

The severe weight loss in individuals with anorexia nervosa affects most of the endocrine glands. Hypothalamic amenorrhea—with low serum concentrations of luteinizing hormone, follicle-stimulating hormone, and estradiol—is a key component of the diagnosis in females. The hypothalamic gonadotropin-releasing hormone (GnRH) pulse generator is very sensitive to loss of body fat, excessive exercise, and stress. Adequate circulating leptin is a key factor for normal function of the GnRH pulse generator. Serum leptin concentrations are low because of the decreased fat mass. Serum cortisol concentrations and 24-hour urinary free cortisol excretion are increased, but patients with anorexia nervosa lack signs and symptoms of Cushing syndrome. Thyroid hormone test results are consistent with euthyroid sick syndrome, with low levels of free thyroxine, low levels of triiodothyronine (T_3), increased levels of reverse T_3 (rT_3), low-normal or suppressed thyrotropin (thyroid-stimulating hormone), and low basal metabolic rate. The serum growth hormone concentration is usually increased, but insulinlike growth factor 1 levels are low. Bone mineral density is low and related to nutritional deficiencies in vitamin D and calcium and to decreased gonadal steroids.

Plate 7.26

Endocrine System: VOLUME 2

OBESITY

Obesity is a global epidemic, and its prevalence is increasing in children, adolescents, and adults. More than 66% of adults in the United States are overweight or obese. The increased morbidity and mortality in individuals who are obese are a result of the increased prevalence of diabetes mellitus, hypertension, ASCVD, hyperlipidemia, obstructive sleep apnea, and cancer.

The diagnosis of obesity includes measurement of BMI, waist circumference, and hip circumference. BMI is calculated by dividing body weight in kilograms by height in meters squared. BMI correlates with body fat mass; however, BMI may overestimate fat mass in individuals who are very muscular (e.g., professional athletes). BMI-based categories of body weight are:

- Underweight: BMI <18.5 kg/m^2
- Normal weight: BMI ≥18.5–24.9 kg/m^2
- Overweight: BMI ≥25.0–29.9 kg/m^2
- Class I obesity (obese): BMI ≥30.0–34.9 kg/m^2
- Class II obesity (moderately obese): BMI ≥35.0–39.9 kg/m^2
- Class III obesity (severely obese): BMI ≥40.0–49.9 kg/m^2
- Class IV obesity (super morbidly obese): BMI ≥50 kg/m^2

For Asians, a BMI between 23.0 and 29.9 kg/m^2 is considered overweight, and a BMI of 30 kg/m^2 or above is consistent with obesity.

Because excess centrally distributed fat mass is uniquely associated with increased morbidity and mortality (associated with ASCVD, diabetes mellitus, hyperlipidemia, and hypertension), waist circumference measurement is helpful in guiding clinical decision-making. The waist circumference should be measured on a horizontal plane at the level of the iliac crest, which is usually in line with the umbilicus. Waist circumferences greater than 88 cm for females and 102 cm for males are associated with an increased risk of ASCVD, hyperlipidemia, type 2 diabetes mellitus, and hypertension. Waist circumferences more than 80 cm in Asian females and more than 90 cm in Asian males are consistent with abdominal obesity. Waist/hip ratios more than 0.9 in males or more than 0.85 in females are also consistent with abdominal obesity.

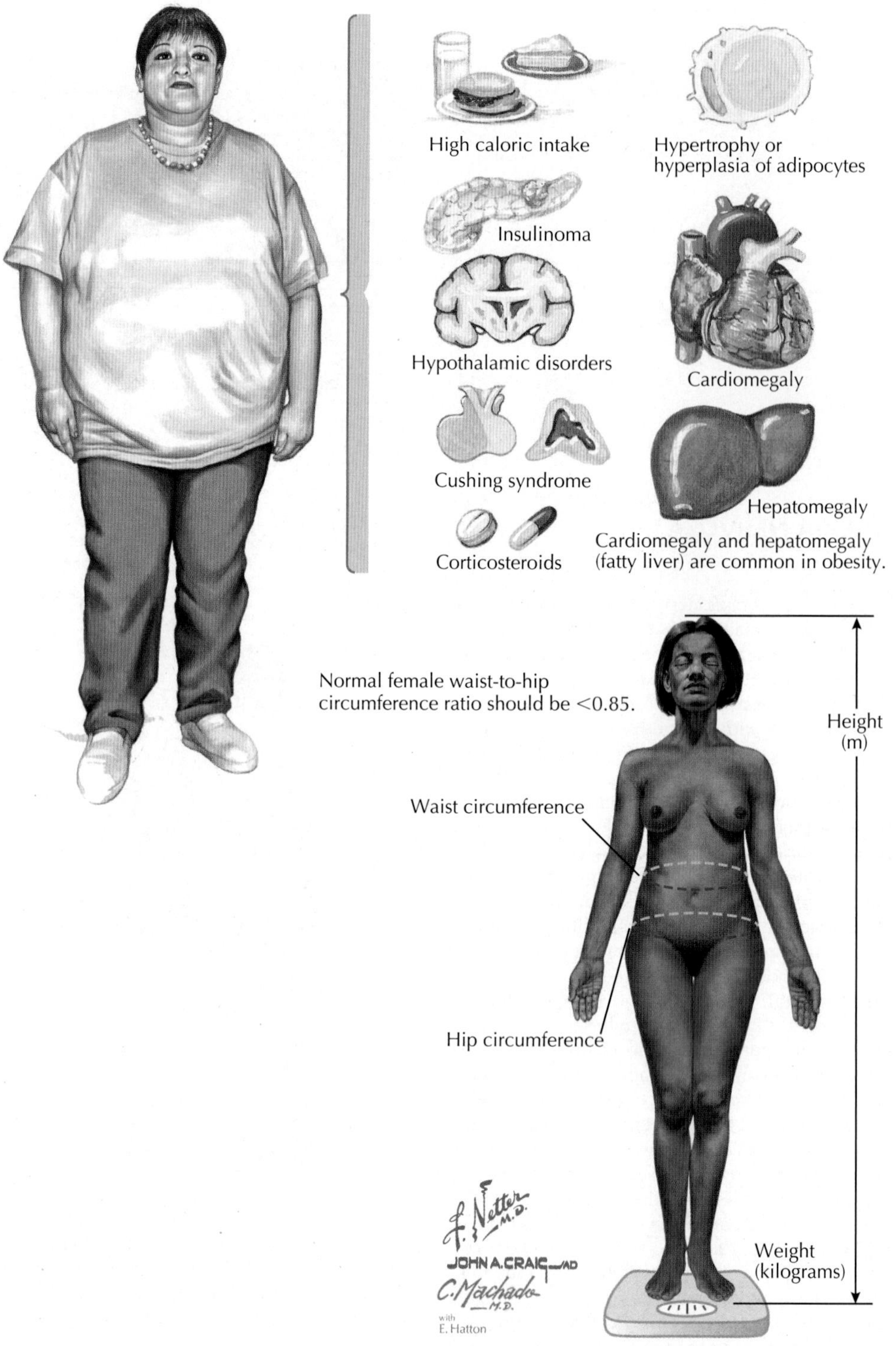

EVALUATION

Obesity is usually the result of increased caloric intake and a sedentary lifestyle. A complete history and physical examination should be performed to exclude secondary causes of obesity. Key pieces of the history include age at onset of weight gain, body weight at different life stages, current and past dietary patterns, exercise habits, details on previous weight loss efforts, current and past medications, patient motivation to lose weight, and history of smoking cessation. Patients should be queried on symptoms of obstructive sleep apnea (loud snoring, apneic episodes while sleeping, feeling not rested on waking in the morning, or daytime hypersomnolence), the presence of cardiovascular risk factors, and the presence of obesity-related comorbidities (e.g., degenerative joint disease). Medications that can contribute to weight gain include corticosteroids, antipsychotics, antidepressants, antiepileptics, thiazolidinediones, and insulin. Very rarely, a patient with new-onset obesity will have a medical disorder that is responsible (e.g., Cushing syndrome, hypothalamic disease, or hypothyroidism). The physical examination should include BP measurement, waist circumference, and an

High caloric intake

Hypertrophy or hyperplasia of adipocytes

Insulinoma

Hypothalamic disorders

Cardiomegaly

Cushing syndrome

Hepatomegaly

Corticosteroids

Cardiomegaly and hepatomegaly (fatty liver) are common in obesity.

Normal female waist-to-hip circumference ratio should be <0.85.

Waist circumference

Hip circumference

Height (m)

Weight (kilograms)

assessment of potential secondary forms of obesity. Laboratory studies should include fasting plasma glucose levels and a lipid profile. Testing (e.g., overnight oximetry) for obstructive sleep apnea is indicated in patients with obesity suspected to have this disorder.

TREATMENT

Weight loss is associated with a decrease in obesity-associated morbidity. Thus the goal of treatment is to improve current obesity-related comorbid conditions and to decrease the risk of developing additional comorbidities in the future. Treatment options include dietary interventions, lifestyle modification, pharmacotherapy (e.g., glucagon-like peptide 1 [GLP-1] receptor agonists and dual-acting GLP-1 and glucose-dependent

insulinotropic polypeptide [GIP] receptor agonists), and surgery (see Plate 7.27). A reasonable initial weight loss target is 10% weight loss over 6 months. The main focus of the diet is to reduce overall caloric intake, a goal that can be achieved by choosing meals with smaller portions, increasing the proportion of fruits and vegetables, decreasing dietary fats (20%–30% of daily calories), increasing dietary fiber, and drinking water instead of calorie-containing beverages. Regular (30 min/d) isotonic exercise is key to maintaining weight loss. Monitoring daily activity with a pedometer can be a useful technique. Cognitive behavioral therapy strategies (journaling, exercise monitoring, stress management, problem-solving, stimulus control, cognitive restructuring) should be used to help reinforce the modified dietary and physical activity plans.

Plate 7.27

Lipids and Nutrition

SURGICAL TREATMENT OPTIONS FOR OBESITY

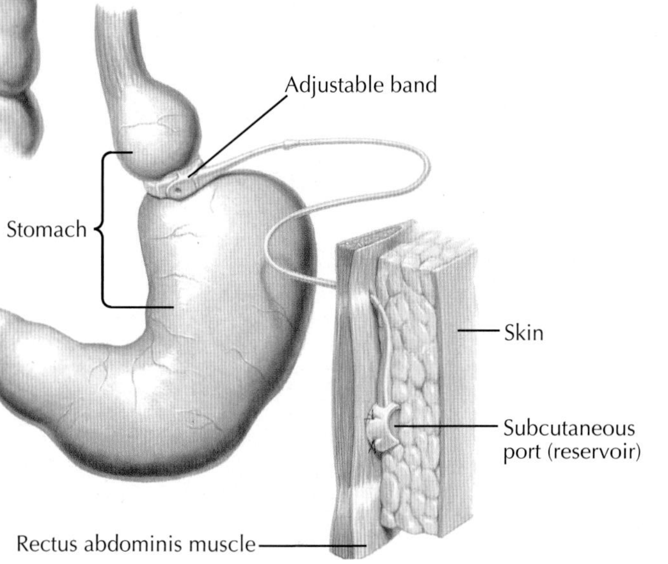

Surgical treatment for obesity can be considered for patients with class IV obesity (super morbidly obese; BMI ≥50 kg/m²), class III obesity (severely obese; BMI ≥40–49.9 kg/m²), or class II obesity (moderately obese; BMI ≥35.0–39.9 kg/m²) who have at least one serious comorbidity and have not met weight loss goals with diet, exercise, and pharmacologic therapy. Bariatric surgery is the most effective currently available treatment option for patients with clinically severe obesity; an average weight loss of 30% to 35% of total body weight is maintained in 60% of patients at 5 years after surgery. This degree of weight loss improves quality of life and cures or improves obesity-related comorbidities (diabetes mellitus, obstructive sleep apnea, hypertension, hyperlipidemia, fatty liver). Evidence supporting a benefit from bariatric surgery is strongest in patients with a BMI more than 40 kg/m². Contraindications for bariatric surgery include patients with binge eating disorders, drug or alcohol abuse, major depression or psychosis, other medical diagnoses associated with prohibitive anesthetic risks, or predicted inability to comply with postoperative nutritional requirements. Bariatric surgery needs to be a component of a larger management program that includes nutritional and behavioral follow-up. The surgical options can be classified as restrictive and combined restrictive-malabsorptive.

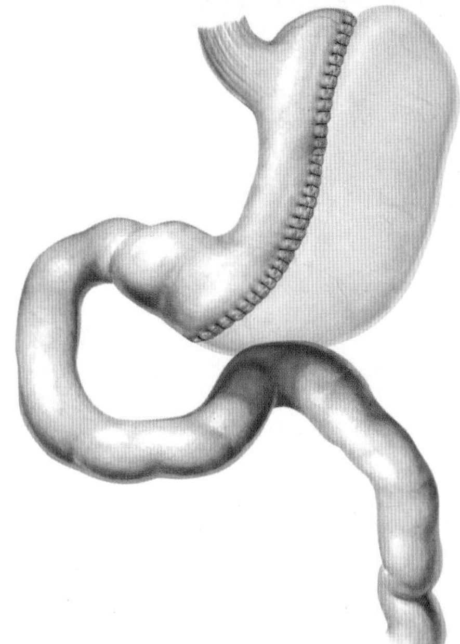

Restrictive surgical options limit the amount of food that can occupy the stomach and slow the rate of gastric emptying. With restrictive procedures, the absorptive function of the small intestine is intact. Gastric stapling (vertical banded gastroplasty) is an example of a restrictive surgical procedure in which the upper part of the stomach is partitioned by a vertical staple line with a tight outlet (stoma) that is wrapped by a band or prosthetic mesh. However, because of limited long-term efficacy and need for revisions (because of stomal stenosis, staple line disruption, band erosion, or pouch dilation), the gastric stapling procedure has been replaced with laparoscopic adjustable gastric banding. A silicone band is placed at the gastric cardia near the gastroesophageal junction to limit food intake. The diameter of the band can be adjusted by injecting or removing saline from a reservoir that is implanted under the skin. Laparoscopic gastric banding has a low complication rate and does not require intestinal resection or division of the stomach. Sleeve gastrectomy consists of laparoscopic partial gastrectomy with removal of the greater curvature of the stomach (creating a tubular stomach with a small capacity and resistance to stretching). Sleeve gastrectomy appears to have an advantage over other restrictive procedures because of better appetite control related to removing the major source of ghrelin.

Restrictive-malabsorptive procedures decrease the efficacy of nutrient absorption by shortening the length of functioning small intestine. Mean weight loss is greater after a combined restrictive-malabsorptive procedure compared with a restrictive bariatric surgical procedure. The most common restrictive-malabsorptive procedure is the roux-en-Y gastric bypass (RYGB) in which a small gastric pouch (e.g., <30 mL) limits oral intake, and the small bowel modification leads to dumping physiology and mild malabsorption. There is a proximal biliopancreatic limb that transports the secretions from the pancreas, liver, and gastric remnant. The alimentary limb (roux limb) is anastomosed

to the gastric pouch. The biliopancreatic limb and roux limb are connected anywhere from 75 to 150 cm distal to the gastrojejunostomy (increasing roux limb length leads to more malabsorption). RYGB can be performed either with an open laparotomy or laparoscopically; the laparoscopic approach is associated with decreased postoperative pain and shorter hospital stays. The two other procedures in the restrictive-malabsorptive category are the biliopancreatic diversion and biliopancreatic diversion with duodenal switch. Biliopancreatic diversion includes a partial gastrectomy and gastroileostomy with a long segment of the roux limb. Biliopancreatic diversion is associated with high rates of stomal

ulceration, anemia, protein malnutrition, and diarrhea. The biliopancreatic diversion with duodenal switch differs by preserving the pylorus, resulting in fewer complications with stomal ulceration and diarrhea.

The bariatric surgery–related mortality rate is less than 1%. The most common complications are stenosis of the stoma and marginal ulcers in approximately 15% of patients; these patients present with nausea, vomiting, and an inability to tolerate solid foods. The combined restrictive-malabsorptive procedures are associated with an increased risk of deficiencies in micronutrients and vitamins (iron, calcium, folate, and vitamins B_{12}, D, and E).

Gastric stapling (vertical banded gastroplasty)
- Esophagus
- Stomach pouch
- Band

Sleeve gastrectomy

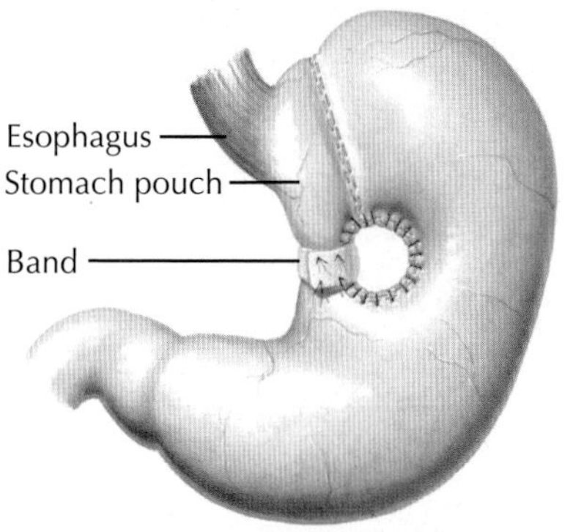

Gastric bypass (roux-en-Y)
- Stomach pouch
- Oversewn staple lines
- End-to-side type anastomosis between the gastric pouch and the roux-en-Y limb
- Duodenum
- Bypassed portion of the stomach
- Jejunum

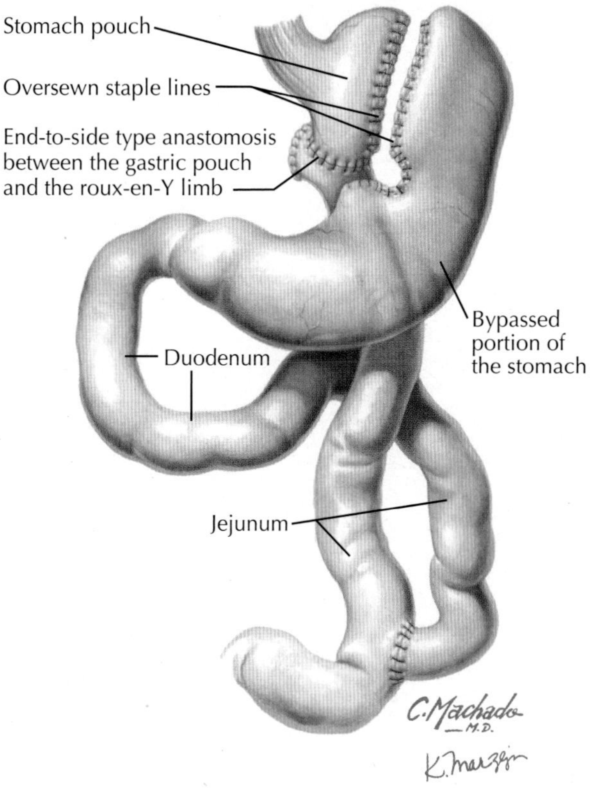

C. Machado M.D.
K. Marzejon

Laparoscopic adjustable gastric banding
- Adjustable band
- Stomach
- Skin
- Subcutaneous port (reservoir)
- Rectus abdominis muscle

GENETICS AND ENDOCRINE NEOPLASIA

Plate 8.1

Endocrine System: VOLUME 2

MULTIPLE ENDOCRINE NEOPLASIA TYPE 1

Multiple endocrine neoplasia type 1 (MEN 1) is a rare (prevalence ~2 per 100,000) autosomal dominant endocrine disorder that is characterized by neoplasms of the pituitary, parathyroid, and pancreas. In addition, neoplasms may arise in the adrenal glands, duodenum (gastrinoma), lung (carcinoid tumor), thymus gland (carcinoid tumor), and esophagus (leiomyoma). An *MEN1* pathogenic variant is highly probable in a patient with two of the three main MEN 1 tumor types (pituitary, parathyroid, or gastroenteropancreatic [GEP] endocrine neoplasms).

Primary hyperparathyroidism is the most common manifestation of MEN 1; the penetrance is 100% by age 50 years. The diagnosis is biochemical with documentation of hypercalcemia and a nonsuppressed serum parathyroid hormone concentration. All four (or occasionally five) of the parathyroid glands are involved, and removing 3.5 of the parathyroid glands is the treatment of choice. Recurrent hypercalcemia may require reoperation or percutaneous ethanol injection.

Pituitary adenomas are found in more than 20% of patients with MEN 1. Prolactinomas are the most common pituitary tumor. However, all pituitary tumor cell types have been identified in MEN 1 kindreds, including growth hormone (GH), corticotropin (adrenocorticotropic hormone [ACTH]), gonadotropin, and null cell. The management of pituitary tumors in patients with MEN 1 is the same as that for patients with sporadic pituitary neoplasms (see Plates 1.19 to 1.24).

The GEP neoplasms are the major life-threatening manifestation of MEN 1. Pancreatic islet cell (often nonfunctioning) and duodenal carcinoid tumors are frequently malignant and may metastasize. Peptic ulcer disease is the most common symptomatic presentation related to GEP tumors and is caused by gastrin-secreting neoplasms (Zollinger-Ellison syndrome). Zollinger-Ellison syndrome is the initial manifestation of MEN 1 in 40% of patients. The gastrinomas are frequently small, multifocal, and localized to the duodenum. The hypercalcemia from primary hyperparathyroidism may aggravate gastrin hypersecretion in Zollinger-Ellison syndrome. Thus normalization of the serum calcium concentration is important in the management of patients with this syndrome. Proton pump inhibitors very effectively control the signs and symptoms related to hypergastrinemia. Removal of the gastrin-secreting duodenal carcinoids may be considered at the time of a pancreatic operation.

The pancreatic islet tumors may hypersecrete insulin, glucagon, human pancreatic polypeptide, chromogranin A, and vasoactive intestinal polypeptide. Insulinomas in MEN 1 may be small and numerous (see Plate 5.23). Cushing syndrome (see Plate 3.9) in individuals with MEN 1 may be caused by a corticotropin-secreting pituitary tumor, a cortisol-secreting adrenal adenoma, or ectopic corticotropin secretion from an islet cell tumor or carcinoid tumor (e.g., bronchial or thymic). Symptomatic islet cell tumors (e.g., insulinomas) should be resected. Pancreatic surgery should also be considered in patients with MEN 1 when a nonfunctioning pancreatic islet cell tumor is approaching 2 cm in diameter; larger islet cell tumors are more likely to be malignant and are prone to metastasize. The hormonal status of the GEP tumors can be monitored by annual measurement of gastrin, glucagon, human pancreatic polypeptide, and chromogranin A.

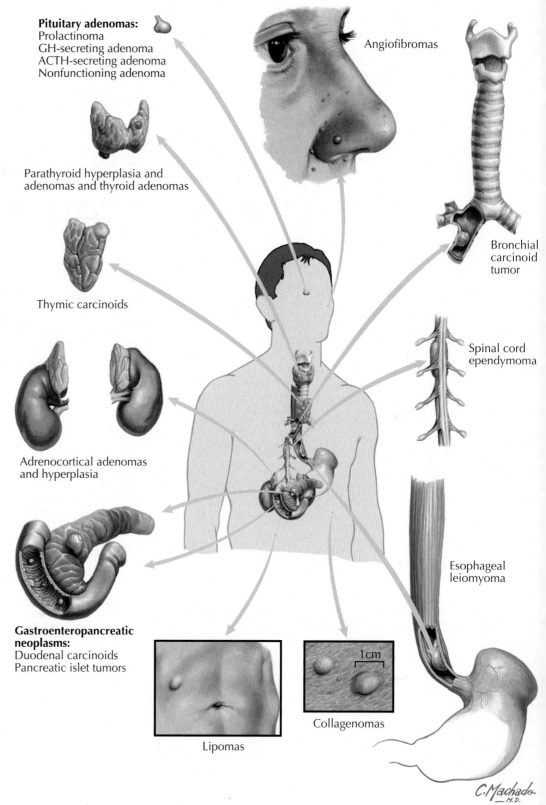

Pituitary adenomas:
Prolactinoma
GH-secreting adenoma
ACTH-secreting adenoma
Nonfunctioning adenoma

Angiofibromas

Parathyroid hyperplasia and adenomas and thyroid adenomas

Bronchial carcinoid tumor

Thymic carcinoids

Spinal cord ependymoma

Adrenocortical adenomas and hyperplasia

Esophageal leiomyoma

Gastroenteropancreatic neoplasms:
Duodenal carcinoids
Pancreatic islet tumors

1 cm

Lipomas

Collagenomas

Patients with MEN 1 may have several skin manifestations. Angiofibromas, collagenomas, and subcutaneous lipomas occur in about 75% of patients with MEN 1. The dermal and subcutaneous lesions are benign and should be removed only if symptomatic. Patients with MEN 1 are also at risk of developing spinal cord ependymomas.

The *MEN1* protein product is menin, and most *MEN1* pathogenic variants inactivate or disrupt menin function. This tumor suppressor gene has no strong genotype-phenotype correlations. Most individuals with MEN 1 inherit one inactivated copy of *MEN1* from a parent who is affected; tumorigenesis requires the subsequent somatic inactivation (e.g., gene deletion) of the remaining normal copy in a cell from a susceptible gland (e.g., parathyroid, pituitary, and pancreas). When an endocrine cell lacks menin tumor suppressor function, it begins the process of proliferation and neoplasia.

Plate 8.2   Genetics and Endocrine Neoplasia

MULTIPLE ENDOCRINE NEOPLASIA TYPE 2

Multiple endocrine neoplasia type 2 (MEN 2) is an autosomal dominant disorder with an estimated prevalence of 2.5 per 100,000 in the general population, and it is classified into three distinct syndromes—MEN 2A, MEN 2B, and familial medullary thyroid carcinoma (FMTC). MEN 2A is characterized by medullary thyroid carcinoma (MTC) in all patients, pheochromocytoma in 50%, primary hyperparathyroidism in 20%, and cutaneous lichen amyloidosis in 5%. MEN 2B is characterized by MTC in all patients, pheochromocytoma in 50%, mucocutaneous neuromas (typically involving the tongue, lips, and eyelids) in most patients, skeletal deformities (kyphoscoliosis or lordosis), joint laxity, myelinated corneal nerves, and intestinal ganglioneuromas (Hirschsprung disease). FMTC is a variant of MEN 2A, and the clinical presentation is limited to MTC.

MEDULLARY THYROID CARCINOMA

MTC is a neuroendocrine tumor of the parafollicular C cells of the thyroid gland and accounts for approximately 3% to 5% of all primary thyroid cancers. C cells—representing 0.1% of thyroid mass and concentrated in the upper third of the thyroid gland—are neuroendocrine cells derived from the ultimobranchial bodies. Multicentric C-cell hyperplasia is found in all patients with MEN 2, and nearly all eventually develop MTC. The C cells produce calcitonin, a 32–amino acid peptide that regulates blood calcium levels in fish. However, a physiologic role for this hormone in humans is unknown. MTC in MEN 2 is multicentric and is concentrated in the upper third of the thyroid gland, reflecting the normal distribution of C cells. Approximately 25% of all patients with MTC have a family history of this disease. In MEN 2A and FMTC the peak incidence of clinical detection of index cases is in the third decade of life, and the typical age of presentation of sporadic MTC is in the fifth to sixth decades of life. When diagnosed as an index case, the clinical presentation (e.g., thyroid nodule) and manifestations (e.g., cervical adenopathy) of MEN 2–associated MTC are similar to those of sporadic MTC. Serum calcitonin concentrations have a positive correlation with tumor mass. MTC in patients with MEN 2B is earlier in onset and more aggressive (e.g., metastatic disease at a young age).

PHEOCHROMOCYTOMA

Pheochromocytomas—affecting approximately 50% of patients with MEN 2A and 2B—frequently involve both adrenal glands and are multicentric. MTC is usually detected before pheochromocytoma in patients with MEN 2. In this patient population, pheochromocytomas are typically diagnosed when asymptomatic because of routine annual case-detection testing. However, patients with MEN 2 who are not followed up regularly or who are new index cases may present with symptoms of pheochromocytoma such as paroxysms of hypertension, forceful heartbeat, hyperhidrosis, headache, and pallor.

PRIMARY HYPERPARATHYROIDISM

Approximately 20% of patients with MEN 2A have primary hyperparathyroidism, and when it occurs, two or more parathyroid glands are involved.

MEN 2A

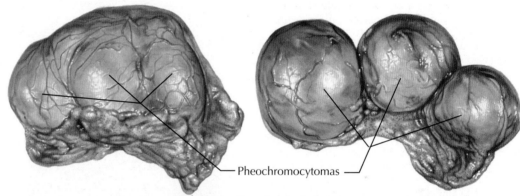

Medullary carcinomas

Multicentric C-cell hyperplasia, which eventually evolves into multicentric medullary thyroid carcinoma.

Normal size parathyroid gland

Approximately 20% of patients with MEN 2A have primary hyperparathyroidism, and when it occurs, two or more parathyroid glands are involved.

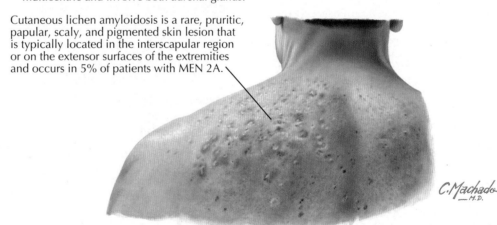

Pheochromocytomas

50% of patients with MEN 2A and 2B are affected with pheochromocytomas that are usually multicentric and involve both adrenal glands.

Cutaneous lichen amyloidosis is a rare, pruritic, papular, scaly, and pigmented skin lesion that is typically located in the interscapular region or on the extensor surfaces of the extremities and occurs in 5% of patients with MEN 2A.

CUTANEOUS LICHEN AMYLOIDOSIS

Cutaneous lichen amyloidosis is a rare skin disorder that may occur in patients with MEN 2A. It is a pruritic, papular, scaly, and pigmented skin lesion that is typically located in the interscapular region or on the extensor surfaces of the extremities.

HIRSCHSPRUNG DISEASE

Hirschsprung disease may occur in individuals with MEN 2B and is characterized by the absence of autonomic ganglion cells within the distal colon parasympathetic plexus, resulting in chronic obstruction and megacolon.

GENETICS

MEN 2A, MEN 2B, and FMTC are inherited in an autosomal dominant pattern with a high degree of penetrance. The pathogenic variants causing these disorders occur in the *RET* protooncogene on chromosome 10. The RET protein is a receptor tyrosine kinase that

Plate 8.3

Endocrine System: VOLUME 2

MULTIPLE ENDOCRINE NEOPLASIA TYPE 2 (Continued)

controls growth and differentiation signals in several tissues, including those derived from the neural crest. Interestingly, there is overlap in the specific *RET* pathogenic variants causing MEN 2A and FMTC; however, MEN 2B is caused by different *RET* pathogenic variants. Most pathogenic variants in MEN 2A kindreds (93%–98%) and in FMTC kindreds (80%–96%) involve one of six cysteine residues in the cysteine-rich region of the RET protein's extracellular domain encoded in *RET* exons 10 (codons 609, 611, 618, and 620) or 11 (codons 630 or 634).

Eighty-five percent of individuals with MEN 2A have a pathogenic variant in codon 634, particularly p.Cys634Arg. These extracellular MEN 2A/FMTC cysteine pathogenic variants lead to constitutive activation of intracellular signaling pathways. Less common pathogenic variants in MEN 2A and FMTC occur in exon 13 (codons 790 and 791). MEN 2B–associated tumors are caused by pathogenic variants in the RET protein's intracellular domain. A single methionine to threonine missense pathogenic variant in exon 16 (p.Met918Thr) is responsible for more than 95% of MEN 2B cases. Another mutation—alanine to phenylalanine at codon 883 in exon 15—has been found in 4% of MEN 2B kindreds. Other infrequent missense pathogenic variants in exons 14, 15, and 16 (codons 804, 806, 904, and 922) have been found in individuals with MEN 2B. Germline pathogenic variants in codons 768 (exon 13), 804 (exon 14), and 891 (exon 15) are found only in FMTC but account for a minority of FMTC cases.

The germline *RET* pathogenic variants causing MEN 2 and FMTC result in a gain-of-function defect; this is different from almost all other inherited neoplasia syndromes, which are caused by heritable "loss-of-function" mutations that inactivate tumor suppressor proteins. Other pathogenic variants in *RET* can produce disorders seemingly unrelated to MEN 2. For example, tissue-specific inactivating pathogenic variants of *RET* have been associated with Hirschsprung disease (congenital megacolon). Thus in some families with a *RET* pathogenic variant, both Hirschsprung disease and MEN 2B are present.

There are genotype–phenotype correlations in MEN 2 that help direct clinical management. For example, the risk of MTC has been stratified into three categories according to *RET* pathogenic variants:

- Children with MEN 2B or *RET* pathogenic variants in codons 883, 918, or 922 have the highest risk of aggressive MTC and should undergo total thyroidectomy with central node dissection within the first 6 months of life.
- Children with *RET* pathogenic variants in codons 611, 618, 620, or 634 have a high risk of MTC. Total thyroidectomy should be performed before age 5 years, with or without central node dissection.
- Children with *RET* pathogenic variants in codons 609, 768, 790, 791, 804, or 891 have a less aggressive and slowly growing MTC and may be operated at a later stage. Some clinicians recommend a prophylactic thyroidectomy by age 5 years, but others suggest thyroidectomy by age 10 years.

For individuals with other known *RET* pathogenic variants, no specific recommendations can be made at present because there is not sufficient experience with these kindreds.

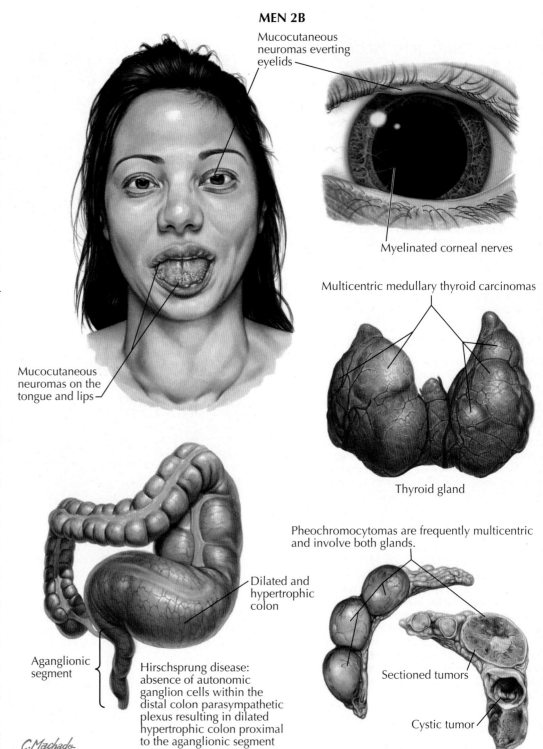

MEN 2B

Mucocutaneous neuromas everting eyelids

Mucocutaneous neuromas on the tongue and lips

Myelinated corneal nerves

Multicentric medullary thyroid carcinomas

Thyroid gland

Dilated and hypertrophic colon

Aganglionic segment

Hirschsprung disease: absence of autonomic ganglion cells within the distal colon parasympathetic plexus resulting in dilated hypertrophic colon proximal to the aganglionic segment

Pheochromocytomas are frequently multicentric and involve both glands.

Sectioned tumors

Cystic tumor

C. Machado
M.D.

Genetic information can also be useful to assess the risk of developing pheochromocytoma. Individuals with *RET* pathogenic variants in codons 609, 611, 618, 620, 630, 634, 790, 883, 918, or 922 (or the specific mutation p.Val804Leu) should have annual biochemical screening. In contrast, it is unlikely that pheochromocytoma will develop in patients with pathogenic variants in codon 768 or in those with the mutation p.Val804Met.

Genetic testing for pathogenic variants in the *RET* protooncogene is commercially available and should be considered for patients with bilateral pheochromocytoma, family history of pheochromocytoma, or cophenotype disorders. More than 95% of patients with MEN 2A and more than 98% of those with MEN 2B have an identifiable pathogenic variant in the *RET* protooncogene. In a family with MEN 2, a family member with a clinical diagnosis of MEN 2 should be tested first. When a *RET* pathogenic variant is found, all family members of unknown status should be offered genotyping. Genetic counseling consultation should be considered before genetic testing is performed. In families with known MEN 2, genetic testing shortly after birth facilitates prompt surgical management of the thyroid gland—an element of care especially important in MEN 2B families in which the thyroid gland should be removed in the first 6 months of life.

Plate 8.4

Genetics and Endocrine Neoplasia

VON HIPPEL-LINDAU SYNDROME

von Hippel-Lindau (VHL) syndrome is an autosomal dominant disorder that may present with a variety of benign and malignant neoplasms, including pheochromocytoma (frequently bilateral), paraganglioma (mediastinal, abdominal, pelvic), hemangioblastoma (involving the cerebellum, spinal cord, or brainstem), retinal angioma, clear cell renal cell carcinoma (RCC), pancreatic neuroendocrine tumors, endolymphatic sac tumors of the middle ear, serous cystadenomas of the pancreas, and papillary cystadenomas of the epididymis and broad ligament. The average age of symptomatic presentation is 26 years. Retinal angiomas and cerebellar hemangioblastomas are usually detected in the third decade of life; RCC is typically detected in the fifth decade. Penetrance is very high; the probability of developing RCC, retinal angiomas, and cerebellar hemangioblastomas is approximately 75%. Pheochromocytoma occurs in 20% of patients with VHL syndrome, and the occurrence depends on the subtype of VHL (see the next paragraph). The most common cause of death in patients with VHL syndrome is RCC.

Patients with VHL syndrome may be divided into two groups: type I and type II. Patients from kindreds with type I syndrome do not develop pheochromocytoma, but patients from kindreds with type II syndrome are at high risk for developing pheochromocytoma. In addition, kindreds with type II VHL syndrome are subdivided into type IIA (low risk for RCC), type IIB (high risk for RCC), and type IIC (pheochromocytomas only).

The prevalence of VHL is approximately 1 in 35,000 persons. The *VHL* tumor suppressor gene, chromosomal location 3p25-26, encodes a protein that regulates hypoxia-induced proteins. More than 300 germline *VHL* pathogenic variants have been identified that lead to loss of function of the VHL protein. Nearly 100% of patients with VHL have an identifiable gene pathogenic variant. Genotype–phenotype correlations have been documented for this disorder, and specific pathogenic variants are associated with particular patterns of tumor formation. In up to 98% of cases, pheochromocytoma is associated with missense mutations, rather than truncating or null mutations, in the *VHL* gene. Certain missense mutations appear to be associated with the type IIC presentation of VHL (pheochromocytomas only). Genetic testing for VHL is commercially available and should be considered for patients with bilateral pheochromocytoma, family history of pheochromocytoma, diagnosis of pheochromocytoma at a young age (i.e., 30 years or younger), or cophenotype disorders.

Pheochromocytomas and paragangliomas occurring in patients with VHL produce predominately norepinephrine and normetanephrine. Patients with VHL should have annual biochemical testing for catecholamine-secreting neoplasms.

Hemangioblastomas are vascular neoplasms that are benign and usually do not invade locally or metastasize. They may be asymptomatic or cause mass-effect symptoms because of pressure on adjacent structures or hemorrhage. Annual or every 2-year imaging surveillance (e.g., magnetic resonance imaging [MRI] of brain and spine) is indicated. However, surgery or stereotactic radiotherapy (or both) is typically reserved for rapidly growing or symptomatic lesions.

RCC is typically multicentric and bilateral and may arise in conjunction with cysts or from noncystic renal parenchyma. Early tumor detection and selective resection with renal-sparing surgery or ablative therapies is the optimal management strategy. Annual imaging

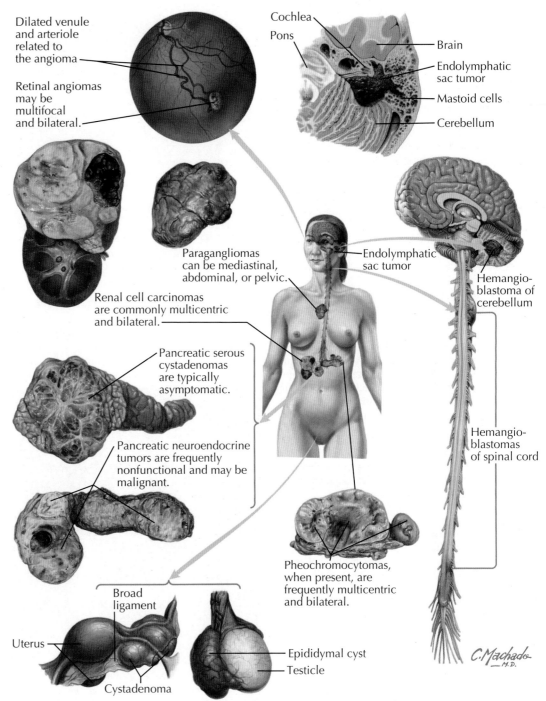

Dilated venule and arteriole related to the angioma

Retinal angiomas may be multifocal and bilateral.

Cochlea
Pons
Brain
Endolymphatic sac tumor
Mastoid cells
Cerebellum

Paragangliomas can be mediastinal, abdominal, or pelvic.

Endolymphatic sac tumor

Hemangioblastoma of cerebellum

Renal cell carcinomas are commonly multicentric and bilateral.

Pancreatic serous cystadenomas are typically asymptomatic.

Pancreatic neuroendocrine tumors are frequently nonfunctional and may be malignant.

Hemangioblastomas of spinal cord

Pheochromocytomas, when present, are frequently multicentric and bilateral.

Broad ligament

Uterus

Epididymal cyst
Testicle

Cystadenoma

C. Machado
M.D.

Papillary cystadenoma of broad ligament (female) and epididymal cysts (male) are benign and frequently bilateral.

(e.g., computed tomography [CT], MRI, or ultrasonography) of the kidneys is indicated.

Retinal angiomas develop in the retina and within the optic nerve and may be multifocal and bilateral. Annual ophthalmologic examinations are indicated. When left untreated, these lesions can hemorrhage and lead to vision loss. Laser photocoagulation and cryotherapy are very effective treatments for angiomas that do not involve the optic nerve.

Pancreatic abnormalities in VHL syndrome are common and include simple cysts (70%), serous cystadenomas (10%), and neuroendocrine tumors (20%). The cysts and serous cystadenomas are typically asymptomatic. The neuroendocrine tumors of

the pancreas are similar to those found in MEN 1, and they are frequently nonfunctional; however, they may cause symptoms related to hormone hypersecretion (e.g., glucagon, insulin, vasoactive intestinal polypeptide), and they can metastasize. The pancreas should be visualized at the time of annual renal imaging.

The epididymal cysts (frequently bilateral) in males and the papillary cystadenomas in the broad ligament in females are benign and usually asymptomatic. Papillary cystadenomas of the endolymphatic sac are vascular lesions arising within the posterior temporal bone, and patients who are affected may present with tinnitus, hearing loss, and vertigo.

Plate 8.5

Endocrine System: VOLUME 2

NEUROFIBROMATOSIS TYPE 1 (VON RECKLINGHAUSEN DISEASE)

Neurofibromatosis is a common neurocutaneous disorder affecting 1 in 3000 individuals. Neurofibromatosis type 1 (NF1), also known as *von Recklinghausen disease*, is the most common form (85%). NF1 is an autosomal dominant disorder characterized by neurofibromas, multiple café au lait spots, axillary and inguinal freckling, iris hamartomas (Lisch nodules), bony abnormalities, central nervous system (CNS) gliomas, pheochromocytoma and paraganglioma, macrocephaly, and cognitive deficits. The expression of these features is variable.

The *NF1* tumor suppressor gene (chromosomal location 17q11.2) spans 350 kb and contains 60 exons encoding a 2818–amino acid protein, neurofibromin. Neurofibromin is a GTPase-activating protein that inhibits Ras activity. Inactivating *NF1* pathogenic variants causes the disorder. More than 95% of *NF1* pathogenic variants can be identified with a multistep testing protocol. Approximately half of newly detected NF1 cases are inherited, and the rest are caused by de novo pathogenic variants. Only one genotype–phenotype correlation has been identified: the c.2970-2972 delAAT (p.990delM) mutation is associated with a lack of cutaneous neurofibromas. This correlation may be because most *NF1* pathogenic variants truncate or prevent neurofibromin formation, but the c.2970-2972 delAAT mutation results in a single amino acid deletion.

At least two of the following clinical features must be present to diagnose NF1: six or more café au lait spots larger than 5 mm in prepubertal individuals and larger than 15 mm in postpubertal individuals, two or more neurofibromas of any type or one plexiform neurofibroma, axillary or inguinal freckling, optic glioma, two or more iris hamartomas (Lisch nodules), osseous lesions (e.g., sphenoid dysplasia), or a first-degree relative with NF1.

Café au lait spots are uniformly hyperpigmented, flat macules that appear during the first year after birth and usually increase in number during early childhood. They have a smooth and regular border described as a "coast of California" border—which contrasts with the "coast of Maine" irregular border of the café au lait macules seen with McCune-Albright syndrome (MAS) (see Plate 8.8). Although up to 25% of healthy individuals have one to three café au lait spots, six or more of these spots is highly suggestive of NF1. Dense axillary and inguinal freckling are rarely found in the absence of NF1. Dense freckling may also be seen on the neck.

Neurofibromas are benign tumors composed of a mixture of Schwann cells, fibroblasts, and mast cells. The four types of neurofibromas are cutaneous, subcutaneous, nodular plexiform, and diffuse plexiform. Cutaneous neurofibromas—the most common type—are soft and fleshy tumors that arise from the peripheral nerve sheath and start to appear during adolescence and increase in size and number with age. Patients may have just a few or may have hundreds, with the trunk being the most common location. Subcutaneous neurofibromas are firm, tender nodules along the course of peripheral nerves. Nodular plexiform neurofibromas are similar to subcutaneous neurofibromas, but they occur in clusters along proximal nerve roots and major

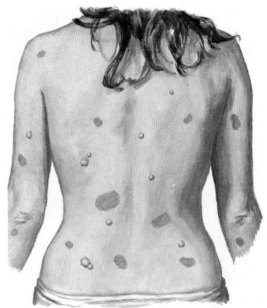

Café-au-lait spots are uniformly hyperpigmented flat macules—six or more café-au-lait spots are highly suggestive of NF1. Cutaneous neurofibromas are soft and fleshy tumors that arise from the peripheral nerve sheath, the trunk being the most common location.

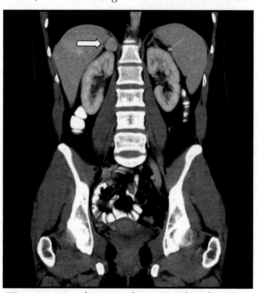

CT scan (coronal image) showing right adrenal pheochromocytoma (*arrow*)

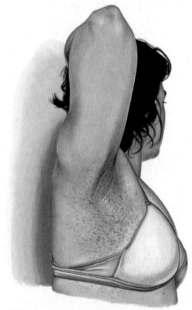

Dense axillary and inguinal freckling is rarely found in the absence of NF1.

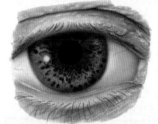

Lisch nodules are hamartomas on the iris. They are raised and frequently pigmented.

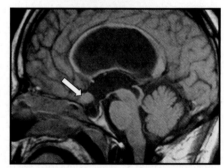

MRI scan (sagittal image) showing optic nerve glioma (*arrow*) and third ventricle hydrocephalus caused by aqueductal stenosis

C. Machado M.D.

nerves. Diffuse plexiform neurofibromas are congenital lesions and are a main cause of morbidity and disfigurement in young children with NF1. In addition, plexiform neurofibromas can undergo malignant transformation to peripheral nerve sheath tumors (neurofibrosarcomas).

Lisch nodules on the iris—identified with an ophthalmoscope if the nodules are large and the iris is light in color or by slit-lamp examination—are raised and frequently pigmented hamartomas.

Bone-related conditions in patients with NF1 include vertebral body scalloping caused by dural ectasia, cortical thinning of the long bones, sphenoid wing dysplasia (causing facial asymmetry), short stature, and kyphoscoliosis.

Patients with NF1 are at increased risk of developing CNS neoplasms, including optic pathway gliomas, astrocytomas, and brainstem gliomas. Patients with

optic gliomas may present with vision loss or mass effect symptoms; MRI typically shows an enlargement of the optic nerve or chiasm. Annual ophthalmologic examination and head MRI every 3 years starting in childhood are indicated. Another CNS finding in NF1 is noncommunicating hydrocephalus caused by aqueductal stenosis (the aqueduct between the third and fourth ventricles is long and narrow, making it vulnerable to internal obstruction and external compression).

Hypertension is common in patients with NF1, and it may be idiopathic or associated with renovascular disease or catecholamine-secreting tumors. Approximately 2% of patients with NF1 develop catecholamine-secreting tumors; the mean age at diagnosis is 42 years. In these patients, the catecholamine-secreting tumor is usually a solitary benign adrenal pheochromocytoma, occasionally a bilateral adrenal pheochromocytoma, and rarely an abdominal paraganglioma.

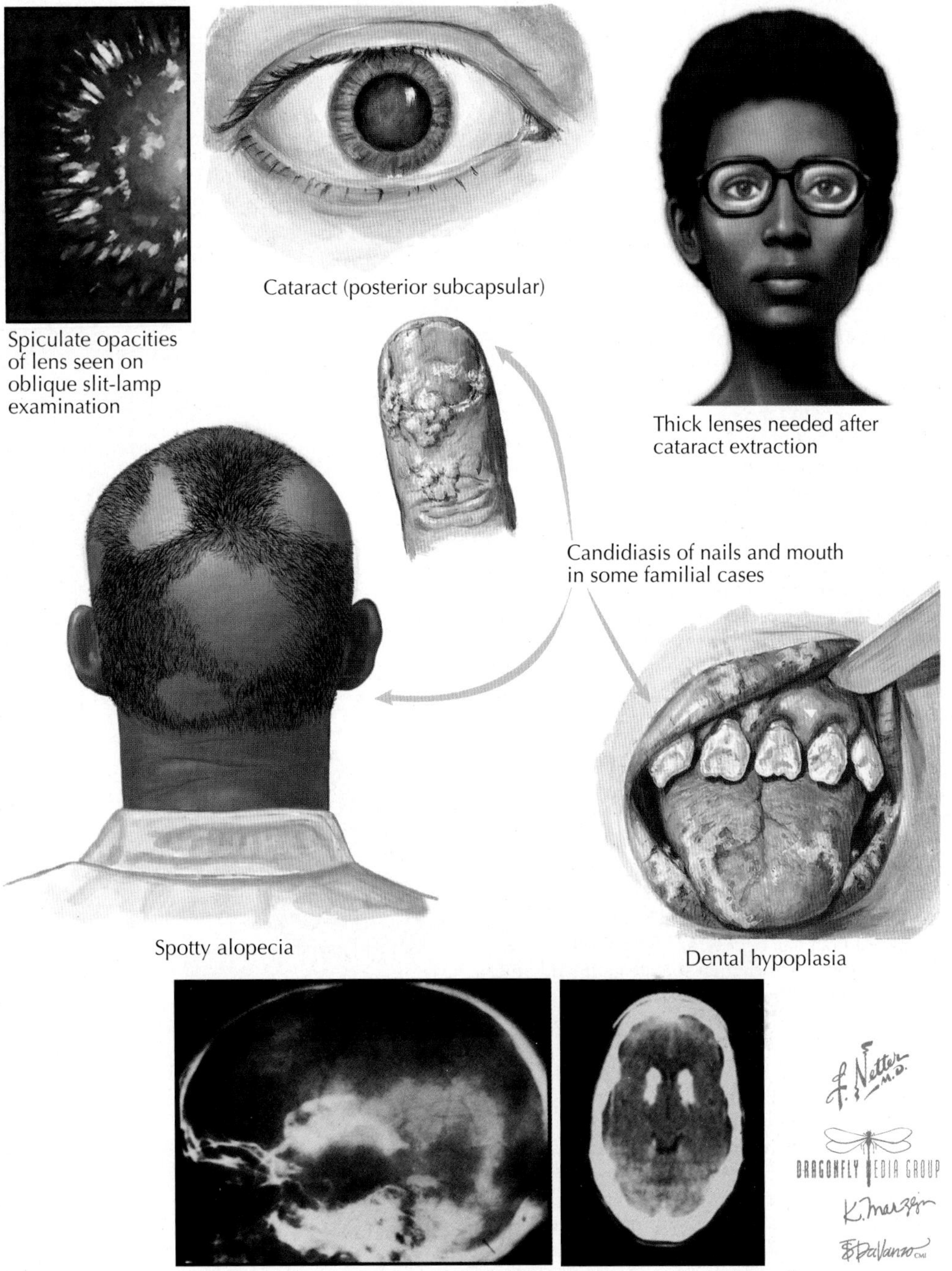

Plate 8.6

Genetics and Endocrine Neoplasia

Clinical Manifestations of Autoimmune Polyglandular Syndrome Type 1

Autoimmune polyglandular syndrome type 1 (APS1) (OMIM 240300), also referred to as *autoimmune polyendocrinopathy-candidiasis-ectodermal dystrophy* (APECED), is a rare autosomal recessive disorder that is most prevalent in individuals of Finnish and Sardinian descent. It is less common than autoimmune polyglandular syndrome APS2 (see later in this section) and is caused by pathogenic variants in the autoimmune regulator (*AIRE*) gene. Hypoparathyroidism or chronic mucocutaneous candidiasis are usually the first manifestations that typically appear during infancy or childhood and are followed shortly thereafter (average age, 15 years) by primary adrenal insufficiency. The candidiasis—typically involving the skin, nail beds, and oral and perianal mucosa—is chronic and recurrent and can be refractory to treatment. Other features of this disorder include primary hypogonadism in 60% of patients, malabsorption in 25%, alopecia totalis or areata in 20%, pernicious anemia in 16%, and vitiligo in 4%. Initially, the alopecia may be spotty before progressing to complete loss of hair (including the eyebrows). Half of patients with APS1 develop all three main components of this syndrome, which are hypoparathyroidism, chronic cutaneous candidiasis, and primary adrenal insufficiency. The presence of at least two of these three components is needed to clinically diagnose APS1; siblings of an individual who is affected need only one of these components to confirm the diagnosis. Diabetes mellitus and autoimmune thyroid disease (e.g., Hashimoto thyroiditis, Graves disease) rarely occur with this disorder. However, the clinical presentation can be variable, probably because of environmental and genetic factors.

The signs and symptoms of chronic hypocalcemia attributable to hypoparathyroidism can be subtle, and it may not be diagnosed until after permanent damage has occurred. The less obvious symptoms of chronic hypocalcemia include mental lassitude, personality changes, sleepiness, or blurred vision. Intellectual disability may result from childhood onset of long-standing, undetected hypocalcemia. In patients with chronic untreated hypoparathyroidism, careful examination of the eye with a slit lamp shows spiculated opacities in the posterior subcapsular area of the lens, which may progress to cataract formation and blindness. The status of the teeth may give a clue as to the time of disease onset. If it began before age 6 years, dental hypoplasia, with poor dental root formation, is usually present. If it began later in childhood, crumbling of the teeth because of poor enamel structure is observed. However, the lamina dura of the teeth may be quite dense. If the disease has been lifelong, a general stunting of growth may occur. Radiographs of the skull may show typical calcification of the basal ganglia.

APS2 (OMIM 269200), previously referred to as *Schmidt syndrome*, typically presents between the ages of 20 and 40 years with primary adrenal insufficiency as the main manifestation. Autoimmune thyroid disease (e.g., Hashimoto thyroiditis, Graves disease) and type 1 diabetes mellitus are common in patients with APS2. This disorder is three times more common in females than in males. The inheritance pattern can be autosomal recessive, autosomal dominant, or polygenic. Primary hypogonadism may also occur in patients with APS2. However, a key distinction is that the hypoparathyroidism and mucocutaneous candidiasis of APS1 do not occur in patients with APS2, but the following have been found with varying frequencies in patients with APS2: alopecia, pernicious anemia, hypopituitarism caused by autoimmune hypophysitis, vitiligo, myasthenia gravis, Sjögren syndrome, and rheumatoid arthritis.

Other rare polyendocrine autoimmune disorders include Hirata disease presenting with hypoglycemia (associated with insulin autoantibodies); immunodysregulation polyendocrinopathy enteropathy X-linked syndrome (IPEX) presenting with type 1 diabetes mellitus (associated with pathogenic variants in the *FOXP3* gene); Kearns-Sayre syndrome presenting with hypoparathyroidism, primary gonadal failure, nonautoimmune diabetes, and hypopituitarism (associated with deletions in mitochondrial DNA); syndrome of polyneuropathy, organomegaly, endocrinopathy (diabetes and primary gonadal failure), M protein spike, and skin changes (POEMS [polyneuropathy, organomegaly, endocrinopathy, edema, M-protein, and skin abnormalities] syndrome) associated with plasma cell dyscrasia and excess cytokine production; thymic tumors presenting with myasthenia gravis, autoimmune thyroid disease, and adrenal insufficiency; type B insulin resistance associated with insulin receptor autoantibodies; and Wolfram syndrome characterized by diabetes insipidus, nonautoimmune diabetes mellitus, bilateral optic atrophy, and sensorineural deafness (associated with pathogenic variants in the *WFS1* gene).

Spiculate opacities of lens seen on oblique slit-lamp examination

Cataract (posterior subcapsular)

Thick lenses needed after cataract extraction

Candidiasis of nails and mouth in some familial cases

Spotty alopecia

Dental hypoplasia

Lateral radiograph and CT scan of skull show calcification of basal ganglia.

Plate 8.7

Endocrine System: VOLUME 2

CARCINOID SYNDROME

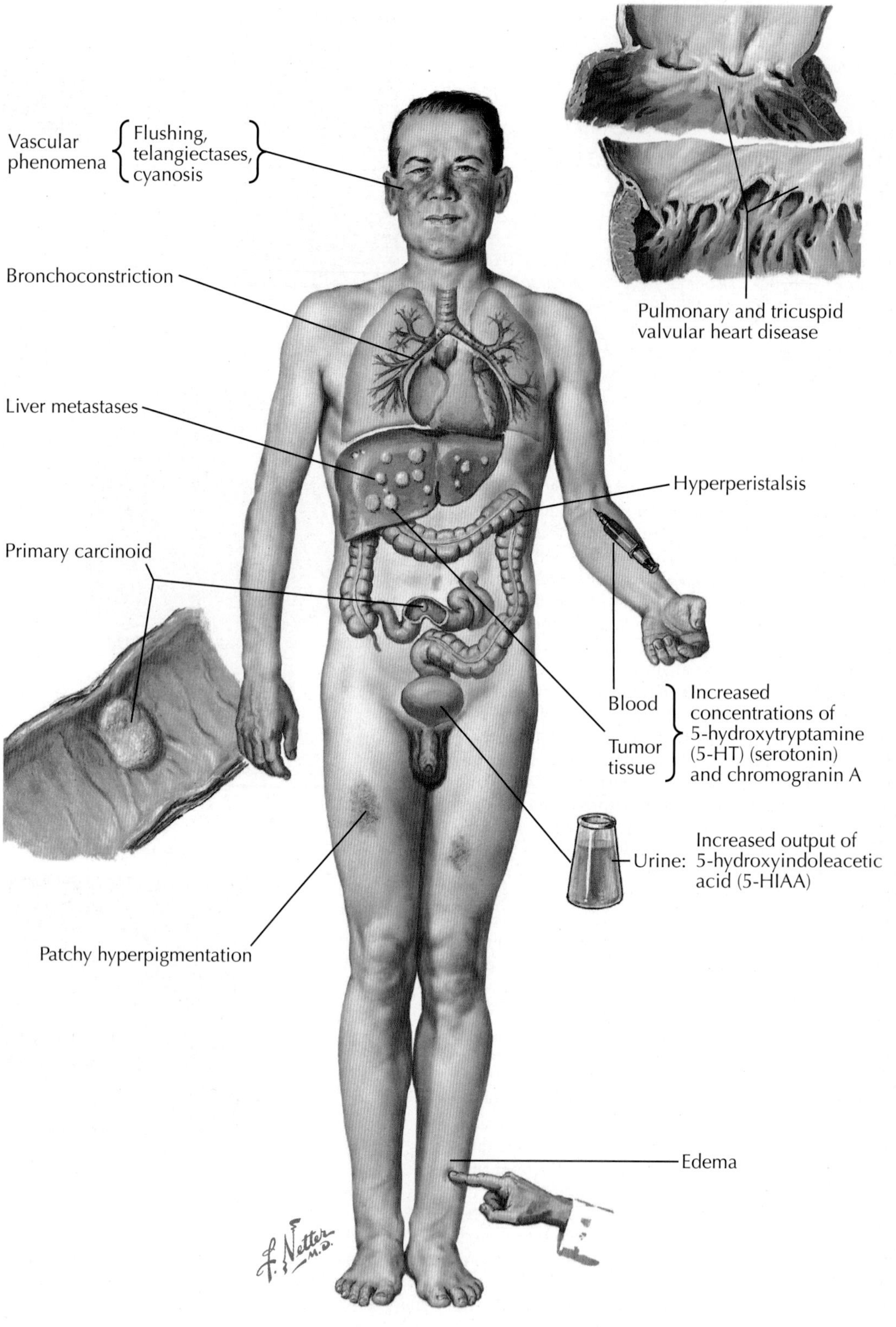

The term *carcinoid* was first used in 1907 to describe tumors that behaved in a more indolent fashion than typical adenocarcinomas. It was not until the 1950s that carcinoid tumors were recognized to be associated with a syndrome of flushing, diarrhea, right-sided valvular heart disease, and increased urinary levels of 5-hydroxyindoleacetic acid (5-HIAA). Seventy-five percent of carcinoid tumors are in the gastrointestinal tract (most commonly in the small intestine with lower frequencies in the rectum and the stomach), and 25% are bronchopulmonary carcinoids. In approximately 15% of patients, metastatic disease is evident at the time of diagnosis. The incidence of carcinoid tumors is 2 per 100,000 people per year. The median age at diagnosis is 55 years, and there is no sex predisposition.

Carcinoid tumors arise from the neuroendocrine cell system that consists of neuronal and epithelial cells; together, they synthesize biogenic amines and peptide hormones. They are distributed diffusely in the mucosa of the lungs and gastrointestinal tract. The underlying pathophysiology of tumorigenesis of these cells is unknown. However, some genetic conditions, such as MEN 1, predispose to carcinoid tumors. When metastatic, these tumors spread primarily to the regional lymph nodes, liver, bone, and the brain. Carcinoid tumor cells retain the capability to produce biogenic amines and peptide hormones, which can result in varying clinical presentations. Chromogranin A is secreted together with hormones and amines; all three secretory products can be used as tumor markers. Neuroendocrine cells often contain somatostatin and other peptide receptors on the cell surface, a finding that may be used diagnostically with somatostatin receptor-based imaging (e.g., Gallium 68 [68-Ga] 1,4,7,10-tetraazacyclododecane-1,4,7,10-tetraacetic acid [DOTA]-octreotate [DOTATATE] positron emission tomography [PET]) or therapeutically with somatostatin analogs.

Pulmonary carcinoids usually have low serotonin content and rarely present with carcinoid syndrome; rather, they often secrete precursors of serotonin such as 5-hydroxytryptophan and many polypeptide hormones that may dominate the clinical presentation. For example, patients with bronchial carcinoid tumors that secrete corticotropin-releasing hormone and corticotropin present with Cushing syndrome. Other hormones that bronchial carcinoids may secrete include growth hormone–releasing hormone, antidiuretic hormone, gastrin, somatostatin, glucagon, tachykinins, and chromogranin A.

Small bowel carcinoids that secrete serotonin and chromogranin A are responsible for most cases of classic carcinoid syndrome. Typical carcinoid syndrome includes flushing, diarrhea, and right-sided valvular heart disease. Less common components include telangiectasia, wheezing caused by bronchoconstriction, patchy hyperpigmentation, and edema. Most patients with the carcinoid syndrome presentation have liver metastases, so that the usual hepatic degradation of amines and peptides is bypassed. The diarrhea is attributable to hyperperistalsis caused by a variety of factors, including serotonin, tachykinins, histamine, kallikrein, and prostaglandins.

Carcinoid heart disease (plaque-like fibrous thickening of the valves) is hemodynamically significant in

Vascular phenomena { Flushing, telangiectases, cyanosis

Bronchoconstriction

Liver metastases

Primary carcinoid

Patchy hyperpigmentation

Pulmonary and tricuspid valvular heart disease

Hyperperistalsis

Blood
Tumor tissue } Increased concentrations of 5-hydroxytryptamine (5-HT) (serotonin) and chromogranin A

Urine: Increased output of 5-hydroxyindoleacetic acid (5-HIAA)

Edema

only 15% of patients. This valvular involvement most commonly results in tricuspid insufficiency; less common outcomes are tricuspid stenosis, pulmonary regurgitation, and pulmonary stenosis. The pathophysiology of this right-sided heart fibrosis is probably related to high serotonin levels. The hypersecretion of tachykinins and bradykinins is the most probable cause of bronchoconstriction.

The biochemical diagnosis of carcinoid syndrome rests primarily on measurement of the serotonin metabolite 5-HIAA in a 24-hour urine collection. Ancillary biochemical diagnostic tests include measurement of blood levels of chromogranin A and serotonin.

The carcinoid tumor is localized with a combination of imaging techniques that include 68-Ga DOTATATE PET CT, CT of the chest and abdomen, CT enterography, rectal ultrasonography, bronchoscopy, upper intestinal endoscopy or endoscopic ultrasonography, and MRI of the liver. The selection of imaging tests and the order in which they are preformed depend on the clinical presentation and the clinical suspicion for pulmonary or gastrointestinal location.

Plate 8.8

Genetics and Endocrine Neoplasia

McCune-Albright Syndrome

MAS (OMIM 174800) is a mosaic disorder caused by postzygotic-activating mutations of the *GNAS1* gene, which encodes the α-subunit of the stimulatory G protein and results in constitutive activation (ligand independent signaling) of adenylyl cyclase in affected tissues. The effects of Gα$_s$ activation are tissue specific and vary in different organ systems. MAS is characterized by the triad of café-au-lait macules, polyostotic fibrous dysplasia (FD), and endocrine hyperactivity.

The café-au-lait macules are found in 66% of patients with MAS. The macules appear at birth or shortly thereafter and are the first manifestation of MAS. Common locations include the chest, neck, and superior aspect of the intergluteal cleft. The café-au-lait macules are caused by cutaneous Gα$_s$ activation and constitutive melanocyte-stimulating hormone receptor signaling, which leads to increased melanin production. The café-au-lait macules have an irregular border described as a "coast of Maine" appearance, which contrasts with the "coast of California" smooth border of the café au lait spots seen with NF1 (see Plate 8.5). The café-au-lait macules are often unilateral, may have a midline demarcation, and follow the lines of Blaschko. In 1901 Alfred Blaschko described the concept of epidermal cell migration patterns and proliferation during the development of the fetus, which are separate from neuronal dermatomes.

Proliferation of undifferentiated skeletal stem cells results in bone being replaced by fibrous connective tissue and poorly formed trabecular bone. FD most commonly presents in the teens or 20s. The clinical presentation varies dramatically based on location and amount of affected bone. It may occur in any bone but is most common in the skull base and proximal femurs. Most patients with FD are asymptomatic. However, it can cause repeated pathologic fractures or severe bone deformity (e.g., coxa vara ["shepherd's crook"] deformity of the proximal femur where there is a decreased angle between the head and neck of the femur and its shaft). With craniofacial involvement, FD may present with asymmetry in frontal, maxillary, or mandibular bones and associated functional impairment. With axial skeleton involvement, scoliosis is common. Fibroblast growth factor 23 (FGF23) overproduction is the result of Gα$_s$ activation in abnormally differentiated osteocytes and results in hypophosphatemia in those patients with severe bony involvement.

Endocrinopathies include gonadotropin-independent gonadal hyperfunction, nonautoimmune hyperthyroidism, GH excess, and neonatal hypercortisolism. Autonomous ovarian activation is common in girls and females with MAS. Approximately 85% of females with MAS have ovarian cysts and associated estradiol secretion, which leads to precocious puberty and intermittent vaginal bleeding. Testicular involvement affects approximately 85% of boys and adult males. However, only 15% of males with MAS have autonomous testosterone secretion. Approximately 66% of patients with MAS have thyroid gland involvement. Hyperthyroidism is due to cyclic adenosine monophosphate–mediated increased deiodinase activity and overproduction of triiodothyronine. Pituitary gland involvement affects 10% to 15% of patients with MAS. When present, pituitary disease is due to increased numbers of mammosomatotroph cells, which cosecrete GH and prolactin. Thus patients can present with acromegaly (see Plate 1.20), secondary hypogonadism, and/or galactorrhea (see Plate 1.21). Corticotropin-independent hypercortisolism occurs in approximately 5% of patients with MAS and presents in the first year of life. The primary adrenocortical hyperplasia is due to Gα$_s$ activation and can result in mild to severe Cushing syndrome (see Plates 3.9 and 3.11).

Other disorders that have been linked to MAS include intramuscular myxomas in 2.2% of patients; intraductal papillary mucinous neoplasms of the pancreas have been found in 50% of patients with MAS; females with MAS have a fourfold increased risk of breast cancer compared with the general population; and there is a risk of malignant transformation of FD to bone cancers (e.g., osteosarcoma, chondrosarcoma, fibrous histiocytoma).

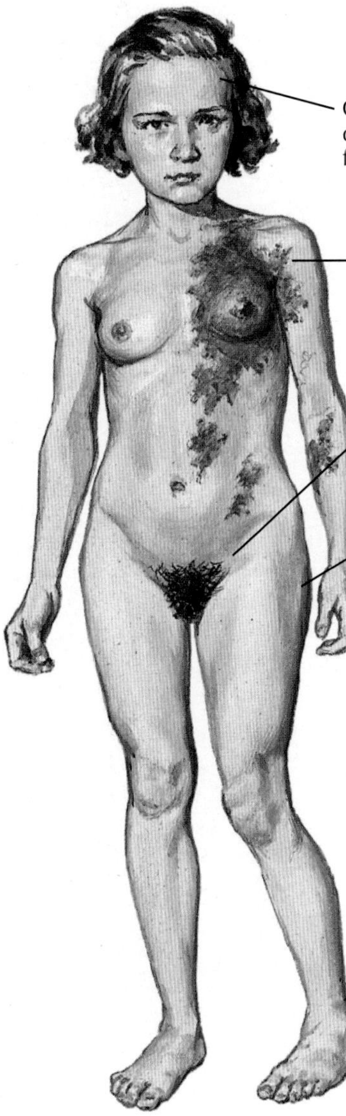

Craniofacial involvement of fibrous dysplasia may show asymmetry in frontal, maxillary, or mandibular bones.

The café-au-lait macules have an irregular border described as a "coast of Maine."

Gonadotropin-independent gonadal hyperfunction leads to precocious puberty and intermittent vaginal bleeding.

Coxa vera deformity of femur makes the leg appear shorter and can lead to a limp.

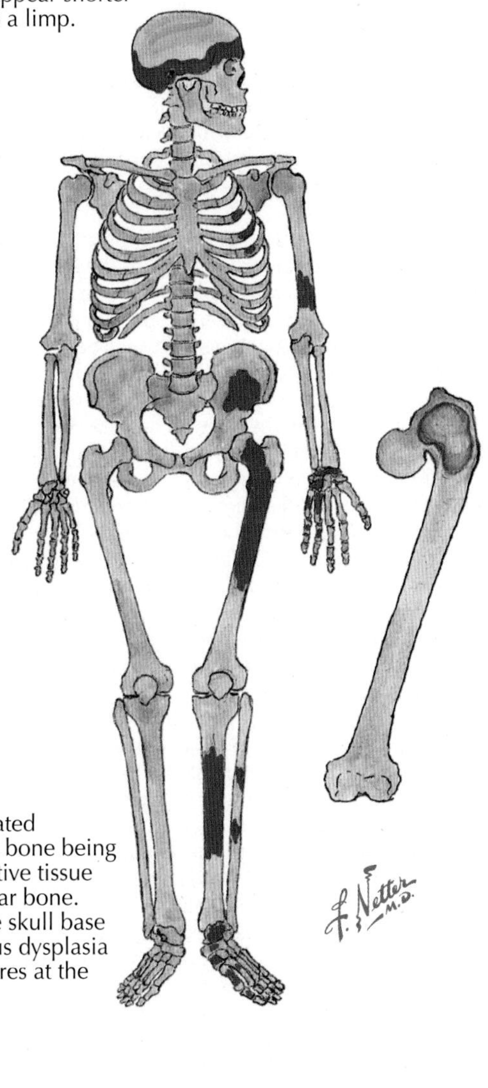

Proliferation of undifferentiated skeletal stem cells results in bone being replaced by fibrous connective tissue and poorly formed trabecular bone. Most commonly seen in the skull base and proximal femurs, fibrous dysplasia can cause pathologic fractures at the hip and elsewhere.

Plate 8.9

Endocrine System: VOLUME 2

CARNEY TRIAD

The Carney triad is a rare (≈200 cases have been described) nonhereditary multitumoral syndrome of unknown etiology. It was described by Aidan Carney in 1977 as "the triad of gastric leiomyosarcoma (gastrointestinal stromal tumor [GIST]), functioning extraadrenal paraganglioma, and pulmonary chondroma." Subsequently, two other tumors, adrenocortical adenoma and esophageal leiomyoma, were added as components—thus Carney triad is actually a "pentad." The disorder occurs primarily in young females. Long-term follow-up shows that the syndrome is a chronic, persistent, and generally indolent condition whose outcome is largely dependent on the behavior of the GIST metastases. The cause of this syndrome is not completely characterized, but epigenetic loss of expression of succinate dehydrogenase, specifically the *SDHC* gene, has been shown to play a role.

The multifocal gastric GISTs, the most common component of the disorder, originate in the interstitial cells of Cajal. They usually occur in the gastric antrum and metastasize early to the liver and lymph nodes. They differ clinically, pathologically, and behaviorally from sporadic, nonsyndromic GISTs. The sporadic gastric GIST is a single tumor with a benign course usually found in an older patient (median age, 65 years) and frequently is caused by a pathogenic variant in the *KIT* gene, and less commonly in the *PDGFRA* gene. In the triad, the gastric GISTs do not exhibit the *KIT* or *PDGFRA* pathogenic variants that are found in sporadic GIST. In the triad, most of the GISTs come to medical attention because of the associated mucosal ulceration, which results in bleeding with consequent anemia, melena, and hematemesis. The mean age at diagnosis of the triad GIST is 20 years. The multifocal GISTs are best treated by total gastrectomy.

Three-fourths of patients with Carney triad have one or more pulmonary chondromas, which are benign lesions composed solely of cartilage. The chondromas may be single or multiple and unilateral or bilateral. The chondromas are often misinterpreted pathologically as pulmonary hamartomas, but they lack bronchial epithelium, an essential component of pulmonary hamartoma. The chondromas cause no symptoms and are usually found during the search for metastases after discovery of the GIST. Chest radiographs show multiple circumscribed tumors scattered in the lungs and often with popcorn-type calcification. When calcified, the appearance of individual tumors is indistinguishable from pulmonary hamartoma. The tumors usually measure several centimeters in diameter and range up to 9 cm. Because they do not cause symptoms or impair lung function and grow very slowly, treatment is usually not needed. The paraganglionic component, the least frequent of the three major components, may occur anywhere in the paraganglionic system, extending from the base of the skull to the scrotum. About half of the patients with the triad have had one or more extraadrenal paragangliomas at a mean age of 26 years. At least six patients with the triad have had

Anatomic locations of paragangliomas and pheochromocytoma

- Secreting norepinephrine
- Secreting epinephrine *and* norepinephrine

Sympathetic trunk

Arch of aorta

Diaphragm

Spleen

Adrenal medulla

Abdominal aorta

Kidney

Organ of Zuckerkandl

Bladder wall

Testis

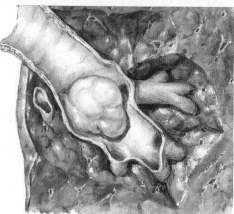

Intraoperative image showing multiple GISTs on the surface of the stomach

Gross pathology image showing multiple GISTs extending from the mucosa of the stomach

Pulmonary chondromas

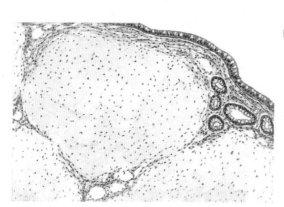

Tumor composed almost entirely of cartilage and covered by bronchial epithelium

Smooth, lobulated growth in a main bronchus

adrenal pheochromocytoma. Most of the triad-related paragangliomas and pheochromocytomas have been catecholamine-secreting and most are resectable after adrenergic blockade (see Plates 3.27 and 3.28).

Adrenocortical adenoma is a more recent addition to the syndrome and is found in about 20% of patients. They are usually lipid-rich on CT and may or may not secrete cortisol autonomously. On pathologic examination, the adrenocortical neoplasms are indistinguishable from sporadic cortical adenomas.

Esophageal leiomyoma is the fifth component of Carney triad. The leiomyomas are small asymptomatic sessile or pedunculated polypoid lesions usually found during upper endoscopy performed for evaluation of the gastric GISTs. The lesions arise from smooth muscle cells of the muscularis propria or muscularis mucosae. Microscopically, they are circumscribed lesions composed of well-differentiated spindle cells arranged in interlacing fascicles and bundles. When asymptomatic, they are simply observed.

1,25[OH]₂D 1,25-dihydroxyvitamin D (calcitriol)
3β-HSD1 3β-hydroxysteroid dehydrogenase type I isozyme
3β-HSD2 3β-hydroxysteroid dehydrogenase type II isozyme
5-HIAA 5-hydroxyindoleacetic acid
11β-HSD1 11β-hydroxysteroid dehydrogenase type 1
11β-HSD2 11β-hydroxysteroid dehydrogenase type 2
17β-HSD1 17β-ketosteroid reductase
17β-HSD2 17β-hydroxysteroid dehydrogenase
17β-HSD3 17β-ketosteroid reductase
17-OHP 17-hydroxyprogesterone
25[OH]D 25-hydroxyvitamin D (calcidiol)
AADC aromatic L-amino acid decarboxylase
ACAT acyl-CoA:cholesterol acyltransferase
ACC adrenocortical carcinoma
ACC American College of Cardiology
ACE angiotensin-converting enzyme
ACTH adrenocorticotropic hormone (corticotropin)
ADH antidiuretic hormone
ADP adenosine diphosphate
AGI α-glucosidase inhibitor
AHA American Heart Association
AIH androgen insensitivity syndrome
AIP aryl hydrocarbon receptor interacting protein
AMH antimüllerian hormone
APA aldosterone-producing adenoma
APECED autoimmune polyendocrinopathy-candidiasis-ectodermal dystrophy
apo apolipoprotein
APS1 autoimmune polyglandular syndrome type I
APS2 autoimmune polyglandular syndrome type II
ARB angiotensin receptor blocker
ASCVD atherosclerotic cardiovascular disease
ATC anaplastic thyroid carcinoma
ATP adenosine triphosphate
ATP III Adult Treatment Panel III
AUS atypia of undetermined significance
AVS adrenal venous sampling
BAAF Bensley acid aniline fuchsin
BMD bone mineral density
BMI body mass index
Ca²⁺ calcium
CAH congenital adrenal hyperplasia
CAIS complete androgen insensitivity syndrome
cAMP cyclic adenosine monophosphate
CaSR calcium-sensing receptor
CBG cortisol-binding globulin
CETP cholesteryl ester transfer protein
CGM continuous glucose monitoring
CHD coronary heart disease
CNS central nervous system
CoA coenzyme A
COMT catechol O-methyltransferase
CRH corticotropin-releasing hormone
CSII continuous subcutaneous insulin infusion
CSF cerebrospinal fluid
CT computed tomography
CTLA4 T-lymphocyte antigen 4 antibody
CTX cerebrotendinous xanthomatosis
CTX c-telopeptide crosslink
CVD cyclophosphamide, vincristine, and dacarbazine
CXR chest radiograph
DA dopamine
DBH dopamine β-hydroxylase
DD disc diameter
DHA docosahexaenoic acid

Dhal-1 dehalogenase 1 isoenzyme
DHEA dehydroepiandrosterone
DHEA-S dehydroepiandrosterone sulfate
DHT dihydrotestosterone
DI diabetes insipidus
DIDMOAD diabetes insipidus, diabetes mellitus, optic atrophy, and deafness
DIT diiodotyrosine
DKA diabetic ketoacidosis
DNA deoxyribonucleic acid
DOC deoxycorticosterone
DPP-IV dipeptidyl peptidase IV
DR diabetic retinopathy
DSD disorder of sex development
DSPN distal symmetric polyneuropathy
DST dexamethasone suppression test
DXA dual energy x-ray absorptiometry
EPA eicosapentaenoic acid
ER endoplasmic reticulum
ESR erythrocyte sedimentation rate
ESRD end-stage renal disease
FAD flavin adenine dinucleotide
FD fibrous dysplasia
FGF23 fibroblast growth factor 23
FH familial hyperaldosteronism
FH familial hypercholesterolemia
FHH familial hypocalciuric hypercalcemia
FISH fluorescence in situ hybridization
FLUS follicular lesions of undetermined significance
FMTC familial medullary thyroid carcinoma
FNA fine-needle aspiration
FRAX fracture risk assessment tool
FSH follicle-stimulating hormone
FTC follicular thyroid carcinoma
Ga-68 DOTATATE PET gallium 68 1,4,7,10-tetraazacyclododecane-1,4,7,10-tetraacetic acid-octreotate positron emission tomography
GABA γ-aminobutyric acid
GAD glutamic acid decarboxylase
GAG glycosaminoglycan
Gb3 globotriaosylceramide
GCT glucose challenge test
GD Gaucher disease
GDM gestational diabetes mellitus
GEP gastroenteropancreatic
GFR glomerular filtration rate
GH growth hormone
GHRH growth hormone-releasing hormone
GI gastrointestinal
GIP gastric inhibitory polypeptide
GIST gastrointestinal stromal tumor
GLP-1 glucagon-like peptide 1
GLUT glucose transporter
GnRH gonadotropin-releasing hormone
GRA glucocorticoid-remediable aldosteronism
GTP guanosine triphosphate
H&E hematoxylin-eosin
HbA₁c hemoglobin A₁c
HCC Hürthle cell carcinoma
hCG human chorionic gonadotropin
HCO₃ bicarbonate
hCS human chorionic somatomammotropin
HDL high-density lipoprotein
Hex A hexosaminidase A
HIF hypoxia-inducible factor
HLA human leukocyte antigen
HMG-CoA 3-hydroxy-3-methylglutaryl coenzyme A

HNF hepatocyte nuclear factor
HPT hyperparathyroidism
HU Hounsfield units
HVA homovanillic acid
I⁻ inorganic iodine
IF intrinsic factor
Ig immunoglobulin
IGF-1 insulin-like growth factor 1
IgG4 immunoglobulin G4
IHA bilateral idiopathic hyperaldosteronism
IP₃ inositol triphosphate
IPEX immunodysregulation polyendocrinopathy enteropathy X-linked syndrome
IPSS inferior petrosal sinus sampling
IRS insulin receptor substrate
IVC inferior vena cava
JNC7 Seventh Report of the Joint National Committee on Prevention, Detection, Evaluation, and Treatment of High Blood Pressure
K⁺ potassium
KClO₄⁻ potassium perchlorate
LCAT lecithin-cholesterol acyltransferase
LDL low-density lipoprotein
LH luteinizing hormone
Lp(a) lipoprotein(a)
LPL lipoprotein lipase
MAO monoamine oxidase
MAPK mitogen-activated protein kinase
MAS McCune-Albright syndrome
MDI multiple daily injections
MEN 1 multiple endocrine neoplasia type 1
MEN 2 multiple endocrine neoplasia type 2
MI myocardial infarction
MIBG metaiodobenzylguanidine
MIT monoiodotyrosine
MLD metachromatic leukodystrophy
MODY maturity-onset diabetes of the young
MR mineralocorticoid receptor
MRI magnetic resonance imaging
MTC medullary thyroid carcinoma
NAD nicotinamide adenine dinucleotide
NADP nicotinamide adenine dinucleotide phosphate
NCEP National Cholesterol Education Program
NF1 neurofibromatosis type 1
NIPHS noninsulinoma pancreatogenous hypoglycemia syndrome
NIS sodium-iodide symporter
NLD necrobiosis diabeticorum
NPD Niemann-Pick disease
NPDR nonproliferative diabetic retinopathy
NPH neutral protamine Hagedorn
NTX N-telopeptide crosslinks
NVD neovascularization at the disc
NVE neovascularization elsewhere
OGTT oral glucose tolerance test
OI osteogenesis imperfecta
P450aro aromatase
P450c11AS aldosterone synthase
P450c11β 11β-hydroxylase
P450c17 17α-hydroxylase
P450c21 21-hydroxylase
P450scc cholesterol side-chain cleavage (desmolase)
PA primary aldosteronism
PAC plasma aldosterone concentration
PAIS partial androgen insensitivity syndrome
PAS periodic acid-Schiff

PBMAH primary bilateral macronodular adrenal hyperplasia
PCOS polycystic ovary syndrome
PCSK9 proprotein convertase subtilisin/kexin type 9 serine protease
PD-1 programmed cell death 1
PD-L1 programmed cell death 1 ligand
PDR proliferative diabetic retinopathy
PHP pseudohypoparathyroidism
PI$_3$ kinase phophatidylinositol-3-kinase
PMDS persistent müllerian duct syndrome
PNMT phenylethanolamine *N*-methyltransferase
POEMS syndrome polyneuropathy, organomegaly, endocrinopathy, edema, M-protein, and skin abnormalities
POMC proopiomelanocortin
PPAR peroxisome proliferator-activated receptor
PPAR α peroxisome proliferator-activated receptor α
PPGL pheochromocytoma and paraganglioma
PPNAD primary pigmented nodular adrenocortical disease
PRA plasma renin activity
PRC plasma renin concentration
PTC papillary thyroid carcinoma
PTH parathyroid hormone

PTHrP parathyroid hormone-related protein
PVN paraventricular nucleus
RAAS renin-angiotensin-aldosterone system
RAE retinol activity equivalents
RANK receptor activator of NF-κB
RANKL nuclear factor κB ligand
RBP retinol-binding proteins
rT$_3$ reverse triiodothyronine
RYGB Roux-en-Y gastric bypass
SD standard deviation
SDH succinate dehydrogenase
SGLT2 sodium-glucose cotransporter 2
SHBG sex hormone-binding globulin
siRNA small interfering mRNA
SMBG self-monitoring of blood glucose
SON supraoptic nucleus
SREBP sterol regulatory element-binding protein
StAR steroidogenic acute regulatory protein
SUR sulfonylurea receptor
T$_2$ diiodothyronine
T$_3$ triiodothyronine
T$_4$ thyroxine
TBG thyroxine-binding globulin
TC transcobalamin
TCA tricarboxylic acid

Tg thyroglobulin
TGRL triglyceride-rich lipoproteins
TH tyrosine hydroxylase
THOX2 thyroid oxidase 2
TPO thyroid peroxidase
TRH thyrotropin-releasing hormone
TSH thyrotropin
TZD thiazolidinedione
UAH unilateral adrenal hyperplasia
UDP uridine diphosphate
UDPGlc uridine diphosphate glucose
UFC urinary free cortisol
U:L ratio upper body to lower body segment ratio
UTI urinary tract infection
UTP uridine triphosphate
VHL von Hippel-Lindau
VLDL very low-density lipoprotein
VMA vanillylmandelic acid
VMAT vesicular monoamine transporter
X-LAG X-linked acro-gigantism
ZF adrenal zona fasciculata
ZG adrenal zona glomerulosa
ZR adrenal zona reticularis

SELECTED REFERENCES

Section 1 Pituitary and Hypothalamus

Abe T. Lymphocytic infundibulo-neurohypophysitis and infundibulo-panhypophysitis regarded as lymphocytic hypophysitis variant. Brain Tumor Pathol. 2008;25(2):59–66.

ACOG Practice Bulletin: Clinical Management Guidelines for Obstetrician-Gynecologists Number 76, October 2006: postpartum hemorrhage. Obstet Gynecol. 2006;108(4):1039–47.

Agrawal D, Mahapatra AK. Visual outcome of blind eyes in pituitary apoplexy after transsphenoidal surgery: a series of 14 eyes. Surg Neurol. 2005;63(1):42–6; discussion 46.

Alatzoglou KS, Dattani MT. Genetic forms of hypopituitarism and their manifestation in the neonatal period. Early Hum Dev. 2009;85(11):705–12.

Alatzoglou KS, Kelberman D, Dattani MT. The role of SOX proteins in normal pituitary development. J Endocrinol. 2009;200(3):245–58.

Albano L, Losa M, Barzaghi LR, Niranjan A, Siddiqui Z, Flickinger JC, et al. Gamma knife radiosurgery for pituitary tumors: a systematic review and meta-analysis. Cancers (Basel). 2021;13(19):4998.

Almeida JP, Sanchez MM, Karekezi C, Warsi N, Fernández-Gajardo R, Panwar J, et al. Pituitary apoplexy: results of surgical and conservative management clinical series and review of the literature. World Neurosurg. 2019;130:e988–99.

Ascoli P, Cavagnini F. Hypopituitarism. Pituitary. 2006;9(4):335–42.

Assie G, Bahurel H, Coste J, Silvera S, Kujas M, Dugue MA, et al. Corticotroph tumor progression after adrenalectomy in Cushing's Disease: a reappraisal of Nelson's Syndrome. J Clin Endocrinol Metab. 2007;92(1):172–9.

Atkinson JL, Young WF Jr, Meyer FB, Davis DH, Nippoldt TB, Erickson D, et al. Sublabial transseptal vs transnasal combined endoscopic microsurgery in patients with Cushing disease and MRI-depicted microadenomas. Mayo Clin Proc. 2008;83(5):550–3.

Atmaca H, Tanriverdi F, Gokce C, Unluhizarci K, Kelestimur F. Posterior pituitary function in Sheehan's syndrome. Eur J Endocrinol. 2007;156(5):563–7.

Barkan AL. Biochemical markers of acromegaly: GH vs. IGF-I. Growth Horm IGF Res. 2004;14(Suppl A):S97–100.

Barzaghi LR, Donofrio CA, Panni P, Losa M, Mortini P. Treatment of empty sella associated with visual impairment: a systematic review of chiasmapexy techniques. Pituitary. 2018;21(1):98–106.

Bell J, Parker KL, Swinford RD, Hoffman AR, Maneatis T, Lippe B. Long-term safety of recombinant human growth hormone in children. J Clin Endocrinol Metab. 2010;95(1):167–77.

Ben-Shlomo A. Pituitary gland: predictors of acromegaly-associated mortality. Nat Rev Endocrinol. 2010;6(2):67–9.

Bhasin S, Cunningham GR, Hayes FJ, Matsumoto AM, Snyder PJ, Swerdloff RS, et al. Testosterone therapy in adult men with androgen deficiency syndromes: an Endocrine Society clinical practice guideline. J Clin Endocrinol Metab. 2006;91(6):1995–2010.

Biller BM, Grossman AB, Stewart PM, Melmed S, Bertagna X, Bertherat J, et al. Treatment of adrenocorticotropin-dependent Cushing's syndrome: a consensus statement. J Clin Endocrinol Metab. 2008;93(7):2454–62.

Blanks AM, Thornton S. The role of oxytocin in parturition. BJOG. 2003;110(Suppl 20):46–51.

Bougneres P, Pantalone L, Linglart A, Rothenbuhler A, Le Stunff C. Endocrine manifestations of the rapid-onset obesity with hypoventilation, hypothalamic, autonomic dysregulation, and neural tumor syndrome in childhood. J Clin Endocrinol Metab. 2008;93(10):3971–80.

Bouligand J, Ghervan C, Tello JA, Brailly-Tabard S, Salenave S, Chanson P, et al. Isolated familial hypogonadotropic hypogonadism and a GNRH1 mutation. N Engl J Med. 2009;360(26):2742–8.

Brewster UC, Hayslett JP. Diabetes insipidus in the third trimester of pregnancy. Obstet Gynecol. 2005;105(5 Pt 2):1173–6.

Brooks EK, Inder WJ. Disorders of salt and water balance after pituitary surgery. J Clin Endocrinol Metab. 2022;108(1):198–208.

Busch W. Die Morphologie der Sella turcica und ihre Beziehungen zur Hypophyse. Virchows Arch Pathol Anat Physiol Klin Med. 1951;320:437–58.

Buurman H, Saeger W. Subclinical adenomas in postmortem pituitaries: classification and correlations to clinical data. Eur J Endocrinol. 2006;154(5):753–8.

Carpinteri R, Patelli I, Casanueva FF, Giustina A. Pituitary tumours: inflammatory and granulomatous expansive lesions of the pituitary. Best Pract Res Clin Endocrinol Metab. 2009;23(5):639–50.

Carrim ZI, Reeks GA, Chohan AW, Dunn LT, Hadley DM. Predicting impairment of central vision from dimensions of the optic chiasm in patients with pituitary adenoma. Acta Neurochir (Wien). 2007;149(3):255–60; discussion 260.

Castinetti F, Saveanu A, Reynaud R, Quentien MH, Buffin A, Brauner R, et al. A novel dysfunctional LHX4 mutation with high phenotypical variability in patients with hypopituitarism. J Clin Endocrinol Metab. 2008;93(7):2790–9.

Cavallo LM, Prevedello D, Esposito F, Laws ER Jr, Dusick JR, Messina A, et al. The role of the endoscope in the transsphenoidal management of cystic lesions of the sellar region. Neurosurg Rev. 2008;31(1):55–64; discussion 64.

Cerbone M, Visser J, Bulwer C, Ederies A, Vallabhaneni K, Ball S, et al. Management of children and young people with idiopathic pituitary stalk thickening, central diabetes insipidus, or both: a national clinical practice consensus guideline. Lancet Child Adolesc Health. 2021;5(9):662–76.

Chahal HS, Stals K, Unterländer M, Balding DJ, Thomas MG, Kumar AV, et al. AIP mutation in pituitary adenomas in the 18th century and today. N Engl J Med. 2011;364(1):43–50.

Chamarthi B, Morris CA, Kaiser UB, Katz JT, Loscalzo J. Clinical problem-solving. Stalking the diagnosis. N Engl J Med. 2010;362(9):834–9.

Chan YM, de Guillebon A, Lang-Muritano M, Plummer L, Cerrato F, Tsiaras S, et al. GNRH1 mutations in patients with idiopathic hypogonadotropic hypogonadism. Proc Natl Acad Sci U S A. 2009;106(28):11703–8.

Chanson P, Salenave S, Kamenicky P, Cazabat L, Young J. Pituitary tumours: acromegaly. Best Pract Res Clin Endocrinol Metab. 2009;23(5):555–74.

Chatterton RT Jr, Hill PD, Aldag JC, Hodges KR, Belknap SM, Zinaman MJ. Relation of plasma oxytocin and prolactin concentrations to milk production in mothers of preterm infants: influence of stress. J Clin Endocrinol Metab. 2000;85(10):3661–8.

Chiamolera MI, Wondisford FE. Minireview: Thyrotropin-releasing hormone and the thyroid hormone feedback mechanism. Endocrinology. 2009;150(3):1091–6.

Chiloiro S, Giampietro A., Bianchi A, Tartaglione T, Capobianco A, Anile C, De Marinis L. Primary empty sella: a comprehensive review. Eur J Endocrinol. 2017;177(6):R275–85.

Choh NA, Choh SA, Jehangir M, Yousuf R. Posterior pituitary ectopia with absent pituitary stalk—a rare cause of hypopituitarism. J Pediatr Endocrinol Metab. 2009;22(5):407–8.

Chow JT, Thompson GB, Grant CS, Farley DR, Richards ML, Young WF Jr. Bilateral laparoscopic adrenalectomy for corticotrophin-dependent Cushing's syndrome: a review of the Mayo Clinic experience. Clin Endocrinol (Oxf). 2008;68(4):513–19.

Christ-Crain M. Diabetes insipidus - An update in diagnosis and management. Best Pract Res Clin Endocrinol Metab. 2020;34(5):101470.

Clark SL, Simpson KR, Knox GE, Garite TJ. Oxytocin: new perspectives on an old drug. Am J Obstet Gynecol. 2009;200(1):35 e31–36.

Colao A, Di Somma C, Savastano S, Rota F, Savanelli MC, Aimaretti G, et al. A reappraisal of diagnosing GH deficiency in adults: role of gender, age, waist circumference, and body mass index. J Clin Endocrinol Metab. 2009;94(11):4414–22.

Colao A, Loche S. Prolactinomas in children and adolescents. Endocr Dev. 2010;17:146–59.

Colvin SC, Mullen RD, Pfaeffle RW, Rhodes SJ. LHX3 and LHX4 transcription factors in pituitary development and disease. Pediatr Endocrinol Rev. 2009;6(Suppl 2):283–90.

Cossu G, Jouanneau E, Cavallo LM, Elbabaa SK, Giammattei L, Starnoni D, et al. Surgical management of craniopharyngiomas in adult patients: a systematic review and consensus statement on behalf of the EANS skull base section. Acta Neurochir (Wien). 2020;162(5):1159–77.

Coya R, Vela A, Perez de Nanclares G, Rica I, Castano L, Busturia MA, et al. Panhypopituitarism: genetic versus acquired etiological factors. J Pediatr Endocrinol Metab. 2007;20(1):27–36.

D'Ambrosio N, Soohoo S, Warshall C, Johnson A, Karimi S. Craniofacial and intracranial manifestations of Langerhans cell histiocytosis: report of findings in 100 patients. AJR Am J Roentgenol. 2008;191(2):589–97.

Darzy KH. Radiation-induced hypopituitarism after cancer therapy: who, how and when to test. Nat Clin Pract Endocrinol Metab. 2009;5(2):88–99.

Darzy KH, Shalet SM. Hypopituitarism following radiotherapy. Pituitary. 2009;12(1):40–50.

De Bellis A, Ruocco G, Battaglia M, Conte M, Coronella C, Tirelli G, et al. Immunological and clinical aspects of lymphocytic hypophysitis. Clin Sci (Lond). 2008;114(6):413–21.

De Marinis L, Bonadonna S, Bianchi A, Maira G, Giustina A. Primary empty sella. J Clin Endocrinol Metab. 2005;90(9):5471–7.

Decaux G, Soupart A, Vassart G. Non-peptide arginine-vasopressin antagonists: the vaptans. Lancet. 2008;371(9624):1624–32.

Dekkers OM, Lagro J, Burman P, Jorgensen JO, Romijn JA, Pereira AM. Recurrence of hyperprolactinemia after withdrawal of dopamine agonists: systematic review and meta-analysis. J Clin Endocrinol Metab. 2010;95(1):43–51.

Delman BN. Imaging of pediatric pituitary abnormalities. Endocrinol Metab Clin North Am. 2009;38(4):673–98.

Desai NR, Cheng S, Nohria A, Halperin F, Giugliano RP. Clinical problem-solving. When past is prologue. N Engl J Med. 2009;360(10):1016–22.

di Iorgi N, Secco A, Napoli F, Calandra E, Rossi A, Maghnie M. Developmental abnormalities of the posterior pituitary gland. Endocr Dev. 2009;14:83–94.

Dubuisson AS, Stevenaert A, Martin DH, Flandroy PP. Intrasellar arachnoid cysts. Neurosurgery. 2007;61(3):505–13; discussion 513.

Dunser MW, Lindner KH, Wenzel V. A century of arginine vasopressin research leading to new therapeutic strategies. Anesthesiology. 2006;105(3):444–5.

Dutta P, Bhansali A, Singh P, Rajput R, Khandelwal N, Bhadada S. Congenital hypopituitarism: clinico-radiological correlation. J Pediatr Endocrinol Metab. 2009;22(10):921–8.

Elliott RE, Hsieh K, Hochm T, Belitskaya-Levy I, Wisoff J, Wisoff JH. Efficacy and safety of radical resection of primary and recurrent craniopharyngiomas in 86 children. J Neurosurg Pediatr. 2010;5(1):30–48.

Ellison DH, Berl T. Clinical practice. The syndrome of inappropriate antidiuresis. N Engl J Med. 2007;356(20):2064–72.

Ersahin Y, Kesikci H, Ruksen M, Aydin C, Mutluer S. Endoscopic treatment of suprasellar arachnoid cysts. Childs Nerv Syst. 2008;24(9):1013–20.

Eugster EA, Pescovitz OH. Gigantism. J Clin Endocrinol Metab. 1999;84(12):4379–84.

Fazio N, Spaggiari L, Pelosi G, Presicci F, Preda L. Langerhans' cell histiocytosis. Lancet. 2005;365(9459):598.

Fenske W, Refardt J, Chifu I, Schnyder I, Winzeler B, Drummond J, et al. Copeptin-based approach in the diagnosis of diabetes insipidus. N Engl J Med. 2018;379(5):428–39.

Fernandez A, Brada M, Zabuliene L, Karavitaki N, Wass JA. Radiation-induced hypopituitarism. Endocr Relat Cancer. 2009;16(3):733–72.

Fewtrell MS, Loh KL, Blake A, Ridout DA, Hawdon J. Randomised, double blind trial of oxytocin nasal spray in mothers expressing breast milk for preterm infants. Arch Dis Child Fetal Neonatal Ed. 2006;91(3):F169–174.

Fleseriu M, Biller BMK, Freda PU, Gadelha MR, Giustina A, Katznelson L, et al. A Pituitary Society update to acromegaly management guidelines. Pituitary. 2021;24(1):1–13.

Fleseriu M, Hashim IA, Karavitaki N, Melmed S, Murad MH, Salvatori R, Samuels MH. Hormonal replacement in hypopituitarism in adults: an Endocrine Society clinical practice guideline. J Clin Endocrinol Metab. 2016;101(11):3888–3921.

Fujimoto N, Saeki N, Miyauchi O, Adachi-Usami E. Criteria for early detection of temporal hemianopia in asymptomatic pituitary tumor. Eye (Lond). 2002;16(6):731–8.

Gaston-Massuet C, Andoniadou CL, Signore M, Sajedi E, Bird S, Turner JM, et al. Genetic interaction between the homeobox transcription factors HESX1 and SIX3 is required for normal pituitary development. Dev Biol. 2008;324(2):322–33.

Geddes JF, Jansen GH, Robinson SF, Gomori E, Holton JL, Monson JP, et al. "Gangliocytomas" of the pituitary: a heterogeneous group of lesions with differing histogenesis. Am J Surg Pathol. 2000;24(4):607–13.

Giustina A, Barkan A, Beckers A, et al. A consensus on the diagnosis and treatment of acromegaly comorbidities: an update. J Clin Endocrinol Metab. 2020;105(4):dgz096.

Goldenberg N, Racine MS, Thomas P, Degnan B, Chandler W, Barkan A. Treatment of pituitary gigantism with the growth hormone receptor antagonist pegvisomant. J Clin Endocrinol Metab. 2008;93(8):2953–6.

Goswami R, Kochupillai N, Crock PA, Jaleel A, Gupta N. Pituitary autoimmunity in patients with Sheehan's syndrome. J Clin Endocrinol Metab. 2002;87(9):4137–41.

Graffeo CS, Perry A, Carlstrom LP, Meyer FB, Atkinson JLD, Erickson D, et al. Characterizing and predicting the Nelson-Salassa syndrome. J Neurosurg. 2017;127(6):1277–87.

Greenman Y, Stern N. How should a nonfunctioning pituitary macroadenoma be monitored after debulking surgery? Clin Endocrinol (Oxf). 2009;70(6):829–32.

Gruber A, Clayton J, Kumar S, Robertson I, Howlett TA, Mansell P. Pituitary apoplexy: retrospective review of 30 patients—is surgical intervention always necessary? Br J Neurosurg. 2006;20(6):379–85.

Guitelman M, Garcia Basavilbaso N, Vitale M, Chervin A, Katz D, Miragaya K, et al. Primary empty sella (PES): a review of 175 cases. Pituitary. 2013;16(2):270–4.

Hamilton BE, Salzman KL, Osborn AG. Anatomic and pathologic spectrum of pituitary infundibulum lesions. AJR Am J Roentgenol. 2007;188(3):W223–232.

Hattori N, Ishihara T, Saiki Y. Macroprolactinaemia: prevalence and aetiologies in a large group of hospital workers. Clin Endocrinol (Oxf). 2009;71(5):702–8.

Herman TE, Siegel MJ. Langerhans cell histiocytosis: radio-graphic images in pediatrics. Clin Pediatr (Phila). 2009;48(2):228–31.
Heshmati HM, Scheithauer BW, Young WF Jr. Metastases to the pituitary gland. Endocrinologist. 2002;12:45–9.
Ishunina TA, Swaab DF. Vasopressin and oxytocin neurons of the human supraoptic and paraventricular nucleus: size changes in relation to age and sex. J Clin Endocrinol Metab. 1999;84(12):4637–44.
Jane JA Jr, Prevedello DM, Alden TD, Laws ER Jr. The transsphenoidal resection of pediatric craniopharyngiomas: a case series. J Neurosurg Pediatr. 2010;5(1):49–60.
Kano H, Niranjan A, Kondziolka D, Flickinger JC, Lunsford LD. Stereotactic radiosurgery for pituitary metastases. Surg Neurol. 2009;72(3):248–55; discussion 255–246.
Karavitaki N, Wass JA. Non-adenomatous pituitary tumours. Best Pract Res Clin Endocrinol Metab. 2009;23(5):651–65.
Kato Y, Ogawa Y, Tominaga T. Treatment and therapeutic strategies for pituitary apoplexy in pregnancy: a case series. J Med Case Rep. 2021;15(1):289.
Kaushal K, Shalet SM. Defining growth hormone status in adults with hypopituitarism. Horm Res. 2007;68(4):185–94.
Kelberman D, Dattani MT. Role of transcription factors in midline central nervous system and pituitary defects. Endocr Dev. 2009; 14:67–82.
Kelberman D, Turton JP, Woods KS, Mehta A, Al-Khawari M, Greening J, et al. Molecular analysis of novel PROP1 mutations associated with combined pituitary hormone deficiency (CPHD). Clin Endocrinol (Oxf). 2009;70(1):96–103.
Kelestimur F. Sheehan's syndrome. Pituitary. 2003;6(4):181–8.
Kelly PA, Samandouras G, Grossman AB, Afshar F, Besser GM, Jenkins PJ. Neurosurgical treatment of Nelson's syndrome. J Clin Endocrinol Metab. 2002;87(12):5465–9.
Kirsch CFE. Imaging of sella and parasellar region. Neuroimaging Clin N Am. 2021;31(4):541–52.
Klibanski A. Clinical practice. Prolactinomas. N Engl J Med. 2010;362 (13):1219–26.
Komninos J, Vlassopoulou V, Protopapa D, Korfias S, Kontogeorgos G, Sakas DE, et al. Tumors metastatic to the pituitary gland: case report and literature review. J Clin Endocrinol Metab. 2004; 89(2):574–80.
Kosmorsky GS, Dupps WJ Jr, Drake RL. Nonuniform pressure generation in the optic chiasm may explain bitemporal hemianopsia. Ophthalmology. 2008;115(3):560–5.
Kovacs K. Sheehan syndrome. Lancet. 2003;361(9356):520–2.
Kristof RA, Rother M, Neuloh G, Klingmuller D. Incidence, clinical manifestations, and course of water and electrolyte metabolism disturbances following transsphenoidal pituitary adenoma surgery: a prospective observational study. J Neurosurg. 2009;111(3):555–62.
Krsmanovic LZ, Hu L, Leung PK, Feng H, Catt KJ. The hypothalamic GnRH pulse generator: multiple regulatory mechanisms. Trends Endocrinol Metab. 2009;20(8):402–8.
Langlois F, Varlamov EV, Fleseriu M. Hypophysitis, the growing spectrum of a rare pituitary disease. J Clin Endocrinol Metab. 2022;107(1):10–28.
Laws ER Jr, Jane JA Jr. Craniopharyngioma. J Neurosurg Pediatr. 2010; 5(1):27–8; discussion 28–29.
Lawson EA, Buchbinder BR, Daniels GH. Hypopituitarism associated with a giant aneurysm of the internal carotid artery. J Clin Endocrinol Metab. 2008;93(12):4616.
Lee MM. Clinical practice. Idiopathic short stature. N Engl J Med. 2006;354(24):2576–82.
Leonidas JC, Guelfguat M, Valderrama E. Langerhans' cell histiocytosis. Lancet. 2003;361(9365):1293–5.
Lloyd RV, Douglas BR, Young WF Jr. Pituitary gland. In: King DW, editor. Atlas of Nontumor Pathology: Endocrine Diseases. American Registry of Pathology and the Armed Forces Institute of Pathology; 2002.
Lury KM. Inflammatory and infectious processes involving the pituitary gland. Top Magn Reson Imaging. 2005;16(4):301–6.
Martin-Grace J, Tomkins M, O'Reilly MW, Thompson CJ, Sherlock M. Approach to the patient: hyponatremia and the Syndrome of Inappropriate Antidiuresis (SIAD). J Clin Endocrinol Metab. 2022;107(8):2362–76.
Mauermann WJ, Sheehan JP, Chernavvsky DR, Laws ER, Steiner L, Vance ML. Gamma Knife surgery for adrenocorticotropic hormone-producing pituitary adenomas after bilateral adrenalectomy. J Neurosurg. 2007;106(6):988–93.
McKenna TJ. Should macroprolactin be measured in all hyperprolactinaemic sera? Clin Endocrinol (Oxf). 2009;71(4):466–9.
McVary KT. Clinical practice. Erectile dysfunction. N Engl J Med. 2007;357(24):2472–81.
Mehta A, Hindmarsh PC, Mehta H, Turton JP, Russell-Eggitt I, Taylor D, et al. Congenital hypopituitarism: clinical, molecular and neuroradiological correlates. Clin Endocrinol (Oxf). 2009;71(3):376–82.
Melmed S. Acromegaly pathogenesis and treatment. J Clin Invest. 2009;119(11):3189–202.
Melmed S. Medical progress: acromegaly. N Engl J Med. 2006; 355(24):2558–73.
Melmed S, Colao A, Barkan A, Molitch M, Grossman AB, Kleinberg D, et al. Guidelines for acromegaly management: an update. J Clin Endocrinol Metab. 2009;94(5):1509–17.
Melmed S, Kaiser UB, Lopes MB, Bertherat J, Syro LV, Raverot G, et al. Clinical biology of the pituitary adenoma. Endocr Rev. 2022;43(6):1003–37.
Milardi D, Giampietro A, Baldelli R, Pontecorvi A, De Marinis L. Fertility and hypopituitarism. J Endocrinol Invest. 2008;31 (9 Suppl):71–4.
Mizukoshi T, Fukuoka H, Takahashi Y. Immune checkpoint inhibitor-related hypophysitis. Best Pract Res Clin Endocrinol Metab. 2022;36(3):101668.
Molitch ME, Clemmons DR, Malozowski S, Merriam GR, Shalet SM, Vance ML, et al. Evaluation and treatment of adult growth hormone deficiency: an Endocrine Society clinical practice guideline. J Clin Endocrinol Metab. 2006;91(5):1621–34.
Muller HL. Childhood craniopharyngioma. Recent advances in diagnosis, treatment and follow-up. Horm Res. 2008;69(4):193–202.
Murad-Kejbou S, Eggenberger E. Pituitary apoplexy: evaluation, management, and prognosis. Curr Opin Ophthalmol. 2009;20(6):456–61.
Nakamoto J. Laboratory diagnosis of multiple pituitary hormone deficiencies: issues with testing of the growth and thyroid axes. Pediatr Endocrinol Rev. 2009;6(Suppl 2):291–7.
Nakhla M, Polychronakos C. Monogenic and other unusual causes of diabetes mellitus. Pediatr Clin North Am. 2005;52(6):1637–50.
Narayanaswamy V, Rettig KR, Bhowmick SK. Excessive growth. Clin Pediatr (Phila). 2008;47(7):705–8.
Nawar RN, AbdelMannan D, Selman WR, Arafah BM. Pituitary tumor apoplexy: a review. J Intensive Care Med. 2008;23(2):75–90.
Nemergut EC, Zuo Z, Jane JA Jr, Laws ER Jr. Predictors of diabetes insipidus after transsphenoidal surgery: a review of 881 patients. J Neurosurg. 2005;103(3):448–54.
Nieman LK. Diagnosis of Cushing's syndrome in the modern era. Endocrinol Metab Clin North Am. 2018;47(2):259–73.
Nieman LK, Biller BM, Findling JW, Newell-Price J, Savage MO, Stewart PM, et al. The diagnosis of Cushing's syndrome: an Endocrine Society clinical practice guideline. J Clin Endocrinol Metab. 2008;93(5):1526–40.
Osamura RY, Grossman A, Korbonits M, Kovacs K, Lopes MBS, Matsuno A, et al. Pituitary adenoma. Lloyd RV, Osamura RY, Kloppel G, Rosai J, editors. World Health Organization Classification of Tumours of Endocrine Organs. IARC Press; 2017.
Ozkan Y, Colak R. Sheehan syndrome: clinical and laboratory evaluation of 20 cases. Neuro Endocrinol Lett. 2005;26(3): 257–60.
Pardanani A, Phyliky RL, Li CY, Tefferi A. 2-Chlorodeoxyadenosine therapy for disseminated Langerhans cell histiocytosis. Mayo Clin Proc. 2003;78(3):301–6.
Pascual JM, Carrasco R, Prieto R, Gonzalez-Llanos F, Alvarez F, Roda JM. Craniopharyngioma classification. J Neurosurg. 2008; 109(6):1180–82; author reply 1182–3.
Patil CG, Prevedello DM, Lad SP, Vance ML, Thorner MO, Katznelson L, et al. Late recurrences of Cushing's disease after initial successful transsphenoidal surgery. J Clin Endocrinol Metab. 2008;93(2):358–62.
Patil CG, Veeravagu A, Prevedello DM, Katznelson L, Vance ML, Laws ER Jr. Outcomes after repeat transsphenoidal surgery for recurrent Cushing's disease. Neurosurgery. 2008;63(2):266–70; discussion 270–261.
Patti G, Napoli F, Fava D, Casalini E, Di Iorgi N, Maghnie M. Approach to the pediatric patient: central diabetes insipidus. J Clin Endocrinol Metab. 2022;107(5):1407–16.
Petersenn S, Buchfelder M, Gerbert B, Franz H, Quabbe HJ, Schulte HM, et al. Age and sex as predictors of biochemical activity in acromegaly: analysis of 1485 patients from the German Acromegaly Register. Clin Endocrinol (Oxf). 2009;71(3):400–5.
Petit JH, Biller BM, Yock TI, Swearingen B, Coen JJ, Chapman P, et al. Proton stereotactic radiotherapy for persistent adrenocorticotropin-producing adenomas. J Clin Endocrinol Metab. 2008;93(2):393–9.
Pitteloud N, Dwyer AA, DeCruz S, Lee H, Boepple PA, Crowley WF Jr, et al. Inhibition of luteinizing hormone secretion by testosterone in men requires aromatization for its pituitary but not its hypothalamic effects: evidence from the tandem study of normal and gonadotropin-releasing hormone-deficient men. J Clin Endocrinol Metab. 2008;93(3):784–91.
Prodam F, Pagano L, Corneli G, Golisano G, Belcastro S, Busti A, et al. Update on epidemiology, etiology, and diagnosis of adult growth hormone deficiency. J Endocrinol Invest. 2008;31(9 Suppl): 6–11.
Quereda V, Malumbres M. Cell cycle control of pituitary development and disease. J Mol Endocrinol. 2009;42(2):75–86.
Raper DM, Besser M. Clinical features, management and recurrence of symptomatic Rathke's cleft cyst. J Clin Neurosci. 2009;16(3): 385–9.
Raverot G, Jacob M, Jouanneau E, Delemer B, Vighetto A, Pugeat M, et al. Secondary deterioration of visual field during cabergoline treatment for macroprolactinoma. Clin Endocrinol (Oxf). 2009; 70(4):588–92.
Raverot G, Wierinckx A, Dantony E, Auger C, Chapas G, Villeneuve L, et al. Prognostic factors in prolactin pituitary tumors: clinical, histological, and molecular data from a series of 94 patients with a long postoperative follow-up. J Clin Endocrinol Metab. 2010; 95(4):1708–16.
Reid TJ, Post KD, Bruce JN, Nabi Kanibir M, Reyes-Vidal CM, Freda PU. Features at diagnosis of 324 patients with acromegaly did not change from 1981 to 2006; acromegaly remains under-recognized and under-diagnosed. Clin Endocrinol (Oxf). 2010;72:203–8.
Reynaud R, Gueydan M, Saveanu A, Vallette-Kasic S, Enjalbert A, Brue T, et al. Genetic screening of combined pituitary hormone deficiency: experience in 195 patients. J Clin Endocrinol Metab. 2006;91(9):3329–36.
Robertson DM, Hale GE, Jolley D, Fraser IS, Hughes CL, Burger HG. Interrelationships between ovarian and pituitary hormones in ovulatory menstrual cycles across reproductive age. J Clin Endocrinol Metab. 2009;94(1):138–44.
Romero CJ, Nesi-Franca S, Radovick S. The molecular basis of hypopituitarism. Trends Endocrinol Metab. 2009;20(10):506–16.
Rudolph T, Frisen L. Influence of ageing on visual field defects due to stable lesions. Br J Ophthalmol. 2007;91(10):1276–8.
Rupp D, Molitch M. Pituitary stalk lesions. Curr Opin Endocrinol Diabetes Obes. 2008;15(4):339–45.
Sailer CO, Refardt J, Blum CA, Schnyder I, Molina-Tijeras JA, Fenske W, et al. Validity of different copeptin assays in the differential diagnosis of the polyuria-polydipsia syndrome. Sci Rep. 2021;11(1):10104.
Saito T, Sato N, Kimoto M, Asano T, Aoki A, Ikoma A, et al. Incomplete deficiency of hypothalamic hormones in hypothalamic hypopituitarism associated with an old traumatic brain injury. Endocr J. 2009;56(8):945–50.
Saleem SN, Said AH, Lee DH. Lesions of the hypothalamus: MR imaging diagnostic features. Radiographics. 2007;27(4):1087–108.
Saraga-Babic M, Bazina M, Vukojevic K, Bocina I, Stefanovic V. Involvement of pro-apoptotic and anti-apoptotic factors in the early development of the human pituitary gland. Histol Histopathol. 2008;23(10):1259–68.
Schlechte JA. Clinical practice. Prolactinoma. N Engl J Med. 2003;349 (21):2035–41.
Schneider HJ, Aimaretti G, Kreitschmann-Andermahr I, Stalla GK, Ghigo E. Hypopituitarism. Lancet. 2007;369(9571):1461–70.
Schulze F, Buhler K, Neubauer A, Kanitsar A, Holton L, Wolfsberger S. Intra-operative virtual endoscopy for image guided endonasal transsphenoidal pituitary surgery. Int J Comput Assist Radiol Surg. 2010;5(2):143–54.
Semple PL, Jane JA, Lopes MB, Laws ER. Pituitary apoplexy: correlation between magnetic resonance imaging and histopathological results. J Neurosurg. 2008;108(5):909–15.
Sharp RJ. Land of the giants. Growth Horm IGF Res. 2009;19(4):291–3.
Sheehan HL. Post-partum necrosis of the anterior pituitary. J Path Bact. 1937;45:189–214.
Sherlock M, Aragon Alonso A, Reulen RC, Ayuk J, Clayton RN, Holder G, et al. Monitoring disease activity using GH and IGF-I in the follow-up of 501 patients with acromegaly. Clin Endocrinol (Oxf). 2009;71(1):74–81.
Shi XE, Wu B, Fan T, Zhou ZQ, Zhang YL. Craniopharyngioma: surgical experience of 309 cases in China. Clin Neurol Neurosurg. 2008;110(2):151–9.
Shou XF, Wang YF, Li SQ, Wu JS, Zhao Y, Mao Y, et al. Microsurgical treatment for typical pituitary apoplexy with 44 patients, according to two pathological stages. Minim Invasive Neurosurg. 2009;52 (5–6):207–11.
Sinha S, Sharma BS. Giant pituitary adenomas—an enigma revisited. Microsurgical treatment strategies and outcome in a series of 250 patients. Br J Neurosurg. 2010;24(1):31–9.
Sklar CA, Antal Z, Chemaitilly W, Cohen LE, Follin C, Meacham LR, Murad MH. Hypothalamic-pituitary and growth disorders in survivors of childhood cancer: an Endocrine Society clinical practice guideline. J Clin Endocrinol Metab. 2018;103(8):2761–84.
Smith ER, Loeffler J, Misra M, Pomerantz SR, Stemmer-Rachamimov A, Post MD. Case records of the Massachusetts General Hospital. Case 37–2008. A 17-year-old boy with a pituitary tumor and skull abnormalities. N Engl J Med. 2008;359(22):2367–77.
Spisek R, Kolouchova E, Jensovsky J, Rusina R, Fendrych P, Plas J, et al. Combined CNS and pituitary involvement as a primary manifestation of Wegener granulomatosis. Clin Rheumatol. 2006; 25(5):739–42.
Tashiro T, Sano T, Xu B, Wakatsuki S, Kagawa N, Nishioka H, et al. Spectrum of different types of hypophysitis: a clinicopathologic study of hypophysitis in 31 cases. Endocr Pathol. 2002;13(3):183–95.
Tomkins M, Lawless S, Martin-Grace J, Sherlock M, Thompson CJ. Diagnosis and management of central diabetes insipidus in adults. J Clin Endocrinol Metab. 2022;107(10):2701–15.
Trainer PJ, Drake WM, Katznelson L, Freda PU, Herman-Bonert V, van der Lely AJ, et al. Treatment of acromegaly with the growth hormone-receptor antagonist pegvisomant. N Engl J Med. 2000; 342(16):1171–7.
Trainer PJ, Ezzat S, D'Souza GA, Layton G, Strasburger CJ. A randomized, controlled, multicentre trial comparing pegvisomant alone with combination therapy of pegvisomant and long-acting octreotide in patients with acromegaly. Clin Endocrinol (Oxf). 2009; 71(4):549–57.
Tritos NA, Fazeli PK, McCormack A, Mallea-Gil SM, Pineyro MM, Christ-Crain M, et al. Pituitary Society Delphi Survey: an international perspective on endocrine management of patients undergoing

transsphenoidal surgery for pituitary adenomas. Pituitary. 2021; 20:1-10.
Trivellin G, Daly AF, Faucz FR, Yuan B, Rostomyan L, Larco DO, et al. Gigantism and acromegaly due to Xq26 microduplications and GPR101 mutation. N Engl J Med. 2014;371(25):2363–74.
Turton JP, Reynaud R, Mehta A, Torpiano J, Saveanu A, Woods KS, et al. Novel mutations within the POU1F1 gene associated with variable combined pituitary hormone deficiency. J Clin Endocrinol Metab. 2005;90(8):4762–70.
Ueda T, Yokoyama Y, Irahara M, Aono T. Influence of psychological stress on suckling-induced pulsatile oxytocin release. Obstet Gynecol. 1994;84(2):259–62.
Unlu E, Puyan FO, Bilgi S, Kemal Hamamcioglu M. Granulomatous hypophysitis: presentation and MRI appearance. J Clin Neurosci. 2006;13(10):1062–6.
Vaidya A, Morris CA, Ross JJ. Interactive medical case. Stalking the diagnosis. N Engl J Med. 2010;362(6):e16.
Valassi E, Biller BM, Swearingen B, Pecori Giraldi F, Losa M, Mortini P, et al. Delayed remission after transsphenoidal surgery in patients with Cushing's disease. J Clin Endocrinol Metab. 2010;95(2):601–10.
Valassi E, Klibanski A, Biller BM. Clinical Review: potential cardiac valve effects of dopamine agonists in hyperprolactinemia. J Clin Endocrinol Metab. 2010;95(3):1025–33.
van Aken MO, Lamberts SW. Diagnosis and treatment of hypopituitarism: an update. Pituitary. 2005;8(3–4):183–91.
Van Gompel JJ, Atkinson JLD, Choby G, Kasperbauer JL, Stokken JK, Janus JR, et al. Pituitary tumor surgery: comparison of endoscopic and microscopic techniques at a single center. Mayo Clin Proc. 2021;96(8):2043–57.
Vandervliet EJ, Vanhoenacker FM, De Praeter G, Vangeneugden J, Parizel PM. Symptomatic Rathke's cleft cyst. JBR-BTR. 2009;92(3): 180–1.
Varan A, Cila A, Akyuz C, Kale G, Kutluk T, Buyukpamukcu M. Radiological evaluation of patients with pituitary Langerhans cell histiocytosis at diagnosis and at follow-up. Pediatr Hematol Oncol. 2008;25(6):567–74.
Vassallo R, Ryu JH, Schroeder DR, Decker PA, Limper AH. Clinical outcomes of pulmonary Langerhans'-cell histiocytosis in adults. N Engl J Med. 2002;346(7):484–90.
Vella A, Young WF Jr. Pituitary apoplexy. Endocrinologist. 2001;11: 282–8.
Verbalis JG, Goldsmith SR, Greenberg A, Schrier RW, Sterns RH. Hyponatremia treatment guidelines 2007: expert panel recommendations. Am J Med. 2007;120(11 Suppl 1):S1–21.
Vieira TC, Boldarine VT, Abucham J. Molecular analysis of PROP1, PIT1, HESX1, LHX3, and LHX4 shows high frequency of PROP1 mutations in patients with familial forms of combined pituitary hormone deficiency. Arq Bras Endocrinol Metabol. 2007;51(7): 1097–103.
Vinchon M, Weill J, Delestret I, Dhellemmes P. Craniopharyngioma and hypothalamic obesity in children. Childs Nerv Syst. 2009; 25(3):347–52.
Viswanathan V, Eugster EA. Etiology and treatment of hypogonadism in adolescents. Endocrinol Metab Clin North Am. 2009;38(4):719–38.
von Stebut E, Schadmand-Fischer S, Brauninger W, Kreft A, Doberauer C, Steinbrink K. Successful treatment of adult multisystemic Langerhans cell histiocytosis with psoralen-UV-A, prednisolone, mercaptopurine, and vinblastine. Arch Dermatol. 2008;144(5):649–53.
Watt A, Pobereskin L, Vaidya B. Pituitary apoplexy within a macroprolactinoma. Nat Clin Pract Endocrinol Metab. 2008;4(11):635–41.
Weiss G, Skurnick JH, Goldsmith LT, Santoro NF, Park SJ. Menopause and hypothalamic-pituitary sensitivity to estrogen. JAMA. 2004; 292(24):2991–6.
Windebank K, Nanduri V. Langerhans cell histiocytosis. Arch Dis Child. 2009;94(11):904–8.
Yong TY, Li JY, Amato L, Mahadevan K, Phillips PJ, Coates PS, et al. Pituitary involvement in Wegener's granulomatosis. Pituitary. 2008; 11(1):77–84.
Young WF Jr, Ospina LF, Wesolowski D, Touma A. The primary empty sella syndrome. Diagnosis with metrizamide cisternography. JAMA. 1981;246(22):2611–2.
Zada G, Ditty B, McNatt SA, McComb JG, Krieger MD. Surgical treatment of Rathke cleft cysts in children. Neurosurgery. 2009;64(6):1132–1137; author reply 1037–138.
Zygmunt-Gorska A, Starzyk J, Adamek D, Radwanska E, Sucharski P, Herman-Sucharska I, et al. Pituitary enlargement in patients with PROP1 gene inactivating mutation represents cystic hyperplasia of the intermediate pituitary lobe. Histopathology and over 10 years follow-up of two patients. J Pediatr Endocrinol Metab. 2009; 22(7):653–60.

Section 2 Thyroid

Asari R, Koperek O, Scheuba C, Riss P, Kaserer K, Hoffmann M, et al. Follicular thyroid carcinoma in an iodine-replete endemic goiter region: a prospectively collected, retrospectively analyzed clinical trial. Ann Surg. 2009;249(6):1023–31.
Balentine CJ, Vanness DJ, Schneider DF. Cost-effectiveness of lobectomy versus genetic testing (Afirma) for indeterminate thyroid nodules: considering the costs of surveillance. Surgery. 2018; 163(1):88–96.
Ball DW. Selectively targeting mutant BRAF in thyroid cancer. J Clin Endocrinol Metab. 2010;95(1):60–1.
Bartalena L, Baldeschi L, Boboridis K, Eckstein A, Kahaly GJ, Marcocci C, et al. The 2016 European Thyroid Association/ European Group on Graves' orbitopathy guidelines for the management of Graves' orbitopathy. Eur Thyroid J. 2016;5(1): 9–26.
Bartalena L, Tanda ML. Clinical practice. Graves' ophthalmopathy. N Engl J Med. 2009;360(10):994–1001.
Biondi B, Cooper DS. Subclinical hyperthyroidism. N Engl J Med. 2018;378(25):2411–19.
Boelaert K, Newby PR, Simmonds MJ, Holder RL, Carr-Smith JD, Heward JM, et al. Prevalence and relative risk of other autoimmune diseases in subjects with autoimmune thyroid disease. Am J Med. 2010;123(2):183 e181–189.
Bradly DP, Reddy V, Prinz RA, Gattuso P. Incidental papillary carcinoma in patients treated surgically for benign thyroid diseases. Surgery. 2009;146(6):1099–104.
Brent GA. Clinical practice. Graves' disease. N Engl J Med. 2008; 358(24):2594–605.
Burch HB. Drug effects on the thyroid. N Engl J Med. 2019;381(8): 749–761.
Chen AX, Leung AM, Korevaar TIM. Thyroid function and conception. N Engl J Med. 2019;381(2):178–81.
Chen H, Nicol TL, Udelsman R. Clinically significant, isolated metastatic disease to the thyroid gland. World J Surg. 1999; 23(2):177–80; discussion 181.
Cheung K, Roman SA, Wang TS, Walker HD, Sosa JA. Calcitonin measurement in the evaluation of thyroid nodules in the United States: a cost-effectiveness and decision analysis. J Clin Endocrinol Metab. 2008;93(6):2173–80.
Chintakuntlawar AV, Rumilla KM, Smith CY, Jenkins SM, Foote RL, Kasperbauer JL, et al. Expression of PD-1 and PD-L1 in anaplastic thyroid cancer patients treated with multimodal therapy: results from a retrospective study. J Clin Endocrinol Metab. 2017 Jun 1;102(6):1943–50.
Cibas ES, Ali SZ. The 2017 Bethesda system for reporting thyroid cytopathology. Thyroid. 2017;27:1341–46.
Cichon S, Anielski R, Konturek A, Barczynski M, Cichon W. Metastases to the thyroid gland: seventeen cases operated on in a single clinical center. Langenbecks Arch Surg. 2006;391(6):581–7.
Corbetta C, Weber G, Cortinovis F, Calebiro D, Passoni A, Vigone MC, et al. A 7-year experience with low blood TSH cutoff levels for neonatal screening reveals an unsuspected frequency of congenital hypothyroidism (CH). Clin Endocrinol (Oxf). 2009;71(5):739–45.
Davies L, Welch HG. Increasing incidence of thyroid cancer in the United States, 1973–2002. JAMA. 2006;295(18):2164–7.
De Groot L, Abalovich M, Alexander EK, Amino N, Barbour L, Cobin RH, et al. Management of thyroid dysfunction during pregnancy and postpartum: an Endocrine Society clinical practice guideline. J Clin Endocrinol Metab. 2012;97(8):2543–65.
De Leo S, Pearce EN. Autoimmune thyroid disease during pregnancy. Lancet Diabetes Endocrinol. 2018;6(7):575–86.
Dierks C, Seufert J, Aumann K, Ruf J, Klein C, Kiefer S, et al. Combination of lenvatinib and pembrolizumab is an effective treatment option for anaplastic and poorly differentiated thyroid carcinoma. Thyroid. 2021;31(7):1076–85.
Diez JJ. Goiter in adult patients aged 55 years and older: etiology and clinical features in 634 patients. J Gerontol A Biol Sci Med Sci. 2005;60(7):920–3.
Douglas RS, Kahaly GJ, Patel A, Sile S, Thompson EHZ, Perdok R, et al. Teprotumumab for the treatment of active thyroid eye disease. N Engl J Med. 2020;382(4):341–52.
Duggan MA, Di Francesco L, Alakija P, Falk V. A pathologic re-review of follicular thyroid neoplasms: the impact of changing the threshold for the diagnosis of the follicular variant of papillary thyroid carcinoma. Surgery. 2009;145(6):687–8; author reply 688–689.
Etit D, Faquin WC, Gaz R, Randolph G, DeLellis RA, Pilch BZ. Histopathologic and clinical features of medullary microcarcinoma and C-cell hyperplasia in prophylactic thyroidectomies for medullary carcinoma: a study of 42 cases. Arch Pathol Lab Med. 2008; 132(11):1767–73.
Fatourechi V, Aniszewski JP, Fatourechi GZ, Atkinson EJ, Jacobsen SJ. Clinical features and outcome of subacute thyroiditis in an incidence cohort: Olmsted County, Minnesota, study. J Clin Endocrinol Metab. 2003;88(5):2100–5.
Few J, Thompson NW, Angelos P, Simeone D, Giordano T, Reeve T. Riedel's thyroiditis: treatment with tamoxifen. Surgery. 1996; 120(6):993–8; discussion 998–999.
Genere N, El Kawkgi OM, Giblon RE, Vaccarella S, Morris JC, Hay ID, Brito JP. Incidence of clinically relevant thyroid cancers remains stable for almost a century: a population-based study. Mayo Clin Proc. 2021;96(11):2823–30.
Ghossein R. Problems and controversies in the histopathology of thyroid carcinomas of follicular cell origin. Arch Pathol Lab Med. 2009;133(5):683–91.
Giles Senyurek Y, Tunca F, Boztepe H, Alagol F, Terzioglu T, Tezelman S. The long term outcome of papillary thyroid carcinoma patients without primary central lymph node dissection: expected improvement of routine dissection. Surgery. 2009;146(6):1188–95.
Gopalakrishnan S, Chugh PK, Chhillar M, Ambardar VK, Sahoo M, Sankar R. Goitrous autoimmune thyroiditis in a pediatric population: a longitudinal study. Pediatrics. 2008;122(3):e670–74.
Grani G, Sponziello M, Pecce V, Ramundo V, Durante C. Contemporary thyroid nodule evaluation and management. J Clin Endocrinol Metab. 2020;105(9):2869–83.
Gulcelik NE, Gulcelik MA, Kuru B. Risk of malignancy in patients with follicular neoplasm: predictive value of clinical and ultrasonographic features. Arch Otolaryngol Head Neck Surg. 2008;134(12):1312–15.
Hanief MR, Igali L, Grama D. Hurthle cell carcinoma: diagnostic and therapeutic implications. World J Surg Oncol. 2004;2:27.
Haugen BR, Kane MA. Approach to the thyroid cancer patient with extracervical metastases. J Clin Endocrinol Metab. 2010;95(3): 987–93.
Haugen BR, Nawaz S, Cohn A, Shroyer K, Bunn PA Jr, Liechty DR, et al. Secondary malignancy of the thyroid gland: a case report and review of the literature. Thyroid. 1994;4(3):297–300.
Hay ID, Hutchinson ME, Gonzalez-Losada T, McIver B, Reinalda ME, Grant CS, et al. Papillary thyroid microcarcinoma: a study of 900 cases observed in a 60-year period. Surgery. 2008;144(6):980–7; discussion 987–988.
Hegedus L. Clinical practice. The thyroid nodule. N Engl J Med. 2004; 351(17):1764–71.
Iraci GS, Fux-Otta C. Images in clinical medicine. Graves' hyperthyroidism. N Engl J Med. 2009;360(24):e31.
Iyer PC, Dadu R, Ferrarotto R, Busaidy NL, Habra MA, Zafereo M, et al. Real-world experience with targeted therapy for the treatment of anaplastic thyroid carcinoma. Thyroid. 2018;28(1):79–87.
Kebebew E, Greenspan FS, Clark OH, Woeber KA, McMillan A. Anaplastic thyroid carcinoma. Treatment outcome and prognostic factors. Cancer. 2005;103(7):1330–5.
Klubo-Gwiezdzinska J, Wartofsky L. Thyrotropin blood levels, subclinical hypothyroidism, and the elderly patient. Arch Intern Med. 2009;169(21):1949–51.
Kushchayeva Y, Duh QY, Kebebew E, Clark OH. Prognostic indications for Hurthle cell cancer. World J Surg. 2004;28(12):1266–70.
Lam KY, Lo CY. Metastatic tumors of the thyroid gland: a study of 79 cases in Chinese patients. Arch Pathol Lab Med. 1998;122(1):37–41.
Leboulleux S, Schroeder PR, Busaidy NL, Auperin A, Corone C, Jacene HA, et al. Assessment of the incremental value of recombinant thyrotropin stimulation before 2-[18F]-Fluoro-2-deoxy-D-glucose positron emission tomography/computed tomography imaging to localize residual differentiated thyroid cancer. J Clin Endocrinol Metab. 2009;94(4):1310–16.
Lloyd RV, Douglas BR, Young WF Jr. Parathyroid gland. In: King DW, editor. Atlas of Nontumor Pathology: Endocrine Diseases. American Registry of Pathology and the Armed Forces Institute of Pathology; 2002.
McDermott MT. In the clinic. Hypothyroidism. Ann Intern Med. 2009;151(11):ITC61.
McLachlan SM, Nagayama Y, Pichurin PN, Mizutori Y, Chen CR, Misharin A, et al. The link between Graves' disease and Hashimoto's thyroiditis: a role for regulatory T cells. Endocrinology. 2007; 148(12):5724–33.
Menon MP, Khan A. Micro-RNAs in thyroid neoplasms: molecular, diagnostic and therapeutic implications. J Clin Pathol. 2009; 62(11):978–85.
Michels AW, Eisenbarth GS. Immunologic endocrine disorders. J Allergy Clin Immunol. 2010;125(2 Suppl 2):S226–237.
Moo-Young TA, Traugott AL, Moley JF. Sporadic and familial medullary thyroid carcinoma: state of the art. Surg Clin North Am. 2009;89(5):1193–204.
Morris JC. How do you approach the problem of TSH elevation in a patient on high-dose thyroid hormone replacement? Clin Endocrinol (Oxf). 2009;70(5):671–3.
Moshynska OV, Saxena A. Clonal relationship between Hashimoto thyroiditis and thyroid lymphoma. J Clin Pathol. 2008;61(4):438–44.
Nakhjavani MK, Gharib H, Goellner Jr, van Heerden JA. Metastasis to the thyroid gland. A report of 43 cases. Cancer. 1997;79(3):574–8.
Nyirenda MJ, Taylor PN, Stoddart M, Beckett GJ, Toft AD. Thyroid-stimulating hormone-receptor antibody and thyroid hormone concentrations in smokers vs nonsmokers with Graves disease treated with carbimazole. JAMA. 2009;301(2):162–4.
Okosieme OE, Chan D, Price SA, Lazarus JH, Premawardhana LD. The utility of radioiodine uptake and thyroid scintigraphy in the diagnosis and management of hyperthyroidism. Clin Endocrinol (Oxf). 2010;72(1):122–7.
O'Neill JP, O'Neill B, Condron C, Walsh M, Bouchier-Hayes D. Anaplastic (undifferentiated) thyroid cancer: improved insight and therapeutic strategy into a highly aggressive disease. J Laryngol Otol. 2005;119(8):585–91.
Pacifico F, Crescenzi E, Mellone S, Iannetti A, Porrino N, Liguoro D, et al. Nuclear factor-{kappa}B contributes to anaplastic thyroid carcinomas through up-regulation of miR-146a. J Clin Endocrinol Metab. 2010;95(3):1421–30.
Pan D, Shin YH, Gopalakrishnan G, Hennessey J, De Groot LJ. Regulatory T cells in Graves' disease. Clin Endocrinol (Oxf). 2009;71(4):587–93.
Papi G, LiVolsi VA. Current concepts on Riedel thyroiditis. Am J Clin Pathol. 2004;121(Suppl):S50–63.

Peter F, Muzsnai A. Congenital disorders of the thyroid: hypo/hyper. Endocrinol Metab Clin North Am. 2009;38(3):491–507.

Pharoah PO. Thyroid hormones and embryogenesis. J Pediatr. 2009; 155(3):455–6; author reply 456–457.

Raef H, Al-Rijjal R, Al-Shehri S, Zou M, Al-Mana H, Baitei EY, et al. Biallelic p.R2223H mutation in the thyroglobulin gene causes thyroglobulin retention and severe hypothyroidism with subsequent development of thyroid carcinoma. J Clin Endocrinol Metab. 2010;95(3):1000–6.

Raymond J, LaFranchi SH. Fetal and neonatal thyroid function: review and summary of significant new findings. Curr Opin Endocrinol Diabetes Obes. 2010;17(1):1–7.

Razvi S, Weaver JU, Vanderpump MP, Pearce SH. The incidence of ischemic heart disease and mortality in people with subclinical hypothyroidism: reanalysis of the Whickham Survey cohort. J Clin Endocrinol Metab. 2010;95(4):1734–40.

Rivkees SA, Mattison DR. Ending propylthiouracil-induced liver failure in children. N Engl J Med. 2009;360(15):1574–5.

Roelfsema F, Pereira AM, Adriaanse R, Endert E, Fliers E, Romijn JA, et al. Thyrotropin secretion in mild and severe primary hypothyroidism is distinguished by amplified burst mass and Basal secretion with increased spikiness and approximate entropy. J Clin Endocrinol Metab. 2010;95(2):928–34.

Roman S, Lin R, Sosa JA. Prognosis of medullary thyroid carcinoma: demographic, clinical, and pathologic predictors of survival in 1252 cases. Cancer. 2006;107(9):2134–42.

Ross DS, Burch HB, Cooper DS, Greenlee MC, Laurberg P, Maia AL, et al. 2016 American Thyroid Association guidelines for diagnosis and management of hyperthyroidism and other causes of thyrotoxicosis. Thyroid. 2016;26(10):1343–21.

Shakoor SK, Aldibbiat A, Ingoe LE, Campbell SC, Sibal L, Shaw J, et al. Endothelial progenitor cells in subclinical hypothyroidism: the effect of thyroid hormone replacement therapy. J Clin Endocrinol Metab. 2010;95(1):319–22.

Sillery JC, Reading CC, Charboneau JW, Henrichsen TL, Hay ID, Mandrekar JN. Thyroid follicular carcinoma: sonographic features of 50 cases. AJR Am J Roentgenol. 2010;194(1):44–54.

Simonsick EM, Newman AB, Ferrucci L, Satterfield S, Harris TB, Rodondi N, et al. Subclinical hypothyroidism and functional mobility in older adults. Arch Intern Med. 2009;169(21):2011–17.

Smith T, Kaufman CS. Ultrasound guided thyroid biopsy. Tech Vasc Interv Radiol. 2021;24(3):100768.

Smith TJ, Hegedüs L. Graves' disease. N Engl J Med. 2016;375(16): 1552–1565.

Song Y, Ruf J, Lothaire P, Dequanter D, Andry G, Willemse E, et al. Association of duoxes with thyroid peroxidase and its regulation in thyrocytes. J Clin Endocrinol Metab. 2010;95(1):375–82.

Stan MN, Sonawane V, Sebo TJ, Thapa P, Bahn RS. Riedel's thyroiditis association with IgG4-related disease. Clin Endocrinol (Oxf). 2017;86(3):425–30.

Stiebel-Kalish H, Robenshtok E, Hasanreisoglu M, Ezrachi D, Shimon I, Leibovici L. Treatment modalities for Graves' ophthalmopathy: systematic review and metaanalysis. J Clin Endocrinol Metab. 2009;94(8):2708–16.

Stoupa A, Kariyawasam D, Nguyen Quoc A, Polak M, Carré A. Approach to the patient with congenital hypothyroidism. J Clin Endocrinol Metab. 2022;107(12):3418–27.

Stucchi CM, Vaccaro V, Magherini A, Di Gregorio C, Greco G, Livolsi VA, et al. Hurthle cell follicular carcinoma of the thyroid gland presenting with diffuse meningeal carcinomatosis and evolving to anaplastic carcinoma. J Clin Pathol. 2007;60(7):831–2.

Suliburk J, Delbridge L. Surgical management of well-differentiated thyroid cancer: state of the art. Surg Clin North Am. 2009; 89(5):1171–91.

Surks MI, Boucai L. Age- and race-based serum thyrotropin reference limits. J Clin Endocrinol Metab. 2010;95(2):496–502.

Taylor PN, Zhang L, Lee RWJ, Muller I, Ezra DG, Dayan CM, et al. New insights into the pathogenesis and nonsurgical management of Graves orbitopathy. Nat Rev Endocrinol. 2020;16(2):104–16.

Tessler FN, Middleton WD, Grant EG, et al. ACR Thyroid Imaging, Reporting and Data System (TI-RADS): white paper of the ACR TI-RADS Committee. J. Am. Coll. Radiol. 2017;14:587–95.

Toft A. Bioequivalence of generic preparations of levothyroxine. Clin Endocrinol (Oxf). 2009;71(4):603; author reply 603–4.

Toft AD. Clinical practice. Subclinical hyperthyroidism. N Engl J Med. 2001;345(7):512–16.

Wang JR, Zafereo ME, Dadu R, Ferrarotto R, Busaidy NL, Lu C, et al. Complete surgical resection following neoadjuvant dabrafenib plus trametinib in BRAFV600E-Mutated Anaplastic Thyroid Carcinoma. Thyroid. 2019;29(8):1036–43.

Wang Y, Tsang R, Asa S, Dickson B, Arenovich T, Brierley J. Clinical outcome of anaplastic thyroid carcinoma treated with radiotherapy of once- and twice-daily fractionation regimens. Cancer. 2006; 107(8):1786–92.

Wolpin BM, Weller PF, Katz JT, Levy BD, Loscalzo J. Clinical problem-solving. The writing on the wall. N Engl J Med. 2009;361(14):1387–92.

Yu Y, Liu J, Yu N, Zhang Y, Zhang S, Li T, Gao Y, et al. IgG4 immunohistochemistry in Riedel's thyroiditis and the recommended criteria for diagnosis: a case series and literature review. Clin Endocrinol (Oxf). 2021;94(5):851–57.

Section 3 Adrenal

Amar L, Pacak K, Steichen O, Akker SA, Aylwin SJB, Baudin E, et al. International consensus on initial screening and follow-up of asymptomatic SDHx mutation carriers. Nat Rev Endocrinol. 2021;17(7):435–44.

Arlt W. The approach to the adult with newly diagnosed adrenal insufficiency. J Clin Endocrinol Metab. 2009;94(4):1059–67.

Armengaud JB, Charkaluk ML, Trivin C, Tardy V, Breart G, Brauner R, et al. Precocious pubarche: distinguishing late-onset congenital adrenal hyperplasia from premature adrenarche. J Clin Endocrinol Metab. 2009;94(8):2835–40.

Assié G, Libé R, Espiard S, Rizk-Rabin M, Guimier A, Luscap W, et al. ARMC5 mutations in macronodular adrenal hyperplasia with Cushing's syndrome. N Engl J Med. 2013;369(22):2105–14.

Baid SK, Lai EW, Wesley RA, Ling A, Timmers HJ, Adams KT, et al. Brief communication: radiographic contrast infusion and catecholamine release in patients with pheochromocytoma. Ann Intern Med. 2009;150(1):27–32.

Baid SK, Rubino D, Sinaii N, Ramsey S, Frank A, Nieman LK. Specificity of screening tests for Cushing's syndrome in an overweight and obese population. J Clin Endocrinol Metab. 2009;94(10):3857–64.

Bancos I, Atkinson E, Eng C, Young WF Jr, Neumann HPH; International Pheochromocytoma and Pregnancy Study Group. Maternal and fetal outcomes in phaeochromocytoma and pregnancy: a multicentre retrospective cohort study and systematic review of literature. Lancet Diabetes Endocrinol. 2021;9(1):13–21.

Bens S, Mohn A, Yuksel B, Kulle AE, Michalek M, Chiarelli F, et al. Congenital lipoid adrenal hyperplasia: functional characterization of three novel mutations in the STAR gene. J Clin Endocrinol Metab. 2010;95(3):1301–8.

Bergthorsdottir R, Leonsson-Zachrisson M, Oden A, Johannsson G. Premature mortality in patients with Addison's disease: a population-based study. J Clin Endocrinol Metab. 2006;91(12):4849–53.

Bertherat J, Horvath A, Groussin L, Grabar S, Boikos S, Cazabat L, et al. Mutations in regulatory subunit type 1A of cyclic adenosine 5′-monophosphate-dependent protein kinase (PRKAR1A): phenotype analysis in 353 patients and 80 different genotypes. J Clin Endocrinol Metab. 2009;94(6):2085–91.

Bessell-Browne R, O'Malley ME. CT of pheochromocytoma and paraganglioma: risk of adverse events with i.v. administration of nonionic contrast material. AJR Am J Roentgenol. 2007;188(4):970–4.

Bidet M, Bellanne-Chantelot C, Galand-Portier MB, Golmard JL, Tardy V, Morel Y, et al. Fertility in women with nonclassical congenital adrenal hyperplasia due to 21-hydroxylase deficiency. J Clin Endocrinol Metab. 2010;95(3):1182–90.

Bidet M, Bellanne-Chantelot C, Galand-Portier MB, Tardy V, Billaud L, Laborde K, et al. Clinical and molecular characterization of a cohort of 161 unrelated women with nonclassical congenital adrenal hyperplasia due to 21-hydroxylase deficiency and 330 family members. J Clin Endocrinol Metab. 2009;94(5):1570–8.

Biller BM, Grossman AB, Stewart PM, Melmed S, Bertagna X, Bertherat J, et al. Treatment of adrenocorticotropin-dependent Cushing's syndrome: a consensus statement. J Clin Endocrinol Metab. 2008;93(7):2454–62.

Bonfig W, Pozza SB, Schmidt H, Pagel P, Knorr D, Schwarz HP. Hydrocortisone dosing during puberty in patients with classical congenital adrenal hyperplasia: an evidence-based recommendation. J Clin Endocrinol Metab. 2009;94(10):3882–8.

Born-Frontsberg E, Reincke M, Rump LC, Hahner S, Diederich S, Lorenz R, et al. Cardiovascular and cerebrovascular comorbidities of hypokalemic and normokalemic primary aldosteronism: results of the German Conn's Registry. J Clin Endocrinol Metab. 2009;94(4):1125–30.

Bornstein SR. Predisposing factors for adrenal insufficiency. N Engl J Med. 2009;360(22):2328–39.

Boscaro M, Arnaldi G. Approach to the patient with possible Cushing's syndrome. J Clin Endocrinol Metab. 2009;94(9):3121–31.

Bouys L, Chiodini I, Arlt W, Reincke M, Bertherat J. Update on primary bilateral macronodular adrenal hyperplasia (PBMAH). Endocrine. 2021;71(3):595–603.

Braun LT, Vogel F, Zopp S, Marchant Seiter T, Rubinstein G, Berr CM, et al. Whom should we screen for Cushing Syndrome? The Endocrine Society Practice Guideline recommendations 2008 revisited. J Clin Endocrinol Metab. 2022;107(9):e3723–30.

Brown ML, Zayas GE, Abel MD, Young WF Jr, Schaff HV. Mediastinal paragangliomas: the mayo clinic experience. Ann Thorac Surg. 2008;86(3):946–51.

Bruynzeel H, Feelders RA, Groenland TH, van den Meiracker AH, van Eijck CH, Lange JF, et al. Risk factors for hemodynamic instability during surgery for pheochromocytoma. J Clin Endocrinol Metab. 2010;95(2):678–85.

Canu L, Van Hemert JAW, Kerstens MN, Hartman RP, Khanna A, Kraljevic I, et al. CT characteristics of pheochromocytoma: relevance for the evaluation of adrenal incidentaloma. J Clin Endocrinol Metab. 2019;104(2):312–18.

Canzanello VJ, Garovic VD. Renal vascular disease: a vexing challenge for the clinician. Prog Cardiovasc Dis. 2009;52(3):181–3.

Carafone LE, Zhang CD, Li D, Lazik N, Hamidi O, Hurtado MD, et al. Diagnostic accuracy of dehydroepiandrosterone sulfate and

corticotropin in autonomous cortisol secretion. Biomedicines. 2021;9(7):741.

Cardoso EM, Arregger AL, Tumilasci OR, Contreras LN. Diagnostic value of salivary cortisol in Cushing's syndrome (CS). Clin Endocrinol (Oxf). 2009;70(4):516–21.

Carney JA, Gordon H, Carpenter PC, Shenoy BV, Go VL. The complex of myxomas, spotty pigmentation, and endocrine overactivity. Medicine (Baltimore). 1985;64(4):270–83.

Carney JA, Libé R, Bertherat J, Young WF. Primary pigmented nodular adrenocortical disease: the original 4 cases revisited after 30 years for follow-up, new investigations, and molecular genetic findings. Am J Surg Pathol. 2014;38(9):1266–73.

Cavalcante IP, Nishi M, Zerbini MCN, Almeida MQ, Brondani VB, Botelho MLAA, Tanno FY, Srougi V, Chambo JL, Mendonca BB, Bertherat J, Lotfi CFP, Fragoso MCBV et al. The role of ARMC5 in human cell cultures from nodules of primary macronodular adrenocortical hyperplasia (PMAH). Mol Cell Endocrinol. 2018;460: 36–46.

Chevalier B, Vantyghem MC, Espiard S. Bilateral adrenal hyperplasia: pathogenesis and treatment. Biomedicines. 2021;9(10):1397.

Chow JT, Thompson GB, Grant CS, Farley DR, Richards ML, Young WF Jr. Bilateral laparoscopic adrenalectomy for corticotrophin-dependent Cushing's syndrome: a review of the Mayo Clinic experience. Clin Endocrinol (Oxf). 2008;68(4):513–19.

Chrysochou C, Kalra PA. Epidemiology and natural history of atherosclerotic renovascular disease. Prog Cardiovasc Dis. 2009;52(3): 184–95.

Claahsen-van der Grinten HL, Speiser PW, Ahmed SF, Arlt W, Auchus RJ, Falhammar H, et al. Congenital adrenal hyperplasia-current insights in pathophysiology, diagnostics, and management. Endocr Rev. 2022;43(1):91–159.

Cooper MS, Stewart PM. 11Beta-hydroxysteroid dehydrogenase type 1 and its role in the hypothalamus-pituitary-adrenal axis, metabolic syndrome, and inflammation. J Clin Endocrinol Metab. 2009; 94(12):4645–54.

Covic A, Gusbeth-Tatomir P. The role of the renin-angiotensin-aldosterone system in renal artery stenosis, renovascular hypertension, and ischemic nephropathy: diagnostic implications. Prog Cardiovasc Dis. 2009;52(3):204–8.

Daunt N. Adrenal vein sampling: how to make it quick, easy, and successful. Radiographics. 2005;25(Suppl 1):S143–58.

Donadille B, Groussin L, Waintrop C, Abbas H, Tenenbaum F, Dugue MA, et al. Management of Cushing's syndrome due to ectopic adrenocorticotropin secretion with 1,ortho-1, para′-dichloro-diphenyl-dichloro-ethane: findings in 23 patients from a single center. J Clin Endocrinol Metab. 2010;95(2):537–44.

Douma S, Petidis K, Doumas M, Papaefthimiou P, Triantafyllou A, Kartali N, et al. Prevalence of primary hyperaldosteronism in resistant hypertension: a retrospective observational study. Lancet. 2008;371(9628):1921–6.

Ebbehoj A, Li D, Kaur RJ, Zhang C, Singh S, Li T, Atkinson E, et al. Epidemiology of adrenal tumours in Olmsted County, Minnesota, USA: a population-based cohort study. Lancet Diabetes Endocrinol. 2020;8(11):894–902.

Eisenhofer G, Bornstein SR, Brouwers FM, Cheung NK, Dahia PL, de Krijger RR, et al. Malignant pheochromocytoma: current status and initiatives for future progress. Endocr Relat Cancer. 2004; 11(3):423–36.

Elfstrom P, Montgomery SM, Kampe O, Ekbom A, Ludvigsson JF. Risk of primary adrenal insufficiency in patients with celiac disease. J Clin Endocrinol Metab. 2007;92(9):3595–8.

Elliott DD, Pitman MB, Bloom L, Faquin WC. Fine-needle aspiration biopsy of Hurthle cell lesions of the thyroid gland: a cytomorphologic study of 139 cases with statistical analysis. Cancer. 2006; 108(2):102–9.

Erichsen MM, Lovas K, Skinningsrud B, Wolff AB, Undlien DE, Svartberg J, et al. Clinical, immunological, and genetic features of autoimmune primary adrenal insufficiency: observations from a Norwegian registry. J Clin Endocrinol Metab. 2009;94(12):4882–90.

Erickson D, Huston J, 3rd Young WF Jr, Carpenter PC, Wermers RA, Bonelli FS, et al. Internal jugular vein sampling in adrenocorticotropic hormone-dependent Cushing's syndrome: a comparison with inferior petrosal sinus sampling. Clin Endocrinol (Oxf). 2004;60(4):413–19.

Erlic Z, Neumann HP. When should genetic testing be obtained in a patient with phaeochromocytoma or paraganglioma? Clin Endocrinol (Oxf). 2009;70(3):354–7.

Freel EM, Stanson AW, Thompson GB, Grant CS, Farley DR, Richards ML, et al. Adrenal venous sampling for catecholamines: a normal value study. J Clin Endocrinol Metab. 2010;95(3):1328–32.

Frisen L, Nordenstrom A, Falhammar H, Filipsson H, Holmdahl G, Janson PO, et al. Gender role behavior, sexuality, and psychosocial adaptation in women with congenital adrenal hyperplasia due to CYP21A2 deficiency. J Clin Endocrinol Metab. 2009;94(9):3432–9.

Funder JW. Aldosterone and mineralocorticoid receptors in the cardiovascular system. Prog Cardiovasc Dis. 2010;52(5):393–400.

Funder JW, Carey RM, Mantero F, Murad MH, Reincke M, Shibata H, et al. The management of primary aldosteronism: case detection, diagnosis, and treatment: an Endocrine Society clinical practice guideline. J Clin Endocrinol Metab. 2016;101(5):1889–916.

Gaal J, Burnichon N, Korpershoek E, Roncelin I, Bertherat J, Plouin PF, et al. Isocitrate dehydrogenase mutations are rare in pheochromocytomas and paragangliomas. J Clin Endocrinol Metab. 2010;95(3):1274–8.

Ghossein RA, Hiltzik DH, Carlson DL, Patel S, Shaha A, Shah JP, et al. Prognostic factors of recurrence in encapsulated Hurthle cell carcinoma of the thyroid gland: a clinicopathologic study of 50 cases. Cancer. 2006;106(8):1669–76.

Gittens PR Jr, Solish AF, Trabulsi EJ. Surgical management of metastatic disease to the adrenal gland. Semin Oncol. 2008;35(2):172–6.

Gruber LM, Hartman RP, Thompson GB, McKenzie TJ, Lyden ML, Dy BM, et al. Pheochromocytoma characteristics and behavior differ depending on method of discovery. J Clin Endocrinol Metab. 2019;104(5):1386–93.

Guerrero MA, Schreinemakers JM, Vriens MR, Suh I, Hwang J, Shen WT, et al. Clinical spectrum of pheochromocytoma. J Am Coll Surg. 2009;209(6):727–32.

Haigh PI, Urbach DR. The treatment and prognosis of Hurthle cell follicular thyroid carcinoma compared with its non-Hurthle cell counterpart. Surgery. 2005;138(6):1152–7; discussion 1157–8.

Hamidi O, Young WF Jr, Gruber L, Smestad J, Yan Q, Ponce OJ, et al. Outcomes of patients with metastatic phaeochromocytoma and paraganglioma: a systematic review and meta-analysis. Clin Endocrinol (Oxf). 2017;87(5):440–50.

Hamidi O, Young WF Jr, Iñiguez-Ariza NM, Kittah NE, Gruber L, Bancos C, et al. Malignant pheochromocytoma and paraganglioma: 272 patients over 55 years. J Clin Endocrinol Metab. 2017;102(9):3296–05.

Havekes B, King K, Lai EW, Romijn JA, Corssmit EP, Pacak K. New imaging approaches to phaeochromocytomas and paragangliomas. Clin Endocrinol (Oxf). 2010;72:137–45.

Karrer-Voegeli S, Rey F, Reymond MJ, Meuwly JY, Gaillard RC, Gomez F. Androgen dependence of hirsutism, acne, and alopecia in women: retrospective analysis of 228 patients investigated for hyperandrogenism. Medicine (Baltimore). 2009;88(1):32–45.

Kempers MJ, Lenders JW, van Outheusden L, van der Wilt GJ, Schultze Kool LJ, Hermus AR, et al. Systematic review: diagnostic procedures to differentiate unilateral from bilateral adrenal abnormality in primary aldosteronism. Ann Intern Med. 2009;151(5):329–37.

Kim SH, Brennan MF, Russo P, Burt ME, Coit DG. The role of surgery in the treatment of clinically isolated adrenal metastasis. Cancer. 1998;82(2):389–94.

Kong MF, Lawden M, Howlett T. The Addison's disease dilemma—autoimmune or ALD? Lancet. 2008;371(9628):1970.

Kudva YC, Sawka AM, Young WF Jr. Clinical review 164: the laboratory diagnosis of adrenal pheochromocytoma: the Mayo Clinic experience. J Clin Endocrinol Metab. 2003;88(10):4533–9.

Lam KY, Lo CY. Metastatic tumours of the adrenal glands: a 30-year experience in a teaching hospital. Clin Endocrinol (Oxf). 2002;56(1):95–101.

Lenders JW, Pacak K, Huynh TT, Sharabi Y, Mannelli M, Bratslavsky G, et al. Low sensitivity of glucagon provocative testing for diagnosis of pheochromocytoma. J Clin Endocrinol Metab. 2010;95(1):238–45.

Lerario AM, Mohan DR, Hammer GD. Update on biology and genomics of adrenocortical carcinomas: rationale for emerging therapies. Endocr Rev. 2022;43(6):1051–73.

Lerman LO, Textor SC, Grande JP. Mechanisms of tissue injury in renal artery stenosis: ischemia and beyond. Prog Cardiovasc Dis. 2009;52(3):196–203.

Li M, Prodanov T, Meuter L, et al. Recurrent disease in patients with sporadic pheochromocytoma and paraganglioma. J Clin Endocrinol Metab. 2023;108(2):397–404.

Lloyd RV, Douglas BR, Young WF Jr. Adrenal gland. In: King DW, editor. Atlas of Nontumor Pathology: Endocrine Diseases. American Registry of Pathology and the Armed Forces Institute of Pathology; 2002.

Lo CY, van Heerden JA, Soreide JA, Grant CS, Thompson GB, Lloyd RV, et al. Adrenalectomy for metastatic disease to the adrenal glands. Br J Surg. 1996;83(4):528–31.

Louiset E, Duparc C, Young J, Renouf S, Tetsi Nomigni M, et al. Intraadrenal corticotropin in bilateral macronodular adrenal hyperplasia. N Engl J Med. 2013;369(22):2115–25.

Louiset E, Stratakis CA, Perraudin V, Griffin KJ, Libe R, Cabrol S, et al. The paradoxical increase in cortisol secretion induced by dexamethasone in primary pigmented nodular adrenocortical disease involves a glucocorticoid receptor-mediated effect of dexamethasone on protein kinase A catalytic subunits. J Clin Endocrinol Metab. 2009;94(7):2406–13.

Lowe KM, Young WF Jr, Lyssikatos C, Stratakis CA, Carney JA. Cushing syndrome in carney complex: clinical, pathologic, and molecular genetic findings in the 17 affected mayo clinic patients. Am J Surg Pathol. 2017;41(2):171–81.

Mandel LR. Endocrine and autoimmune aspects of the health history of John F. Kennedy. Ann Intern Med. 2009;151(5):350–4.

Marik PE, Varon J. Requirement of perioperative stress doses of corticosteroids: a systematic review of the literature. Arch Surg. 2008;143(12):1222–6.

McMahon GT, Blake MA, Wu CL. Case records of the Massachusetts General Hospital. Case 1–2010. A 75-year-old man with hypertension, hyperglycemia, and edema. N Engl J Med. 2010;362(2):156–66.

Melck A, Bugis S, Baliski C, Irvine R, Anderson DW, Wilkins G, et al. Hemithyroidectomy: the preferred initial surgical approach for management of Hurthle cell neoplasm. Am J Surg. 2006;191(5):593–7.

Merke DP. Approach to the adult with congenital adrenal hyperplasia due to 21-hydroxylase deficiency. J Clin Endocrinol Metab. 2008;93(3):653–60.

Metherell LA, Naville D, Halaby G, Begeot M, Huebner A, Nurnberg G, et al. Nonclassic lipoid congenital adrenal hyperplasia masquerading as familial glucocorticoid deficiency. J Clin Endocrinol Metab. 2009;94(10):3865–71.

Miller WL, White PC. History of adrenal research: from ancient anatomy to contemporary molecular biology. Endocr Rev. 2023;44(1):70–116.

Mulatero P, Bertello C, Sukor N, Gordon R, Rossato D, Daunt N, et al. Impact of different diagnostic criteria during adrenal vein sampling on reproducibility of subtype diagnosis in patients with primary aldosteronism. Hypertension. 2010;55(3):667–73.

Mulatero P, Bertello C, Veglio F, Monticone S. Approach to the patient on antihypertensive therapy: screen for primary aldosteronism. J Clin Endocrinol Metab. 2022;107(11):3175–81.

Mulatero P, Stowasser M, Loh KC, Fardella CE, Gordon RD, Mosso L, et al. Increased diagnosis of primary aldosteronism, including surgically correctable forms, in centers from five continents. J Clin Endocrinol Metab. 2004;89(3):1045–50.

Neumann HP, Bausch B, McWhinney SR, Bender BU, Gimm O, Franke G, et al. Germ-line mutations in nonsyndromic pheochromocytoma. N Engl J Med. 2002;346(19):1459–66.

Neumann HPH, Young WF Jr, Eng C. Pheochromocytoma and Paraganglioma. N Engl J Med. 2019;381(6):552–65.

New MI. Extensive clinical experience: nonclassical 21-hydroxylase deficiency. J Clin Endocrinol Metab. 2006;91(11):4205–14.

Nieman LK. Molecular Derangements and the diagnosis of ACTH-dependent Cushing's syndrome. Endocr Rev. 2022;43(5):852–77.

Nieman LK, Biller BM, Findling JW, Newell-Price J, Savage MO, Stewart PM, et al. The diagnosis of Cushing's syndrome: an Endocrine Society clinical practice guideline. J Clin Endocrinol Metab. 2008;93(5):1526–40.

Parajes S, Loidi L, Reisch N, Dhir V, Rose IT, Hampel R, et al. Functional consequences of seven novel mutations in the CYP11B1 gene: four mutations associated with nonclassic and three mutations causing classic 11{beta}-hydroxylase deficiency. J Clin Endocrinol Metab. 2010;95(2):779–88.

Pereira AM, Hes FJ, Horvath A, Woortman S, Greene E, Bimpaki E, et al. Association of the M1V PRKAR1A mutation with primary pigmented nodular adrenocortical disease in two large families. J Clin Endocrinol Metab. 2010;95(1):338–42.

Perry CG, Sawka AM, Singh R, Thabane L, Bajnarek J, Young WF Jr. The diagnostic efficacy of urinary fractionated metanephrines measured by tandem mass spectrometry in detection of pheochromocytoma. Clin Endocrinol (Oxf). 2007;66(5):703–8.

Petri BJ, van Eijck CH, de Herder WW, Wagner A, de Krijger RR. Phaeochromocytomas and sympathetic paragangliomas. Br J Surg. 2009;96(12):1381–92.

Pham TH, Moir C, Thompson GB, Zarroug AE, Hamner CE, Farley D, et al. Pheochromocytoma and paraganglioma in children: a review of medical and surgical management at a tertiary care center. Pediatrics. 2006;118(3):1109–17.

Pitsava G, Zhu C, Sundaram R, Mills JL, Stratakis CA. Predicting the risk of cardiac myxoma in Carney complex. Genet Med. 2021;23(1):80–5.

Porterfield Jr, Thompson GB, Young WF Jr, Chow JT, Fryrear RS, van Heerden JA, et al. Surgery for Cushing's syndrome: an historical review and recent ten-year experience. World J Surg. 2008;32(5):659–77.

Powell AC, Stratakis CA, Patronas NJ, Steinberg SM, Batista D, Alexander HR, et al. Operative management of Cushing syndrome secondary to micronodular adrenal hyperplasia. Surgery. 2008;143(6):750–8.

Raff H. Utility of salivary cortisol measurements in Cushing's syndrome and adrenal insufficiency. J Clin Endocrinol Metab. 2009;94(10):3647–55.

Reincke M, Rump LC, Quinkler M, Hahner S, Diederich S, Lorenz R, et al. Risk factors associated with a low glomerular filtration rate in primary aldosteronism. J Clin Endocrinol Metab. 2009;94(3):869–75.

Rossi GP, Belfiore A, Bernini G, Fabris B, Caridi G, Ferri C, et al. Body mass index predicts plasma aldosterone concentrations in overweight-obese primary hypertensive patients. J Clin Endocrinol Metab. 2008;93(7):2566–71.

Rossi GP, Bernini G, Caliumi C, Desideri G, Fabris B, Ferri C, et al. A prospective study of the prevalence of primary aldosteronism in 1,125 hypertensive patients. J Am Coll Cardiol. 2006;48(11):2293–300.

Savas M, Mehta S, Agrawal N, van Rossum EFC, Feelders RA. Approach to the patient: diagnosis of Cushing syndrome. J Clin Endocrinol Metab. 2022;107(11):3162–74.

Sechi LA, Di Fabio A, Bazzocchi M, Uzzau A, Catena C. Intrarenal hemodynamics in primary aldosteronism before and after treatment. J Clin Endocrinol Metab. 2009;94(4):1191–7.

Sechi LA, Novello M, Lapenna R, Baroselli S, Nadalini E, Colussi GL, et al. Long-term renal outcomes in patients with primary aldosteronism. JAMA. 2006;295(22):2638–45.

Shariq OA, Bancos I, Cronin PA, Farley DR, Richards ML, Thompson GB, et al. Contralateral suppression of aldosterone at adrenal venous sampling predicts hyperkalemia following adrenalectomy for primary aldosteronism. Surgery. 2018;163(1):183–90.

Shulman DI, Palmert MR, Kemp SF. Adrenal insufficiency: still a cause of morbidity and death in childhood. Pediatrics. 2007;119(2):e484–94.

Sjoqvist F, Garle M, Rane A. Use of doping agents, particularly anabolic steroids, in sports and society. Lancet. 2008;371(9627):1872–82.

Speiser PW, Arlt W, Auchus RJ, Baskin LS, Conway GS, Merke DP, et al. Congenital adrenal hyperplasia due to steroid 21-hydroxylase deficiency: an Endocrine Society clinical practice guideline. J Clin Endocrinol Metab. 2018;103(11):4043–88.

Strajina V, Al-Hilli Z, Andrews JC, Bancos I, Thompson GB, Farley DR, et al. Primary aldosteronism: making sense of partial data sets from failed adrenal venous sampling-suppression of adrenal aldosterone production can be used in clinical decision making. Surgery. 2018;163(4):801–06.

Stratakis CA, Kirschner LS, Carney JA. Clinical and molecular features of the Carney complex: diagnostic criteria and recommendations for patient evaluation. J Clin Endocrinol Metab. 2001;86(9):4041–6.

Stratakis CA, Sarlis N, Kirschner LS, Carney JA, Doppman JL, Nieman LK, et al. Paradoxical response to dexamethasone in the diagnosis of primary pigmented nodular adrenocortical disease. Ann Intern Med. 1999;131(8):585–91.

Sukor N, Kogovsek C, Gordon RD, Robson D, Stowasser M. Improved quality of life, blood pressure, and biochemical status following laparoscopic adrenalectomy for unilateral primary aldosteronism. J Clin Endocrinol Metab. 2010;95(3):1360–4.

Swain JM, Grant CS, Schlinkert RT, Thompson GB, vanHeerden JA, Lloyd RV, et al. Corticotropin-independent macronodular adrenal hyperplasia: a clinicopathologic correlation. Arch Surg. 1998;133(5):541–5; discussion 545–546.

Tardy V, Menassa R, Sulmont V, Lienhardt-Roussie A, Lecointre C, Brauner R, et al. Phenotype-genotype correlations of 13 rare CYP21A2 mutations detected in 46 patients affected with 21-hydroxylase deficiency and in one carrier. J Clin Endocrinol Metab. 2010;95(3):1288–300.

Textor SC. Current approaches to renovascular hypertension. Med Clin North Am. 2009;93(3):717–32.

Timmers HJ, Chen CC, Carrasquillo JA, Whatley M, Ling A, Havekes B, et al. Comparison of 18F-fluoro-L-DOPA, 18F-fluoro-deoxyglucose, and 18F-fluorodopamine PET and 123I-MIBG scintigraphy in the localization of pheochromocytoma and paraganglioma. J Clin Endocrinol Metab. 2009;94(12):4757–67.

Todd GR, Acerini CL, Ross-Russell R, Zahra S, Warner JT, McCance D. Survey of adrenal crisis associated with inhaled corticosteroids in the United Kingdom. Arch Dis Child. 2002;87(6):457–61.

Turcu AF, Auchus R. Approach to the patient with primary aldosteronism: utility and limitations of adrenal vein sampling. J Clin Endocrinol Metab. 2021;106(4):1195–1208.

Vaidya A, Hundemer GL, Nanba K, Parksook WW, Brown JM. Primary aldosteronism: state-of-the-art review. Am J Hypertens. 2022;35(12):967–988.

Valassi E, Swearingen B, Lee H, Nachtigall LB, Donoho DA, Klibanski A, et al. Concomitant medication use can confound interpretation of the combined dexamethasone-corticotropin releasing hormone test in Cushing's syndrome. J Clin Endocrinol Metab. 2009;94(12):4851–9.

Van Helvoort-Postulart D, Dirksen CD, Nelemans PJ, Kroon AA, Kessels AG, de Leeuw PW, et al. Renal artery stenosis: cost-effectiveness of diagnosis and treatment. Radiology. 2007;244(2):505–13.

Van Zaane B, Nur E, Squizzato A, Dekkers OM, Twickler MT, Fliers E, et al. Hypercoagulable state in Cushing's syndrome: a systematic review. J Clin Endocrinol Metab. 2009;94(8):2743–50.

Vanderveen KA, Thompson SM, Callstrom MR, Young WF Jr, Grant CS, Farley DR, et al. Biopsy of pheochromocytomas and paragangliomas: potential for disaster. Surgery. 2009;146(6):1158–66.

Venkatesan AM, Locklin J, Lai EW, Adams KT, Fojo AT, Pacak K, et al. Radiofrequency ablation of metastatic pheochromocytoma. J Vasc Interv Radiol. 2009;20(11):1483–90.

Whaley-Connell A, Johnson MS, Sowers JR. Aldosterone: role in the cardiometabolic syndrome and resistant hypertension. Prog Cardiovasc Dis. 2010;52(5):401–9.

Wolff AS, Erichsen MM, Meager A, Magitta NF, Myhre AG, Bollerslev J, et al. Autoimmune polyendocrine syndrome type 1 in Norway: phenotypic variation, autoantibodies, and novel mutations in the autoimmune regulator gene. J Clin Endocrinol Metab. 2007;92(2):595–603.

Young AL, Baysal BE, Deb A, Young WF Jr. Familial malignant catecholamine-secreting paraganglioma with prolonged survival associated with mutation in the succinate dehydrogenase B gene. J Clin Endocrinol Metab. 2002;87(9):4101–5.

Young WF. Metastatic pheochromocytoma: in search of a cure. Endocrinology. 2020;161(3):bqz019.

Young WF. Primary aldosteronism: renaissance of a syndrome. Clin Endocrinol (Oxf). 2007;66(5):607–18.

Young WF, Stanson AW. What are the keys to successful adrenal venous sampling (AVS) in patients with primary aldosteronism? Clin Endocrinol (Oxf). 2009;70(1):14–7.

Young WF, Stanson AW, Thompson GB, Grant CS, Farley DR, van Heerden JA. Role for adrenal venous sampling in primary aldosteronism. Surgery. 2004;136(6):1227–35.

Young WF Jr. Clinical practice. The incidentally discovered adrenal mass. N Engl J Med. 2007;356(6):601–10.

Young WF Jr. Diagnosis and treatment of primary aldosteronism: practical clinical perspectives. J Intern Med. 2019;285(2):126–48.

Young WF Jr. Paragangliomas: clinical overview. Ann N Y Acad Sci. 2006;1073:21–9.

Young WF Jr. Primary aldosteronism—one picture is not worth a thousand words. Ann Intern Med. 2009;151(5):357–8.

Young WF Jr, Carney JA, Musa BU, Wulffraat NM, Lens JW, Drexhage HA. Familial Cushing's syndrome due to primary pigmented nodular adrenocortical disease. Reinvestigation 50 years later. N Engl J Med. 1989;321(24):1659–64.

Young WF Jr, du Plessis H, Thompson GB, Grant CS, Farley DR, Richards ML, et al. The clinical conundrum of corticotropin-independent autonomous cortisol secretion in patients with bilateral adrenal masses. World J Surg. 2008;32(5):856–62.

Yu K, Ebbehøj AL, Obeid H, Vaidya A, Else T, Wachtel H, et al. Presentation, management, and outcomes of urinary bladder paraganglioma: results from a multicenter study. J Clin Endocrinol Metab. 2022;107(10):2811–21.

Zarnegar R, Young WF Jr, Lee J, Sweet MP, Kebebew E, Farley DR, et al. The aldosteronoma resolution score: predicting complete resolution of hypertension after adrenalectomy for aldosteronoma. Ann Surg. 2008;247(3):511–18.

Zhang L, Smyrk TC, Young WF Jr, Stratakis CA, Carney JA. Gastric stromal tumors in Carney triad are different clinically, pathologically, and behaviorally from sporadic gastric gastrointestinal stromal tumors: findings in 104 cases. Am J Surg Pathol. 2010; 34(1):53–64.

Section 4   Reproduction

Acién P, Acién M. Disorders of sex development: classification, review, and impact on fertility. J Clin Med. 2020;9(11):3555.

Al Wattar BH, Fisher M, Bevington L, Talaulikar V, Davies M, Conway G, Yasmin E. Clinical practice guidelines on the diagnosis and management of polycystic ovary syndrome: a systematic review and quality assessment study. J Clin Endocrinol Metab. 2021;106(8):2436–46.

American College of Obstetricians and Gynecologists' Committee on Practice Bulletins—Gynecology. ACOG Practice Bulletin No. 194: Polycystic Ovary Syndrome. Obstet Gynecol. 2018;131(6):e157–71.

Armengaud JB, Charkaluk ML, Trivin C, Tardy V, Breart G, Brauner R, et al. Precocious pubarche: distinguishing late-onset congenital adrenal hyperplasia from premature adrenarche. J Clin Endocrinol Metab. 2009;94(8):2835–40.

Audi L, Fernandez-Cancio M, Carrascosa A, Andaluz P, Toran N, Piro C, et al. Novel (60%) and recurrent (40%) androgen receptor gene mutations in a series of 59 patients with a 46,XY disorder of sex development. J Clin Endocrinol Metab. 2010;95(4):1876–88.

Azziz R. Polycystic ovary syndrome. Obstet Gynecol. 2018;132(2): 321–336.

Bannink EM, van Sassen C, van Buuren S, de Jong FH, Lequin M, Mulder PG, et al. Puberty induction in Turner syndrome: results of oestrogen treatment on development of secondary sexual characteristics, uterine dimensions and serum hormone levels. Clin Endocrinol (Oxf). 2009;70(2):265–73.

Bhasin S, Brito JP, Cunningham GR, Hayes FJ, Hodis HN, Matsumoto AM, Snyder PJ, Swerdloff RS, Wu FC, Yialamas MA. Testosterone therapy in men with hypogonadism: an Endocrine Society clinical practice guideline. J Clin Endocrinol Metab. 2018;103(5): 1715–1744.

Bradley SH, Lawrence N, Steele C, Mohamed Z. Precocious puberty. BMJ. 2020;368:l6597.

Braunstein GD. Clinical practice. Gynecomastia. N Engl J Med. 2007; 357(12):1229–37.

Carel JC, Leger J. Clinical practice. Precocious puberty. N Engl J Med. 2008;358(22):2366–77.

Colin JF. Gynaecomastia: drugs and surgical concerns. BMJ. 2008; 336(7648):790.

Cosma M, Swiglo BA, Flynn DN, Kurtz DM, Labella ML, Mullan RJ, et al. Clinical review: insulin sensitizers for the treatment of hirsutism: a systematic review and metaanalyses of randomized controlled trials. J Clin Endocrinol Metab. 2008;93(4):1135–42.

Davenport ML. Approach to the patient with Turner syndrome. J Clin Endocrinol Metab. 2010;95(4):1487–95.

Dayner JE, Lee PA, Houk CP. Medical treatment of intersex: parental perspectives. J Urol. 2004;172(4 Pt 2):1762–5; discussion 1765.

De Boer H, van Gastel P, van Sorge A. Luteinizing hormone-releasing hormone and postmenopausal flushing. N Engl J Med. 2009;361(12):1218–19.

De Vries L, Guz-Mark A, Lazar L, Reches A, Phillip M. Premature thelarche: age at presentation affects clinical course but not clinical characteristics or risk to progress to precocious puberty. J Pediatr. 2010;156(3):466–71.

Donadille B, Christin-Maitre S. Heart and Turner syndrome. Ann Endocrinol (Paris). 2021;82(3-4):135–40.

El-Mansoury M, Barrenas ML, Bryman I, Hanson C, Landin-Wilhelmsen K. Impaired body balance, fine motor function and hearing in women with Turner syndrome. Clin Endocrinol (Oxf). 2009;71(2):273–8.

Elzaiat M, McElreavey K, Bashamboo A. Genetics of 46,XY gonadal dysgenesis. Best Pract Res Clin Endocrinol Metab. 2022;36(1):101633.

Euling SY, Selevan SG, Pescovitz OH, Skakkebaek NE. Role of environmental factors in the timing of puberty. Pediatrics. 2008;121 (Suppl 3):S167–71.

Ferriman D, Gallwey JD. Clinical assessment of body hair growth in women. J Clin Endocrinol Metab. 1961;21:1440–7.

Finkielstain GP, Vieites A, Bergadá I, Rey RA. Disorders of sex development of adrenal origin. Front Endocrinol (Lausanne). 2021; 12:770782.

Gomes NL, Batista RL, Nishi MY, Lerário AM, Silva TE, de Moraes Narcizo A, et al. Contribution of clinical and genetic approaches for diagnosing 209 index cases with 46,XY Differences of sex development. J Clin Endocrinol Metab. 2022;107(5):e1797–806.

Gordon CM, Ackerman KE, Berga SL, Kaplan JR, Mastorakos G, Misra M, Murad MH, Santoro NF, Warren MP. Functional hypothalamic amenorrhea: an Endocrine Society clinical practice guideline. J Clin Endocrinol Metab. 2017;102(5):1413–39.

Grady D. Clinical practice. Management of menopausal symptoms. N Engl J Med. 2006;355(22):2338–47.

Gravholt CH, Viuff MH, Brun S, Stochholm K, Andersen NH. Turner syndrome: mechanisms and management. Nat Rev Endocrinol. 2019;15(10):601–14.

Growth KA, Skakkebæk A, Høst C, Gravholt CH, Bojesen A. Clinical review: Klinefelter syndrome–a clinical update. J Clin Endocrinol Metab. 2013;98(1):20–30.

Harrington J, Palmert MR. An approach to the patient with delayed puberty. J Clin Endocrinol Metab. 2022;107(6):1739–50.

Hembree WC, Cohen-Kettenis PT, Gooren L, Hannema SE, Meyer WJ, Murad MH, Rosenthal SM, Safer JD, Tangpricha V, T'Sjoen GG. Endocrine treatment of gender-dysphoric/gender-incongruent persons: an Endocrine Society clinical practice guideline. J Clin Endocrinol Metab. 2017;102(11):3869–3903.

Himes JH, Park K, Styne D. Menarche and assessment of body mass index in adolescent girls. J Pediatr. 2009;155(3):393–7.

Hindmarsh PC. How do you initiate oestrogen therapy in a girl who has not undergone puberty? Clin Endocrinol (Oxf). 2009;71(1): 7–10.

Hines SL, Tan W, Larson JM, Thompson KM, Jorn HK, Files JA. A practical approach to guide clinicians in the evaluation of male patients with breast masses. Geriatrics. 2008;63(6):19–24.

Hirschberg AL. Approach to investigation of hyperandrogenism in a postmenopausal woman. J Clin Endocrinol Metab. 2023; 108(5):1243–53.

Hoeger KM, Dokras A, Piltonen T. Update on PCOS: consequences, challenges, and guiding treatment. J Clin Endocrinol Metab. 2021;106(3):e1071–83.

Hyun G, Kolon TF. A practical approach to intersex in the newborn period. Urol Clin North Am. 2004;31(3):435–43:viii.

Joham AE, Norman RJ, Stener-Victorin E, Legro RS, Franks S, Moran LJ, Boyle J, Teede HJ. Polycystic ovary syndrome. Lancet Diabetes Endocrinol. 2022;10(9):668–80.

Johnson RE, Murad MH. Gynecomastia: pathophysiology, evaluation, and management. Mayo Clin Proc. 2009;84(11):1010–15.

Jorgensen KT, Rostgaard K, Bache I, Biggar RJ, Nielsen NM, Tommerup N, et al. Autoimmune diseases in women with Turner's syndrome. Arthritis Rheum. 2010;62(3):658–66.

Kanakis GA, Nieschlag E. Klinefelter syndrome: more than hypogonadism. Metabolism. 2018;86:135–44.

Kanakis GA, Nordkap L, Bang AK, Calogero AE, Bártfai G, Corona G, Forti G, Toppari J, Goulis DG, Jørgensen N. EAA clinical practice guidelines-gynecomastia evaluation and management. Andrology. 2019;7(6):778–93.

Karrer-Voegeli S, Rey F, Reymond MJ, Meuwly JY, Gaillard RC, Gomez F. Androgen dependence of hirsutism, acne, and alopecia in women: retrospective analysis of 228 patients investigated for hyperandrogenism. Medicine (Baltimore). 2009;88(1):32–45.

Karthikeyan A. Precocious puberty. Clin Pediatr (Phila). 2008; 47(7):718.

Kaunitz AM. Clinical practice. Hormonal contraception in women of older reproductive age. N Engl J Med. 2008;358(12):1262–70.

Koulouri O, Conway GS. Management of hirsutism. BMJ. 2009; 338:b847.

Kumar R, St John J, Devendra D. Hirsutism. BMJ. 2009;339:b3090.

Laimon W, El-Hawary A, Aboelenin H, Elzohiri M, Abdelmaksoud S, Megahed N, Salem N. Prepubertal gynecomastia is not always idiopathic: case series and review of the literature. Eur J Pediatr. 2021; 180(3):977–82.

Lanfranco F, Kamischke A, Zitzmann M, Nieschlag E. Klinefelter's syndrome. Lancet. 2004;364(9430):273–83.

Latronico AC, Brito VN, Carel JC. Causes, diagnosis, and treatment of central precocious puberty. Lancet Diabetes Endocrinol. 2016; 4(3):265–74.

Lee JM, Kaciroti N, Appugliese D, Corwyn RF, Bradley RH, Lumeng JC. Body mass index and timing of pubertal initiation in boys. Arch Pediatr Adolesc Med. 2010;164(2):139–44.

Lopez L, Arheart KL, Colan SD, Stein NS, Lopez-Mitnik G, Lin AE, et al. Turner syndrome is an independent risk factor for aortic dilation in the young. Pediatrics. 2008;121(6):e1622–7.

Marshall WA, Tanner JM. Variations in pattern of pubertal changes in girls. Arch Dis Child. 1969;44(235):291–303.

Marshall WA, Tanner JM. Variations in the pattern of pubertal changes in boys. Arch Dis Child. 1970;45(239):13–23.

Martin KA, Anderson RR, Chang RJ, Ehrmann DA, Lobo RA, Murad MH, Pugeat MM, Rosenfield RL. Evaluation and treatment of hirsutism in premenopausal women: an Endocrine Society clinical practice guideline. J Clin Endocrinol Metab. 2018; 103(4):1233–1257.

Matura LA, Ho VB, Rosing DR, Bondy CA. Aortic dilatation and dissection in Turner syndrome. Circulation. 2007;116(15):1663–70.

Mendonca BB, Domenice S, Arnhold IJ, Costa EM. 46,XY disorders of sex development (DSD). Clin Endocrinol (Oxf). 2009;70(2):173–87.

Mimoto MS, Oyler JL, Davis AM. Evaluation and treatment of hirsutism in premenopausal women. JAMA. 2018;319(15):1613–14.

Nelson LM. Clinical practice. Primary ovarian insufficiency. N Engl J Med. 2009;360(6):606–14.

Ogilvy-Stuart AL, Brain CE. Early assessment of ambiguous genitalia. Arch Dis Child. 2004;89(5):401–7.

Papadimitriou A, Pantsiotou S, Douros K, Papadimitriou DT, Nicolaidou P, Fretzayas A. Timing of pubertal onset in girls: evidence for non-Gaussian distribution. J Clin Endocrinol Metab. 2008;93(11):4422–5.

Pawlowski EJ, Nield LS. Gynecomastia and hypogonadism. Clin Pediatr (Phila). 2008;47(3):313–5; comment 314–315.

Poomthavorn P, Stargatt R, Zacharin M. Psychosexual and psychosocial functions of anorchid young adults. J Clin Endocrinol Metab. 2009;94(7):2502–5.

Rosenfield RL. Clinical practice. Hirsutism. N Engl J Med. 2005;353 (24):2578–88.

Sachdev V, Matura LA, Sidenko S, Ho VB, Arai AE, Rosing DR, et al. Aortic valve disease in Turner syndrome. J Am Coll Cardiol. 2008; 51(19):1904–9.

Sathyapalan T, Atkin SL. Investigating hirsutism. BMJ. 2009;338:b912.

Swiglo BA, Cosma M, Flynn DN, Kurtz DM, Labella ML, Mullan RJ, et al. Clinical review: Antiandrogens for the treatment of hirsutism: a systematic review and metaanalyses of randomized controlled trials. J Clin Endocrinol Metab. 2008;93(4):1153–60.

Van Dongen H, Janssen CA, Smeets MJ, Emanuel MH, Jansen FW. The clinical relevance of hysteroscopic polypectomy in premenopausal women with abnormal uterine bleeding. BJOG. 2009; 116(10):1387–90.

Verkauskas G, Jaubert F, Lortat-Jacob S, Malan V, Thibaud E, Nihoul-Fekete C. The long-term followup of 33 cases of true hermaphroditism: a 40-year experience with conservative gonadal surgery. J Urol. 2007;177(2):726–31; discussion 731.

Viuff MH, Just J, Brun S, Dam TV, Hansen M, Melgaard L, Hougaard DM, Lappe M, Gravholt CH. Women with Turner syndrome are both estrogen and androgen deficient: the impact of hormone replacement therapy. J Clin Endocrinol Metab. 2022;107(7): 1983–1993.

Wood CL, Lane LC, Cheetham T. Puberty: Normal physiology (brief overview). Best Pract Res Clin Endocrinol Metab. 2019;33(3):101265.

Zacharin M. Disorders of ovarian function in childhood and adolescence: evolving needs of the growing child. An endocrine perspective. BJOG. 2010;117(2):156–62.

Zeger MP, Zinn AR, Lahlou N, Ramos P, Kowal K, Samango-Sprouse C, et al. Effect of ascertainment and genetic features on the phenotype of Klinefelter syndrome. J Pediatr. 2008;152(5):716–22.

Section 5   Pancreas

American Diabetes Association. Diagnosis and classification of diabetes mellitus. Diabetes Care. 2010;33(Suppl 1):S62–9.

Balsells M, Garcia-Patterson A, Gich I, Corcoy R. Maternal and fetal outcome in women with type 2 versus type 1 diabetes mellitus: a systematic review and metaanalysis. J Clin Endocrinol Metab. 2009;94(11):4284–91.

Barnett AH. New treatments in type 2 diabetes: a focus on the incretin-based therapies. Clin Endocrinol (Oxf). 2009;70(3):343–53.

Besirli CG, Johnson MW. Proliferative diabetic retinopathy. Mayo Clin Proc. 2009;84(12):1054.

Bingley PJ. Clinical applications of diabetes antibody testing. J Clin Endocrinol Metab. 2010;95(1):25–33.

Boulton AJ, Kirsner RS, Vileikyte L. Clinical practice. Neuropathic diabetic foot ulcers. N Engl J Med. 2004;351(1):48–55.

Broome DT, Pantalone KM, Kashyap SR, Philipson LH. Approach to the patient with MODY-monogenic diabetes. J Clin Endocrinol Metab. 2021;106(1):237–50.

Bustan RS, Wasim D, Yderstræde KB, Bygum A. Specific skin signs as a cutaneous marker of diabetes mellitus and the prediabetic state – a systematic review. Dan Med J. 2017;64(1):A5316.

Camilleri M. Clinical practice. Diabetic gastroparesis. N Engl J Med. 2007;356(8):820–9.

Ceriello A, Prattichizzo F, Phillip M, Hirsch IB, Mathieu C, Battelino T. Glycaemic management in diabetes: old and new approaches. Lancet Diabetes Endocrinol. 2022;10(1):75–84.

Cheer K, Shearman C, Jude EB. Managing complications of the diabetic foot. BMJ. 2009;339:b4905.

Cheung BM, Ong KL, Cherny SS, Sham PC, Tso AW, Lam KS. Diabetes prevalence and therapeutic target achievement in the United States, 1999 to 2006. Am J Med. 2009;122(5):443–53.

Chun SH, Li AH. Association of proliferative diabetic retinopathy with insulin use and microalbuminuria. Arch Ophthalmol. 2010;128(1):146; author reply 146–7.

Conway BN, Miller RG, Klein R, Orchard TJ. Prediction of proliferative diabetic retinopathy with hemoglobin level. Arch Ophthalmol. 2009;127(11):1494–9.

Cryer PE, Axelrod L, Grossman AB, Heller SR, Montori VM, Seaquist ER, et al. Evaluation and management of adult hypoglycemic disorders: an Endocrine Society clinical practice guideline. J Clin Endocrinol Metab. 2009;94(3):709–28.

Currie CJ, Peters Jr, Tynan A, Evans M, Heine RJ, Bracco OL, et al. Survival as a function of HbA(1c) in people with type 2 diabetes: a retrospective cohort study. Lancet. 2010;375(9713):481–9.

DeFronzo RA. Current issues in the treatment of type 2 diabetes. Overview of newer agents: where treatment is going. Am J Med. 2010;123(3 Suppl):S38–48.

Dluhy RG, McMahon GT. Intensive glycemic control in the ACCORD and ADVANCE trials. N Engl J Med. 2008;358(24):2630–3.

Duckworth W, Abraira C, Moritz T, Reda D, Emanuele N, Reaven PD, et al. Glucose control and vascular complications in veterans with type 2 diabetes. N Engl J Med. 2009;360(2):129–39.

Fante RJ, Durairaj VD, Oliver SC. Diabetic retinopathy: an update on treatment. Am J Med. 2010;123(3):213–16.

Ferrannini E, Mari A, Nofrate V, Sosenko JM, Skyler JS. Progression to diabetes in relatives of type 1 diabetic patients: mechanisms and mode of onset. Diabetes. 2010;59(3):679–85.

Finfer S, Chittock DR, Su SY, Blair D, Foster D, Dhingra V, et al. Intensive versus conventional glucose control in critically ill patients. N Engl J Med. 2009;360(13):1283–97.

Frye RL, August P, Brooks MM, Hardison RM, Kelsey SF, MacGregor JM, et al. A randomized trial of therapies for type 2 diabetes and coronary artery disease. N Engl J Med. 2009;360(24):2503–15.

Gerstein HC, Miller ME, Byington RP, Goff DC Jr, Bigger JT, Buse JB, et al. Effects of intensive glucose lowering in type 2 diabetes. N Engl J Med. 2008;358(24):2545–59.

Ghetti S, Lee JK, Sims CE, Demaster DM, Glaser NS. Diabetic ketoacidosis and memory dysfunction in children with type 1 diabetes. J Pediatr. 2010;156(1):109–14.

Goldfine AB. Assessing the cardiovascular safety of diabetes therapies. N Engl J Med. 2008;359(11):1092–5.

Hashemi DA, Brown-Joel ZO, Tkachenko E, et al. Clinical features and comorbidities of patients with necrobiosis lipoidica with or without diabetes. JAMA Dermatol. 2019;155:455.

Hedderson MM, Gunderson EP, Ferrara A. Gestational weight gain and risk of gestational diabetes mellitus. Obstet Gynecol. 2010; 115(3):597–604.

Holman RR, Farmer AJ, Davies MJ, Levy JC, Darbyshire JL, Keenan JF, et al. Three-year efficacy of complex insulin regimens in type 2 diabetes. N Engl J Med. 2009;361(18):1736–47.

Holman RR, Paul SK, Bethel MA, Matthews DR, Neil HA. 10-year follow-up of intensive glucose control in type 2 diabetes. N Engl J Med. 2008;359(15):1577–89.

Holman RR, Paul SK, Bethel MA, Neil HA, Matthews DR. Long-term follow-up after tight control of blood pressure in type 2 diabetes. N Engl J Med. 2008;359(15):1565–76.

Horvath K, Koch K, Jeitler K, Matyas E, Bender R, Bastian H, et al. Effects of treatment in women with gestational diabetes mellitus: systematic review and meta-analysis. BMJ. 2010;340:c1395.

Inzucchi SE. Clinical practice. Management of hyperglycemia in the hospital setting. N Engl J Med. 2006;355(18):1903–11.

Inzucchi SE, Peixoto AJ, Testani JM. Glucose-lowering drugs to reduce cardiovascular risk in type 2 diabetes. N Engl J Med. 2021;385(7):669–70.

Inzucchi SE, Siegel MD. Glucose control in the ICU—how tight is too tight? N Engl J Med. 2009;360(13):1346–9.

Jessen L, D'Alessio D. The incretins and beta-cell health: contrasting glucose-dependent insulinotropic polypeptide and glucagon-like peptide-1 as a path to understand islet function in diabetes. Gastroenterology. 2009;137(6):1891–4.

Kao SL, Chan CL, Tan B, Lim CC, Dalan R, Gardner D, et al. An unusual outbreak of hypoglycemia. N Engl J Med. 2009;360(7):734–6.

Katavetin P, Katavetin P. Renal and retinal effects of enalapril and losartan in type 1 diabetes. N Engl J Med. 2009;361(14):1410–11; author reply 1411.

Kitabchi AE, Umpierrez GE, Fisher JN, Murphy MB, Stentz FB. Thirty years of personal experience in hyperglycemic crises: diabetic ketoacidosis and hyperglycemic hyperosmolar state. J Clin Endocrinol Metab. 2008;93(5):1541–52.

Korytkowski MT, Muniyappa R, Antinori-Lent K, Donihi AC, Drincic AT, Hirsch IB, et al. Management of Hyperglycemia in hospitalized adult patients in non-critical care settings: an Endocrine Society clinical practice guideline. J Clin Endocrinol Metab. 2022;107(8):2101–2128.

Kosaka S, Kawana S. Case of necrobiosis lipoidica diabeticorum successfully treated by photodynamic therapy. J Dermatol. 2012; 39:497.

Koul PB. Diabetic ketoacidosis: a current appraisal of pathophysiology and management. Clin Pediatr (Phila). 2009;48(2):135–44.

Landon MB, Spong CY, Thom E, Carpenter MW, Ramin SM, Casey B, et al. A multicenter, randomized trial of treatment for mild gestational diabetes. N Engl J Med. 2009;361(14):1339–48.

LeRoith D, Biessels GJ, Braithwaite SS, Casanueva FF, Draznin B, Halter JB, Hirsch IB, McDonnell ME, Molitch ME, Murad MH, Sinclair AJ. Treatment of diabetes in older adults: an Endocrine Society clinical practice guideline. J Clin Endocrinol Metab. 2019; 104(5):1520–74.

Lloyd RV, Douglas BR, Young WF Jr. Diffuse neuroendocrine system. In: King DW, editor. Atlas of Nontumor Pathology: Endocrine Diseases. American Registry of Pathology and the Armed Forces Institute of Pathology; 2002.

Ludvigsson J, Faresjo M, Hjorth M, Axelsson S, Cheramy M, Pihl M, et al. GAD treatment and insulin secretion in recent-onset type 1 diabetes. N Engl J Med. 2008;359(18):1909–20.

Malik VS, Popkin BM, Bray GA, Despres JP, Hu FB. Sugar-sweetened beverages, obesity, type 2 diabetes mellitus, and cardiovascular disease risk. Circulation. 2010;121(11):1356–64.

Mathur A, Gorden P, Libutti SK. Insulinoma. Surg Clin North Am. 2009;89(5):1105–21.

Mauer M, Zinman B, Gardiner R, Suissa S, Sinaiko A, Strand T, et al. Renal and retinal effects of enalapril and losartan in type 1 diabetes. N Engl J Med. 2009;361(1):40–51.

McCall AL, Lieb DC, Gianchandani R, et al. Management of individuals with diabetes at high risk for hypoglycemia: an Endocrine Society clinical practice guideline. J Clin Endocrinol Metab. 2023; 108(3):529–62.

Meltzer SJ. Treatment of gestational diabetes. BMJ. 2010;340:c1708.

Miller ME, Bonds DE, Gerstein HC, Seaquist ER, Bergenstal RM, Calles-Escandon J, et al. The effects of baseline characteristics, glycaemia treatment approach, and glycated haemoglobin concentration on the risk of severe hypoglycaemia: post hoc epidemiological analysis of the ACCORD study. BMJ. 2010;340:b5444.

Mudaliar S, Henry RR. Effects of incretin hormones on beta-cell mass and function, body weight, and hepatic and myocardial function. Am J Med. 2010;123(3 Suppl):S19–27.

Muller SA, Winkelmann RK. Necrobiosis lipoidica diabeticorum. A clinical and pathological investigation of 171 cases. Arch Dermatol. 1966; 93:272.

Murphy-Chutorian B, Han G, Cohen SR. Dermatologic manifestations of diabetes mellitus: a review. Endocrinol Metab Clin North Am. 2013;42(4):869–98.

Nakagawa T, Kosugi T, Haneda M, Rivard CJ, Long DA. Abnormal angiogenesis in diabetic nephropathy. Diabetes. 2009;58(7):1471–8.

Nathan DM. Clinical practice. Initial management of glycemia in type 2 diabetes mellitus. N Engl J Med. 2002;347(17):1342–9.

Nathan DM, Zinman B, Cleary PA, Backlund JY, Genuth S, Miller R, et al. Modern-day clinical course of type 1 diabetes mellitus after 30 years' duration: the diabetes control and complications trial/epidemiology of diabetes interventions and complications and Pittsburgh epidemiology of diabetes complications experience (1983–2005). Arch Intern Med. 2009;169(14):1307–16.

Oyibo SO, Jude EB, Tarawneh I, Nguyen HC, Harkless LB, Boulton AJ. A comparison of two diabetic foot ulcer classification systems: the Wagner and the University of Texas wound classification systems. Diabetes Care. 2001;24(1):84–8.

Packer M, Anker SD, Butler J, Filippatos G, Pocock SJ, Carson P, et al. Cardiovascular and renal outcomes with empagliflozin in heart failure. N Engl J Med. 2020;383(15):1413–24.

Parving HH, Persson F, Lewis JB, Lewis EJ, Hollenberg NK. Aliskiren combined with losartan in type 2 diabetes and nephropathy. N Engl J Med. 2008;358(23):2433–46.

Pascuzzi RM. Peripheral neuropathy. Med Clin North Am. 2009;93(2):317–42:vii–viii.

Patel A, MacMahon S, Chalmers J, Neal B, Billot L, Woodward M, et al. Intensive blood glucose control and vascular outcomes in patients with type 2 diabetes. N Engl J Med. 2008;358(24):2560–72.

Perkins BA, Aiello LP, Krolewski AS. Diabetes complications and the renin-angiotensin system. N Engl J Med. 2009;361(1):83–5.

Peters A. Incretin-based therapies: review of current clinical trial data. Am J Med. 2010;123(3 Suppl):S28–37.

Peters AL, Ahmann AJ, Hirsch IB, Raymond JK. Advances in glucose monitoring and automated insulin delivery: supplement to Endocrine Society clinical practice guidelines. J Endocr Soc. 2018;2(11):1214–1225.

Pirkola J, Pouta A, Bloigu A, Miettola S, Hartikainen AL, Jarvelin MR, et al. Prepregnancy overweight and gestational diabetes as determinants of subsequent diabetes and hypertension after 20-year follow-up. J Clin Endocrinol Metab. 2010;95(2):772–8.

Placzkowski KA, Vella A, Thompson GB, Grant CS, Reading CC, Charboneau JW, et al. Secular trends in the presentation and management of functioning insulinoma at the Mayo Clinic, 1987–2007. J Clin Endocrinol Metab. 2009;94(4):1069–73.

Proia AD, Caldwell MC. Intraretinal neovascularization in diabetic retinopathy. Arch Ophthalmol. 2010;128(1):142–4.

Raffel A, Krausch MM, Anlauf M, Wieben D, Braunstein S, Kloppel G, et al. Diffuse nesidioblastosis as a cause of hyperinsulinemic hypoglycemia in adults: a diagnostic and therapeutic challenge. Surgery. 2007;141(2):179–84; discussion 185–176.

Rahier J, Guiot Y, Sempoux C. Persistent hyperinsulinaemic hypoglycaemia of infancy: a heterogeneous syndrome unrelated to nesidioblastosis. Arch Dis Child Fetal Neonatal Ed. 2000;82(2):F108–112.

Reaven PD, Emanuele NV, Wiitala WL, Bahn GD, Reda DJ, McCarren M, Duckworth WC, Hayward RA; VADT Investigators. Intensive glucose control in patients with type 2 diabetes – 15-year follow-up. N Engl J Med. 2019;380(23):2215–24.

Remuzzi G, Schieppati A, Ruggenenti P. Clinical practice. Nephropathy in patients with type 2 diabetes. N Engl J Med. 2002;346(15):1145–51.

Retnakaran R, Qi Y, Connelly PW, Sermer M, Zinman B, Hanley AJ. Glucose intolerance in pregnancy and postpartum risk of metabolic syndrome in young women. J Clin Endocrinol Metab. 2010;95(2):670–7.

Rishi P, Bhende PS. Images in clinical medicine. Proliferative diabetic retinopathy. N Engl J Med. 2009;360(9):912.

Robinson AH, Pasapula C, Brodsky JW. Surgical aspects of the diabetic foot. J Bone Joint Surg Br. 2009;91(1):1–7.

Roden M. Optimal insulin treatment in type 2 diabetes. N Engl J Med. 2009;361(18):1801–3.

Rosenzweig JL, Bakris GL, Berglund LF, Hivert MF, Horton ES, Kalyani RR, Murad MH, Vergès BL. Primary prevention of ASCVD and T2DM in patients at metabolic risk: an Endocrine Society clinical practice guideline. J Clin Endocrinol Metab. 2019;104(9):3939–85.

Rostambeigi N, Thompson GB. What should be done in an operating room when an insulinoma cannot be found? Clin Endocrinol (Oxf). 2009;70(4):512–15.

Rostène W, De Meyts P. Insulin: a 100-year-old discovery with a fascinating history. Endocr Rev. 2021;42(5):503–27.

Selvin E, Steffes MW, Zhu H, Matsushita K, Wagenknecht L, Pankow J, et al. Glycated hemoglobin, diabetes, and cardiovascular risk in nondiabetic adults. N Engl J Med. 2010;362(9):800–11.

Service FJ. Hypoglycemic disorders. N Engl J Med. 1995;332(17):1144–52.

Service FJ, Natt N, Thompson GB, Grant CS, van Heerden JA, Andrews JC, et al. Noninsulinoma pancreatogenous hypoglycemia: a novel syndrome of hyperinsulinemic hypoglycemia in adults independent of mutations in Kir6.2 and SUR1 genes. J Clin Endocrinol Metab. 1999;84(5):1582–9.

Service FJ, O'Brien PC. Increasing serum betahydroxybutyrate concentrations during the 72-hour fast: evidence against hyperinsulinemic hypoglycemia. J Clin Endocrinol Metab. 2005;90(8):4555–8.

Service GJ, Thompson GB, Service FJ, Andrews JC, Collazo-Clavell ML, Lloyd RV. Hyperinsulinemic hypoglycemia with nesidioblastosis after gastric-bypass surgery. N Engl J Med. 2005;353(3):249–54.

Shoag JE, Al Hussein Al Awamlh B, Rajagopalan S. Diabetes treatment and control in U.S. adults. N Engl J Med. 2021;385(10):e30.

Smith RJ, Nathan DM, Arslanian SA, Groop L, Rizza RA, Rotter JI. Individualizing therapies in type 2 diabetes mellitus based on patient characteristics: what we know and what we need to know. J Clin Endocrinol Metab. 2010;95(4):1566–74.

Staels B. A review of bile acid sequestrants: potential mechanism(s) for glucose-lowering effects in type 2 diabetes mellitus. Postgrad Med. 2009;121(3 Suppl 1):25–30.

Stanley CA. Hyperinsulinism in infants and children. Pediatr Clin North Am. 1997;44(2):363–74.

Stolar M. Glycemic control and complications in type 2 diabetes mellitus. Am J Med. 2010;123(3 Suppl):S3–11.

Sweeting A, Wong J, Murphy HR, Ross GP. A clinical update on gestational diabetes mellitus. Endocr Rev. 2022;43(5):763–93.

Tamborlane WV, Beck RW, Bode BW, Buckingham B, Chase HP, Clemons R, et al. Continuous glucose monitoring and intensive treatment of type 1 diabetes. N Engl J Med. 2008;359(14):1464–76.

Thompson GB, Service FJ, Andrews JC, Lloyd RV, Natt N, van Heerden JA, et al. Noninsulinoma pancreatogenous hypoglycemia syndrome: an update in 10 surgically treated patients. Surgery. 2000;128(6):937–44; discussion 944–935.

Thrower SL, Bingley PJ. Strategies to prevent type 1 diabetes. Diabetes Obes Metab. 2009;11(10):931–8.

Torn C, Mueller PW, Schlosser M, Bonifacio E, Bingley PJ. Diabetes Antibody Standardization Program: evaluation of assays for autoantibodies to glutamic acid decarboxylase and islet antigen-2. Diabetologia. 2008;51(5):846–52.

Wagner FW Jr. The dysvascular foot: a system for diagnosis and treatment. Foot Ankle. 1981;2(2):64–122.

Willcox A, Richardson SJ, Bone AJ, Foulis AK, Morgan NG. Analysis of islet inflammation in human type 1 diabetes. Clin Exp Immunol. 2009;155(2):173–81.

Yeh HC, Duncan BB, Schmidt MI, Wang NY, Brancati FL. Smoking, smoking cessation, and risk for type 2 diabetes mellitus: a cohort study. Ann Intern Med. 2010;152(1):10–7.

Yogev, Chen, Hod, Coustan, Oats, McIntyre, Metzger, Lowe, Dyer, Dooley, Trimble, McCance, Hadden, Persson, Rogers; Hyperglycemia and Adverse Pregnancy Outcome (HAPO) Study Cooperative

Research Group. Hyperglycemia and Adverse Pregnancy Outcome (HAPO) study: preeclampsia. Am J Obstet Gynecol. 2010;202(3), 255:e251–257.

Section 6 Bone and Calcium

Ackah SA, Imel EA. Approach to hypophosphatemic rickets. J Clin Endocrinol Metab. 2022;108(1):209–20.

Adams JS, Hewison M. Update in vitamin D. J Clin Endocrinol Metab. 2010;95:471–8.

American Geriatrics Society Workgroup on Vitamin D Supplementation for Older Adults. Recommendations abstracted from the American Geriatrics Society Consensus Statement on vitamin D for Prevention of Falls and Their Consequences. J Am Geriatr Soc. 2014; 62:147.

Asari R, Passler C, Kaczirek K, Scheuba C, Niederle B. Hypoparathyroidism after total thyroidectomy: a prospective study. Arch Surg. 2008;143(2):132–7; discussion 138.

Astrom E, Jorulf H, Soderhall S. Intravenous pamidronate treatment of infants with severe osteogenesis imperfecta. Arch Dis Child. 2007;92(4):332–8.

Bachrach LK, Ward LM. Clinical review 1: bisphosphonate use in childhood osteoporosis. J Clin Endocrinol Metab. 2009;94(2):400–9.

Barnes AM, Carter EM, Cabral WA, Weis M, Chang W, Makareeva E, et al. Lack of cyclophilin B in osteogenesis imperfecta with normal collagen folding. N Engl J Med. 2010;362(6):521–8.

Barrett-Connor E, Nielson CM, Orwoll E, Bauer DC, Cauley JA. Epidemiology of rib fractures in older men: Osteoporotic Fractures in Men (MrOS) prospective cohort study. BMJ. 2010;340:c1069.

Bastin S, Bird H, Gamble G, Cundy T. Paget's disease of bone—becoming a rarity? Rheumatology (Oxford). 2009;48(10):1232–5.

Bikle D. Nonclassic actions of vitamin D. J Clin Endocrinol Metab. 2009;94(1):26–34.

Bilezikian JP. Hypoparathyroidism. J Clin Endocrinol Metab. 2020; 105(6):1722–36.

Bilezikian JP, Silverberg SJ. Clinical practice. Asymptomatic primary hyperparathyroidism. N Engl J Med. 2004;350(17):1746–51.

Bitzan M, Goodyer PR. Hypophosphatemic rickets. Pediatr Clin North Am. 2019;66(1):179–207.

Bolland MJ, Grey A. Disparate outcomes from applying U.K. and U.S. osteoporosis treatment guidelines. J Clin Endocrinol Metab. 2010;95(4):1856–60.

Bolland MJ, Grey AB, Gamble GD, Reid IR. Effect of osteoporosis treatment on mortality: a meta-analysis. J Clin Endocrinol Metab. 2010;95(3):1174–81.

Buchbinder R, Osborne RH, Ebeling PR, Wark JD, Mitchell P, Wriedt C, et al. A randomized trial of vertebroplasty for painful osteoporotic vertebral fractures. N Engl J Med. 2009;361(6):557–68.

Bumpous JM, Goldstein RL, Flynn MB. Surgical and calcium outcomes in 427 patients treated prospectively in an image-guided and intraoperative PTH (IOPTH) supplemented protocol for primary hyperparathyroidism: outcomes and opportunities. Laryngoscope. 2009;119(2):300–6.

Cahill RA, Wenkert D, Perlman SA, Steele A, Coburn SP, McAlister WH, et al. Infantile hypophosphatasia: transplantation therapy trial using bone fragments and cultured osteoblasts. J Clin Endocrinol Metab. 2007;92(8):2923–30.

Canalis E. Update in new anabolic therapies for osteoporosis. J Clin Endocrinol Metab. 2010;95(4):1496–504.

Cheng S, Massaro JM, Fox CS, Larson MG, Keyes MJ, McCabe EL, et al. Adiposity, cardiometabolic risk, and vitamin D status: the Framingham Heart Study. Diabetes. 2010;59(1):242–8.

Clarke BL. New and emerging treatments for osteoporosis. Clin Endocrinol (Oxf). 2009;71(3):309–21.

Cook MJ, Pye SR, Lunt M, Dixon WG, Ashcroft DM' O'Neill TW. Incidence of Paget's disease of bone in the UK: evidence of a continuing decline. Rheumatology (Oxford). 2021;60(12):5668–76.

Cooper M. Bone protective therapy in the young patient with fractures and chronic disease: what drug(s) should be given and for how long? Clin Endocrinol (Oxf). 2009;70(2):188–91.

Cooper MS, Gittoes NJ. Diagnosis and management of hypocalcaemia. BMJ. 2008;336(7656):1298–302.

Cox G, Einhorn TA, Tzioupis C, Giannoudis PV. Bone-turnover markers in fracture healing. J Bone Joint Surg Br. 2010;92(3): 329–34.

Cummings SR, San Martin J, McClung MR, Siris ES, Eastell R, Reid IR, et al. Denosumab for prevention of fractures in postmenopausal women with osteoporosis. N Engl J Med. 2009;361(8):756–65.

Dahir KM, Seefried L, Kishnani PS, Petryk A, Högler W, Linglart A, et al. Clinical profiles of treated and untreated adults with hypophosphatasia in the Global HPP Registry. Orphanet J Rare Dis. 2022;17(1):277.

Drake MT, Clarke BL, Khosla S. Bisphosphonates: mechanism of action and role in clinical practice. Mayo Clin Proc. 2008;83(9): 1032–45.

Eastell R, Arnold A, Brandi ML, Brown EM, D'Amour P, Hanley DA, et al. Diagnosis of asymptomatic primary hyperparathyroidism: proceedings of the third international workshop. J Clin Endocrinol Metab. 2009;94(2):340–50.

Eastell R, Rosen CJ, Black DM, Cheung AM, Murad MH, Shoback D. Pharmacological management of osteoporosis in postmenopausal women: an Endocrine Society clinical practice guideline. J Clin Endocrinol Metab. 2019;104(5):1595–1622.

Ebeling PR. Approach to the patient with transplantation-related bone loss. J Clin Endocrinol Metab. 2009;94(5):1483–90.

Ebeling PR. Clinical practice. Osteoporosis in men. N Engl J Med. 2008;358(14):1474–82.

Fernandez-Rebollo E, Barrio R, Perez-Nanclares G, Carcavilla A, et al. New mutation type in pseudohypoparathyroidism type Ia. Clin Endocrinol (Oxf). 2008;69(5):705–12.

Fernandez-Rebollo E, Garcia-Cuartero B, Garin I, Largo C, Martinez F, Garcia-Lacalle C, et al. Intragenic GNAS deletion involving exon A/B in pseudohypoparathyroidism type 1A resulting in an apparent loss of exon A/B methylation: potential for misdiagnosis of pseudohypoparathyroidism type 1B. J Clin Endocrinol Metab. 2010; 95(2):765–71.

Finkelstein JS, Wyland JJ, Lee H, Neer RM. Effects of teriparatide, alendronate, or both in women with postmenopausal osteoporosis. J Clin Endocrinol Metab. 2010;95(4):1838–45.

Fraser WD. Hyperparathyroidism. Lancet. 2009;374(9684):145–58.

Glorieux FH. Experience with bisphosphonates in osteogenesis imperfecta. Pediatrics. 2007;119(Suppl 2):S163–5.

Goasguen N, Chirica M, Roger N, Munoz-Bongrand N, Zohar S, Noullet S, et al. Primary hyperparathyroidism from parathyroid microadenoma: specific features and implications for a surgical strategy in the era of minimally invasive parathyroidectomy. J Am Coll Surg. 2010;210(4):456–62.

Goji K, Ozaki K, Sadewa AH, Nishio H, Matsuo M. Somatic and germline mosaicism for a mutation of the PHEX gene can lead to genetic transmission of X-linked hypophosphatemic rickets that mimics an autosomal dominant trait. J Clin Endocrinol Metab. 2006;91(2):365–70.

Hannan FM, Babinsky VN, Thakker RV. Disorders of the calcium-sensing receptor and partner proteins: insights into the molecular basis of calcium homeostasis. J Mol Endocrinol. 2016;57(3):R127–42.

Harrison B. What steps should be considered in the patient who has had a negative cervical exploration for primary hyperparathyroidism? Clin Endocrinol (Oxf). 2009;71(5):624–7.

Hartley IR, Miller CB, Papadakis GZ, Bergwitz C, Del Rivero J, Blau JE, et al. Targeted FGFR blockade for the treatment of tumor-induced osteomalacia. N Engl J Med. 2020;383(14):1387–89.

Hofmann CE, Harmatz P, Vockley J, Högler W, Nakayama H, Bishop N, et al. Efficacy and safety of asfotase alfa in infants and young children with hypophosphatasia: a phase 2 open-label study. J Clin Endocrinol Metab. 2019;104(7):2735–47.

Holick MF. High prevalence of vitamin D inadequacy and implications for health. Mayo Clin Proc. 2006;81(3):353–73.

Holmes J, Lazarus A. Sarcoidosis: extrathoracic manifestations. Dis Mon. 2009;55(11):675–92.

Husebye ES. Functional autoantibodies cause hypoparathyroidism. J Clin Endocrinol Metab. 2009;94(12):4655–7.

Ichikawa S, Sorenson AH, Imel EA, Friedman NE, Gertner JM, Econs MJ. Intronic deletions in the SLC34A3 gene cause hereditary hypophosphatemic rickets with hypercalciuria. J Clin Endocrinol Metab. 2006;91(10):4022–7.

Imanishi Y, Ito N, Rhee Y, Takeuchi Y, Shin CS, Takahashi Y, et al. Interim analysis of a phase 2 open-label trial assessing burosumab efficacy and safety in patients with tumor-induced osteomalacia. J Bone Miner Res. 2021;36(2):262–70.

Imel EA, Peacock M, Pitukcheewanont P, Heller HJ, Ward LM, Shulman D, et al. Sensitivity of fibroblast growth factor 23 measurements in tumor-induced osteomalacia. J Clin Endocrinol Metab. 2006;91(6):2055–61.

Jan de Beur SM. Tumor-induced osteomalacia. JAMA. 2005;294(10): 1260–7.

Jehan F, Gaucher C, Nguyen TM, Walrant-Debray O, Lahlou N, Sinding C, et al. Vitamin D receptor genotype in hypophosphatemic rickets as a predictor of growth and response to treatment. J Clin Endocrinol Metab. 2008;93(12):4672–82.

Joshi D, Center Jr, Eisman JA. Investigation of incidental hypercalcaemia. BMJ. 2009;339:b4613.

Jovanovic M, Guterman-Ram G, Marini JC. Osteogenesis imperfecta: mechanisms and signaling pathways connecting classical and rare OI types. Endocr Rev. 2022;43(1):61–90.

Kallmes DF, Comstock BA, Heagerty PJ, Turner JA, Wilson DJ, et al. A randomized trial of vertebroplasty for osteoporotic spinal fractures. N Engl J Med. 2009;361(6):569–79.

Khosla S. Increasing options for the treatment of osteoporosis. N Engl J Med. 2009;361(8):818–20.

Khosla S. Update in male osteoporosis. J Clin Endocrinol Metab. 2010;95(1):3–10.

Khosla S, Melton LJ, 3rd. Clinical practice. Osteopenia. N Engl J Med. 2007;356(22):2293–300.

Khosla S, Westendorf JJ, Oursler MJ. Building bone to reverse osteoporosis and repair fractures. J Clin Invest. 2008;118(2):421–8.

Kishnani PS, Rockman-Greenberg C, Rauch F, Bhatti MT, Moseley S, Denker AE, et al. Five-year efficacy and safety of asfotase alfa therapy for adults and adolescents with hypophosphatasia. Bone. 2019;121:149–62.

Kitanaka S, Murayama A, Sakaki T, Inouye K, Seino Y, Fukumoto S, et al. No enzyme activity of 25-hydroxyvitamin D3 1alpha-hydroxylase gene product in pseudovitamin D deficiency rickets, including that with mild clinical manifestation. J Clin Endocrinol Metab. 1999; 84(11):4111–17.

Kitanaka S, Takeyama K, Murayama A, Sato T, Okumura K, Nogami M, et al. Inactivating mutations in the 25-hydroxyvitamin D3 1alpha-hydroxylase gene in patients with pseudovitamin D-deficiency rickets. N Engl J Med. 1998;338(10):653–61.

Lew JI, Solorzano CC. Surgical management of primary hyperparathyroidism: state of the art. Surg Clin North Am. 2009;89(5):1205–25.

Linglart A, Menguy C, Couvineau A, Auzan C, Gunes Y, Cancel M, et al. Recurrent PRKAR1A mutation in acrodysostosis with hormone resistance. N Engl J Med. 2011;364(23):2218–26.

Lloyd RV, Douglas BR, Young WF Jr. Parathyroid gland. In: King DW, editor. Atlas of Nontumor Pathology: Endocrine Diseases. American Registry of Pathology and the Armed Forces Institute of Pathology; 2002.

Lopes MP, Kliemann BS, Bini IB, Kulchetscki R, Borsani V, Savi L, et al. Hypoparathyroidism and pseudohypoparathyroidism: etiology, laboratory features and complications. Arch Endocrinol Metab. 2016; 60(6):532–36.

Ma RC, Cockram CS. Pseudopseudohypoparathyroidism. Lancet. 2009;374(9707):2090.

Management of Postmenopausal Osteoporosis: ACOG Clinical Practice Guideline No. 2. Obstet Gynecol. 2022;139(4):698–717.

Mantovani G, de Sanctis L, Barbieri AM, Elli FM, Bollati V, Vaira V, et al. Pseudohypoparathyroidism and GNAS epigenetic defects: clinical evaluation of Albright hereditary osteodystrophy and molecular analysis in 40 patients. J Clin Endocrinol Metab. 2010;95(2):651–8.

Marom R, Rabenhorst BM, Morello R. Osteogenesis imperfecta: an update on clinical features and therapies. Eur J Endocrinol. 2020; 183(4):R95–106.

Medarov BI. Milk-alkali syndrome. Mayo Clin Proc. 2009;84(3):261–7.

Mei Y, Zhang H, Zhang Z. Comparing clinical and genetic characteristics of de novo and inherited COL1A1/COL1A2 variants in a large chinese cohort of osteogenesis imperfecta. Front Endocrinol (Lausanne). 2022;13:935905

Menezes AH. Osteogenesis imperfecta. J Neurosurg. 2006;105(3):359; discussion 359–60.

Milkman LA. Pseudofractures (hunger osteopathy, late rickets, osteomalacia): Report of a case. Am J Roentgenol. 1930;24:29–37.

Minisola S, Fukumoto S, Xia W, Corsi A, Colangelo L, Scillitani A, et al. Tumor-induced osteomalacia: a comprehensive review. Endocr Rev. 2023;44(2):323–53.

Mornet E. Hypophosphatasia. Best Pract Res Clin Rheumatol. 2008; 22(1):113–27.

Nayak S, Greenspan SL. Bisphosphonate drug holidays. Osteoporos Int. 2019;30(12):2525.

Pasieka JL, Parsons L, Jones J. The long-term benefit of parathyroidectomy in primary hyperparathyroidism: a 10-year prospective surgical outcome study. Surgery. 2009;146(6):1006–13.

Peach CA, Zhang Y, Wordsworth BP. Mutations of the tissue non-specific alkaline phosphatase gene (TNAP) causing a non-lethal case of perinatal hypophosphatasia. Rheumatology (Oxford). 2007;46(6):1037–40.

Perrier ND, Balachandran D, Wefel JS, Jimenez C, Busaidy N, Morris GS, et al. Prospective, randomized, controlled trial of parathyroidectomy versus observation in patients with "asymptomatic" primary hyperparathyroidism. Surgery. 2009;146(6):1116–22.

Petje G, Meizer R, Radler C, Aigner N, Grill F. Deformity correction in children with hereditary hypophosphatemic rickets. Clin Orthop Relat Res. 2008;466(12):3078–85.

Pilz S, Dobnig H, Nijpels G, Heine RJ, Stehouwer CD, Snijder MB, et al. Vitamin D and mortality in older men and women. Clin Endocrinol (Oxf). 2009;71(5):666–72.

Prockop DJ. Targeting gene therapy for osteogenesis imperfecta. N Engl J Med. 2004;350(22):2302–4.

Qaseem A, Forciea MA, McLean RM, Denberg TD; Clinical Guidelines Committee of the American College of Physicians, Barry MJ, et al. Treatment of low bone density or osteoporosis to prevent fractures in men and women: a clinical practice guideline update from the American College of Physicians. Ann Intern Med. 2017;166(11):818–39.

Raisz LG. Clinical practice. Screening for osteoporosis. N Engl J Med. 2005;353(2):164–71.

Ralston SH, Corral-Gudino L, Cooper C, Francis RM, Fraser WD, Gennari L, et al. Diagnosis and management of Paget's disease of bone in adults: a clinical guideline. J Bone Miner Res. 2019;34(4): 579–604.

Ralston SH, Langston AL, Reid IR. Pathogenesis and management of Paget's disease of bone. Lancet. 2008;372(9633):155–63.

Rauch F, Glorieux FH. Osteogenesis imperfecta. Lancet. 2004; 363(9418):1377–85.

Ray D, Goswami R, Gupta N, Tomar N, Singh N, Sreenivas V. Predisposition to vitamin D deficiency osteomalacia and rickets in females is linked to their 25(OH)D and calcium intake rather than vitamin D receptor gene polymorphism. Clin Endocrinol (Oxf). 2009;71(3):334–40.

Rendina D, Abate V, Cacace G, et al. Tumor-induced osteomalacia: a systematic review and individual patient's data analysis. J Clin Endocrinol Metab. 2022;107(8):e3428–36.

Riches PL, McRorie E, Fraser WD, Determann C, van't Hof R, Ralston SH. Osteoporosis associated with neutralizing autoantibodies against osteoprotegerin. N Engl J Med. 2009;361(15):1459–65.

Rosen CJ. Clinical practice. Postmenopausal osteoporosis. N Engl J Med. 2005;353(6):595–603.

Ruda JM, Hollenbeak CS, Stack BC Jr. A systematic review of the diagnosis and treatment of primary hyperparathyroidism from 1995 to 2003. Otolaryngol Head Neck Surg. 2005;132(3):359–72.

Saintonge S, Bang H, Gerber LM. Implications of a new definition of vitamin D deficiency in a multiracial us adolescent population: the National Health and Nutrition Examination Survey III. Pediatrics. 2009;123(3):797–803.

Saul D, Khosla S. Fracture healing in the setting of endocrine diseases, aging, and cellular senescence. Endocr Rev. 2022;43(6):984–1002.

Sawamura K, Kitoh H, Kaneko H, Kitamura A, Hattori T. Prognostic factors for mobility in children with osteogenesis imperfecta. Medicine (Baltimore). 2022;101(36):e30521.

Shoback D. Clinical practice. Hypoparathyroidism. N Engl J Med. 2008;359(4):391–403.

Shoback D. Update in osteoporosis and metabolic bone disorders. J Clin Endocrinol Metab. 2007;92(3):747–53.

Shoback D, Rosen CJ, Black DM, Cheung AM, Murad MH, Eastell R. Pharmacological management of osteoporosis in postmenopausal women: an Endocrine Society Guideline Update. J Clin Endocrinol Metab. 2020;105(3):dgaa048.

Singer FR, Bone HG 3rd, Hosking DJ, Lyles KW, Murad MH, Reid IR, et al. Paget's disease of bone: an Endocrine Society clinical practice guideline. J Clin Endocrinol Metab. 2014;99(12):4408–22.

Singh Ospina N, Thompson GB, Lee RA, Reading CC, Young WF Jr. Safety and efficacy of percutaneous parathyroid ethanol ablation in patients with recurrent primary hyperparathyroidism and multiple endocrine neoplasia type 1. J Clin Endocrinol Metab. 2015;100(1):E87–90.

Stewart AF. Clinical practice. Hypercalcemia associated with cancer. N Engl J Med. 2005;352(4):373–9.

Sun L, Hu J, Liu J, Zhang Q, Wang O, Jiang Y, et al. Relationship of pathogenic mutations and responses to zoledronic acid in a cohort of osteogenesis imperfecta children. J Clin Endocrinol Metab. 2022;107(9):2571–79.

Tay YD, Tabacco G, Cusano NE, Williams J, Omeragic B, Majeed R, et al. Therapy of hypoparathyroidism with rhPTH(1-84): a prospective, 8-year investigation of efficacy and safety. J Clin Endocrinol Metab. 2019;104(11):5601–10.

Tencza AL, Ichikawa S, Dang A, Kenagy D, McCarthy E, Econs MJ, et al. Hypophosphatemic rickets with hypercalciuria due to mutation in SLC34A3/type IIc sodium-phosphate cotransporter: presentation as hypercalciuria and nephrolithiasis. J Clin Endocrinol Metab. 2009;94(11):4433–8.

Thacher TD, Obadofin MO, O'Brien KO, Abrams SA. The effect of vitamin D2 and vitamin D3 on intestinal calcium absorption in Nigerian children with rickets. J Clin Endocrinol Metab. 2009;94(9):3314–21.

Unnanuntana A, Gladnick BP, Donnelly E, Lane JM. The assessment of fracture risk. J Bone Joint Surg Am. 2010;92(3):743–53.

Wagner CL, Greer FR. Prevention of rickets and vitamin D deficiency in infants, children, and adolescents. Pediatrics. 2008;122(5):1142–52.

Watts NB, Diab DL. Long-term use of bisphosphonates in osteoporosis. J Clin Endocrinol Metab. 2010;95(4):1555–65.

Weinstein RS, Roberson PK, Manolagas SC. Giant osteoclast formation and long-term oral bisphosphonate therapy. N Engl J Med. 2009;360(1):53–62.

Whyte MP. Clinical practice. Paget's disease of bone. N Engl J Med. 2006;355(6):593–600.

Whyte MP, Greenberg CR, Salman NJ, Bober MB, McAlister WH, Wenkert D, et al. Enzyme-replacement therapy in life-threatening hypophosphatasia. N Engl J Med. 2012;366(10):904–13.

Winer KK. Advances in the treatment of hypoparathyroidism with PTH 1-34. Bone. 2019;120:535–41.

Yu N, Donnan PT, Murphy MJ, Leese GP. Epidemiology of primary hyperparathyroidism in Tayside, Scotland, UK. Clin Endocrinol (Oxf). 2009;71(4):485–93.

Section 7 Lipids and Nutrition

Aasheim ET, Hofso D, Sovik TT. Vitamin supplements after bariatric surgery. Clin Endocrinol (Oxf). 2010;72(1):134–5.

Abel LA, Walterfang M, Fietz M, Bowman EA, Velakoulis D. Saccades in adult Niemann-Pick disease type C reflect frontal, brainstem, and biochemical deficits. Neurology. 2009;72(12):1083–6.

Alberti KG, Eckel RH, Grundy SM, Zimmet PZ, Cleeman JI, Donato KA, et al. Harmonizing the metabolic syndrome: a joint interim statement of the International Diabetes Federation Task Force on Epidemiology and Prevention; National Heart, Lung, and Blood Institute; American Heart Association; World Heart Federation; International Atherosclerosis Society; and International Association for the Study of Obesity. Circulation. 2009;120(16):1640–5.

Ambrose JA, Srikanth S. Vulnerable plaques and patients: improving prediction of future coronary events. Am J Med. 2010;123(1):10–6.

Anagnostis P, Athyros VG, Tziomalos K, Karagiannis A, Mikhailidis DP. Clinical review: the pathogenetic role of cortisol in the metabolic syndrome: a hypothesis. J Clin Endocrinol Metab. 2009;94(8):2692–701.

Angelidi AM, Belanger MJ, Kokkinos A, Koliaki CC, Mantzoros CS. Novel noninvasive approaches to the treatment of obesity: from pharmacotherapy to gene therapy. Endocr Rev. 2022;43(3):507–557.

Arnlov J, Ingelsson E, Sundstrom J, Lind L. Impact of body mass index and the metabolic syndrome on the risk of cardiovascular disease and death in middle-aged men. Circulation. 2010;121(2):230–6.

Ashen MD, Blumenthal RS. Clinical practice. Low HDL cholesterol levels. N Engl J Med. 2005;353(12):1252–60.

Ashourian N, Mousdicas N. Images in clinical medicine. Pellagra-like dermatitis. N Engl J Med. 2006;354(15):1614.

Attia E, Walsh BT. Behavioral management for anorexia nervosa. N Engl J Med. 2009;360(5):500–6.

August GP, Caprio S, Fennoy I, Freemark M, Kaufman FR, Lustig RH, et al. Prevention and treatment of pediatric obesity: an Endocrine Society clinical practice guideline based on expert opinion. J Clin Endocrinol Metab. 2008;93(12):4576–99.

Authors/Task Force Members; ESC Committee for Practice Guidelines (CPG); ESC National Cardiac Societies. 2019 ESC/EAS guidelines for the management of dyslipidaemias: Lipid modification to reduce cardiovascular risk. Atherosclerosis. 2019;290:140–205.

Bahardoust M, Eghbali F, Shahmiri SS, Alijanpour A, Yarigholi F, Valizadeh R, et al. B1 vitamin deficiency after bariatric surgery, prevalence, and symptoms: a systematic review and meta-analysis. Obes Surg. 2022;32(9):3104–12.

Batsis JA, Lopez-Jimenez F, Collazo-Clavell ML, Clark MM, Somers VK, Sarr MG. Quality of life after bariatric surgery: a population-based cohort study. Am J Med. 2009;122(11):1055 e1051–1055 e1010.

Belfort R, Berria R, Cornell J, Cusi K. Fenofibrate reduces systemic inflammation markers independent of its effects on lipid and glucose metabolism in patients with the metabolic syndrome. J Clin Endocrinol Metab. 2010;95(2):829–36.

Berberich AJ, Hegele RA. A modern approach to dyslipidemia. Endocr Rev. 2022;43(4):611–53.

Brabin B. Infant vitamin A supplementation: consensus and controversy. Lancet. 2007;369(9579):2054–6.

Braegger CP, Belli DC, Mentha G, Steinmann B. Persistence of the intestinal defect in abetalipoproteinaemia after liver transplantation. Eur J Pediatr. 1998;157(7):576–8.

Briel M, Ferreira-Gonzalez I, You JJ, Karanicolas PJ, Akl EA, Wu P, et al. Association between change in high density lipoprotein cholesterol and cardiovascular disease morbidity and mortality: systematic review and meta-regression analysis. BMJ. 2009;338:b92.

Brooks AM, Paisey RB, Waterson MJ, Smith JC. Diagnostic difficulties with a lipaemic blood sample. BMJ. 2010;340:b5530.

Brown TM, Voeks JH, Bittner V, Safford MM. Variations in prevalent cardiovascular disease and future risk by metabolic syndrome classification in the REasons for Geographic and Racial Differences in Stroke (REGARDS) study. Am Heart J. 2010;159(3):385–91.

Brunzell JD. Clinical practice. Hypertriglyceridemia. N Engl J Med. 2007;357(10):1009–17.

Buch A, Marcus Y, Shefer G, Zimmet P, Stern N. Approach to obesity in the older population. J Clin Endocrinol Metab. 2021;106(9):2788–2805.

Califf RM, Harrington RA, Blazing MA. Premature release of data from clinical trials of ezetimibe. N Engl J Med. 2009;361(7):712–17.

Carlsson LMS, Sjöholm K, Jacobson P, Andersson-Assarsson JC, Svensson PA, Taube M, et al. Life expectancy after bariatric surgery in the Swedish Obese Subjects study. N Engl J Med. 2020;383(16):1535–1543.

Carpenter KJ. The history of scurvy and vitamin C. Cambridge University Press; 1986.

Cheng TO. Lind's SCURVY trial. J Lab Clin Med. 2004;144(1):53.

Chillaron JJ, Goday A, Flores-Le-Roux JA, Benaiges D, Carrera MJ, Puig J, et al. Estimated glucose disposal rate in assessment of the metabolic syndrome and microvascular complications in patients with type 1 diabetes. J Clin Endocrinol Metab. 2009;94(9):3530–4.

Cho NH, Chan JC, Jang HC, Lim S, Kim HL, Choi SH. Cigarette smoking is an independent risk factor for type 2 diabetes: a four-year community-based prospective study. Clin Endocrinol (Oxf). 2009;71(5):679–85.

Choh CT, Rai S, Abdelhamid M, Lester W, Vohra RK. Unrecognised scurvy. BMJ. 2009;339:b3580.

Chou R, Dana T, Blazina I, Daeges M, Jeanne TL. Statins for prevention of cardiovascular disease in adults: evidence report and systematic review for the US Preventive Services Task Force. JAMA. 2016;316(19):2008.

Civeira F, Jarauta E, Cenarro A, Garcia-Otin AL, Tejedor D, Zambon D, et al. Frequency of low-density lipoprotein receptor gene mutations in patients with a clinical diagnosis of familial combined hyperlipidemia in a clinical setting. J Am Coll Cardiol. 2008;52(19):1546–53.

Civeira F, Ros E, Jarauta E, Plana N, Zambon D, Puzo J, et al. Comparison of genetic versus clinical diagnosis in familial hypercholesterolemia. Am J Cardiol. 2008;102(9):1187–93.

Cole RP. Heparin treatment for severe hypertriglyceridemia in diabetic ketoacidosis. Arch Intern Med. 2009;169(15):1439–41.

Comabella M, Canton A, Montalban X, Codina A. Iatrogenic fulminant beriberi. Lancet. 1995;346(8968):182–3.

Crane AM. Anorexia nervosa. Awareness is key. BMJ. 2010;340:c295.

Crow SJ, Peterson CB, Swanson SA, Raymond NC, Specker S, Eckert ED, et al. Increased mortality in bulimia nervosa and other eating disorders. Am J Psychiatry. 2009;166(12):1342–6.

Davidson MH, Rosenson RS. Novel targets that affect high-density lipoprotein metabolism: the next frontier. Am J Cardiol. 2009;104 (10 Suppl):52E–7E.

Davis HR Jr, Murgolo NJ, Graziano MP. Simvastatin with or without ezetimibe in familial hypercholesterolemia. N Engl J Med. 2008;359(5):531; author reply 532–3.

Deedwania P, Singh V, Davidson MH. Low high-density lipoprotein cholesterol and increased cardiovascular disease risk: an analysis of statin clinical trials. Am J Cardiol. 2009;104(10 Suppl):3E–9E.

Di Sabatino A, Corazza GR. Coeliac disease. Lancet. 2009;373(9673):1480–93.

Diagnostic and Statistical Manual of Mental Disorders: DSM-5-TR. 5th ed. American Psychiatric Association; 2022.

Dietz WH, Robinson TN. Clinical practice. Overweight children and adolescents. N Engl J Med. 2005;352(20):2100–9.

Ding EL, Smit LA, Hu FB. The metabolic syndrome as a cluster of risk factors: is the whole greater than the sum of its parts?: comment on "The metabolic syndrome, its component risk factors, and progression of coronary atherosclerosis." Arch Intern Med. 2010;170(5):484–5.

Dod HS, Bhardwaj R, Sajja V, Weidner G, Hobbs GR, Konat GW, et al. Effect of intensive lifestyle changes on endothelial function and on inflammatory markers of atherosclerosis. Am J Cardiol. 2010;105 (3):362–7.

Donnino M. Gastrointestinal beriberi: a previously unrecognized syndrome. Ann Intern Med. 2004;141(11):898–9.

Doosti M, Najafi M, Reza JZ, Nikzamir A. The role of ATP-binding-cassette-transporter-A1 (ABCA1) gene polymorphism on coronary artery disease risk. Transl Res. 2010;155(4):185–90.

Duggan CP, Westra SJ, Rosenberg AE. Case records of the Massachusetts General Hospital. Case 23–2007. A 9-year-old boy with bone pain, rash, and gingival hypertrophy. N Engl J Med. 2007;357(4):392–400.

Eckel RH. Clinical practice. Nonsurgical management of obesity in adults. N Engl J Med. 2008;358(18):1941–50.

Eckel RH, Alberti KG, Grundy SM, Zimmet PZ. The metabolic syndrome. Lancet. 2010;375(9710):181–3.

Fasano A, Leonard MM, Mitchell DM, Eng G. Case 1-2020: an 11-year-old boy with vomiting and weight loss. N Engl J Med. 2020;382(2):180–89.

Fazio S, Guyton Jr, Polis AB, Adewale AJ, Tomassini JE, Ryan NW, et al. Long-term safety and efficacy of triple combination ezetimibe/simvastatin plus extended-release niacin in patients with hyperlipidemia. Am J Cardiol. 2010;105(4):487–94.

Fletcher RH, Fairfield KM. Vitamins for chronic disease prevention in adults: clinical applications. JAMA. 2002;287(23):3127–9.

Ford ES, Li C, Zhao G, Pearson WS, Mokdad AH. Hypertriglyceridemia and its pharmacologic treatment among US adults. Arch Intern Med. 2009;169(6):572–8.

Franks PW, Hanson RL, Knowler WC, Sievers ML, Bennett PH, Looker HC. Childhood obesity, other cardiovascular risk factors, and premature death. N Engl J Med. 2010;362(6):485–93.

Fredrickson DS. The inheritance of high density lipoprotein deficiency (Tangier disease). J Clin Invest. 1964;43:228–36.

Garcia-Otin AL, Cofan M, Junyent M, Recalde D, Cenarro A, Pocovi M, et al. Increased intestinal cholesterol absorption in autosomal dominant hypercholesterolemia and no mutations in the low-density lipoprotein receptor or apolipoprotein B genes. J Clin Endocrinol Metab. 2007;92(9):3667–73.

Gencer B, Marston NA, Im K, Cannon CP, Sever P, Keech A, Braunwald E, Giugliano RP, Sabatine MS. Efficacy and safety of lowering LDL cholesterol in older patients: a systematic review and meta-analysis of randomised controlled trials. Lancet. 2020;396 (10263):1637–43.

Ghali WA, Rodondi N. HDL cholesterol and cardiovascular risk. BMJ. 2009;338:a3065.

Girish MP, Gupta MD. Xanthomatous pseudospectacles in familial hypercholesterolemia. N Engl J Med. 2005;352(23):2424.

Goldberger J. The etiology of pellagra. 1914. Public Health Rep. 2006;121(Suppl 1):77–9; discussion 76.

Gottlieb MG. V, Mancia da Cruz IB, Duarte MM.F, Moresco RN, Wiehe M, Schwanke CH.A, Bodanese LC. Associations among metabolic syndrome, ischemia, inflammatory, oxidatives, and lipids biomarkers. J Clin Endocrinol Metab. 2010;95:586–91.

Grabowski GA. Phenotype, diagnosis, and treatment of Gaucher's disease. Lancet. 2008;372(9645):1263–71.

Graham GG. Starvation in the modern world. N Engl J Med. 1993;328 (14):1058–61.

Grundy SM, Stone NJ, Bailey AL, Beam C, Birtcher KK, Blumenthal RS, et al. 2018 AHA/ACC/AACVPR/AAPA/ABC/ACPM/ADA/AGS/APhA/ASPC/NLA/PCNA Guideline on the management of blood cholesterol: a report of the American College of Cardiology/American Heart Association Task Force on Clinical Practice Guidelines. Circulation. 2019;139(25):e1082–143.

Guardamagna O, Restagno G, Rolfo E, Pederiva C, Martini S, Abello F, et al. The type of LDLR gene mutation predicts cardiovascular risk in children with familial hypercholesterolemia. J Pediatr. 2009;155(2):199–204 e192.
Gull AT. On certain affection of the skin, vitilogoidea—(a) plana: (b) tubersosa with remarks. Guy's Hosp Rep. 1851;7.
Gustafson JK, Yanoff LB, Easter BD, Brady SM, Keil MF, Roberts MD, et al. The stability of metabolic syndrome in children and adolescents. J Clin Endocrinol Metab. 2009;94(12):4828–34.
Hayes BB, Boyd AS. Eruptive xanthomas. Papules may indicate underlying lipid disorder. Postgrad Med. 2005;118(2):11–2.
Hiatt WR, Smith RJ. Assessing the clinical benefits of lipid-disorder drugs. N Engl J Med. 2014;370(5):396–9.
Houston MC, Fazio S, Chilton FH, Wise DE, Jones KB, Barringer TA, et al. Nonpharmacologic treatment of dyslipidemia. Prog Cardiovasc Dis. 2009;52(2):61–94.
Höybye C, Tauber M. Approach to the patient with Prader-Willi syndrome. J Clin Endocrinol Metab. 2022;107(6):1698–1705.
Kamanna VS, Kashyap ML. Mechanism of action of niacin. Am J Cardiol. 2008;101(8A):20B–6B.
Karthiga S, Dubey S, Garber S, Watts R. Scurvy: MRI appearances. Rheumatology (Oxford). 2008;47(7):1109.
Kastelein JJ, Bots ML. Statin therapy with ezetimibe or niacin in high-risk patients. N Engl J Med. 2009;361(22):2180–3.
Kim BK, Hong SJ, Lee YJ, Hong SJ, Yun KH, Hong BK, et al. Long-term efficacy and safety of moderate-intensity statin with ezetimibe combination therapy versus high-intensity statin monotherapy in patients with atherosclerotic cardiovascular disease (RACING): a randomised, open-label, non-inferiority trial. Lancet. 2022;400(10349):380–90.
Ladenson PW, Kristensen JD, Ridgway EC, Olsson AG, Carlsson B, Klein I, et al. Use of the thyroid hormone analogue eprotirome in statin-treated dyslipidemia. N Engl J Med. 2010;362(10):906–16.
Lawson EA, Donoho D, Miller KK, Misra M, Meenaghan E, Lydecker J, et al. Hypercortisolemia is associated with severity of bone loss and depression in hypothalamic amenorrhea and anorexia nervosa. J Clin Endocrinol Metab. 2009;94(12):4710–16.
Leff DR, Heath D. Surgery for obesity in adulthood. BMJ. 2009;339: b3402.
Leggett J, Convery R. Images in clinical medicine. Scurvy. N Engl J Med. 2001;345(25):1818.
Lewington S, Clarke R, Qizilbash N, Peto R, Collins R; Prospective Studies Collaboration. Age-specific relevance of usual blood pressure to vascular mortality: a meta-analysis of individual data for one million adults in 61 prospective studies. Lancet. 2002; 360(9349):1903–13.
Li SG. Images in clinical medicine. Familial hypercholesterolemia. N Engl J Med. 2009;360(18):1885.
Libby P, Ridker PM, Hansson GK. Inflammation in atherosclerosis: from pathophysiology to practice. J Am Coll Cardiol. 2009;54 (23):2129–38.
Livingston EH. Surgical treatment of obesity in adolescence. JAMA. 2010;303(6):559–60.
Logue J, Thompson L, Romanes F, Wilson DC, Thompson J, Sattar N. Management of obesity: summary of SIGN guideline. BMJ. 2010; 340:c154.
Ludvigsson JF, Montgomery SM, Ekbom A, Brandt L, Granath F. Small-intestinal histopathology and mortality risk in celiac disease. JAMA. 2009;302(11):1171–8.
Malinowski SS. Nutritional and metabolic complications of bariatric surgery. Am J Med Sci. 2006;331(4):219–25.
Mantaring M, Rhyne J, Ho Hong S, Miller M. Genotypic variation in ATP-binding cassette transporter-1 (ABCA1) as contributors to the high and low high-density lipoprotein-cholesterol (HDL-C) phenotype. Transl Res. 2007;149(4):205–10.
Marston NA, Giugliano RP, Im K, Silverman MG, O'Donoghue ML, Wiviott SD, et al. Association between triglyceride lowering and reduction of cardiovascular risk across multiple lipid-lowering therapeutic classes: a systematic review and meta-regression analysis of randomized controlled trials. Circulation. 2019;140(16): 1308–17.
Martins AM, Valadares ER, Porta G, Coelho J, Semionato Filho J, Pianovski MA, et al. Recommendations on diagnosis, treatment, and monitoring for Gaucher disease. J Pediatr. 2009;155(4 Suppl):S10–18.
Masana L, Ibarretxe D, Plana N. Reasons why combination therapy should be the new standard of care to achieve the LDL-cholesterol targets: lipid-lowering combination therapy. Curr Cardiol Rep. 2020; 22(8):66.
Mathieu P, Lemieux I, Despres JP. Obesity, inflammation, and cardiovascular risk. Clin Pharmacol Ther. 2010;87(4):407–16.
Matrana MR, Vasireddy S, Davis WE. The skinny on a growing problem: dry beriberi after bariatric surgery. Ann Intern Med. 2008;149(11):842–4.
McGowan KE, Castiglione DA, Butzner JD. The changing face of childhood celiac disease in North America: impact of serological testing. Pediatrics. 2009;124(6):1572–8.
McKnight R, Boughton N. A patient's journey. Anorexia nervosa. BMJ. 2009;339:b3800.
Mehler PS. Clinical practice. Bulimia nervosa. N Engl J Med. 2003; 349(9):875–81.
Mitchell JE, Peterson CB. Anorexia nervosa. N Engl J Med. 2020; 382(14):1343–51.
Moreno PR, Sanz J, Fuster V. Promoting mechanisms of vascular health: circulating progenitor cells, angiogenesis, and reverse cholesterol transport. J Am Coll Cardiol. 2009;53(25):2315–23.
Mulleman D, Goupille P. Medical mystery: extensive ecchymosis—the answer. N Engl J Med. 2006;354(4):419–20.
Mziray-Andrew CH, Sentongo TA. Nutritional deficiencies in intestinal failure. Pediatr Clin North Am. 2009;56(5):1185–200.
Natarajan P, Ray KK, Cannon CP. High-density lipoprotein and coronary heart disease: current and future therapies. J Am Coll Cardiol. 2010;55(13):1283–99.
National Cholesterol Education Program (NCEP) Expert Panel on Detection Evaluation, and Treatment of High Blood Cholesterol in Adults (Adult Treatment Panel III). Third Report of the National Cholesterol Education Program (NCEP) Expert Panel on Detection, Evaluation, and Treatment of High Blood Cholesterol in Adults (Adult Treatment Panel III) final report. Circulation. 2002;106 (25):3143–421.
Navab M, Anantharamaiah GM, Reddy ST, Van Lenten BJ, Fogelman AM. HDL as a biomarker, potential therapeutic target, and therapy. Diabetes. 2009;58(12):2711–17.
Nayak KR, Daly RG. Images in clinical medicine. Eruptive xanthomas associated with hypertriglyceridemia and new-onset diabetes mellitus. N Engl J Med. 2004;350(12):1235.
Newman CB, Blaha MJ, Boord JB, Cariou B, Chait A, Fein HG, Ginsberg HN, Goldberg IJ, Murad MH, Subramanian S, Tannock LR. Lipid management in patients with endocrine disorders: an Endocrine Society clinical practice guideline. J Clin Endocrinol Metab. 2020;105(12):dgaa674.
Nichols GA, Ambegaonkar BM, Sazonov V, Brown JB. Frequency of obtaining national cholesterol education program adult treatment panel III goals for all major serum lipoproteins after initiation of lipid altering therapy. Am J Cardiol. 2009;104(12):1689–94.
O'Brien PE, Sawyer SM, Laurie C, Brown WA, Skinner S, Veit F, et al. Laparoscopic adjustable gastric banding in severely obese adolescents: a randomized trial. JAMA. 2010;303(6):519–26.
O'Connell J, Murray JA, Kaukinen K. Uncertain diagnosis of celiac disease and implications for management. N Engl J Med. 2021; 384(24):2346–48.
O'Mahony C, Elliott P. Anderson-Fabry disease and the heart. Prog Cardiovasc Dis. 2010;52(4):326–35.
Ouchi Y, Sasaki J, Arai H, Yokote K, Harada K, Katayama Y, et al. Ezetimibe lipid-lowering trial on prevention of atherosclerotic cardiovascular disease in 75 or older (EWTOPIA 75): a randomized, controlled trial. Circulation. 2019;140(12):992–1003.
Pasquali R, Casanueva F, Haluzik M, van Hulsteijn L, Ledoux S, Monteiro MP, Salvador J, Santini F, Toplak H, Dekkers OM. European Society of Endocrinology Clinical Practice Guideline: endocrine work-up in obesity. Eur J Endocrinol. 2020;182(1):G1-G32.
Pemberton J. Unrecognised scurvy. Signs and requirements. BMJ. 2010; 340:c590.
Penniston KL, Tanumihardjo SA. The acute and chronic toxic effects of vitamin A. Am J Clin Nutr. 2006;83(2):191–201.
Pournaras DJ, le Roux CW. After bariatric surgery, what vitamins should be measured and what supplements should be given? Clin Endocrinol (Oxf). 2009;71(3):322–5.
Preiss D, Sattar N. Lipids, lipid modifying agents and cardiovascular risk: a review of the evidence. Clin Endocrinol (Oxf). 2009;70(6): 815–28.
Rader DJ, Brewer HB Jr. Abetalipoproteinemia. New insights into lipoprotein assembly and vitamin E metabolism from a rare genetic disease. JAMA. 1993;270(7):865–9.
Rajakumar K. Infantile scurvy: a historical perspective. Pediatrics. 2001;108(4):E76.
Rajakumar K. Pellagra in the United States: a historical perspective. South Med J. 2000;93(3):272–7.
Ray KK, Bays HE, Catapano AL, et al. Safety and efficacy of bempedoic acid to reduce LDL cholesterol. N Engl J Med. 2019;380: 1022–1032.
Richey R, Howdle P, Shaw E, Stokes T. Recognition and assessment of coeliac disease in children and adults: summary of NICE guidance. BMJ. 2009;338:b1684.
Ridker PM, Danielson E, Fonseca FA, Genest J, Gotto AM Jr, Kastelein JJ, et al. Reduction in C-reactive protein and LDL cholesterol and cardiovascular event rates after initiation of rosuvastatin: a prospective study of the JUPITER trial. Lancet. 2009; 373(9670):1175–82.
Robinson JG, Farnier M, Krempf M, Bergeron J, Luc G, Averna M, et al. Efficacy and safety of alirocumab in reducing lipids and cardiovascular events. N Engl J Med. 2015;372(16):1489–99.
Rosenzweig JL, Ferrannini E, Grundy SM, Haffner SM, Heine RJ, Horton ES, et al. Primary prevention of cardiovascular disease and type 2 diabetes in patients at metabolic risk: an Endocrine Society clinical practice guideline. J Clin Endocrinol Metab. 2008;93(10): 3671–89.
Rubino F, Kaplan LM, Schauer PR, Cummings DE. The Diabetes Surgery Summit consensus conference: recommendations for the evaluation and use of gastrointestinal surgery to treat type 2 diabetes mellitus. Ann Surg. 2010;251(3):399–405.
Sampietro T, Puntoni M, Bigazzi F, Pennato B, Sbrana F, Dal Pino B, et al. Images in cardiovascular medicine. Tangier disease in severely progressive coronary and peripheral artery disease. Circulation. 2009;119(20):2741–2.
Sattar N, Preiss D, Murray HM, Welsh P, Buckley BM, de Craen AJ, et al. Statins and risk of incident diabetes: a collaborative meta-analysis of randomised statin trials. Lancet. 2010;375(9716):735–42.
Schippling S, Orth M, Beisiegel U, Rosenkranz T, Vogel P, Munchau A, et al. Severe Tangier disease with a novel ABCA1 gene mutation. Neurology. 2008;71(18):1454–5.
Schuppan D, Junker Y, Barisani D. Celiac disease: from pathogenesis to novel therapies. Gastroenterology. 2009;137(6):1912–33.
Seidah NG, Prat A. The multifaceted biology of PCSK9. Endocr Rev. 2022;43(3):558–82.
Sen Sarma M, Tripathi PR. Natural history and management of liver dysfunction in lysosomal storage disorders. World J Hepatol. 2022 Oct 27;14(10):1844–61.
Shah AS, Dolan LM, Kimball TR, Gao Z, Khoury PR, Daniels SR, et al. Influence of duration of diabetes, glycemic control, and traditional cardiovascular risk factors on early atherosclerotic vascular changes in adolescents and young adults with type 2 diabetes mellitus. J Clin Endocrinol Metab. 2009;94(10):3740–5.
Shai I, Spence JD, Schwarzfuchs D, Henkin Y, Parraga G, Rudich A, et al. Dietary intervention to reverse carotid atherosclerosis. Circulation. 2010;121(10):1200–8.
Sharma M, Ansari MT, Abou-Setta AM, Soares-Weiser K, Ooi TC, Sears M, et al. Systematic review: comparative effectiveness and harms of combination therapy and monotherapy for dyslipidemia. Ann Intern Med. 2009;151(9):622–30.
Singh IM, Shishehbor MH, Ansell BJ. High-density lipoprotein as a therapeutic target: a systematic review. JAMA. 2007;298(7):786–98.
Siri-Tarino PW, Sun Q, Hu FB, Krauss RM. Saturated fat, carbohydrate, and cardiovascular disease. Am J Clin Nutr. 2010;91(3):502–9.
Skinner AC, Perrin EM, Moss LA, Skelton JA. Cardiometabolic risks and severity of obesity in children and young adults. N Engl J Med. 2015;373(14):1307–17.
Stalenhoef AF. Images in clinical medicine. Phytosterolemia and xanthomatosis. N Engl J Med. 2003;349(1):51.
Staretz-Chacham O, Lang TC, LaMarca ME, Krasnewich D, Sidransky E. Lysosomal storage disorders in the newborn. Pediatrics. 2009; 123(4):1191–207.
Stone NJ, Robinson JG, Lichtenstein AH, Goff DC Jr, Lloyd-Jones DM, Smith SC Jr, et al. Treatment of blood cholesterol to reduce atherosclerotic cardiovascular disease risk in adults: synopsis of the 2013 American College of Cardiology/American Heart Association cholesterol guideline. Ann Intern Med. 2014;160(5):339–43.
Strang AC, Hovingh GK, Stroes ES, Kastelein JJ. The genetics of high-density lipoprotein metabolism: clinical relevance for therapeutic approaches. Am J Cardiol. 2009;104(10 Suppl):22E–31E.
Styne DM, Arslanian SA, Connor EL, Farooqi IS, Murad MH, Silverstein JH, Yanovski JA. Pediatric obesity-assessment, treatment, and prevention: an Endocrine Society clinical practice guideline. J Clin Endocrinol Metab. 2017;102(3):709–57.
Subramanian S. Approach to the patient with moderate hypertriglyceridemia. J Clin Endocrinol Metab. 2022;107(6):1686–97.
Superko HR. Cardiovascular event risk: high-density lipoprotein and paraoxonase. J Am Coll Cardiol. 2009;54(14):1246–8.
Suskind DL. Nutritional deficiencies during normal growth. Pediatr Clin North Am. 2009;56(5):1035–53.
Tall AR. The effects of cholesterol ester transfer protein inhibition on cholesterol efflux. Am J Cardiol. 2009;104(10 Suppl):39E–45E.
Tanigawa H, Billheimer JT, Tohyama J, Fuki IV, Ng DS, Rothblat GH, et al. Lecithin: cholesterol acyltransferase expression has minimal effects on macrophage reverse cholesterol transport in vivo. Circulation. 2009;120(2):160–9.
Towbin A, Inge TH, Garcia VF, Roehrig HR, Clements RH, Harmon CM, et al. Beriberi after gastric bypass surgery in adolescence. J Pediatr. 2004;145(2):263–7.
Treasure J, Claudino AM, Zucker N. Eating disorders. Lancet. 2010; 375(9714):583–93.
US Preventive Services Task Force, Mangione CM, Barry MJ, Nicholson WK, Cabana M, Chelmow D, et al. Statin use for the primary prevention of cardiovascular disease in adults: US Preventive Services Task Force Recommendation Statement. JAMA. 2022; 328(8):746–53.
van der Graaf A, Fouchier SW, Vissers MN, Defesche JC, Wiegman A, Sankatsing RR, et al. Familial defective apolipoprotein B and familial hypobetalipoproteinemia in one family: two neutralizing mutations. Ann Intern Med. 2008;148(9):712–14.
Vega GL, Barlow CE, Grundy SM. Prevalence of the metabolic syndrome as influenced by the measure of obesity employed. Am J Cardiol. 2010;105(9):1306–12.
Ward H, Mitrou PN, Bowman R, Luben R, Wareham NJ, Khaw KT, et al. APOE genotype, lipids, and coronary heart disease risk: a prospective population study. Arch Intern Med. 2009;169(15):1424–9.
Weiner M, Van Eys J. The discovery of nicotinic acid as a nutrient: clinical pharmacology. In: Weiner M, editor. Nicotinic acid: Nutrient-cofactor-drug. New York: Marcel Dekker; 1983. p. 3.
Whelton PK, Carey RM, Aronow WS, Casey DE Jr, Collins KJ, Dennison Himmelfarb C, et al. 2017 ACC/AHA/AAPA/ABC/ACPM/

AGS/APhA/ASH/ASPC/NMA/PCNA guideline for the prevention, detection, evaluation, and management of high blood pressure in adults: a report of the American College of Cardiology/American Heart Association Task Force on Clinical Practice Guidelines. Circulation. 2018 Oct 23;138(17):e484–594.

Yager J, Andersen AE. Clinical practice. Anorexia nervosa. N Engl J Med. 2005;353(14):1481–8.

Zarate YA, Hopkin RJ. Fabry's disease. Lancet. 2008;372(9647): 1427–35.

Zhang Y, McGillicuddy FC, Hinkle CC, O'Neill S, Glick JM, Rothblat GH, et al. Adipocyte modulation of high-density lipoprotein cholesterol. Circulation. 2010;121(11):1347–55.

Section 8   Genetics and Endocrine Neoplasia

Akerstrom G, Stalberg P. Surgical management of MEN-1 and -2: state of the art. Surg Clin North Am. 2009;89(5):1047–68.

Alimohammadi M, Bjorklund P, Hallgren A, Pontynen N, Szinnai G, Shikama N, et al. Autoimmune polyendocrine syndrome type 1 and NALP5, a parathyroid autoantigen. N Engl J Med. 2008;358(10): 1018–28.

Anderson MS. Update in endocrine autoimmunity. J Clin Endocrinol Metab. 2008;93(10):3663–70.

Bhattacharyya S, Davar J, Dreyfus G, Caplin ME. Carcinoid heart disease. Circulation. 2007;116(24):2860–5.

Blansfield JA, Choyke L, Morita SY, Choyke PL, Pingpank JF, Alexander HR, et al. Clinical, genetic and radiographic analysis of 108 patients with von Hippel-Lindau disease (VHL) manifested by pancreatic neuroendocrine neoplasms (PNETs). Surgery. 2007;142(6):814–8; discussion 818 e811–12.

Boedeker CC, Erlic Z, Richard S, Kontny U, Gimenez-Roqueplo AP, Cascon A, et al. Head and neck paragangliomas in von Hippel-Lindau disease and multiple endocrine neoplasia type 2. J Clin Endocrinol Metab. 2009;94(5):1938–44.

Boyce AM, Collins MT. Fibrous Dysplasia/McCune-Albright syndrome: a rare, mosaic disease of Gα$_s$ activation. Endocr Rev. 2020;41(2):345–70.

Bratslavsky G, Liu JJ, Johnson AD, Sudarshan S, Choyke PL, et al. Salvage partial nephrectomy for hereditary renal cancer: feasibility and outcomes. J Urol. 2008;179(1):67–70.

Burgess J. How should the patient with multiple endocrine neoplasia type 1 (MEN 1) be followed? Clin Endocrinol (Oxf). 2010;72(1): 13–6.

Butman JA, Linehan WM, Lonser RR. Neurologic manifestations of von Hippel-Lindau disease. JAMA. 2008;300(11):1334–42.

Carney JA. Gastric stromal sarcoma, pulmonary chondroma, and extra-adrenal paraganglioma (Carney Triad): natural history, adrenocortical component, and possible familial occurrence. Mayo Clin Proc. 1999;74(6):543–52.

Carney JA, Sheps SG, Go VL, Gordon H. The triad of gastric leiomyosarcoma, functioning extra-adrenal paraganglioma and pulmonary chondroma. N Engl J Med. 1977;296(26):1517–8.

Carney JA, Stratakis CA, Young WF Jr. Adrenal cortical adenoma: the fourth component of the Carney triad and an association with subclinical Cushing syndrome. Am J Surg Pathol. 2013 Aug;37 (8):1140–9.

Clark PE, Cookson MS. The von Hippel-Lindau gene: turning discovery into therapy. Cancer. 2008;113(7 Suppl):1768–78.

Dittmar M, Kahaly GJ. Polyglandular autoimmune syndromes: immunogenetics and long-term follow-up. J Clin Endocrinol Metab. 2003;88(7):2983–92.

Elisei R, Romei C, Cosci B, Agate L, Bottici V, Molinaro E, et al. RET genetic screening in patients with medullary thyroid cancer and their relatives: experience with 807 individuals at one center. J Clin Endocrinol Metab. 2007;92(12):4725–9.

Gaal J, van Nederveen FH, Erlic Z, Korpershoek E, Oldenburg R, Boedeker CC, et al. Parasympathetic paragangliomas are part of the Von Hippel-Lindau syndrome. J Clin Endocrinol Metab. 2009;94 (11):4367–71.

Gauger PG, Doherty GM, Broome JT, Miller BS, Thompson NW. Completion pancreatectomy and duodenectomy for recurrent MEN-1 pancreaticoduodenal endocrine neoplasms. Surgery. 2009;146(4):801–6; discussion 807–808.

Gavalas NG, Kemp EH, Krohn KJ, Brown EM, Watson PF, Weetman AP. The calcium-sensing receptor is a target of autoantibodies in patients with autoimmune polyendocrine syndrome type 1. J Clin Endocrinol Metab. 2007;92(6):2107–14.

Goudet P, Murat A, Binquet C, Cardot-Bauters C, Costa A, et al. Risk factors and causes of death in MEN1 disease. A GTE (Groupe d'Etude des Tumeurs Endocrines) cohort study among 758 patients. World J Surg. 2010;34(2):249–55.

Haller F, Moskalev EA, Faucz FR, et al. Aberrant DNA hypermethylation of SDHC: a novel mechanism of tumor development in Carney triad. Endocr Relat Cancer. 2014;21(4):567–77.

Jagannathan J, Lonser RR, Smith R, DeVroom HL, Oldfield EH. Surgical management of cerebellar hemangioblastomas in patients with von Hippel-Lindau disease. J Neurosurg. 2008;108(2):210–22.

Javaid MK, Boyce A, Appelman-Dijkstra N, et al. Best practice management guidelines for fibrous dysplasia/McCune-Albright syndrome: a consensus statement from the FD/MAS international consortium. Orphanet J Rare Dis. 2019;14(1):139.

Jensen RT, Berna MJ, Bingham DB, Norton JA. Inherited pancreatic endocrine tumor syndromes: advances in molecular pathogenesis, diagnosis, management, and controversies. Cancer. 2008;113(7 Suppl):1807–43.

Juskewich JE, Carney JA, Alexander MP. The case of index patient of Carney Triad: a clinical puzzle and an epigenetic solution. Am J Surg Pathol: Reviews and Reports. 2017;22:54–7.

Kamaoui I, De-Luca V, Ficarelli S, Mennesson N, Lombard-Bohas C, Pilleul F. Value of CT enteroclysis in suspected small-bowel carcinoid tumors. AJR Am J Roentgenol. 2010;194(3):629–33.

Krauss T, Ferrara AM, Links TP, Wellner U, Bancos I, Kvachenyuk A, et al. Preventive medicine of von Hippel-Lindau disease-associated pancreatic neuroendocrine tumors. Endocr Relat Cancer. 2018;25 (9):783–93.

Lloyd RV, Douglas BR, Young WF Jr. Diffuse neuroendocrine system. In: King DW, editor. Atlas of Nontumor Pathology: Endocrine Diseases. American Registry of Pathology and the Armed Forces Institute of Pathology; 2002.

Messiaen L, Yao S, Brems H, Callens T, Sathienkijkanchai A, et al. Clinical and mutational spectrum of neurofibromatosis type 1-like syndrome. JAMA. 2009;302(19):2111–18.

Morrow EH, Norton JA. Surgical management of Zollinger-Ellison syndrome; state of the art. Surg Clin North Am. 2009;89(5): 1091–103.

Neumann HP, Vortmeyer A, Schmidt D, Werner M, Erlic Z, et al. Evidence of MEN-2 in the original description of classic pheochromocytoma. N Engl J Med. 2007;357(13):1311–15.

Nunley KS, Gao F, Albers AC, Bayliss SJ, Gutmann DH. Predictive value of cafe au lait macules at initial consultation in the diagnosis of neurofibromatosis type 1. Arch Dermatol. 2009;145(8):883–7.

Pasieka JL. Carcinoid tumors. Surg Clin North Am. 2009;89(5): 1123–37.

Pitsava G, Settas N, Faucz FR, Stratakis CA. Carney triad, Carney-Stratakis syndrome, 3PAS and other tumors due to SDH deficiency. Front Endocrinol (Lausanne). 2021;12:680609.

Powell AC, Libutti SK. Multiple endocrine neoplasia type 1: clinical manifestations and management. Cancer Treat Res. 2010;153: 287–302.

Quayle FJ, Fialkowski EA, Benveniste R, Moley JF. Pheochromocytoma penetrance varies by RET mutation in MEN 2A. Surgery. 2007;142(6):800–5; discussion 805 e801.

Robinson C, Collins MT, Boyce AM. Fibrous Dysplasia/McCune-Albright syndrome: clinical and translational perspectives. Curr Osteoporos Rep. 2016;14(5):178–86.

Shariq OA, Lines KE, English KA, Jafar-Mohammadi B, Prentice P, Casey R, et al. Multiple endocrine neoplasia type 1 in children and adolescents: clinical features and treatment outcomes. Surgery. 2022;171(1):77–87.

Skinner MA, Moley JA, Dilley WG, Owzar K, Debenedetti MK, Wells SA Jr. Prophylactic thyroidectomy in multiple endocrine neoplasia type 2A. N Engl J Med. 2005;353(11):1105–13.

Su MA, Giang K, Zumer K, Jiang H, Oven I, Rinn JL, et al. Mechanisms of an autoimmunity syndrome in mice caused by a dominant mutation in Aire. J Clin Invest. 2008;118(5):1712–26.

Taieb A, Picardo M. Clinical practice. Vitiligo. N Engl J Med. 2009; 360(2):160–9.

Tham E, Grandell U, Lindgren E, Toss G, Skogseid B, Nordenskjold M. Clinical testing for mutations in the MEN1 gene in Sweden: a report on 200 unrelated cases. J Clin Endocrinol Metab. 2007; 92(9):3389–95.

Turner JJ, Christie PT, Pearce SH, Turnpenny PD, Thakker RV. Diagnostic challenges due to phenocopies: lessons from Multiple Endocrine Neoplasia type1 (MEN1). Hum Mutat. 2010;31(1):E1089–101.

Weinstein LS, Shenker A, Gejman PV, Merino MJ, Friedman E, Spiegel AM. Activating mutations of the stimulatory G protein in the McCune-Albright syndrome. N Engl J Med. 1991;325 (24):1688–95.

Williams VC, Lucas J, Babcock MA, Gutmann DH, Korf B, Maria BL. Neurofibromatosis type 1 revisited. Pediatrics. 2009;123(1):124–33.

Wilson SD, Krzywda EA, Zhu YR, Yen TW, Wang TS, Sugg SL, et al. The influence of surgery in MEN-1 syndrome: observations over 150 years. Surgery. 2008;144(4):695–701; discussion 701–692.

You YN, Thompson GB, Young WF Jr, Larson D, Farley DR, Richards M, et al. Pancreatoduodenal surgery in patients with multiple endocrine neoplasia type 1: operative outcomes, long-term function, and quality of life. Surgery. 2007;142(6):829–36; discussion 836; e821.

Cirrhosis, 127, 127f
Citric acid cycle, 136
Clavicle, 36f
Clear cell hyperplasia, primary, 164
Cleft, 2f, 3f
Clinically nonfunctioning pituitary tumor, 25, 25f
Clitoris
    body, 104f
    enlarged, 113f
    enlargement, 84f
    hypertrophy, 123f
Clivus, 7f
Clubbing, in Graves disease, 43, 43f
Cobalamin, 201, 201f, 201t
Coelomic epithelium, 102f
Cole-Carpenter syndrome, 181
Colic (splenic) flexure, left, 67f
Collagen fibrils, 156f
Collagen matrix, in bone, 158
Collagen space, 9f
Colles fracture, in osteoporosis, 170
Colloid goiter, 54, 54f
Colon, 130f
Coma, diabetic, 138, 138f, 139f
Common bile duct, 130f
Common iliac vein, 87f
Communicating vein, 36f
Complete androgen insensitivity syndrome (CAIS), 116
Complete testicular feminization, 116
Compression fractures, osteoporotic vertebral, clinical
    manifestations of, 172, 172f
Computed tomography (CT)
    in atherosclerosis, 196
    of catecholamine-secreting tumors, 96
    in Cushing syndrome, 76
    of pheochromocytoma, 95f
    in renal artery stenosis, 88f
Computed tomography angiogram, in atherosclerosis, 146f
Congenital adrenal hyperplasia (CAH), 80f, 84f, 115
Congenital adrenal hypoplasia, 90f
Congenital anomalies, of thyroid gland, 40, 40f
Congenital hypoparathyroidism, 165
Conjugation, 105f
Connective tissue, glucocorticoid effects on, 74, 74f
Contrasexual gonadotropin-independent precocious
    puberty, 111
Contrasexual precocious puberty, 110
Corneal thinning, in vitamin A deficiency, 205
Coronary heart disease
    diabetes mellitus and, 146
    risk factors for, 197f
Corpus callosum, 5f
Cortical atrophy, autoimmune with, 90f
Cortical capillaries, 70f
Cortical primordium, 66f
Corticosteroid, obesity and, 210f
Corticosterone, 72f, 80f
Corticotropin
    adrenal gland structure and function of, 70
    Cushing syndrome associated with, 77
    deficiency, 14
    pituitary tumor secreting, 77
    secretion of, 71
Corticotropin-releasing hormone (CRH), secretion, 72f
Corticotropin-secreting pituitary tumor, 23, 23f
Cortisol, 72f, 78f, 80f, 82f, 91f
    biosynthesis of, 71
        major blocks in, 80
    circulatory collapse caused by, 82f
    metabolism of, 71
    in primary pigmented nodular adrenocortical disease, 79
    salivary, in Cushing syndrome, 76
    secretion of, 70
    serum
        in anorexia nervosa, 209, 209f
        in Cushing syndrome, 76, 76f, 77
    urinary free, in Cushing syndrome, 71, 76f
Cortisone, 71, 72f, 73t
Coxa vera deformity, 221f

Cranial nerve, palsy of, in diabetes mellitus, 145f
Craniopharyngeal canal, 2
Craniopharyngioma, 11, 11f
Craniotomy, 34
Cricoid cartilage, 37f
Cricothyroid ligament, 37f
Cricothyroid muscle, 37f
Crooke hyaline change, 77
Cryptorchidism, 121f
Cushing disease, 77
Cushing syndrome, 75, 75f
    ACTH-dependent, 77, 84
    ACTH-independent, 77
    clinical findings in, 75
    diagnostic testing in, 76
    evaluation of, 76f
    obesity and, 210f
    pathophysiology of, 77
    tests used in, 76, 76f
Cutaneous lichen amyloidosis, in multiple endocrine
    neoplasia type 2, 215, 215f
Cyanosis, in adrenal crisis, 89f
Cyclic adenosine monophosphate (cAMP),
    pseudohypoparathyroidism type 1 and, 167
Cyst
    epididymal, in von Hippel-Lindau syndrome, 217
    thyroglossal, 40f
    uterine bleeding and, 126f
Cystadenoma, in von Hippel-Lindau syndrome, 217, 217f
Cystic tumor, 216f

D

Dark chief cell, 156
Decalcification, of skull, 160
Defective bone remodeling, 158
Deformities, rickets and, 176
Dementia, in pellagra, 203, 203f
Dense stroma, 118f
Dental anomalies, acute hypocalcemia and, 166
Dental hypoplasia, in autoimmune polyglandular syndrome
    type I, 219f
11-Deoxycorticosterone, 80f
11-Deoxycortisol, 72f
Dermatitis herpetiformis, celiac disease and, 206
Dermopathy
    diabetic, 147, 147f
    infiltrative, in Graves disease, 43f, 44, 44f
Desmolase, 73t
Desmosome, 156f
Dexamethasone, low-dose, in Cushing syndrome, 76
Dexamethasone suppression test, in Cushing syndrome, 76
Dextrose, for adrenal crisis, 89
DHA. see Docosahexaenoic acid
DHEA (dehydroepiandrosterone), 72f, 105, 105f
DHEA (dehydroepiandrosterone) sulfate
    adrenal synthesis and metabolism of, 71, 83
    biologic actions of, 83
Diabetes insipidus, 92f
    central, 28, 28f
Diabetes mellitus
    atherosclerosis in, 146, 146f, 197, 197f
    in autoimmune polyglandular syndrome type II, 219
    celiac disease and, 206
    dermatologic manifestations of, 147
    foot ulcers in, 148, 148f
    gestational, 149, 149f
    histopathology of, 140, 140f
    ketoacidosis in, 139, 139f
    maturity onset, of young, 141
    in metabolic syndrome, 198
    nephropathy in, 144, 144f
    neuropathy in, 145, 148
    in pregnancy, 149, 149f
    retinopathy in, 142, 142f, 143, 143f
    type 1, 140, 140f
        intensive diabetes therapy of, 151, 151f
    type 2, 141, 141f
        treatment of, 150, 150f
    vascular insufficiency in, 148

Diaphoresis, 95f
Diaphragm, 96f, 222f
Diaphragma sellae, 5f, 6f
Diarrhea, 90f
    in carcinoid syndrome, 220
Diet
    gluten-free, 206
    in hyperlipidemia, 200, 200f
    in metabolic syndrome, 198
    for osteoporosis, 170
Digastric muscle, 36f
Direct transnasal transsphenoidal surgical approach, 34, 34f
Disorders of sex development (DSD), 113–116, 113f–116f,
    123f
    46,XX, 82f, 113, 113f, 115, 115f
    46,XY, 82f, 113, 114f, 116
    47,XXY karyotype, 118f
Diurnal rhythms, 8
Diverticulum, 32f
Docosahexaenoic acid (DHA), 199
Dopamine
    biologic actions of, 93f
    metabolism of, 94f
    synthesis of, 94f
Dorsal mesentery, 66f
Dorsal spinal ganglion, 66f
Dorsocervical ("buffalo hump") supraclavicular, 75f
Dorsum sellae, 7f
Dowager's hump, in osteoporosis, 170
Down syndrome, celiac disease and, 206
DSD. see Disorders of sex development
Ductus epididymidis, 102f
Duodenal carcinoids, 214f
Duodenal switch, biliopancreatic diversion with, 211
Duodenojejunal flexure, 67f
Duodenum, topographic relationships of, 67f, 130f
Dwarfism, 92f
Dysbetalipoproteinemia, familial, 186, 192
Dyslipidemia
    in diabetes mellitus, 141
    in metabolic syndrome, 198f

E

Ecchymoses
    in Cushing syndrome, 75, 75f
    in scurvy, 204f
Ectoderm, 66f
Ectopic posterior pituitary, 9
Ectopic pregnancy, 126f
Edema, 220f
    macular, in diabetic retinopathy, 142, 143
    periorbital
        in Graves disease, 45
        in hypothyroidism, 49, 49f
Efferent ductules, 102f
Efferent hypophysial vein, 4f
Ehlers-Danlos syndrome, 181
Eicosapentaenoic acid (EPA), 199
Elbow, xanthoma of, 189f
Emaciation, 90f
Empty sella, 32, 32f
Encephalopathy, in pellagra, 203
Endocervical polyps, 126f
Endocervix, cancer of, 126f
Endocrine neoplasia, 213–222
Endolymphatic sac tumor, 217f
Endometriosis, 126f
Endometritis, 126f
Endometrium, 125f
Endoplasmic reticulum, 156f
Endothelial cell, 156f
Endothelium, 9f
Enterokinase, 131, 131f
Enteropathy, gluten-sensitive, 206
Eosinophilic granuloma, 29
Epididymal cyst, in von Hippel-Lindau syndrome, 217, 217f
Epididymis, 103f
Epigastric pain, 95f

Gums, bleeding, in scurvy, 204f
Gut, 66f, 105f
Gynecomastia, 127, 127f

H
Hair
    in adrenal insufficiency, 90
    axillary, development of, 83, 83f
    darkening of, 90f
    growth, 122
    in hypothyroidism, 49, 49f, 50, 50f
    male-pattern
        adrenal androgen effects on, 84
    pubic, development of, 83f
    thinning of, in Cushing syndrome, 75f
Hair line, receding, 84f
Hand-Schüller-Christian disease, 29
Hashimoto thyroiditis, 51, 56, 56f, 219
Head trauma, 13
Headache, 95f
Heart, enlarged, in hypothyroidism, 49, 49f
Heart disease
    carcinoid, 220
    coronary
        diabetes mellitus and, 146
        risk factors for, 197f
    valvular, in carcinoid tumors, 220f
Heart failure, in Graves disease, 44, 44f
Hemangioblastoma, in von Hippel-Lindau syndrome, 217, 217f
Hemorrhage
    of adrenal glands, 89
    perifollicular, in scurvy, 204f
Hepatomegaly, obesity and, 210f
Hepatosplenomegaly, in hypertriglyceridemia, 193, 193f
Hereditary vitamin D-resistant rickets, 174
Herpes zoster, 128f
Herring bodies, 9f
HIFs. see Hypoxia-inducible factors
Hilum cell, 123f
Hirata disease, 219
Hirschsprung disease, 215, 216f
Hirsutism, 84, 122–123, 122f, 123f
    in Cushing syndrome, 75f
    facial, 84f
    generalized, 84f
Histiocytosis-X, 29
HLA. see Human leukocyte antigen
HMG-CoA reductase, 184
Homocystinuria, 169
Homovanillic acid (HVA), 94f
Hormonal events, in female and male puberty, 109f
Human leukocyte antigen (HLA), in diabetes mellitus, 140
Hürthle cell thyroid carcinoma, 61, 61f
Hydatidiform mole, 126f
Hydrocephalus, in neurofibromatosis type 1, 218
Hydrocortisone
    for adrenal crisis, 89
    for adrenal insufficiency, 92
3-Hydroxy-3-methylglutaryl coenzyme A (HMG-CoA), 184
5-Hydroxyindole acetic acid, in carcinoid tumors, 220f
11β-Hydroxylase, 73t
    deficiency of, 80, 81
17α-Hydroxylase, 73t
    deficiency of, 80, 81
21-Hydroxylase, 73t
    deficiency, 80, 81
17α-Hydroxypregnenolone, 72f, 80f
17-Hydroxyprogesterone, 72f, 80f
3β-Hydroxysteroid dehydrogenase, 73t
    deficiency of, 80, 81
    late-onset, 84
11β-Hydroxysteroid dehydrogenase, 73t
17β-Hydroxysteroid dehydrogenase, 73t
5-hydroxytryptamine, 220f
Hyoid bone, 36f, 37f
Hyperalgesia, in diabetes mellitus, 145, 145f

Hyperapobetalipoproteinemia, familial, 188
Hypercalcemia, 160
    apparent, 161
    causes of, differential diagnosis of, 161, 161f
    non-parathyroid hormone-mediated, 161
    parathyroid hormone-mediated, 161
Hypercholesterolemia, 188
    atherosclerosis and, 197, 197f
    familial, 186, 188, 189, 192
    guidelines on, 188
    multifactorial causes of, 188f
    polygenic, 186
    xanthomatosis in, 189–190
Hypercortisolism
    in Cushing syndrome, 75, 77
    in primary pigmented nodular adrenocortical disease, 79
Hyperglycemia
    in diabetes mellitus, 140, 141, 149
    maternal, 149
    treatment of, 150f
Hyperinsulinemia, in diabetes mellitus, 141
Hyperinsulinism, congenital, 153
Hyperkalemia, 85f
    in adrenal insufficiency, 91
Hyperkeratinization, in vitamin A deficiency, 205f
Hyperlipemia retinalis, 194f
Hyperlipidemia
    atherosclerosis and, 197
    familial combined, 188, 192
Hyperlipoproteinemia
    classification of, 192
    type I, 192
    type II, 192
    type III, 186, 192
    type IV, 192
    type V, 192
Hyperparathyroidism
    in multiple endocrine neoplasia, 215
    parathyroid glands in, histology of, 164, 164f
    primary, 215f
        clinical manifestations of, 160, 160f
        pathology of, 160, 160f
        pathophysiology of, 159, 159f
Hyperperistalsis, 220f
Hyperpigmentation
    in adrenal insufficiency, 90
    in carcinoid tumors, 220, 220f
Hyperplasia, 104f, 214f
    obesity and, 210f
Hyperprolactinemia, 22
    in prolactin-secreting pituitary tumor, 128f
Hypertension, 95f
    in aldosteronism, 86
    in atherosclerosis, 197, 197f
    in diabetic nephropathy, 144
    in hypothyroidism, 49f
    in neurofibromatosis type 1, 218
    renovascular, in renal artery stenosis, 88
Hypertensive syndrome, 82f
Hyperthecosis, 122–123
Hyperthyroidism, 126f
    in Graves disease, 43
    in toxic adenoma and toxic multinodular goiter, 47, 47f, 48, 48f
Hypertriglyceridemia, 192
    apolipoprotein CII deficiency, 192f, 193
    borderline, 192
    clinical manifestations of, 193–194
    familial, 192, 194
    in lipoprotein lipase deficiency, 193–194, 193f
    mixed, 192
    risk factors for, 192f
    treatment of, 194, 200
Hypertrophic colon, 217f
Hypertrophy, obesity and, 210f
Hyperventilation, diabetic ketoacidosis and, 139f
Hypesthesia, in diabetes mellitus, 145, 145f

Hypocalcemia
    acute, clinical manifestations of, 166, 166f
    in autoimmune polyglandular syndrome type I, 219
Hypoglycemia
    for adrenal insufficiency, 92
    differential diagnosis of, 153
    from insulinoma, 152
    from islet-cell hyperplasia, 153
    noninsulinoma pancreatogenous, 153
    post-gastric bypass, 153
Hypogonadism, 127
    primary, in autoimmune polyglandular syndrome type I and II, 219
    secondary, 14
Hypokalemia, in aldosteronism, 86, 86f
Hypokalemic alkalosis, 86f
Hyponatremia, in adrenal insufficiency, 92
Hypoparathyroidism
    autoimmune, 165
    in autoimmune polyglandular syndrome type I, 219
    genetic causes of, 165
    pathophysiology of, 165, 165f
Hypophosphatasia, 177, 182, 182f
Hypophosphatemic rickets, 175, 175f
Hypophysial fossa, 7, 7f
Hypophysial portal system
    primary plexus of, 4f
    secondary plexus of, 4f
Hypophysial stalk, 3f
Hypophysis. see Pituitary gland
Hypopituitarism, 13
Hypoplasia, 13
Hypospadiac phallus, 121f
Hypotension, 90f, 91f
    in adrenal crisis, 89f
    in adrenal insufficiency, 90
Hypothalamic area, 3f
Hypothalamic disorders, obesity and, 210f
Hypothalamic-pituitary-adrenal (HPA) axis, 71
Hypothalamic sulcus, 3f, 5f
Hypothalamic vessels, 4f
Hypothalamohypophysial tract, 3f
Hypothalamus, 1–34, 72f, 105f, 125f
    craniopharyngioma compressing, 11f
    pituitary, relationship to, 3
Hypothyroidism, 92f, 126f
    in adults, 49, 49f, 51, 51f
    central (hypothalamic or pituitary), 51f
    congenital, 52, 52f
    etiology of, 50
    signs and symptoms of, 49
    treatment of, 51, 51f
Hypoxia-inducible factors (HIFs), regulation of, 136

I
Idiopathic gynecomastia, 127
Idiopathic hirsutism, 123
IgA deficiency, 206
Immune checkpoint inhibitor-induced hypophysitis, 13
Incomplete precocious puberty, 111
Incomplete testicular feminization, 116
Incretin effect, 133
Incretin-related agents, for diabetes mellitus, 150, 150f
Infarction, myocardial, diabetes mellitus and, 146
Infections, chronic primary adrenal failure, 90f
Inferior adrenal artery, 67f
Inferior hypophysial artery, 4f, 9f
Inferior petrosal sinus sampling (IPSS), 76f
Inferior phrenic artery, 67f, 68f, 69f
Inferior phrenic plexus, 69f
Inferior phrenic vein, 68f, 87f
Inferior renal artery, 68f
Inferior vena cava, 67f, 68f, 87f
Infradian rhythms, 8
Infundibular arteries, 4
Infundibular process, 2f, 3f
    capillary plexus of, 4f
Infundibular stem, 3f

Thyroid gland *(Continued)*
  Hürthle cell, 61, 61f
  medullary, 60, 60f, 215
  in multiple endocrine neoplasia type 2, 60, 215–216
  papillary, 58, 58f
  development of, 38, 38f, 39, 39f
  dysgenesis of, 52
  hyperplasia of, goiter after, 55, 55f
  metastatic disease to, 64, 64f
  pathology of, in Graves disease, 46, 46f
  pyramidal lobe of, 39
  thyrotropin effects on, 41, 41f
Thyroid hormones
  in anorexia nervosa, 209, 209f
  deficiency of, 55, 55f
  physiology of, 42, 42f
  reduced sensitivity to, 55, 55f
Thyroid isthmus, 38f
Thyroid peroxidase
  antibodies to, in Hashimoto thyroiditis, 56f
  inhibition of, 55f
Thyroid tissue, aberrant, 40, 40f
Thyroid vein, 37f
Thyroidectomy
  for follicular thyroid carcinoma, 59
  for Hürthle cell thyroid carcinoma, 61
  for medullary thyroid carcinoma, 60
  for papillary thyroid carcinoma, 58
Thyroiditis
  acute nonsuppurative, 57
  chronic lymphocytic (Hashimoto), 51, 51f, 56, 56f
  fibrous (Riedel), 56, 56f
  subacute (de Quervain), 57
Thyrotropic hormone, 92f
Thyrotropin
  effects of, on thyroid gland, 41, 41f
  in hypothyroidism, 51
  pituitary tumor secreting, 41
  in subacute thyroiditis, 57
Thyrotropin receptor, 43
  mutations of, goiter from, 47, 55, 55f
Thyrotropin-releasing hormone (TRH), 41
Thyroxine, 41
  physiology of, 42
  in subacute thyroiditis, 57
Tongue, 38, 38f
  in hypothyroidism, 49f
  in pellagra, 203, 203f
Tonsil, in Tangier disease, 191f
Tooth (teeth)
  in autoimmune polyglandular syndrome type I, 219
  malocclusion of, in acromegaly, 21f
  opalescent, in osteogenesis imperfecta, 180f
Toxic adenoma, 47, 47f, 48, 48f
Toxic multinodular goiter, 47, 47f, 48, 48f
Trabecula, 3f, 4f
  artery of, 4f
Trachea, 36, 36f, 38f
  compression of, by anaplastic thyroid carcinoma, 62, 62f
Transabdominal adrenalectomy, open, 68
Transsphenoidal surgery
  for clinically nonfunctioning pituitary tumor, 25
  for pituitary-dependent Cushing syndrome, 23
Transverse mesocolon, attachment of, 130f
Trauma, 126f
Tremor
  in Graves disease, 43f
  in pheochromocytoma, 95f
Tricarboxylic acid cycle, 136
Trigeminal nerve (V), 5f, 6f
Triglycerides
  dietary, 185
  gastrointestinal absorption of, 185, 185f
  metabolism of, 192
  serum of, 192
Triiodothyronine, 41
  physiology of, 42, 42f
Triple X syndrome, 117, 117f
Trisomy X, 117
Trochlear nerve (IV), 5f, 6f

Trousseau sign, acute hypocalcemia and, 166
True hermaphroditism, 115, 116f
Trypsinogen, 131, 131f
Tubal inflammation, 126f
Tuber cinereum, 5f
Tuberculosis, of adrenal glands, 90f
Tuberculum sellae, 7f
Tuberohypophysial tract, 3f
Tuberous xanthoma, 189, 189f, 190f
Tumor-induced osteomalacia, 175
Tumors
  of ovary, 123f
  of thymus gland, 214
Tunica albuginea, 102f
Tunica vaginalis, 102f
Turner syndrome, 113, 114, 117, 117f, 119–121, 119f–121f
Type 1 pseudovitamin D-deficient rickets, 174
Type 2 pseudovitamin D-deficient rickets, 174
Tyrosine, 94f

U
Ulcer, neuropathic, in diabetes mellitus, 145, 145f, 148
Ultradian rhythms, 8
Uncinate process, 130, 130f
Undifferentiated skeletal stem cells, 221f
Unicornuate uterus, 116f
Unilateral primary adrenal disease, 78f
Unilateral renal artery stenosis, 88f
Upper body to lower body segment ratio (U:L), 107
Ureter, 66f
Urethra, 103f, 113f
Urethral fold, 104f
Urethral groove, 104f
Urethral meatus, 104f
Urethral slit, 104f
Urogenital sinus, 103f, 113f
Urogenital slit, 104, 104f
Uterine bleeding, functional and pathologic causes of, 126, 126f
Uterine disorders, local, 126f
Uterine mucosa, 126
Uterus, 103f, 113f
  infantile, 115f, 119f, 120f

V
Vagal trunk, anterior, 69f
Vagina, 103f, 104, 104f, 113f
Vaginal mucosa, 125f
Vaginal smear, 125f
Vagus fibers, 131f
Vagus nerve, 36f, 37f
Valvular heart disease, in carcinoid tumors, 220
Vanillylmandelic acid, 93, 94f
Vas deferens, 102f, 103f, 115f
Vasa efferentia, 103f
Vascular insufficiency, in diabetes mellitus, 148
Vascular phenomena, 220f
Vasoconstriction, 88f, 95f
Vasopressin, 9, 27f
  absorption, site of, 9f
  action of, 27
  secretion of, 27
Vena cava
  inferior, 67f, 68f, 87f, 130f
  superior, 37f
Venous drainage, of posterior lobe, 9f
Vertebral body, 36f
Vestibule, 104f
VHL tumor suppressor gene, in von Hippel-Lindau syndrome, 217
Vibration sense, loss of, in diabetes mellitus, 145f
Virchow nodes, 37f
Virilization, 122–123, 122f–123f
  definition of, 81, 84
Virilizing tumor, 113f
Vitamin A
  absorption of, 201, 201t
  deficiency of, 205, 205f
  recommended dietary allowance for, 205, 205f
Vitamin B, in tricarboxylic acid cycle, 136

Vitamin B$_1$ (thiamine)
  absorption of, 201, 201t
  deficiency of, 202
  recommended dietary allowance for, 202
Vitamin B$_2$ (riboflavin), 201, 201t
Vitamin B$_3$ (niacin)
  absorption of, 201
  deficiency of, 203
  recommended dietary allowance for, 203
Vitamin B$_5$ (pantothenic acid), 201
Vitamin B$_6$ (pyridoxine), 201, 201t
Vitamin B$_{12}$ (cobalamin), 201, 201f, 201t
Vitamin C (ascorbic acid)
  absorption of, 201, 201t
  deficiency of, 204
  recommended dietary allowance for, 204
Vitamin D (calciferol)
  absorption of, 201, 201t
  deficiency, 160
    osteomalacia and, 163
  in nutritional-deficiency rickets, 173
Vitamin D-deficient rickets, 173
Vitamin E, 201, 201t
Vitamin K, 201, 201t
Vitamins, absorption of, 201, 201f, 201t
Vitiligo
  in Addison disease, 90f
  in autoimmune polyglandular syndrome type I, 219
Vitreal contraction, in diabetic retinopathy, 143, 143f
Vitreous hemorrhage, in diabetic retinopathy, 143, 143f
Voice changes, in hypothyroidism, 49f
Volume repletion
  for adrenal crisis, 89
  for diabetic ketoacidosis, 139
Vomer, 7f
Vomiting, 90f
Von Hippel-Lindau syndrome, 217, 217f
Von Recklinghausen disease, 218, 218f

W
Water-soluble vitamins, 201, 201f, 201t
Waterhouse-Friderichsen syndrome, 89
Weakness, 95f
Weight loss
  in Addison disease, 90f
  in anorexia nervosa, 209
  in Graves disease, 44
  from insulin deprivation, 138, 138f
  for obesity, 210
Wernicke encephalopathy, 202
Wernicke-Korsakoff syndrome, 202, 202f
Whipple procedure, for insulinoma, 152
Whipple triad, in insulinoma, 152, 152f
Wirsung, duct of, 130, 130f
Wolffian body, 103f
Wolffian duct, 102f, 103, 103f
Wolfram syndrome, 28, 219
Wound healing, in Cushing syndrome, 75f
Wrist drop, in diabetes mellitus, 145, 145f

X
X chromosome, 102
X-linked acro-gigantism, 20
X-linked hypophosphatemic rickets, 175
Xanthoma
  hypercholesterolemic, 189–190
  in hypertriglyceridemia, 193, 193f, 194f
Xanthoma disseminatum, 31
Xanthomatosis, cerebrotendinous, 190
Xerophthalmia, in vitamin A deficiency, 205, 205f

Y
Y chromosome, 102

Z
Zona fasciculata, 70, 70f
Zona glomerulosa, 70, 70f
Zona reticularis, 70f
Zuckerkandl organ, 66, 96f, 222f